BRADY

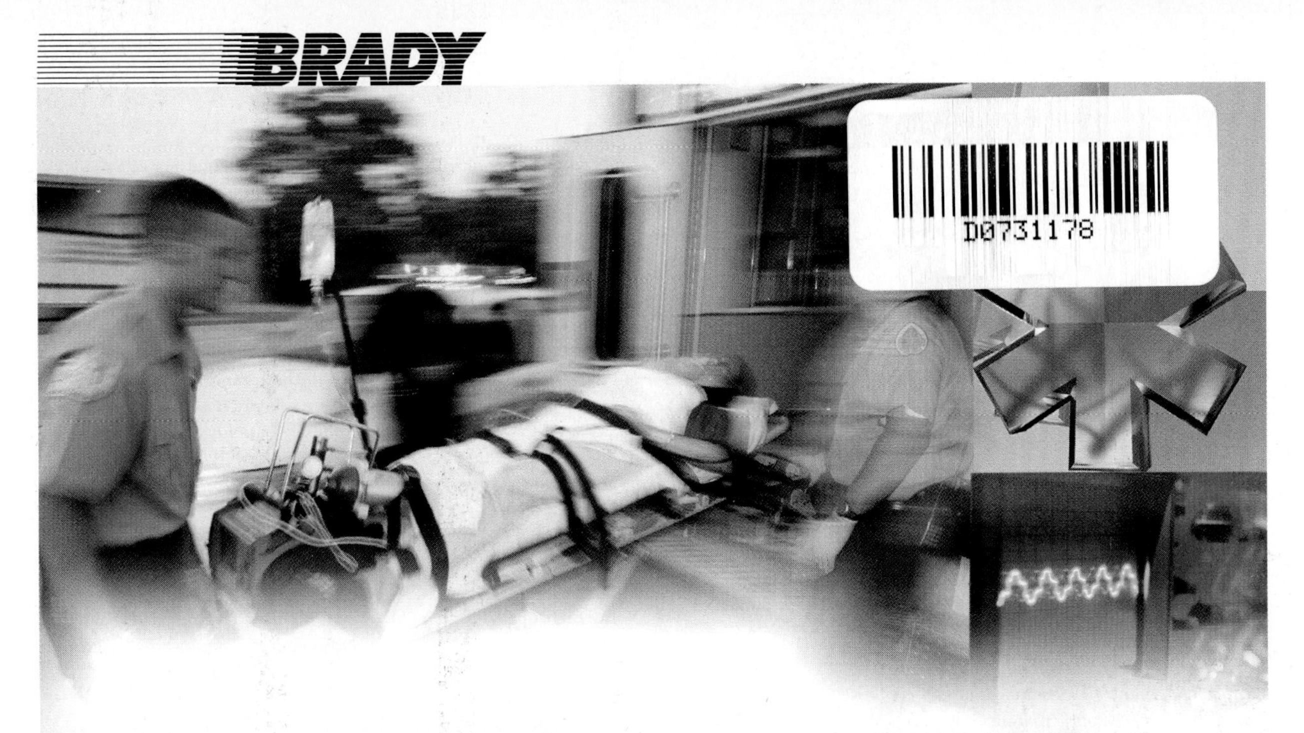

ADVANCED MEDICAL LIFE SUPPORT

A PRACTICAL APPROACH TO ADULT MEDICAL EMERGENCIES

THIRD EDITION

Alice L. Dalton, RN, MS, NREMT-P
Director, EMS Division, Mountain View Fire Protection District, Longmont, Colorado

Daniel Limmer, AS, EMT-P
Southern Maine Community College, South Portland, Maine
Kennebunk Fire and Rescue, Kennebunk, Maine

Joseph J. Mistovich, MEd, NREMT-P
Chairperson, Department of Health Professions;
Professor of Health Professions, Youngstown State University, Youngstown, Ohio

Howard A. Werman, MD, FACEP
Professor of Emergency Medicine,
The Ohio State University College of Medicine, Columbus, Ohio

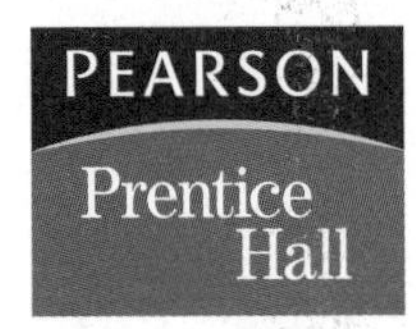

Upper Saddle River, New Jersey 07458

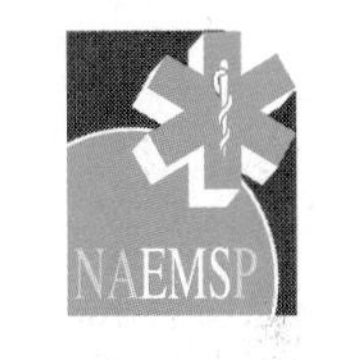

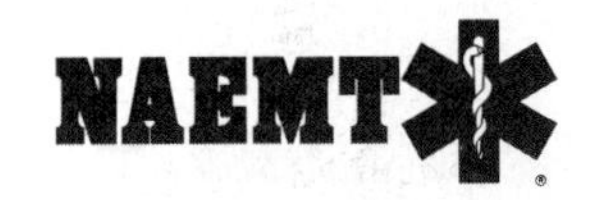

Library of Congress Cataloging-in-Publication Data
Advanced medical life support : a practical approach
to adult medical emergencies / Alice L. Dalton ...
[et al.]. -- 3rd ed.
p. ; cm.
Includes bibliographical references and index.
ISBN 0-13-172340-5
1. Medical emergencies. 2. Emergency medical
technicians. I. Dalton, Alice.
[DNLM: 1. Emergencies. 2. Emergency Medical
Services. 3. Life Support Care--methods.
WB 105 A2445 2007]
R86.7.A343 2007
616.02′5--dc22 2006019000

Publisher: *Julie Levin Alexander*
Publisher's Assistant: *Regina Bruno*
Senior Acquisitions Editor: *Stephen Smith*
Senior Managing Editor for Development: *Lois Berlowitz*
Project Manager: *Sandy Breuer*
Editorial Assistant: *Diane Edwards*
Associate Editor: *Monica Moosang*
Director of Marketing: *Karen Allman*
Executive Marketing Manager: *Katrin Beacom*
Marketing Coordinator: *Michael Sirinides*
Marketing Assistant: *Wayne Celia, Jr.*
Director of Production and Manufacturing: *Bruce Johnson*
Managing Production Editor: *Patrick Walsh*
Production Liaison: *Julie Li*
Production Editor: *Peggy Hood, Techbooks*
Media Product Manager: *John Jordan*
Manager of Media Production: *Amy Peltier*
New Media Project Manager: *Tina Rudowski*
Manufacturing Manager: *Ilene Sanford*
Manufacturing Buyer: *Pat Brown*
Senior Design Coordinator: *Christopher Weigand*
Interior Designer: *Lee Goldstein*
Cover Designer: *Lee Goldstein*
Cover Image: *Fotosearch*
Director, Image Resource Center: *Melinda Reo*
Manager, Rights and Permissions: *Zina Arabia*
Manager, Visual Research: *Beth Brenzel*
Manager, Cover Visual Research and Permissions: *Karen Sanatar*
Image Permission Coordinator: *Carolyn Gauntt*
Composition: *Techbooks*
Printing and Binding: *The Banta Company*
Cover Printer: *Phoenix Color Corporation*
Managing Photography Editor: *Michal Heron*
Photographer: *Carl Leet, Photographic Specialist, Youngstown State University*

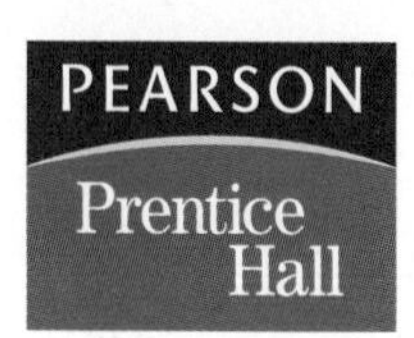

Notice on Care Procedures: The authors and the publisher of this book have taken care to make certain that equipment, procedures, and treatments, including recommended drugs, dosages, and routes of administration, are correct and compatible with the standards generally accepted at the time of publication. Nevertheless, as new information becomes available, changes in equipment, procedures, and treatments become necessary. The reader is advised to carefully consult the instructions and information provided for each piece of equipment, device, drug, or other substance before use. *Readers are also warned that the use of any technique, procedure, treatment, drug, or other substance must be authorized by their medical direction through standing orders or protocols or by online consultation and direction and must also, where appropriate, be in accord with local, state, and federal laws and regulations.* The publisher disclaims any liability, loss, injury, or damage incurred as a consequence, directly or indirectly, of the use or application of any of the contents of this book.

Notice on Scope and Intended Audience: *This text addresses advanced care for adult medical emergencies in the prehospital environment.* To understand what this text is about, it helps to read between the lines (or between the words) of the foregoing statement. "Advanced care" indicates that the text is intended primarily for students who are pursuing or have completed advanced-level training. Much of the text assumes that the student is already familiar with advanced concepts and terminology. "Adult" indicates that the text focuses on adult emergencies and, therefore, does not address pediatric care. "Medical emergencies" indicates that trauma is not the focus of the text and is mentioned only as necessary to differentiate medical from traumatic conditions and etiologies. "Prehospital" indicates that the text focuses on assessment, differential diagnosis, and care that are appropriate in the field. In-hospital emergency care is occasionally mentioned only to indicate how the patient's care may be continued after the patient has been transferred to the care of the emergency department staff.

Notice on Gender Usage: In English, masculine pronouns such as "he" and "his" have historically been used to refer to both male and female genders. Society evolves faster than language, and no broadly accepted neutral-gender alternative to this use of masculine-gender pronouns has yet developed. The authors and publisher recognize that there are both female and male patients and care providers. We have made the choice to use masculine pronouns to refer to both genders simply because the language offers no alternative that does not become annoyingly awkward in the course of a long text. We wish to assure our readers that no disrespect to women is intended by this choice.

Pearson Education Ltd., *London*
Pearson Education Australia Pty. Limited, *Sydney*
Pearson Education Singapore, Pte. Ltd.
Pearson Education North Asia Ltd., *Hong Kong*
Pearson Education Canada, Ltd., *Toronto*
Pearson Educación de Mexico, S.A. de C.V.
Pearson Education—Japan, *Tokyo*
Pearson Education Malaysia, Pte. Ltd
Pearson Education, Upper Saddle River, New Jersey

10 9 8 7 6 5 4
ISBN: 0-13-172340-5

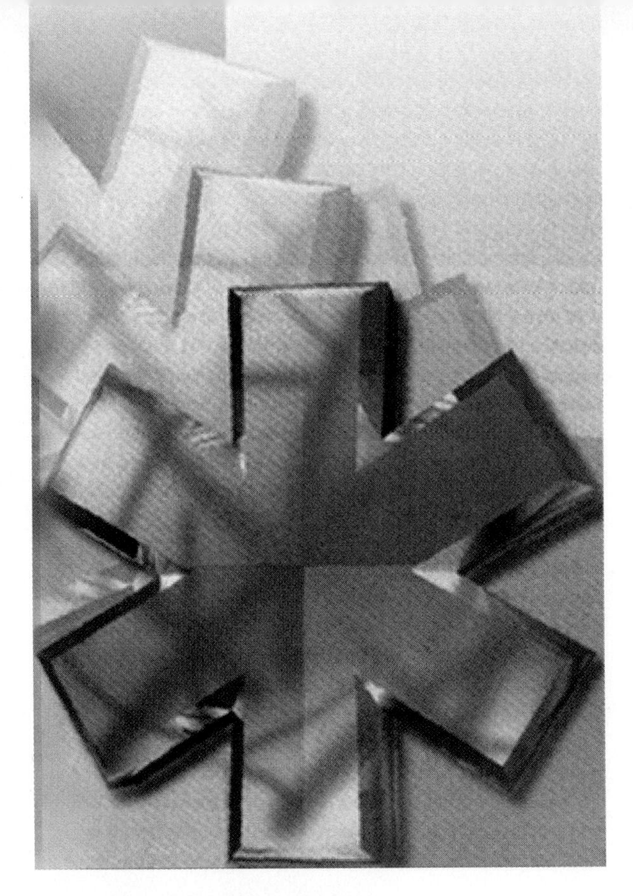

CONTENTS

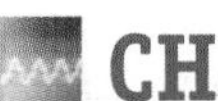

CHAPTER 13

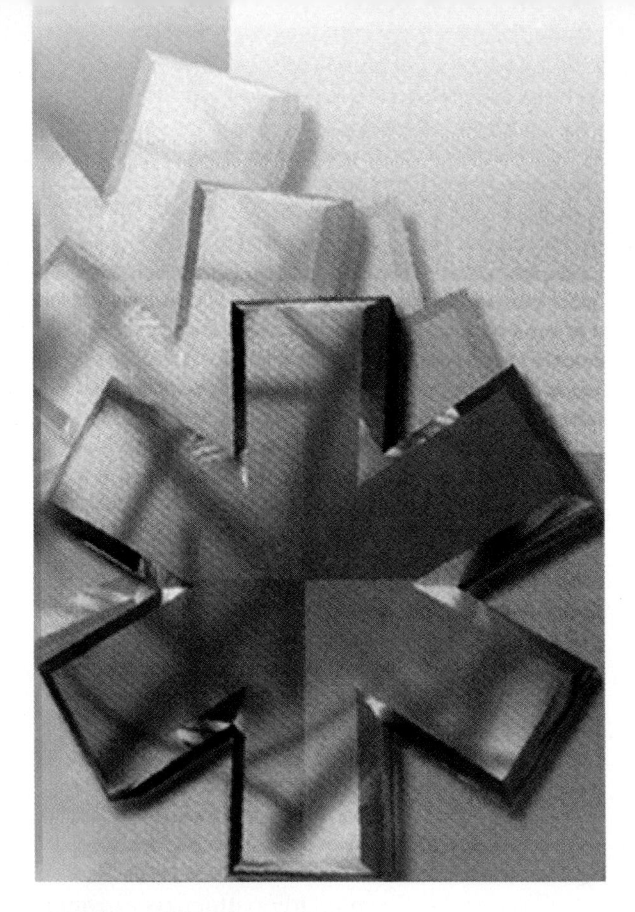

PREFACE

This third edition of *Advanced Medical Life Support,* offering a practical approach to adult medical emergencies, is newly updated and revised to conform to the 2005 American Heart Association Guidelines for Cardiopulmonary Resuscitation and Emergency Cardiovascular Care. The authors assume that the students who use this textbook are currently taking or have completed paramedic or other advanced-level training. They are assumed to have a familiarity with anatomy, physiology, and pathophysiology, as well as an overall understanding of the nature of medical emergencies. *Advanced Medical Life Support* offers pragmatic approaches to applying this knowledge to common medical emergencies.

After introductory chapters on assessment, airway management/oxygenation/ventilation, and venous access/medication administration, the text includes chapters on such common medical complaints and presentations as shock, dyspnea, chest discomfort or pain, altered mental status, acute abdominal pain, gastrointestinal bleeding, seizures, syncope, and headache, nausea, and vomiting. Each chapter presents an integrated, practical approach to the care of the patient who has that complaint or presentation—the kind of realistic approach a seasoned veteran would use. Each chapter moves from assessment- and complaint-based initial assessment (identifying and controlling immediate life threats) to field diagnosis and management of immediately treatable underlying diseases.

Several features of the chapters are designed to help with study and review:

- "Possibilities to Probabilities" in Chapter 1 walks students through a reasoning process of patient assessment (new to this edition).
- A scenario with an end-of-chapter follow-up presents chapter content in a realistic context.
- Terms and definitions are highlighted in the margins.
- "Clinical Insights" provide special perspectives on assessing and managing the patient (new to this edition).
- Summaries of important information appear in boxes.
- Typical findings associated with various etiologies are summarized in tables.

- A "Treatment Pathway" in algorithm format appears at the end of each complaint-based chapter.
- A "Further Reading" bibliography suggests sources to consult for additional information.

A final "Scenarios" chapter presents 10 patients with typical complaints. The cases require that students use critical thinking skills to bring together information from the prior chapters and apply it to the patient at hand. On the basis of the information given about each patient, the student is challenged at various points during each case to identify and manage life threats, form a field impression of the underlying etiology, and determine appropriate treatment.

Four appendices provide valuable reference information:

- Pharmacology Index
- Electrocardiographic Interpretation (new to this edition)
- Anatomy and Physiology Illustrations
- Normal Laboratory Values

An instructor's course guide and slide program that accompany the text are available.

New in the Third Edition

- *Throughout:* Updated to conform to the 2005 American Heart Association Guidelines for Cardiopulmonary Resuscitation and Emergency Cardiovascular Care.

New text on many topics. Examples:

- *Chapter 1 Assessment of the Medical Patient:* Acts of terrorism; respiratory rate effects on tidal volumes; testing for light touch and pain.
- *Chapter 2 Airway Management, Ventilation, and Oxygen Therapy:* Use of the gum elastic bougie; use of the LMA Fastrach® (intubating) airway.
- *Chapter 3 IV Access and Medication Administration:* Intraosseous (IO) infusions in adults.
- *Chapter 4 Hypoperfusion (Shock):* Pulmonary emboli on effects on cardiac and pulmonary function; drugs for anaphylactic shock; waveform and numerical value end-tidal CO_2.
- *Chapter 5 Dyspnea:* BiPAP and CPAP to avoid intubation in acute COPD exacerbations; cardiomyopathy as a factor in congestive heart failure and dysrhythmia.
- *Chapter 6 Chest Discomfort and Pain:* "Chest discomfort" replaces and includes "chest pain"; the spectrum of acute coronary syndromes (unstable angina, non-ST segment elevation MI, ST segment elevation MI).
- *Chapter 7 Altered Mental Status:* Blood glucose readings in relation to last oral intake; updated guidelines on ventilation of patients with increased intracranial pressure.
- *Chapter 8 Acute Abdominal Pain:* Three types of aortic aneurysm (fusiform, saccular, dissecting).
- *Chapter 9 Gastrointestinal Bleeding:* Gastric-esophageal reflux disease (GERD).
- *Chapter 10 Seizures and Seizure Disorders:* The implanted vagus nerve stimulator (VNS) device used to control seizure activity.
- *Chapter 11 Syncope:* idiopathic hypertrophic subaortic stenosis (IHSS) as a cause of syncope.
- *Chapter 12 Headache, Nausea, and Vomiting:* Primary and secondary headache classifications; symptoms that require transport of a patient with headache; cyclic vomiting syndrome (CVS).
- *Chapter 13 Putting It All Together—The Scenarios:* "Sudden-Onset Paraplegia" and "Unconscious Woman" scenarios added; ECG tracings added to some scenarios.
- *Pharmacology Index:* Adds drugs that are newly discussed in various chapters.

Comments and Suggestions

We encourage you to send your suggestions and comments about the text. Please send them to

Brady Marketing Department
Brady/Prentice Hall
One Lake Street
Upper Saddle River, NJ 07548

You can also reach the authors via e-mail:

twinkers@juno.com
danlimmer@earthlink.net
jjmistovich@ysu.edu
hwerman@medflight.com

Visit Brady's website at **www.bradybooks.com.**

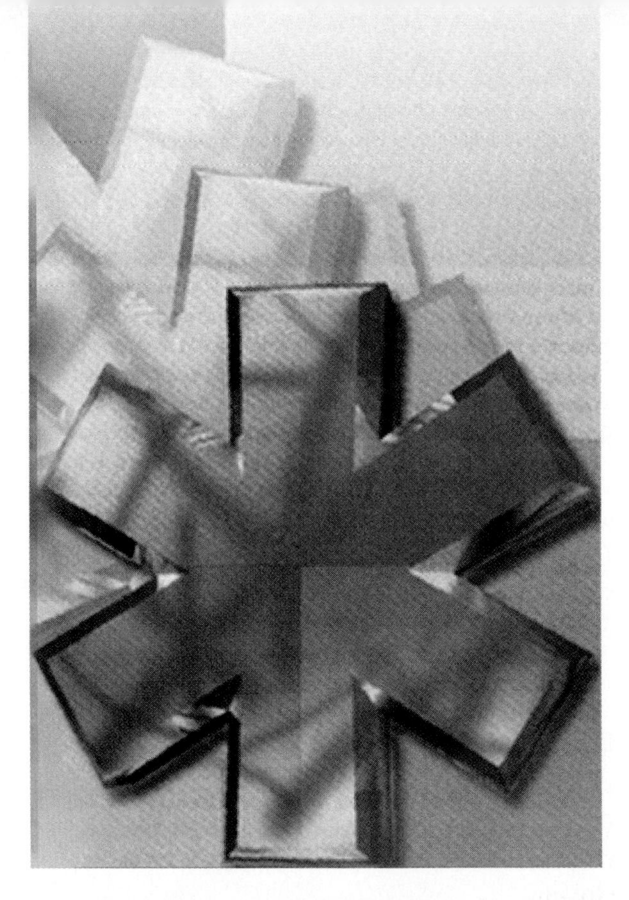

ACKNOWLEDGMENTS

The authors are grateful to fellow author and friend Dr. Howard A. Werman for his contributions as Medical Editor to *Advanced Medical Life Support.* His medical knowledge and understanding of prehospital issues are impressive and have added significantly to the development of this program.

The authors also thank the following people who have made important contributions to this program:

Contributing Writers

Melissa Alexander, MS, NREMT-P
Assistant Professor/Clinical Coordinator
Emergency Health Services Program
Department of Emergency Medicine
The George Washington University
Washington, DC

James W. Drake, BS, NREMT-P
Instructor
Department of Emergency Medical Technology
School of Health Related Professions
University of Mississippi Medical Center
Jackson, MS

William S. Krost, NREMT-P
Operations Manager and Flight Paramedic
St. Vincent/Medical University of Ohio/St. Rita's
Critical Care Transport Network
Toledo, OH

Keith A. Monosky, MPM, EMT-P
Assistant Professor
Emergency Health Services Program
The George Washington University
Washington, DC

Matthew S. Zavarella, BSAS, NREMT-P, CCTEMT-P
Director of Prehospital Education
Medical College of Ohio
Toledo, OH

Medical Reviewers

Our special thanks to Dr. Robert De Lorenzo and Dr. Edward T. Dickinson for their thoughtful reviews of text material in early stages of development.

Robert De Lorenzo, MD, FACEP
Lieutenant Colonel, Medical Corps
United States Army
Associate Clinical Professor of Military and Emergency Medicine
Uniformed Services University of the Health Sciences
Bethesda, MD

Edward T. Dickinson, MD, NREMT-P, FACEP
Associate Professor
Director of EMS Field Operations
Department of Emergency Medicine
University of Pennsylvania Medical Center
Philadelphia, PA

Technical Advisor for Photography

Randall W. Benner, MEd, NREMT-P
Program Director, Emergency Medical Technology
Instructor, Department of Health Professions
Youngstown State University
Youngstown, OH

Instructor Reviewers

We want to thank the following reviewers for providing invaluable feedback and suggestions in preparation of the third edition of *Advanced Medical Life Support.*

Douglas J. Boles, MPA, MICP, NREMT-P
Administrative Director
MICU and Emergency Care Education Center
Englewood Hospital and Medical Center
Englewood, NJ

Brian K. Bugbee
FF/Paramedic, Perrysburg Township Fire
Flight Paramedic, St. Vincent's Medical Center
Medical College of Ohio, St. Rita's Medical Center
Critical Care Network
Perrysburg, OH

Robin C. Goede, NREMT-P, AAS, BA
St. John's Mercy Medical Center
St. Louis, MO

Attila J. Hertelendy, MHSM, CCEMT-P, NREMT-P
Department of Emergency Medical Technology
School of Health Related Professions
University of Mississippi Medical Center
Jackson, MS

Arthur Hsieh, MA, NREMT-P
Chief Operating Officer
San Francisco Paramedic Association
San Francisco, CA

Rod Kimble, BA, EMT-P
WVU Center for Rural Emergency Medicine
Morgantown, WV

Janice T. Posey, EMT-P
Northeast LA Ambulance
LA Technical College
Winnsboro, LA

Virginia Riedy, RN, NREMT-P
EMS Education Manager
Columbus Division of Fire
Columbus, OH

Carol Vining, EMSI, REMT-P
Adjunct Faculty
Mercy Hospitals
Batavia, OH

We also want to thank the following instructors who reviewed earlier editions of *Advanced Medical Life Support.* They helped make this program a successful teaching tool.

Brenda M. Beasley, RN, BS, EMT-P
Department Chair, Allied Health
Calhoun Community College
Decatur, AL

Dan Silver, BSEMS, NRPM
EMS Faculty
Omaha Fire Department
Omaha, NE

Sandy Hunter, MA Ed, MREMT-P
Assistant Professor, Emergency Medical Care Program
Eastern Kentucky University
Richmond, KY

Scott Garrett
Director of Education
Upstate EMS Council, Inc.
Greenville, SC

Shawn Salter, RN, NREMT-P, CFP
Flight Paramedic
San Antonio AirLife
San Antonio, TX

Beth Lothrop Adams, MA, RN, NREMT-P
EMS Quality Manager
Inova Health System
Fairfax County Fire Department
Fairfax, VA

Robert R. Bass, MD
National Association of EMS Physicians

Jeffrey L. Beinke, BS, REMT
Lead Paramedic Instructor
Montgomery Community College
Troy, NC

Michael D. Berg
Medical Liaison Officer
Travis County Department of Emergency Services
Austin, TX

Bruce K. Bowling, NREMT-P
Careflight Air Medical Service
Saint Joseph Hospital
Lexington, KY

Kenneth O. Bradford, EMT-P
Santa Rosa Jr. College
Emergency Medical Care Programs
Petaluma, CA

Jeffrey A. Brown
Education Director
Richmond Lenox EMS
Richmond, MI

Chuck Carter, RN, CEN, NREMT-P NAEMT
Clinton, MS

Heather Davis, MS, NREMT-P
Clinical Coordinator
UCLA-DFH Paramedic Education
Inglewood, CA

Garry L. DeJong
Captain, Albuquerque Fire Department
Albuquerque, NM

Terry DeVito
Coordinator, Paramedic Education
Capital Community Technical College
Hartford, CT

Ralph J. Diamato
Center for Emergency Care Training, Inc.
East Meadow, NY

Ned Fowler, MEd, EMT-P
Department Chair
Emergency Medical Science
Asheville-Buncombe Technical Community College
Asheville, NC

Don Hampton, CIC NREMT-I
Director of Linch Ambulance Service
Linch, WY

Paul L. Hillers, EMT-P, ERT, EMSI
Iowa Valley Continued Education
Iowa Valley Community College District
Marshalltown, IA

Linda K. Honeycutt, EMT-P, I/C
Healthstream, Inc.
Nashville, TN

Raymond J. Hughes, III
Division Commander
Department of Emergency Medical Services
Town of Colonie, NY

David Huskey
Clinical Instructor
Educational Services
Hutcheson Medical Center
Ft. Oglethorpe, GA

Dave Jackson, BAAS, EMT-P
Del Mar College
EMS Professions Program
Corpus Christi, TX

Jerry W. Jones, MPA, BA, EMT-IV
Columbia State Community College
Paramedic Program
Columbia, TN

Joseph Jones, AS, EMT-P
Broward Community College
Paramedic Instructor
Coconut Creek, FL

Kristine Kern, EMT-P
EMS Education Clinical Director
San Antonio College
San Antonio, TX

William R. Kerney, BES, EMTP-A
Professor of Emergency Medicine
Community College of Southern Nevada
Henderson, NV

Thomas J. McGuire
Berkeley Fire Department
Oakland, CA

Ronald G. Pirrallo, MD, MHSA, FACEP
Assistant Professor, Emergency Medicine
Director of Medical Services
Milwaukee County EMS
Milwaukee, WI

Janice T. Posey, EMT-P
Northeast LA Technical College
Winnsboro, LA

Keven Roles, NREMT-P
The Victoria College
Program in Emergency Medical Technology
Victoria, TX

Marlene A. Shengle, EMT-P
Colorado Springs, CO

David C. Spaulding, EMT-P
Director of Training
TLC EMS, Inc.
Cortland, NY

Patricia Stafford, EMT-P
Education Director
Gateway Ambulance
St. Louis, MO

Gail A. Stewart, BS, EMT-P
Santa Fe Community College
EMS Programs
Gainesville, FL

Steven Stokely
Lamar University
Institute of Technology
Regional Fire Training Academy
Beaumont, TX

Richard Stump, EMT-P
New Hanover County EMS
Wilmington, NC

Glenn Susskind, BS, NREMT-P
Flight Paramedic
Life Force Air Medical Services
Erlanger Health System
Chattanooga, TN

William F. Toon, BS, NREMT-P
Education Supervisor

Johnson County EMS/MED-ACT
Olathe, KS

Pauline Van Meurs, BA, EMT-P
Associate Professor
Emergency Medical Services Technology
Austin Community College
Austin, TX

Phyllis R. Vinson
Adjunct Faculty
University of South Alabama
Mobile, AL

Carl Voskamp
Program Coordinator
The Victoria College
Victoria, TX

Polli S. Williams
McLennan Community College
EMS Programs
Waco, TX

The authors want to thank the National Association of EMS Physicians for their review of this program and the endorsement they have provided. We are pleased that our textbook has met the standards of this respected organization. We would specifically like to thank Robert Bass, MD; Ronald Pirrallo, MD; Robert M. Domeier, MD; and Vincent N. Mosesso, Jr., MD, for their careful review of this program when it was first developed.

We want to thank the following members of National Association of Emergency Medical Technicians (NAEMT) for their work in developing the Advanced Medical Life Support (AMLS) course: James B. Allen, BS, NREMT-P; Ann Bellows, PhD, RN, EMT-P; Dan Gerard, RN, EMT-P; Keith Holtermann; Deborah Knight-Smith, EMT; Jim Paturas; Michael D. Sturgill; and Matthew S. Zavarella, BSAS, NREMT-P, CCTEMT-P.

The *Advanced Medical Life Support* text is an integral part of the AMLS course offered by the NAEMT. For information about the NAEMT AMLS course, visit NAEMT online at **www.NAEMT.org.**

Photo Acknowledgments

All photographs not credited adjacent to the photograph were photographed on assignment for Brady Prentice Hall Pearson Education.

Organizations

We want to thank the following organizations for their assistance in creating the photo program for this third edition:

Youngstown State University
College of Health and Human Services
Department of Health Professions
Youngstown, OH

Youngstown State University
Media & Academic Computing
Youngstown, OH

Beaver Township Fire and Rescue
Chief Gary Borman
North Lima, OH

Technical Advisors

Thanks to Randy Benner for providing technical support during the photo shoots for the third edition:

Randall Benner, MEd, MICP, NREMT-P
Director, Emergency Medical Technology
Youngstown State University
Youngstown, OH

Models

Our appreciation to the following people who provided locations or portrayed patients and EMS providers in our photographs:

Richard Barnes, Robert Benson, Julie Brown, Will Cohen, Margie Davidson, Jack Martin, Christy Morgan-McMillan, Renee Vivacqua

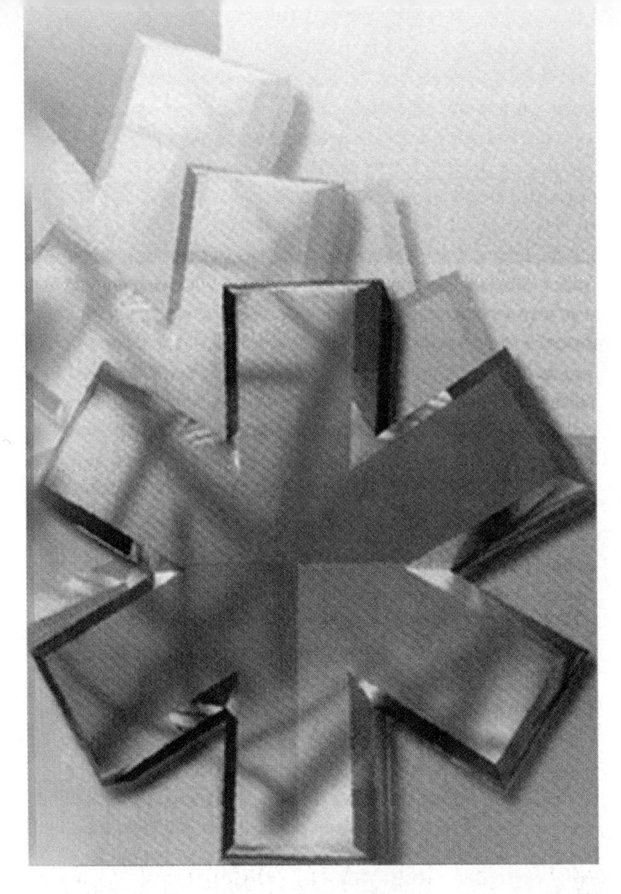

ABOUT THE AUTHORS

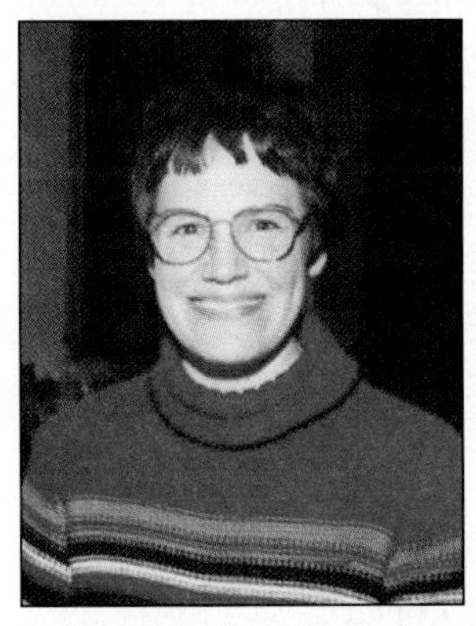

Alice L. (Twink) Dalton, RN, MS, NREMT-P

Alice Dalton, more commonly known as Twink, has been in the emergency care field since 1974, when she started as an emergency department nurse. She was a faculty member of Creighton University's Prehospital Education Program for 13 years, teaching all levels of EMTs and serving as Omaha Fire Department's Paramedic Nurse Coordinator. After functioning as the Trauma Nurse Coordinator at St. Joseph Hospital, she returned to the Omaha Fire Department and served as their EMS Education Coordinator prior to accepting a position as Clinical Educator with Pridemark Paramedic Services. She is now the Director of the EMS Division of the Mountain View Fire Protection District in Longmont, Colorado.

Mrs. Dalton received her Master of Science in Nursing degree from Creighton University in 1998; her Bachelor of Science in Nursing degree from Midland College in Fremont, Nebraska, in 1990; and her RN diploma from Immanuel Hospital School of Nursing in Omaha in 1974. She is also certified as a Nationally Registered Paramedic.

Mrs. Dalton has more than 17 years of experience in both teaching prehospital care providers and providing patient care. She has authored many articles and several chapters in textbooks, and is a frequent speaker at local, state, and national conferences.

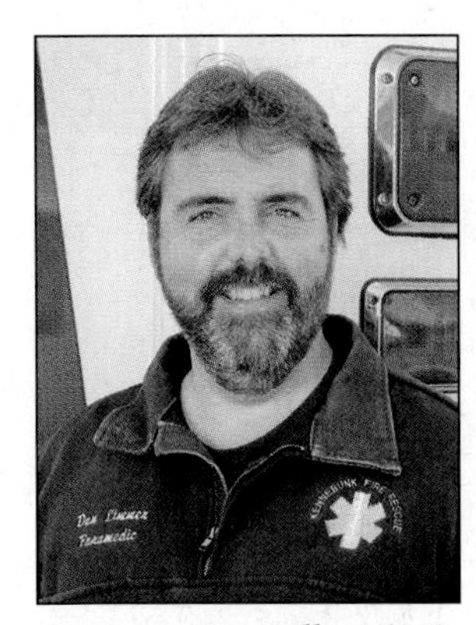

Daniel Limmer, AS, EMT-P

Dan Limmer has been involved in EMS for 28 years, serving as a field provider and educator. He is a paramedic with Kennebunk Fire Rescue in Kennebunk, Maine. He currently instructs at the Southern Maine Community College in South Portland, Maine. He is a coauthor of several EMS textbooks, including *Emergency Care: Essentials of Emergency Care* and *First Responder: A Skills Approach,* and is a frequent speaker at EMS conferences across the United States.

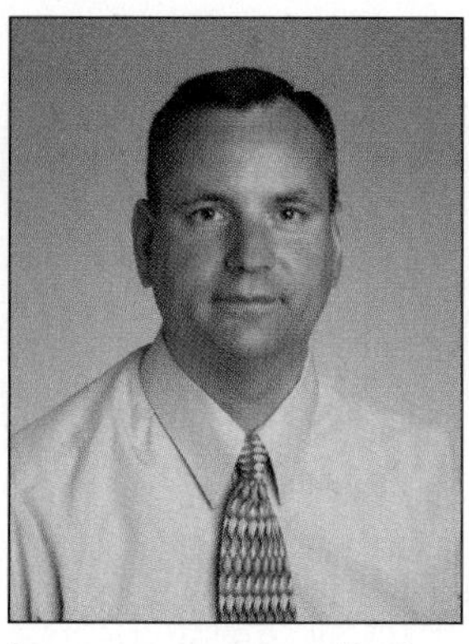

Joseph J. Mistovich, MEd, NREMT-P

Joseph Mistovich is the Chairperson of the Department of Health Professions and a Professor at Youngstown State University in Youngstown, Ohio. He has more than 22 years of experience as an educator in emergency medical services.

Mr. Mistovich received his Master of Education degree in Community Health Education from Kent State University in 1988. He completed a Bachelor of Science in Applied Science degree with a major in Allied Health in 1985 and an Associate in Applied Science degree in Emergency Medical Technology in 1982 from Youngstown State University.

He is a coauthor of several textbooks, including *Prehospital Emergency Care, Prehospital Advanced Cardiac Life Support, EMT-Basic Self-Assessment Review Manual, EMT-Intermediate 85 Self-Assessment Review Manual, EMT-Intermediate 99 Self-Assessment Review Manual, First Responder Self-Assessment Review Manual, EMT-Paramedic Self-Assessment Review Manual,* and an online self-assessment product titled *Paramedic Achieve.*

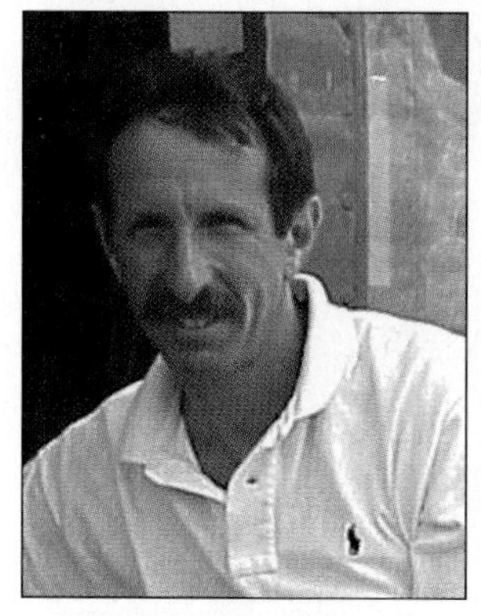

Howard A. Werman, MD, FACEP

Howard A. Werman, MD, is Professor of Emergency Medicine at The Ohio State University. He is an active teacher of medical students in the College of Medicine and the residency training program in Emergency Medicine at The Ohio State University Medical Center. He has been a member of the faculty at Ohio State since 1984, and has been a contributing author to several prehospital and emergency medicine texts. He is past Chairman of the Board of the National Registry of Emergency Medical Technicians.

Dr. Werman has been active in medical direction of several emergency medical services and is currently Medical Director of MedFlight of Ohio, a critical care transport service that offers fixed-wing, helicopter, and mobile ICU services.

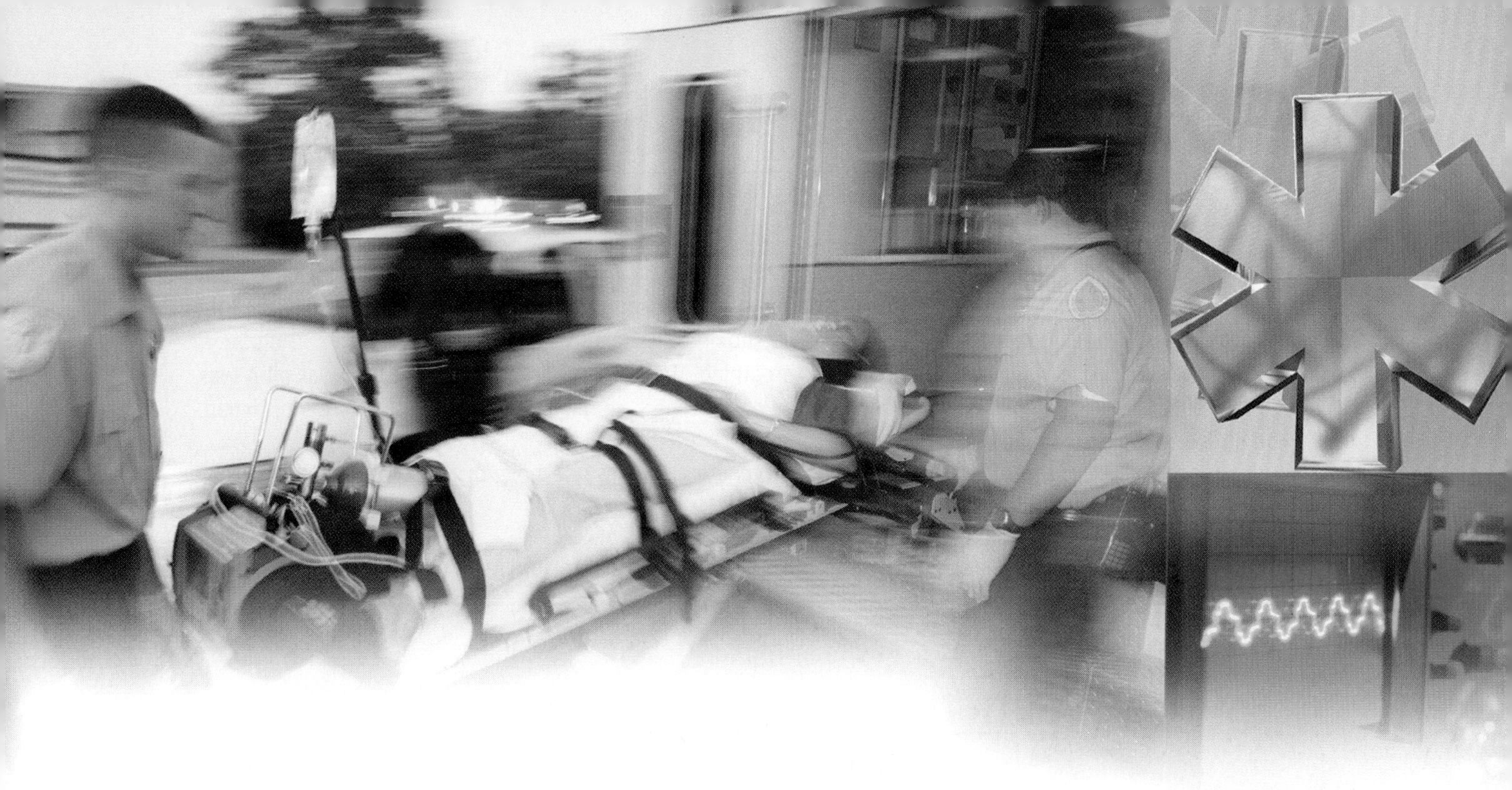

ASSESSMENT OF THE MEDICAL PATIENT

1

An accurate and reliable patient assessment is one of the most important skills that is performed in the prehospital environment. The EMS professional must rely primarily on information gathered in the patient history and on physical assessment findings to develop an appropriate approach to the patient, identify priorities, and establish an emergency care plan. Developing a systematic assessment routine that you follow for every patient will increase your confidence in your assessment skills and ensure that life-threatening conditions will be managed prior to other, non-life threats that may present more dramatically.

Topics that are covered in this chapter are

- Components of the Medical Assessment
- Dispatch Information
- Scene Size-Up
- Physiologically Stable or Unstable Criteria
- Initial Assessment
- Focused History and Physical Exam
- Possibilities to Probabilities: Forming a Differential Field Diagnosis
- Detailed Physical Exam
- Ongoing Assessment

SCENARIO

You are dispatched to an elderly patient for "respiratory distress for the past several days." You arrive on the scene and are greeted at the door by the patient's daughter. As you walk in, you scan the scene for safety hazards. You find the 86-year-old patient, who does not appear to be alert, lying supine on the couch. His daughter tells you, "He started complaining last week that he was having some trouble breathing. He had a cold, and I thought that was all it was. But it's gotten much worse over the last few days. He wouldn't let me take him to the doctor or emergency department." You notice an oxygen tank in the corner of the room.

As you approach the patient, you note that he appears cyanotic. He does not move or respond when you call his name.

How would you proceed with the assessment and management of this patient?

INTRODUCTION

When responding to an emergency scene, many questions enter the mind of the EMS professional. What are the possible conditions the patient might be suffering from? Will there be key information available that will allow me to determine the condition the patient is most probably suffering from? What treatment will be required? How quickly will I need to proceed with the treatment? Will critical interventions be necessary, such as tracheal intubation or drug therapy? Will I need to change the treatment based on additional information gained in the history or physical examination? Will I need to transport the patient rapidly?

Categorize the Patient: Medical versus Trauma

A decision the EMS professional must try to make very early in the assessment is whether this is a medical or a trauma patient. You can usually do this on the basis of the dispatch information and as part of your scene size-up. However, some scenes are very confusing and lack a wealth of overt clues as to whether the patient was injured or is ill. You may not be able to determine the real nature of the patient's problem until you do the focused history and physical exam. You must always be prepared to change your direction of thought and focus based on further assessment findings. Dispatch information can be erroneous, or the patient's real complaint can turn out to be something other than what you suspected when you formed your first impression.

Furthermore, you must categorize the patient not only by mechanism of injury or nature of illness, but also—based on some very objective clinical indicators in the initial assessment—you must determine if the patient is physiologically stable or unstable. The unstable patient will require immediate intervention, as well as a much more aggressive and rapid management plan. Categorizing the patient by degree of stability will allow you to manage immediately life-threatening conditions before proceeding to form a differential field diagnosis as the basis for advanced patient management.

Based on this assessment model, any immediately life-threatening conditions will be managed very early in the assessment process. Once these conditions are managed effectively, you will move on to further assessment to attempt to determine the actual cause of the patient's condition.

In essence, you will move from an assessment-based approach aimed at identifying and abolishing immediate life threats to a diagnostic-based approach where you are looking to provide further care for a specific problem or etiology. During this process, you will be using information gained from the scene, the history, and the physical examination to move from "possible" conditions the patient could be suffering from to "probable" conditions the patient could be suffering from. This dynamic process is based on your ability to "rule out" or "rule in" conditions through linking and processing findings throughout the patient contact.

Assessing a medical patient is quite different from assessing a trauma patient. The trauma patient typically presents with observable signs of injury. Thus, when you assess a suspected trauma patient, you inspect and palpate for clues to injury. The signs are usually objective and can be well documented. Complaints by the patient should lead to more thorough assessment of the relevant body cavity, region, or organ system; however, in the trauma patient, you can usually get more information from the physical exam than from the chief complaint and medical history.

In the medical patient, by contrast, evidence is usually not as obvious. The condition may correlate more closely with the patient's complaints than with overt signs of the condition. For this reason, in the medical patient, the patient interview and medical history usually take precedence over the physical exam. However, objective physical signs may reveal the severity of the condition. So you must view patient complaints and physical exam findings as a whole—as interrelated components—in order to develop an effective field diagnosis and emergency care plan.

A medical patient who is unresponsive or has an altered mental status and cannot provide the necessary information to direct your assessment and treatment is a confounding problem. In this patient, you must rely on your physical exam findings, plus information from family or bystanders, to provide evidence of the suspected condition and severity.

Keep in mind that the prehospital provider usually has the best access to this information. Hospital personnel are remote from the scene and from the time of the incident. It is important that you obtain as much information as you can, as accurately as you can, and provide a thorough report to the hospital staff.

Hospital personnel are remote from the incident. Gather as much information as accurately as you can to report to the hospital staff.

It is imperative that, initially, you focus on identifying and managing immediate life threats—without regard to the possible cause of these conditions. As an example, whether respiratory failure occurs in an exhausted asthma patient or in one who has suffered a stroke, you must immediately recognize the respiratory failure and begin ventilating the patient. It is not necessary to identify the asthma, stroke, or other cause prior to your intervention.

To summarize, you initially take an assessment-based approach to the patient (identifying and correcting life threats), as opposed to a diagnostic-based approach (identifying and treating the underlying cause). Once life threats are properly managed, you rely on the history and physical exam findings to formulate a differential impression of the problem, based on the presenting complaint, and provide more advanced emergency medical care. If you have not managed the airway or ventilated the patient from the beginning of your assessment, however, administering drugs to correct the underlying condition will be futile.

Components of the Medical Assessment
Scene size-up
Initial assessment
Focused history and physical exam
Detailed physical exam
Ongoing assessment

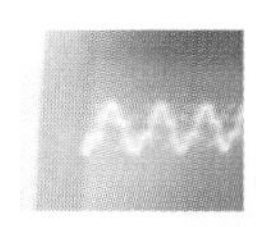

COMPONENTS OF THE MEDICAL ASSESSMENT

The medical assessment is comprised of several components that are integrated into one systematic approach to the patient. The components are

- Scene size-up
- Initial assessment
- Focused history and physical exam
- Detailed physical exam (condition and time dependent)
- Ongoing assessment

Every patient contact requires a scene size-up, initial assessment, focused history and physical exam, and ongoing assessment. However, as is discussed later, the detailed physical exam is of limited use in many medical patients and should be conducted only if time and the patient's condition allow. It is more important to conduct a continuous ongoing assessment so you can effectively monitor and manage life-threatening conditions. Thus, you may never perform a detailed physical exam on some patients.

Each component has a specific purpose for gathering information about the patient and directing emergency medical care. In general, the purposes of the patient assessment are

- ***To categorize the patient as injured or ill.*** This information is primarily gathered from the scene size-up and the general impression you form during the initial assessment. However, you may need to change your thinking as the assessment proceeds. For example, you arrive on the scene to find a patient in a car in a shallow ditch. Based on your scene size-up, you categorize him as a trauma patient. However, on further assessment, you find no evidence of trauma, question the mechanism of injury, and begin to note signs and symptoms of hypoglycemia. You change the direction of your assessment, obtain a blood glucose level of 37 mg/dl, and, based on the clinical findings, administer 50 percent dextrose to the patient. You must always remain flexible and remember that the assessment is a dynamic process.

Clinical Insight

Assessment is a dynamic process. Always be prepared to adjust your thinking as the assessment progresses.

- ***To identify and manage immediate life threats.*** Regardless of whether the patient is a trauma or a medical patient, certain life-threatening compromises to the airway, breathing, and circulation will lead to certain death. The initial assessment is designed to identify these life threats.
- ***To determine the patient's priority status.*** At the conclusion of the initial assessment, you must determine the patient's priority status—whether the patient is a high priority for immediate intervention and expeditious transport or whether more time should be spent with the patient on the scene. Assessment and emergency care will continue in either event.
- ***To gather a patient history.*** Vital to assessment of the medical patient, a history is gathered as early as possible. Most of the information that will direct assessment and emergency medical care is gained from the history. Unresponsive patients pose a special problem because they are unable to provide information. Look for alternative history sources, such as bystanders, family, or medication containers found in bathrooms, nightstands, and refrigerators.
- ***To conduct a physical exam and measure vital signs.*** The physical exam and vital signs will help establish the severity of the patient's condition. Physical

exam findings and vital signs may be the only clues to the condition of an unresponsive medical patient.

- *To assess for other life-threatening conditions.* Use information from the history and physical exam to identify any additional life threats.
- *To provide continued and advanced medical care.* Your initial goal is to abolish immediate life threats. However, as you progress in your assessment, you are looking to form differential diagnoses—seeking clues to help you differentiate the underlying cause of this patient's condition from other etiologies with similar presentations. Based on your differential field diagnosis, you may provide advanced emergency care, such as drug therapy. You will base your differential field diagnosis primarily on information gathered during the focused history and physical exam and the detailed physical exam, if any. This, too, is a dynamic process, based on limited information—that is, without the access to sources of information available at the hospital, such as laboratory data or advanced diagnostic equipment.
- *To continuously monitor the patient's condition and assess the effectiveness of your interventions.* The ongoing assessment is designed to help you continuously monitor for changes in the patient's condition and evaluate the effectiveness of the emergency medical care that has already been provided.
- *To communicate and document information.* The information gathered from the scene and the assessment must be communicated to the hospital staff and accurately documented.

DISPATCH INFORMATION

Dispatch information can be extremely useful. It may tell you whether the patient is injured or ill and the preliminary mechanism of injury or nature of the illness. The proper body substance isolation, need for additional resources, potential for more than one patient, possible hazards at the scene, and other vital information may be available simply from the dispatch. You can begin to form an assessment approach and develop an initial management plan while you are responding to the scene.

Based on the dispatch information, you should begin to develop a mental list of "possible" patient conditions. Your list should include all possibilities, including medical and trauma conditions. For example, simply because you are responding to a residential neighborhood for an elderly male complaining of chest pain does not preclude the possibility of trauma. The chest pain may be associated with a pneumothorax the patient suffered when he fell and struck his chest on the table. Do not develop tunnel vision. Keep all "possibilities" open. This is a dynamic process.

Although dispatch information is usually very helpful, it may also lead to a great deal of confusion. Sometimes the public provides inaccurate information to the call-taker, either inadvertently, out of ignorance or excitement, or intentionally. You may get called to the scene for chest pain, as reported by the caller. You go through scenarios in your mind and develop an assessment and management plan to deal with a medical patient complaining of chest pain. You think to yourself that scene hazards will more than likely be minimal. You elect to put on only disposable gloves as body substance isolation protection because you expect blood and other body fluid exposure to be limited. Also, you assume there will be no need for additional resources unless you find the patient in cardiac arrest.

Sometimes the public provides inaccurate information to the call-taker, either inadvertently, out of ignorance or excitement, or intentionally.

However, when you arrive on the scene and walk into the house, you find a young male patient with multiple gunshot wounds to the anterior body. Blood is pooled on the floor and splattered around the kitchen. You have gloves on but no eye protection; you are prepared to deal with a medical patient, not trauma; and you are now in a potentially violent scene without the proper law enforcement presence. Immediately, you have to change your direction of thought and develop a completely new plan of action.

This type of situation may occur in high-crime areas. The caller knows that if a shooting is reported, the police will be sent and EMS will wait outside the scene until it is made safe; therefore, he reports a common complaint, such as chest pain, that will not induce a police response.

Also, in some situations, the severity of the complaint is downplayed. "He just needs to go to the hospital to get checked out" is a common statement. You typically respond in a nonemergency mode and may approach the scene with a complacent attitude. Unfortunately, many of these patients turn out to be in severe distress, suffering a critical medical crisis. Again, you need to change direction immediately to deal with a critical patient instead of a routine nonemergency transfer. Throughout, you must always remain alert and realize that prehospital care is a dynamic process.

SCENE SIZE-UP

The scene size-up is the initial evaluation of the scene and of the patient in relationship to his environment. This is the first phase of patient assessment, and it can provide you with valuable information that is not available to the remainder of the health care team who have not been at the scene. Thus, it is imperative to pay close attention to the scene and its characteristics not only for how these will affect on-scene care decisions but also so you can convey this information to the hospital staff.

There are three main purposes to the scene size-up. First, the environment in which the patient is found will usually provide some clues as to what body substance isolation precautions are necessary. Next, you must identify any potential hazards so you can take steps to ensure your own safety and that of your partner, the patient, and bystanders. The last purpose is to categorize the patient as either trauma or nontrauma—a patient with injuries or a medical patient suffering an illness.

As emphasized earlier, the scene size-up is never finished; it is a dynamic, ongoing process. You need to continuously reevaluate the patient and the scene and be ready to change your direction of thought, assessment, management, and scene control at any time.

Body Substance Isolation

Body substance isolation precautions are a safety measure that reduces the incidence of infectious disease transmission. Most often the nature of the call, as relayed by the dispatcher, provides clues as to what type of equipment you will need to protect yourself.

Clinical Insight

All body fluids, not just blood, are potentially infectious. Appropriate body substance isolation precautions must be taken for medical calls and for trauma.

Your first instinct may be that trauma calls, which are usually more dramatic and have a high potential for exposure to blood, require more protection than medical calls, which are less dramatic and have minimal risk of exposure to blood. However, blood is not the only body fluid that can transmit infectious disease. In addition to blood, oral, and respiratory secretions, other body substances are also potentially infectious. These include vomitus, urine, feces, sweat, tears, pus, and vaginal, seminal, synovial, pleural, peritoneal, pericardial, and amniotic fluid. So you must protect yourself against all body fluids, not just blood, and take body substance isolation precautions as seriously for medical calls as for trauma.

Dispatch information may be most helpful when responding to a patient with a known infectious disease, such as tuberculosis (TB), vancomycin-resistant *enterococcus* (VRE), or methicillin-resistant *Staphylococcus aureus* (MRSA). The information-taker may be able to determine the potential for infectious disease exposure, especially for calls to nursing homes and long-term care facilities where diseases of this type are fairly common.

Often the clues will be subtle, but they should increase your index of suspicion that you may be dealing with a potentially infectious patient. For example, if dispatched for a patient complaining of a headache, fever, stiff neck, and vomiting, you may suspect meningitis and should take precautions before entering the scene. Once you are at the patient's side and have come in contact with his secretions, exposure has occurred, and your risk of contracting the disease has already drastically increased. You have no way of gauging the infectivity or virulence of the disease, so you need to take the maximal precautions.

Protective equipment will prevent body fluid contact with the skin, eyes, mouth, mucous membranes, and clothing. The decision as to which equipment is appropriate is based on the potential for body fluid exposure, contamination, and disease transmission. In general, be very aggressive in applying BSI precautions. Items can always be removed if the risk of exposure is not as great as expected.

Gloves

Because the prehospital environment is so uncontrolled, the risk of exposure to body fluids is high. You will need to perform a physical exam on every patient, so the potential to come in contact with body fluids is always present. Gloves will reduce the risk of unexpected exposure. Therefore, they must be considered standard protective equipment for all patient contacts, regardless of whether body fluids are visible or suspected. Be sure that the gloves you wear are designed for medical purposes and meet the standards for protection against transmission of infectious disease (Figure 1-1).

One consideration regarding the use of latex examination gloves is the possibility of the patient or EMS responder having a latex allergy. If known, use exam gloves made from a nonlatex material such as vinyl. If the patient exhibits evidence of a local reaction or systemic signs of an allergic reaction, manage him accordingly.

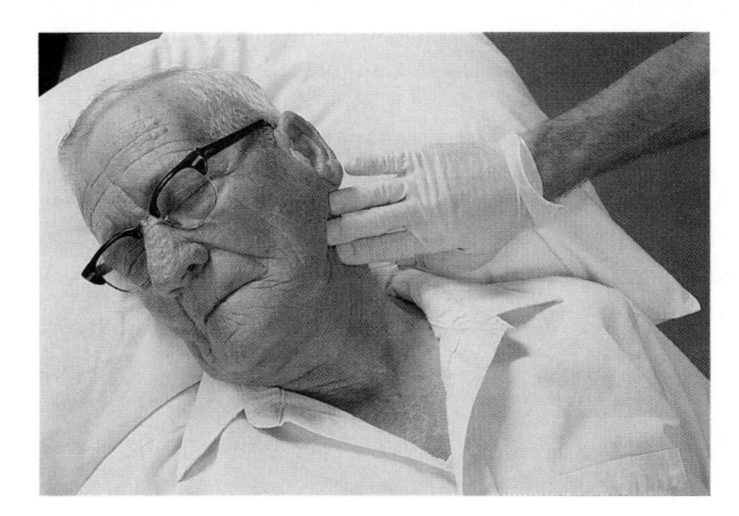

FIGURE 1-1
Gloves are considered standard protective equipment for all patient contacts.

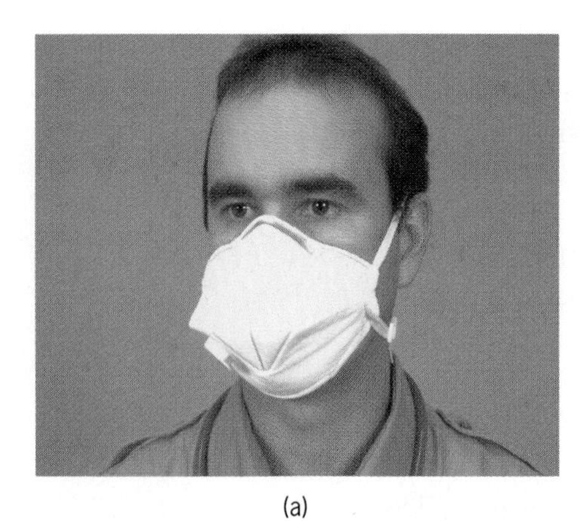

(a)

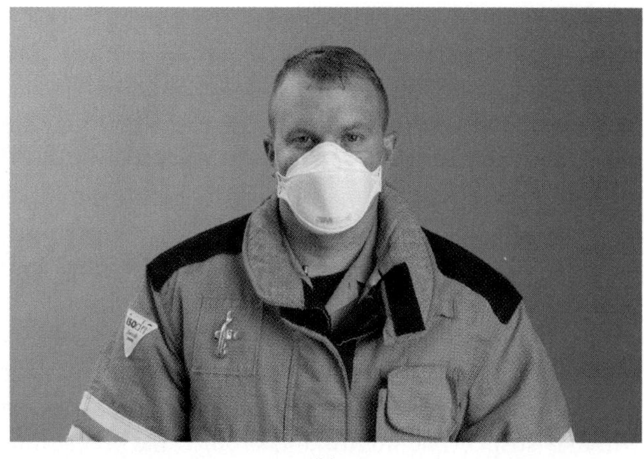

(b)

FIGURE 1-2
Whenever a patient is suspected of having tuberculosis (TB), you must wear (a) a high-efficiency particulate air (HEPA) respirator or (b) an N-95 respirator.
(© Scott Metcalfe)

Protective Eyewear

Wear protective eyewear on all calls that may involve splattering of blood or other body fluids. If you already wear glasses, attach side shields to your regular glasses. Face shields, which provide protection to the entire face, can also be worn. Some face shields have a surgical-type mask incorporated into the shield. These are ideal when splatters of blood are possible, suction is to be performed, or the patient is coughing.

HEPA or N-95 Respirator

Wear a high-efficiency particulate air (HEPA) or N-95 respirator (Figure 1-2) whenever you are in contact with a patient who potentially has infectious TB. Most often, by the time you can determine at the scene that the patient exhibits typical signs and symptoms of TB, it is too late and exposure has already occurred. So pay special attention to any clues from the dispatch that indicate a potential case of TB. Signs and symptoms of TB are cough, weakness, fever, night sweats, and weight loss. Those who are at most risk for TB infection include patients from a nursing home or institutional setting; HIV-positive, transplant, and cancer chemotherapy patients who are immunosuppressed (thus vulnerable to infections of all types); alcoholics; immigrants from areas where TB is prevalent; and any patient living in a poor environment and lacking in health care.

Surgical Mask

Wear a standard surgical mask to protect your oral and nasal mucous membranes from exposure to blood and other body fluids, especially respiratory droplets, which can be spread by a cough, sneeze, or secretions that are being suctioned. It may also be prudent to place a mask over the patient's nose and mouth to reduce the number of respiratory droplets emitted into the ambient atmosphere. Be sure to explain to the patient the reason why it is necessary for both him and you to wear a mask.

If you place a mask on a suspected TB patient, however, you must still wear a HEPA or N-95 respirator because the filtration of a surgical mask is not efficient enough to prevent TB bacteria from escaping. Be sure the HEPA or N-95 mask was properly fit, tested, and replaced following an exposure. Do not place a HEPA mask with an exhalation valve on the patient because this type of mask does not filter exhaled gases.

Gown

Where copious blood or body fluids are present, such as in emergency childbirth, and contact with your clothing and undergarments is possible, you should wear a gown. Use your judgment. Gowns are sometimes worn inappropriately when no blood or body fluid exposure is expected; conversely, there are often situations where a gown should have been worn but was not, and blood and body fluids have contaminated clothing. The driver should remove his gown and gloves before entering the cab so as not to contaminate the driver and passenger compartments.

Scene Safety

Scene safety is the phase of the scene size-up where you assess for any real or perceived hazards to you, your partner, the patient, or bystanders. Personal protection is your number one priority, taking precedence even over patient care.

Situation Awareness

A major consideration in scene safety is maintaining an awareness of the surroundings at all times while on the scene—not just having a heightened sense of awareness initially when entering and making first contact with the patient.

Fighter pilots are taught "situation awareness." That is, no matter what circumstances they are in, whether a dog fight or a training flight, they must maintain a heightened awareness of all aspects of their aircraft and surroundings at all times. EMS personnel have a tendency to be aware of the scene surroundings initially. Subsequently, however, they tend to lose this sense and develop "patient awareness," focusing solely on the patient once contact is made. This leaves them vulnerable. EMS personnel, similar to fighter pilots, must vigilantly maintain a "scene awareness" at all times. Be sure to keep track of who is in the house, where they are, how they are postured, where the exits are, where the potential weapons are, and the mood of the family and bystanders.

Protect Yourself

As a general rule, if the scene is unsafe, either make it safe or retreat until it can be made safe by others, such as the fire department, hazardous materials team, or law enforcement. If you are going to participate in making the scene safe, be sure you have the necessary knowledge, skills, and tools. It may be as simple as dragging a patient who is lying under, but not in contact with, electrical wires to a safe place, or it may be as complex as making a rescue from a rushing stream, which requires special equipment and training. Attempting a swift-water rescue without the proper equipment and training will most likely end with tragic results for both you and the patient.

Medical patients typically do not present in such dramatic situations, but the same rules hold true. If your patient is attempting to commit suicide by inhaling toxic fumes, you are not going to charge into the room to save him without taking some precautions. Entering the scene of an aggressive overdose patient may require the assistance of law enforcement. Always follow your intuition. If the scene does not feel right, do not enter it without the proper back-up or resources.

Scene safety evaluation never ends. You must continuously assess the environment you are in and be ready to react or retreat. An object you do not necessarily think of as dangerous, such as a letter opener, can easily become a weapon in the hands of an irate, agitated, or aggressive person. Just because you are not dealing with a violent crime does not mean that weapons, such as guns and knives, are not close at hand at the scene. It is not unusual to walk into a patient's bedroom and find a loaded pistol on the nightstand. Be especially cautious when entering a scene involving potential drug

Scene safety evaluation never ends. You must continuously assess the environment you are in and be ready to react or retreat.

Clinical Insight

Patients who require restraints must be restrained in a supine or lateral position, never a prone position. A supine or lateral position allows for adequate assessment of the patient. It puts less strain on the diaphragm and does not impinge on the ventilatory volume.

use, alcohol intoxication, or drug overdose. The patients or bystanders may not be rational and may become aggressive and violent.

A major misconception among EMS personnel is that most violent injuries to EMS providers occur at crime scenes, such as shootings and stabbings. In fact, however, most violent acts against EMS personnel occur at scenes that involve sudden behavior changes. These scenes typically involve alcohol, drugs, or behaviorally disturbed patients or bystanders.

Be Aware of Scene Characteristics

You leave a relatively safe environment when you exit your ambulance or rescue vehicle and enter a potentially unstable environment. Study the scene. Each scene is dynamic and unique. You must tailor your approach to accommodate the specific characteristics. When approaching a scene, follow these basic principles:

- Do not enter a scene that is potentially hazardous or unstable.
- Take the extra time and precautions at crime scenes, suspected crime scenes, and scenes involving alcohol, drugs, or behaviorally disturbed patients or bystanders, volatile crowds, or aggressive patients (Figure 1-3). Wait for the police before entering, or retreat if the situation becomes threatening.
- Always carry your portable radio into the scene so you can call for help if necessary.
- Realize your own limitations and do not exceed your abilities to manage a hazardous scene.
- Retreat from the scene if it becomes unstable and you cannot control it.
- An EMS career involves a certain amount of risk. However, do not take unnecessary risks.

Protect the Patient

Many medical emergencies occur outside the home and can expose the patient to environmental conditions that may cause discomfort or exacerbate the patient's problem. Also, the public's curiosity may increase the patient's stress. You must have a sense of what factors would affect the patient and alter them to keep your patient safe and comfortable.

Remove patients from extremely hot environments, especially patients with possible heat cramps, heat exhaustion, or heat stroke. Leaving a patient exposed to a high ambient temperature can easily lead to further deterioration and extreme discomfort. For example, you respond to a patient who was running the peace race

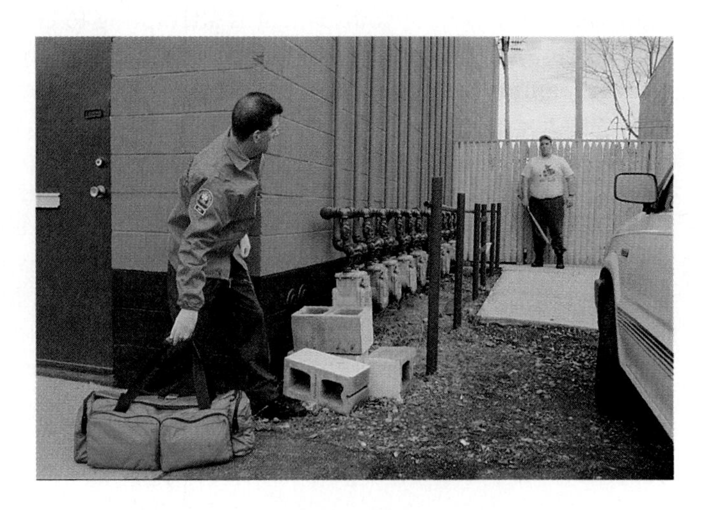

FIGURE 1-3
Wait for the police before entering a potentially hazardous scene.

in the local park and has suffered a syncopal episode from what you suspect to be heat exhaustion. The ambient temperature is 95 degrees Fahrenheit, and the relative humidity is 97 percent. You perform your initial assessment and rapid medical assessment, and then quickly move the patient to the back of the ambulance with the air conditioning on high. You can easily continue your assessment and emergency care in the ambulance while providing not only a more comfortable environment but also, by using the air conditioning to help cool the patient, taking a vital emergency management step.

Similarly, in a cold environment, move the patient quickly into the back of the heated ambulance. Again, this is both a comfort measure and part of your emergency care for a potentially hypothermic patient. When transporting a patient from a heated home or building to the ambulance, be sure to cover the patient, leaving as little skin exposed as possible and covering the patient's head with a blanket or towel.

When dealing with patients in the public's view, keep the patient's modesty in mind. If clothing must be removed, do it discreetly and cover the patient with a sheet. You may want to position yourself and others to block the view of onlookers. Or you might ask police or fire personnel to move the crowd back out of view to lessen the patient's anxiety. Verbal communication and continuous reassurance provide a great deal of therapeutic benefit in these situations.

Protect Bystanders

Emergencies have a tendency to draw crowds. This can be a serious distraction when you need to direct your attention to the patient. Also, you are responsible for ensuring the safety of the bystanders because they are part of the scene. It may be necessary to have the police keep the crowd out of your way and under control. Dispersing the crowd or directing them to another area may be the most appropriate method in situations where bystanders could also become patients, such as in a chemical spill or toxic inhalation incident.

Nature of the Illness

Once scene safety has been assured, the next priority is to categorize your patient as being either injured or ill. As noted earlier, the trauma patient often exhibits objective signs of injury, whereas observable signs may be subtle or absent in the medical patient. Later in the assessment, you will rely heavily on the patient's chief complaint and history, but during the scene size-up, dispatch information may be the first indication of a medical problem.

You must try to determine the real reason you were called to the scene. Sometimes you will have to actually ask the patient, "Why did you call us today?" Relatives, bystanders, or the physical environment may provide you with clues to what the patient is suffering from. However, the patient, if he is responsive and alert, will be the most reliable source of information as you attempt to determine the nature of the illness.

When performing the scene size-up, it is important to recognize clues to the medical problem. Also, do not forget that you are probably the only person who will be able to provide information about the scene to others who will assume care of the patient later on. Scan the scene for relevant information (Figure 1-4).

For example, an oxygen concentrator usually indicates that the patient has preexisting respiratory problems. A bucket next to the bed or couch may be a clue that the patient was nauseated and vomiting. Finding a patient in pajamas at 3 o'clock in the afternoon may indicate that the patient has been ill all day. A hospital bed should make you suspect that the patient has a chronic condition.

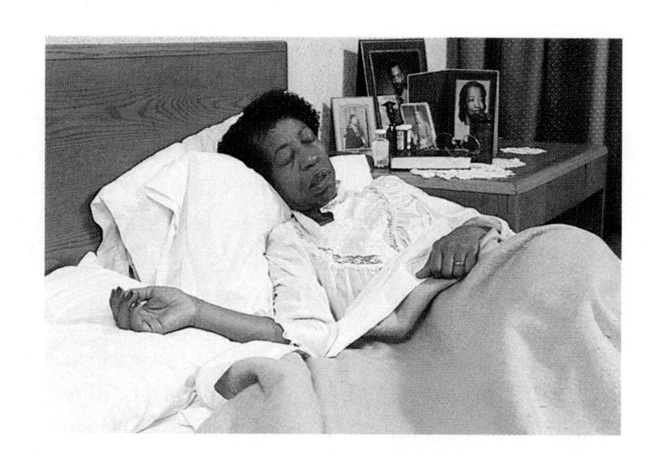

FIGURE 1-4
Scan the scene for relevant information.

Clinical Insight

Pure alcohol has very little odor. You cannot rule out alcoholic-related conditions in patients who do not necessarily smell of alcoholic beverages. However, suspect other medical conditions in patients with an altered mental status who present with a strong smell of alcohol.

Other potential sources of information regarding the etiology of the current condition or past medical history may be medications found at the scene or on the patient, medical identification tags, and medical information cards. Items such as syringes, drug paraphernalia, and alcohol containers may raise your index of suspicion. For example, syringes may cause you to suspect potential intravenous drug abuse or insulin injection associated with diabetes mellitus. Alcohol containers may also explain an altered mental status etiology.

Use a clue like this as only one piece of the puzzle. Do not lose sight of other potential etiologies of the medical condition. As your assessment proceeds, you will also rely heavily on any patient complaints and the patient history and physical exam findings. Consider all information you gather as a whole as you progress toward forming a field diagnosis.

Number of Patients

The scene size-up is also used to determine the number of patients who require medical attention. It is more common to have more than one patient in traumatic situations than in medical ones. However, the possibility of having more than one medical patient definitely exists.

For example, you are dispatched on a call for weakness, headache, tinnitus, and nausea. On arrival at the scene, you note that three others in the same home are complaining of similar symptoms, some more severe than others. Recognizing the signs of carbon monoxide poisoning, you know that you have to manage all patients. You would probably need to call for additional resources to provide efficient medical care.

Events that take place in hot, humid weather may provide you with large numbers of patients exhibiting signs and symptoms of heat exhaustion. You may need to set up a system similar to a mass casualty incident in order to manage every patient effectively.

Thus, just because it is a medical call, do not rule out the possibility of having more than one patient. You may be required to triage and make priority transport decisions in situations like these.

Additional Resources

Some medical situations require additional resources at the scene. These may include the fire department, law enforcement, crisis intervention team, or other agencies. Some situations may require additional resources before you even enter the scene. You would not walk into a garage with a pesticide all over the patient and the floor without having the proper protective clothing; the hazardous materials team and fire department would need to control the scene first. A potentially violent person who is threatening suicide will require law enforcement to establish scene safety before the EMS crew goes into the scene.

Be cautious when approaching the scene. Medical calls can produce the same types of violence, injury, and death to EMS providers as trauma scenes. Do not become complacent and end up injured or dead from what was "only" a medical call at what you assumed would be a nonthreatening scene.

Agents of Terrorism

Because of recent domestic and international terrorist attacks and the possibility of future such attacks, EMS personnel must be prepared to recognize and manage patients who have been exposed to biological, chemical, and nuclear agents used by terrorists. In addition, as an EMS provider, your first priority is to protect yourself from these deadly agents. The following material provides a brief overview of common signs and symptoms that may be seen in some of these exposures. The intent is to create awareness of these chemical and infectious agents, as well as the syndromes they produce, so you may consider the conditions resulting from exposure to these agents as a "possibility" in the critical analysis that goes into your differential field diagnosis. It is very possible that the EMS crew may be the first line of health care provider assessing and treating patients who have been exposed to these agents. Your awareness may assist public health and emergency management officials in responding quickly to an incident that may involve chemical or biological agents. However, it is beyond the scope of this book to discuss treatment and personal protection associated with exposure to these agents.

Terrorists may use chemical, biological, or nuclear agents to cause social panic in addition to loss of life and property. Exposure to chemical agents may cause immediate reactions in patients, who will quickly exhibit myriad signs and symptoms, depending on the agent of exposure. Patients exposed to bacterial agents, however, may take days to weeks to present with signs and symptoms. Nuclear agents may cause both immediate signs and symptoms and delayed syndromes. Chemical and biological agents are much more readily available and accessible to terrorists than nuclear materials; thus, we focus on chemical and biological agents.

Chemical agents include nerve agents such as Sarin, Tabun, and VX, which inhibit acetylcholinesterase and bind with acetylcholine, preventing nerve transmission. They affect both sympathetic and parasympathetic nervous systems. Patients exposed to nerve agents may present with the typical SLUDGE signs (Salivation, Lacrimation, Urination, Defecation, and Emesis), pinpoint pupils, bronchoconstriction, laryngospasm, respiratory failure or arrest, altered mental status, and seizures. The patient may complain of muscle cramps, eye pain, visual disturbances, tremors, rhinorrhea, or diaphoresis. If the exposure occurred as a result of aerosols, the onset of signs and symptoms will take seconds to minutes, whereas if the route of exposure was contact with liquid agents, signs and symptoms may take minutes to hours to present.

Cyanide agents, which include hydrogen cyanide and cyanogen chloride, typically produce a very rapid onset of signs and symptoms and may result in death within 1 to 15 minutes if the person is exposed to a high level of the agent. Patients may present with respiratory distress, hyperpnea, seizures, palpitations, dizziness, nausea, vomiting, altered mental status, coma, and eye irritation.

Blister or vesicant agents include sulfur mustard, nitrogen mustard, phosgene oxime, and lewisite. These agents typically cause severe irritation to the lungs, eyes, and mucous membranes. Most of the signs appear as cutaneous lesions; however, the respiratory and gastrointestinal tract may also suffer injury. The skin becomes erythematous (red) and progresses to bullae (serous fluid-filled vesicles) with burning and itching. The eyes may become red and irritated with tearing. The patient may also suffer respiratory distress, nausea, vomiting, cough, and hemoptysis (bloody sputum). Lewisite may produce signs and symptoms within minutes after exposure, whereas sulfur mustard may take hours to days.

Pulmonary or choking agents produce severe irritation of the upper and lower respiratory tract. Agents may include phosgene, chlorine, diphosgene, chloropicrin, and sulfur dioxide. The patient will typically present with respiratory distress, chest tightness or discomfort, coughing, wheezing, stridor, mucosal irritation, hoarseness, and signs of pulmonary edema. Onset of signs and symptoms may take 1 to 24 hours.

Ricin is another chemical agent that may cause pulmonary, gastrointestinal, and cardiovascular deterioration. If the ricin is ingested, the patient may complain of nausea, vomiting, diarrhea, abdominal pain, and fever. If it is inhaled, the patient may have chest discomfort, respiratory distress, crackles, weakness, nausea, and fever. If ricin is ingested, the onset of signs and symptoms may take 18 to 24 hours. If it is inhaled, the patient may exhibit signs and symptoms within 8 to 36 hours.

Dispersion of a biological agent may go unrecognized for a period of time. Exposure to the agent may not be apparent until long after the dispersion, following the incubation period. It would be important for you, as an EMS provider, to recognize typical patterns of patient complaints and presentations. Infectious biological agents may be viruses, bacteria, protozoa, or fungi. They may include anthrax, botulinum toxin, *Yersinia pestis*, and variola virus (smallpox). Other agents include *Brucella*, Venezuelan equine encephalitis (VEE), *Coxiella buirnetii* (Q fever), Rift valley fever, and *Francisella tularensis*.

Anthrax infection is caused by *Bacillus anthracis*. It can be inhaled, absorbed through the skin, or ingested. Signs and symptoms of inhaled anthrax include headache, fever, fatigue, muscle aches, dyspnea, nonproductive cough, and chest discomfort. The patient commonly believes he has the flu. He may improve for 1 to 2 days and then suddenly deteriorate to respiratory failure and shock. Skin exposure produces intense itching followed by development of nonpainful papular lesions (elevated palpable lesons) that then become vesicular (fluid filled). Ingestion of anthrax toxin typically produces abdominal pain, nausea, vomiting, diarrhea, evidence of gastrointestinal bleeding, and fever.

Botulinum poisoning commonly presents as progressive symmetric weakness and paralysis descending down the body. Respiratory failure eventually occurs. The patient typically maintains a normal mental status and is afebrile. The patient may complain of excessive mucus, dry mouth, dizziness, and difficulty in moving the eyelids. Other signs include papillary dilation, nystagmus, cranial nerve palsies, speech disturbance, unsteady gait, and weakness leading to flaccid paralysis. If the poison is inhaled, the onset of signs and symptoms may occur within 12 to 80 hours after exposure. If it is ingested, the incubation time is 12 to 72 hours.

The pneumonic plague results from exposure to *Y. pestis*. It presents most often as pneumonia but then commonly leads to respiratory failure and cardiovascular collapse. The patient typically presents with high fever, cough, hemoptysis, chest discomfort, productive cough (purulent or watery sputum), nausea, and vomiting. The skin may have purpuric lesions (red blotches). The onset of signs and symptoms is typically 2 to 3 days following exposure.

Smallpox infection is caused by the variola virus. The patient usually complains of fever, vomiting, headache, backache, and malaise. After 2 to 4 days, macules (flat, nonpalpable lesions) appear on the skin that progress to papules (elevated, palpable lesions), then vesicles (elevated lesions filled with serous fluid), and finally to pustules (elevated lesion filled with purulent fluid). Lesions are typically all in the same stage of development. The lesions are most commonly found on the face, the neck, the palms of the hands, and the soles of the feet, then typically progress to the trunk of the body. The incubation period for smallpox infection is usually 12 to 14 days.

Entering the Scene

If you do not take charge, someone else will.

On arrival, it is necessary to take charge of the scene and establish rapport, not only with the patient, relatives, and bystanders, but also with first responders and other health care professionals who may be providing initial care. You must always convey confidence and competence when making this transition. If you do not take charge of the scene, someone else will. This may be a firefighter, a police officer, another health care professional, a family member, or the patient himself.

When you arrive on the scene, gather information from the first responders. If the patient is alert and talking, you may have time to ascertain what information the first responders have already gathered and what care they have provided before you begin your own patient assessment and care. However, if the patient has an altered mental status, you may need to start patient assessment and interventions immediately while you or your partner collects information from the first responders.

Also when arriving on the scene, take steps to reduce the patient's anxiety as much as possible. Simply reducing the anxiety of a patient who is suffering from a myocardial infarction may reduce myocardial workload and myocardial oxygen demand, thus limiting the size and extent of the infarction. You can reduce the patient's anxiety by bringing order to the environment, introducing yourself, gaining patient consent, positioning yourself, using communication skills, being courteous, and using touch when appropriate.

As quickly as possible after you arrive on the scene, gain control and bring order to the environment. It may be necessary to turn off a television or radio, remove children from the room, or have a family member place a dog in a closed room for safety and to lessen distractions. However, avoid the possibility of violent confrontations. For example, do not just walk up and turn off the television when someone is watching it, no matter how serious the situation. A person may become outraged and violent very quickly over something that, to you, seems so appropriate to do. Be calm and nonconfrontational when bringing the scene to order. Be firm and clear that you were called to deliver emergency medical care, and you are in charge.

Always introduce yourself to the patient. Also, if the patient's condition permits, ask what the patient would like you to call him. During this introductory phase, gain consent from the patient for emergency care. This is legally necessary before you assess the patient and provide emergency care. It may be as simple as asking, "Is it all right for me to help you?" to gain the patient's expressed consent. If the patient has an altered mental status or is unable to make or communicate a rational decision, as with some strokes, you will have to proceed under implied consent. If the patient refuses care, do not immediately accept that decision. He may really need medical attention but is going through a denial phase. If you offer some explanation to help the patient make an informed decision, then he may readily provide the necessary consent.

Your body position and posture are nonverbal modes of communication. Position yourself, if possible, so your eye level is somewhat the same as the patient's. This translates into equality. If you stand over the patient, you exhibit authority and control. This may set the wrong tone for the scene, making the patient more anxious and uncomfortable and lessening the patient's cooperation. Standing with your arms crossed over your chest is a closed communication posture that implies disinterest or even hostility. Relax your posture to communicate a sense of confidence, openness, and willingness to help. Do not yell or scream at the scene; talk to your partner calmly and confidently.

Maintain eye contact with the patient as much as possible. This will establish rapport and convey a sense of concern. Speak calmly and deliberately so the patient can process the information. Raise your voice only if the patient appears to be hearing impaired. Also, actively listen to what your patient is telling you. This prevents unnecessary repetition of questions and shows concern on your part. Do not allow your attention to wander while you gather information from the patient.

Touch is a very powerful comfort measure to most people. Use eye contact to allay the patient's perception of touching as encroachment. Hold a hand, touch a shoulder, or lay your hand on a forearm. Be sincere in your gestures of touch. However, some patients may be extremely uncomfortable with any touch. This is sometimes rooted in culture, or it may be a personal preference of the patient.

Remember that the emergency scene can be very stressful for the patient, family, bystanders, friends, and emergency care providers. People are typically at their worst when an emergency arises. They may often seem hostile, rude, or argumentative. Attempt to understand these as responses to the stress of the situation and not as a direct attack on you. Remain firm, but professional and courteous.

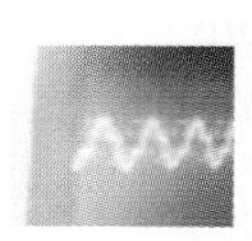

PHYSIOLOGICALLY STABLE OR UNSTABLE CRITERIA

Once you have categorized the patient as trauma or medical, the next step in your assessment plan should be to determine whether the patient is physiologically stable or physiologically unstable. Obviously, the unstable patient would require the most immediate intervention.

Clinical Insight

Categorizing your patient as physiologically stable or unstable will provide you with a basis to determine further assessment and develop an aggressive management plan.

Categorizing your patient as stable or unstable is basically what the seasoned EMS professional does subconsciously, through years of experience. He determines whether the medical patient is "sick" or "not sick." The physiologically unstable patient is "sick" or "ill" and in need of immediate intervention. Without adequate intervention, this patient will deteriorate rapidly. The physiologically stable patient, however, has no immediate life threats, so you can devote more time to assessment and management. Thus, categorizing your patient as physiologically stable or unstable will provide you with a basis to determine further assessment and develop an aggressive management plan.

To categorize your patient as physiologically stable or unstable, you need to assess specific critical criteria. You will also need to identify the potential presence of high-risk medical conditions that would warrant more aggressive assessment and intervention. You will identify these criteria and conditions primarily during the initial assessment and the focused history and physical exam. Also, you must continuously reassess the patient during the ongoing assessment to determine whether the patient's condition has improved or deteriorated and to make appropriate additional interventions.

The critical criteria you must assess will identify the "red flags" that immediately indicate physiological instability. Most can be found during the initial assessment of the patient while you are evaluating the airway, breathing, circulation, and central nervous system. Each "red flag" is a potential indication of a poor patient

TABLE 1-1 Indicators of Physiological Instability

Assessment Phase	Red Flags
General Impression	■ Compromised airway ■ Apnea or inadequate breathing ■ Pulselessness
Mental Status/Neurologic Assessment	■ No spontaneous eye movement ■ No spontaneous movement or response to painful stimulus ■ Not oriented to year ■ Unable to move fingers and toes to commands
Airway Assessment	■ Altered mental status with inability to protect the airway ■ Obstructive sounds such as stridor, snoring, or gurgling ■ Obstruction due to tongue, vomitus, secretions, blood, or foreign bodies
Breathing Assessment	■ Apnea ■ Respiratory rate < 8 or > 30 ■ Absent or diminished breath sounds ■ Little to no detectable air movement or irregular pattern ■ Retractions of intercostal spaces, suprasternal notch, or supraclavicular spaces
Circulation Assessment	■ Weak or absent peripheral or central pulses ■ Pulse rate < 60 or > 100 ■ Irregular pulse ■ Pale or cyanotic nails, skin, or palms ■ Cool, diaphoretic skin

condition. Each flag raises your suspicion, and some may require immediate and aggressive intervention and consideration of expeditious transport.

The "red flags," or indicators of physiological instability (also see Table 1-1), are

- *Airway*
  - Obstructive sounds such as snoring (sonorous), gurgling, stridor, or crowing
  - Obstruction due to vomitus, secretions, blood, or foreign bodies
- *Breathing*
  - Apnea
  - Respiratory rate less than 8 breaths per minute
  - Respiratory rate greater than 30 breaths per minute
  - Irregular respiratory pattern
  - Absent or diminished breath sounds
  - Little to no detectable air movement
  - Retractions of the intercostal spaces, suprasternal notch, supraclavicular spaces, or subcostal area
- *Circulation*
  - Absent central pulses
  - Absent peripheral pulses
  - Weak peripheral or central pulses
  - Bradycardia
  - Tachycardia
  - Irregular pulse

  - Pale or cyanotic nail or skin/palm color
  - Cool, diaphoretic skin
- *Central Nervous System*
  - No spontaneous eye opening
  - Not oriented to year
  - Unable to move fingers and toes to commands
  - No spontaneous movement or no response to a pinch to the nail bed, earlobe, or web between the thumb and first finger, or other painful stimulus

These criteria constitute a brief assessment of the status of the airway, breathing effort and effectiveness, perfusion status, motor function, sensory function, and cognition level. Although these criteria are elementary, they are good indicators of the potential severity of the patient's condition. Some are designed to be extreme indicators. For example, if your patient is unable to say what year it is, you would not expect him to be oriented to the day or time.

INITIAL ASSESSMENT

Once the scene has been secured, you must rapidly move to performing an initial assessment. This assessment is designed to identify and manage immediate life threats to the airway, breathing, or circulation. Other obvious life threats are also managed during the initial assessment. An immediate life threat is defined as one that may lead to rapid patient deterioration or death within a brief period of time. Any life-threatening condition must be managed immediately before continuing in the assessment process. The initial assessment should only take about 60 seconds to perform; however, if any interventions are required, it may take longer.

Clinical Insight

Any life-threatening condition must be managed immediately before continuing in the assessment process.

The steps of the initial assessment are conducted in the following sequence:

- Form a general impression.
- Assess mental status.
- Assess the airway.
- Assess breathing.
- Assess circulation.
- Establish patient priorities.

Form a General Impression

Your initial assessment begins as soon as you approach the patient. Experienced EMS professionals can gain a lot of valuable information from their first impression about the patient. Consider the patient's general appearance, speech pattern, and posture (Figure 1-5).

Initial Assessment
Form a general impression.
Assess mental status.
Assess the airway.
Assess the adequacy of breathing.
Assess circulation.
Establish patient priorities.

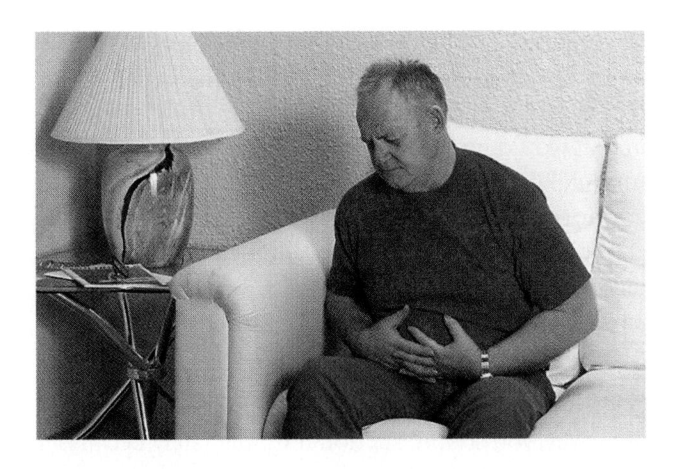

FIGURE 1-5
In forming a general impression, consider the patient's general appearance, speech pattern, and posture.

Some patients have the general appearance of being "ill" without any specific signs or symptoms on initial inspection. The intuition that identifies which patients are "ill" or "sick" develops with experience.

Speech patterns may indicate degree of cognitive impairment or severity of respiratory distress. A patient who has an altered mental status is likely not to be making much sense, or may not be speaking at all. A patient with severe respiratory distress will speak in short, broken sentences with frequent gasps for air.

Posture may also be an indicator of the severity of illness. If you are called to the scene for respiratory distress and find the patient lying flat, you can come to one of two conclusions. The first is that the patient is so exhausted from working hard to breathe that he can no longer support himself in the typical tripod position. This patient most likely will require immediate positive-pressure ventilation. The second is that the patient's respiratory distress is not very severe because he is able to lie flat. Also, nonpurposeful posturing, such as flexion (decorticate) or extension (decerebrate) (described later), may indicate a significant increase in intracranial pressure from a stroke or other structural lesion. Significant abdominal pain usually causes the patient to draw his legs up and lie very still. So arriving on the scene for abdominal pain and finding the patient walking around the house or sitting in the recliner may indicate that the pain and the condition itself are not very severe or that the patient may be suffering from renal calculi.

You may also note abnormal odors, skin color, disarrayed clothing, and other potential clues as you form your general impression. For example, the odor of alcoholic beverages may help explain an altered mental status. Likewise, an acetone or fruity odor on the breath may make you suspect diabetic ketoacidosis. Putrid smells may indicate infection. Severe cyanosis usually indicates a significant cardiac or pulmonary compromise, whereas pallor is typical of hypoperfusion associated with blood loss or volume depletion. Red skin may indicate a heat emergency or other condition related to significant vasodilation. Jaundice would make you suspect an acute or chronic liver disease.

Clinical Insight

A patient with a pericardial effusion will typically sit up and lean forward, and will present with engorged jugular veins.

Clinical Insight

Patients with peritonitis are normally very still and avoid any movement. Patients with an intestinal obstruction are typically restless.

Identify the Chief Complaint

The chief complaint is the patient's answer to the question "Why did you call the ambulance today?" It usually is a symptom (chest pain), a sign (bloody diarrhea), an abnormal function (slurred speech), or an observation you make (altered mental function). The chief complaint is typically sought and identified during the general impression phase of initial assessment.

In the unresponsive medical patient, the chief complaint is difficult to determine. You must rely on others at the scene. You will need to ask what the patient was complaining of or about any unusual behavior prior to becoming unresponsive.

Clinical Insight

The complaint of fatigue in an elderly patient may be an indication of a serious health condition.

Family, friends, or bystanders may be able to provide pertinent clues as to the nature of the illness. For example, a bystander might indicate that the patient complained of "the worst headache I've had in my life" before collapsing to the ground. This is important information that would not be available otherwise, and it sets the tone of the entire call and continued care.

In addition to bystander information, you must rely on the scene characteristics, general impression, and physical assessment findings in the process of forming a field diagnosis in a patient with an altered mental status.

Identify Immediate Life Threats

The general impression is also the phase of the initial assessment where obvious immediate life threats are managed. For example, if you arrive on the scene and find the patient with vomitus in his airway, you should suction it immediately because it may compromise the airway and lead to rapid patient deterioration and, potentially, to death. Do not wait to suction until the airway phase of the initial assessment; by that time, the patient may have aspirated and become severely hypoxic.

Common life threats to the medical patient that need immediate attention and management are

- A compromised airway from vomitus, blood, secretions, the tongue, or other objects or substances
- Apnea or inadequate breathing
- Pulselessness

Position the Patient for Assessment

If you find the patient in a prone position, you will need to immediately log roll him into a supine position in order to perform an accurate assessment and control the airway and breathing adequately. If there is a possibility of spine injury, be sure to maintain manual in-line stabilization while log rolling the patient. A patient who presents with a significant amount of vomitus, blood, or secretions may need to be placed in a lateral recumbent position (recovery or coma position) to facilitate drainage and to assist in keeping the airway patent.

Evaluate Other Information

Other information that is routinely gained during the general impression phase includes the patient's age, gender, and apparent race. Most often, this information is of limited relevance in managing the patient. However, in some conditions, such as sickle cell anemia, hemophilia, and ectopic pregnancy, it is important to consider such things as race and gender.

Assess Mental Status

Cognitive impairment is a potential indicator of some type of intracranial pathology such as intracranial bleeding, stroke, infections, neoplasms, seizures, hypoxia, hypertension, or metabolic encephalopathies such as hypoglycemia, diabetic ketoacidosis, and uremia. Environmental causes such as heat stroke and hypothermia and conditions such as thiamine deficiency may also be involved. (See Chapter 7, Altered Mental Status.)

Use the AVPU mnemonic to quickly ascertain a baseline mental status in the patient (Figure 1-6). This assessment should begin as you form your general impression of the patient when you are looking at whether the patient opens his eyes spontaneously, representing an **A**lert patient. If no spontaneous eye opening is present, you should speak to the patient and instruct him to open his eyes or perform another function, such as moving his fingers or toes, to determine if he obeys your **V**erbal commands. If there is no response, you should then employ a **P**ainful stimulus, such as

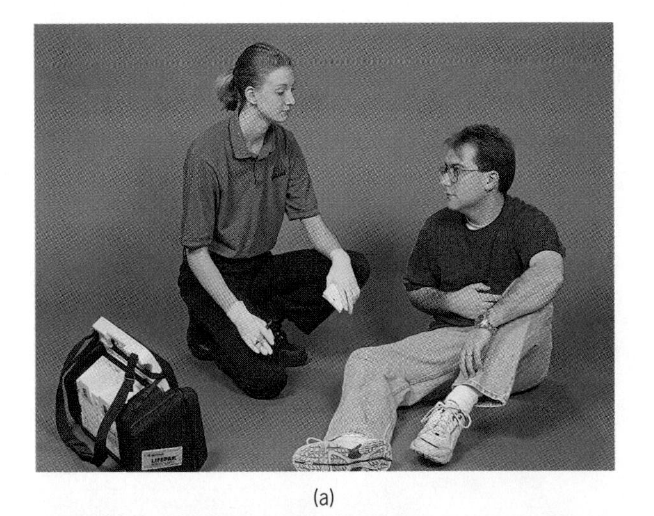

(a)

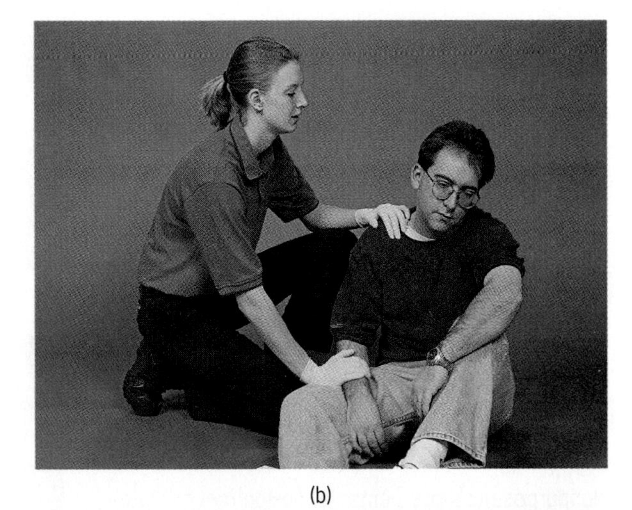

(b)

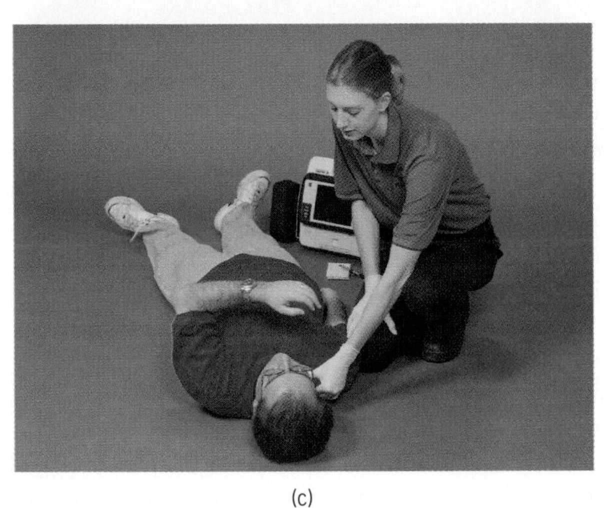

(c)

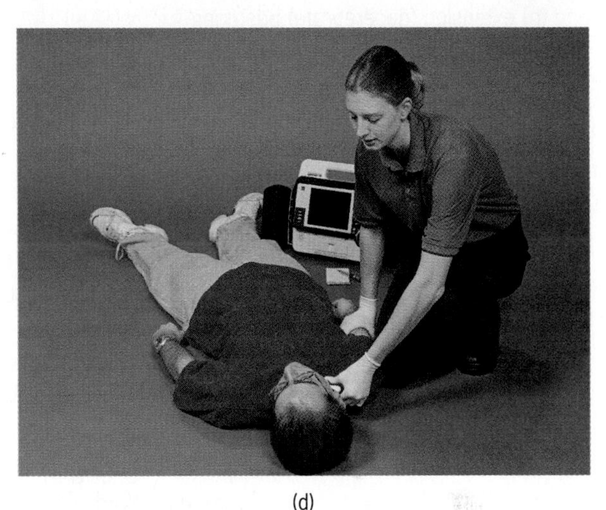

(d)

FIGURE 1-6
The AVPU levels of responsiveness: (a) Alert—eyes are open spontaneously, (b) Verbal—patient responds to verbal stimuli with eye opening or with verbal or motor response; (c) Painful—patient responds to painful stimuli with eye opening or with verbal or motor response; and (d) Unresponsive—patient has no response to external stimuli.

a trapezius pinch or an earlobe pinch, to elicit eye opening or some other motor function. If the patient still does not respond, he would then be considered **U**nresponsive.

Some providers may use a nail bed pinch or may pinch the web between the index finger and the thumb as a painful stimulus to elicit a response. Any pain applied to the extremities is considered to be a peripheral painful stimulus. A peripheral painful stimulus may not provide the most accurate assessment results because the pain reception must be picked up and transmitted by peripheral nerve tracts. If there is an interruption in the peripheral nerve tract that carries the pain impulse, the patient will not respond. You may misinterpret this as a failure of the brain to respond even though the problem was interrupted nerve transmission. Therefore, if there is no patient response to a peripheral painful stimulus, you must assess for response to a central painful stimulus, one that is applied to the core of the body. A trapezius pinch, an earlobe pinch, or supraorbital pressure is an appropriate central painful stimulus.

A sternal rub or pressure applied to the sternum is no longer considered to be a good distinguishing painful stimulus. Pain applied to the sternum may elicit a spinal reflex response rather than an interpretation and response from the brain.

AVPU

A - Patient is alert.
V - Patient responds to verbal stimuli.
P - Patient responds to painful stimuli.
U - Patient is unresponsive.

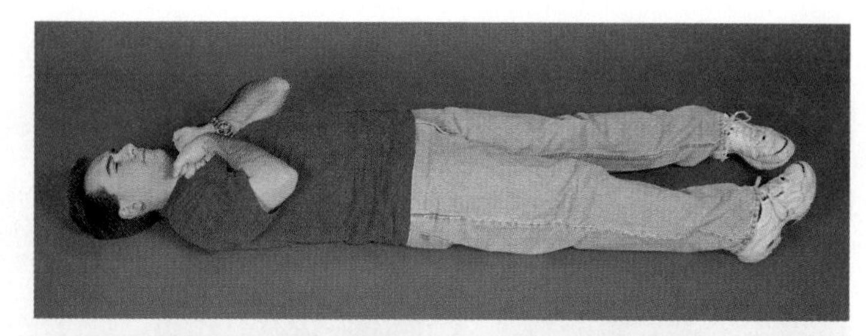

(a)

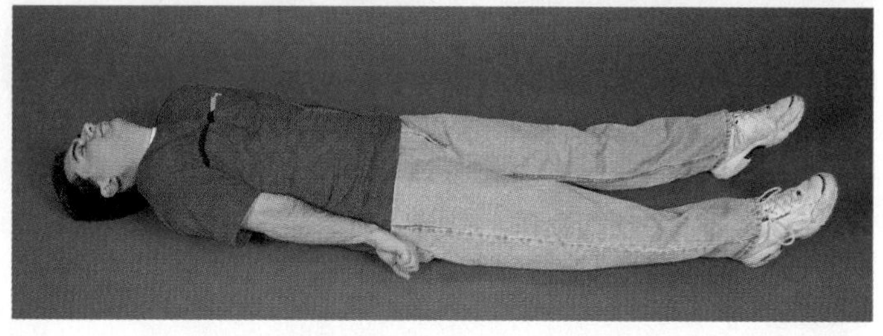

(b)

FIGURE 1-7
Nonpurposeful movements: (a) flexion (decorticate) and (b) extension (decerebrate) posturing.

In other words, motor function associated with a sternal rub may result not from higher-level brain function but rather from a reflex arc in the spinal column.

During the AVPU assessment, it is important to note how the patient actually responds. This is not the phase where a detailed account of orientation or neuromuscular function is made; however, it is essential to note particular responses to determine baseline cognitive impairment and then be able to note trends in deterioration or improvement in the patient's condition. Note the quality of verbal responses to stimuli, such as confusion, disorientation, inappropriate words or sounds, or incomprehensible sounds. Also note the nature of any motor responses to stimuli. Patients who attempt to remove the stimuli have a much higher level of function than those who display nonpurposeful movement such as flexion or extension posturing (Figure 1-7). Flexion, also known as decorticate posturing (rigid body, arms flexed, fists clenched, legs extended), typically indicates a low cerebral cortex or high brainstem injury or compression. Extension, also known as decerebrate posturing (rigid body, arms and legs extended, head retracted), carries a poor prognosis because it most often indicates lower brainstem injury or compression.

The two indicators of physiological instability associated with the AVPU assessment are no spontaneous eye opening and no spontaneous movement or no response to an earlobe pinch or other painful stimulus. Both of these indicators represent a patient who has serious cognitive impairment and a potential injury or insult involving the central nervous system.

Considerations at this point should include aggressive airway management, because these patients typically cannot protect their airway due to relaxation and loss of muscular control of the upper airway. If adequate suctioning is not immediately available or effective, log roll the patient to the recovery (lateral recumbent, or coma) position as early as possible to prevent aspiration of secretions or vomitus. If the patient has no protective reflex, such as a gag or cough reflex, consider early tracheal intubation. Also, because cerebral hypoxia may be the etiology of the altered mental status, consider administration of high-concentration oxygen by nonrebreather mask if the rate and tidal volume are adequate or by positive-pressure ventilation if rate or tidal volume is inadequate.

Assess the Airway

Once you have assessed the patient's level of responsiveness, you must immediately progress to airway assessment. A partially or completely blocked airway is an immediately life-threatening condition. Without a patent airway, regardless of any other emergency care, the patient will not survive. Thus, this is one of the most vital components of the assessment. If the airway is not open, you must immediately take the necessary steps to open it, using manual maneuvers, mechanical devices, or transtracheal techniques, as necessary. (See Chapter 2, Airway Management, Ventilation, and Oxygen Therapy.)

Clinical Insight

Without a patent airway, regardless of any other emergency care, the patient will not survive.

Alert Patient

If the patient is responsive, alert, and talking with you in a normal tone and pattern of speech, assume the airway is open and proceed to assessment of breathing. In some situations, although the patient is alert, he may still have an airway that is partially occluded by foreign objects or edema. Note the speech pattern, hoarseness, or the inability to speak altogether. A patient who can only say a few words before gasping for a breath, or one who cannot speak at all, needs to be assessed closely for an occluded airway. Inspect inside the mouth, looking for objects or edema to the tongue, uvula, and other upper airway structures.

Patient with an Altered Mental Status

You must assume that a patient with an altered mental status cannot effectively maintain his own airway. This is typically due to relaxation of the submandibular muscles that control the tongue and epiglottis. The tongue may fall posteriorly and completely or partially occlude the airway at the level of the hypopharynx.

Thus, in a patient with an altered mental status, it is vital that you open the mouth; inspect the oral cavity for blood, vomitus, or other secretions; suction if necessary; and perform a manual maneuver to open the airway. The airway may need to be maintained with a mechanical adjunct such as an oropharyngeal airway or a more advanced technique such as tracheal intubation or insertion of a laryngeal mask airway. As a rule, if the patient accepts an oropharyngeal airway, he has a significantly compromised airway from lack of a protective reflex and should be intubated with a tracheal tube for definitive protection of the airway.

Also note any abnormal upper airway sounds such as stridor, snoring, or gurgling. Stridor indicates partial upper airway occlusion with resistance of air movement through the hypopharynx and larynx. Sonorous, or snoring-type, sounds are produced when the tongue relaxes and partially occludes the upper airway at the level of the hypopharynx. Gurgling indicates collection of fluid in the upper airway, such as blood, secretions, or vomitus. *Keep in mind that obstructive sounds or actual obstruction of the airway by vomitus, blood, or secretions is an indicator of physiological instability.*

Open the Airway

If the airway is closed or partially obstructed, immediately intervene to open it with manual maneuvers, mechanical devices, or transtracheally.

You should begin with manual maneuvers, performing the head-tilt, chin-lift maneuver (Figure 1-8), or performing the jaw-thrust maneuver on the patient with a suspected spine injury. If this is not effective or is difficult to maintain, you will need to go to an airway adjunct such as an oropharyngeal, nasopharyngeal, or laryngeal mask airway or tracheal intubation. Discussion of alternative devices that are available is found in Chapter 2.

If you cannot open and manage the airway by manual or mechanical means, you may have to establish an airway using transtracheal techniques and equipment. A needle or surgical cricothyroidotomy should be performed in patients who present with airway problems that cannot be effectively managed with tracheal intubation. A patient with severe laryngeal edema from an anaphylactic reaction may be a candidate for transtracheal jet ventilation. (These techniques are also discussed in Chapter 2.)

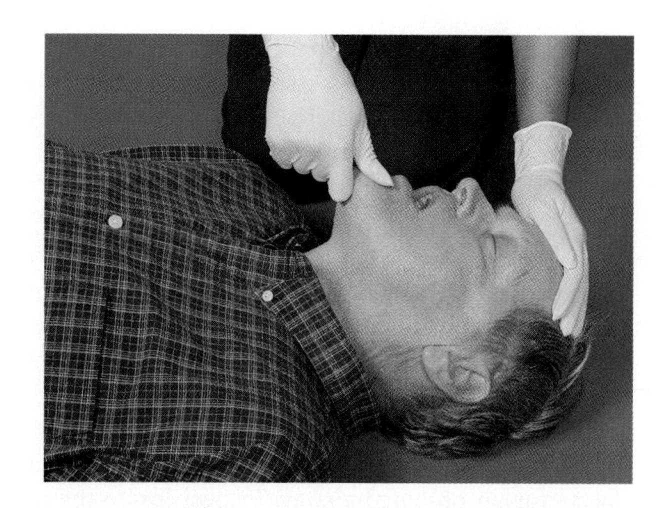

FIGURE 1-8
Open the airway with a head-tilt, chin-lift (as shown here) or a jaw-thrust maneuver.

Transtracheal techniques are not to be performed just because you lack the skill to intubate the patient; rather, they should be reserved for the patient in whom you cannot pass a tracheal tube due to severe distortion of the anatomical structures and closure from upper airway edema and who cannot be ventilated by other means. Also remember that to use surgical techniques, you must have prior authorization by the local medical director.

Assess Breathing

As soon as you have cleared and opened the airway, assess the patient's breathing, determining the following:

- Is the breathing adequate or inadequate?
- Is there a need for oxygen therapy?

To determine the breathing status, it is necessary to assess the minute ventilation (V_E), which is comprised of both the rate of ventilation (f) and the tidal volume (V_T). Assessing only one of these components will provide you with an inadequate evaluation and may fail to prompt you to intervene when necessary. For example, the patient's respiratory rate may be 16 breaths per minute, which would fall into a normal range. However, each breath may be extremely shallow, and the volume of air inhaled may be inadequate to sustain normal oxygenation of the cells. If you assess only the rate, and not the tidal volume, you may fail to realize that this patient needs positive-pressure ventilation, which may lead to deleterious results.

An average-size patient has a tidal volume of 500 ml per breath. If this patient is breathing at 12 times per minute, his respiratory minute volume (V_E) is approximately 6,000 ml or 6.0 liters per minute:

$$\begin{aligned} V_E &= f \times V_T \\ &= 12 \text{ (breaths per minute)} \times 500 \text{ ml (volume of air breathed each minute)} \\ &= 6{,}000 \text{ ml per minute or } 6.0 \text{ liters per minute} \end{aligned}$$

An increase in the frequency (respiratory rate) or depth (tidal volume) would increase the respiratory minute ventilation. Your assumption would be that the patient is moving more air and is breathing adequately. Thus, if you encounter a patient who has a respiratory rate that is increased, even though the tidal volume may be lower (shallow breathing), the patient should compensate and have a higher respiratory minute ventilation and adequate breathing. As an example, the average-size patient is now breathing at 20 times per minute; however, the tidal volume (depth) has decreased to approximately 350 ml per breath. Based on the calculation of respiratory minute ventilation, the patient is now breathing at 7,000 ml or 7.0 liters per minute.

$$V_E = f \times V_T$$
$$= 20 \text{ (breaths per minute)} \times 350 \text{ ml (volume of air breathed each minute)}$$
$$= 7{,}000 \text{ ml per minute or } 7.0 \text{ liters per minute}$$

This reflects an increased respiratory minute ventilation. One would assume that this puts the patient in a better physiological status than when previously breathing at 6,000 ml or 6.0 liters per minute and that the rate is compensating well for the decreased tidal volume. Most EMS practitioners would consider this breathing as adequate.

A major consideration in the assessment of adequacy of ventilation, however, is the alveolar ventilation. Alveolar ventilation takes into account the amount of air that actually reaches the alveoli and, therefore, is functional in gas exchange. The respiratory minute ventilation (V_E) measures pulmonary ventilation and indicates how much air is moving in and out of the respiratory tract. However, not all of the air breathed in (tidal volume) reaches the alveoli and provides for functional gas exchange.

A major consideration in the assessment of adequacy of ventilation is the alveolar ventilation.

Approximately 350 ml of inhaled air in the average-size adult actually reaches the alveolar exchange surfaces. The remaining 150 ml never gets farther than the large conducting airways. These spaces are referred to as the anatomic dead space (V_D). Thus, alveolar ventilation (V_A) measures the amount of air reaching the alveoli for functional gas exchange each minute. The alveolar ventilation, which plays a much more important role in determining hypoxia because it is most related to gas exchange, is less than the respiratory minute ventilation because it eliminates the dead-space air that does not reach the alveolar surfaces and plays no role in gas exchange. To calculate alveolar ventilation (V_A), subtract the dead space from the tidal volume:

$$V_A = f \times (V_T - V_D)$$
$$= 12 \times (500 - 150 \text{ ml})$$
$$= 12 \times 350 \text{ ml}$$
$$= 4{,}200 \text{ ml or } 4.2 \text{ liters per minute reach the alveoli for gas exchange}$$

Alterations in the tidal volume have a much more significant effect on the alveolar ventilation as compared to the respiratory minute ventilation. An increase in respiratory rate does not compensate as well as one might think it does to produce or maintain adequate breathing. Take the average-size patient in the second example who had an increased respiratory rate of 20 breaths per minute and a tidal volume of 350 ml. Originally, it was assumed that the breathing status was still adequate because the respiratory minute ventilation actually increased from 6,000 ml to 7,000 ml. One may actually believe that, in a sense, the patient has a better ventilatory status now as compared to his normal ventilatory status. In this patient, the dead space does not change and will continue to be filled regardless of the tidal volume. Therefore, calculate the patient's alveolar ventilation, accounting for the increased respiratory rate and decreased tidal volume:

$$V_A = f \times (V_T - V_D)$$
$$= 20 \times (350 - 150 \text{ ml})$$
$$= 20 \times 200 \text{ ml}$$
$$= 4{,}000 \text{ ml or } 4.0 \text{ liters per minute reach the alveoli for gas exchange}$$

Unlike the respiratory minute volume, which increased above normal with the increased respiratory rate, the alveolar ventilation dropped below the patient's normal level, even with the increased respiratory rate. So the increased rate does not necessarily compensate for the decrease in tidal volume. Thus, just because a patient has an increased respiratory rate and potentially an increased minute ventilation, this does not equate to better alveolar ventilation or, worse yet, to adequate breathing. In addition, an increase in the respiratory rate reduces the time allowed for each inhalation, which reduces the tidal volume. Typically, an adult patient with a respiratory rate of 40 breaths per minute or greater will have a significant reduction in tidal volume resulting from inadequate inhalation time. Even though the respiratory rate is excessively elevated, the alveolar ventilation is severely disturbed, leading to hypoxia.

This illustrates the need to very carefully assess the tidal volume of the patient, because a reduction in tidal volume affects the alveolar ventilation more drastically and leads to poor gas exchange sooner than rate disturbances. However, you are not trying to determine an actual number value; rather, you are merely attempting to determine whether the tidal volume is adequate. Also, as we have pointed out, do not assume that an increased rate will compensate for lower tidal volumes.

Remember: The dead space is filled with each breath regardless of the volume breathed in. If the average-size patient is only breathing in a tidal volume of 200 ml of air with each breath, only 50 ml will reach the alveoli. This translates to severely inadequate breathing. A patient with an inadequate respiratory rate—or a poor tidal volume regardless of the respiratory rate—needs positive-pressure ventilation.

Look, listen, and feel to determine the tidal volume (Figure 1-9). You must look at the chest; inadequate tidal volumes will produce very little chest rise and fall. Listen and feel for air escape from the nose and mouth; with poor tidal volumes, little air is heard or felt with each breath.

To summarize: Adequate minute ventilation will consist of a rate of breathing typically between 8 and 24 breaths per minute, good tidal volume evidenced by adequate chest rise and fall, and good air escape from the nose and mouth with each breath. Adequate alveolar ventilation will rely heavily on adequate tidal volumes and is not well compensated by an increase in the respiratory rate.

Also, look for the following additional signs of poor or inadequate breathing:

- Retractions of the suprasternal notch, intercostal spaces, supraclavicular spaces, and subcostal area
- Nasal flaring (rare in adults but common in children)
- Excessive abdominal muscle use

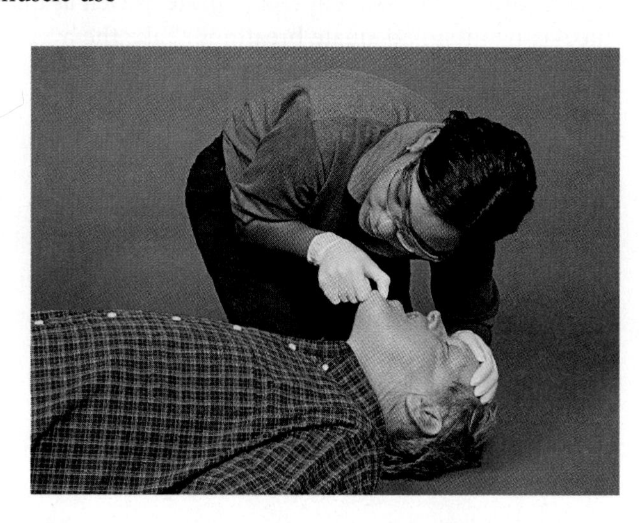

FIGURE 1-9
Look, listen, and feel to determine an estimate of tidal volume.

- Tracheal tugging exhibited by a pendulum motion at the anterior neck during inhalation
- Cyanosis
- Asymmetric chest wall movement

Once you determine that the breathing is adequate, consider the administration of oxygen. Oxygen should be considered in patients with any state of hypoxia, suspected hypoxia, the potential to become hypoxic, shock, or if an unknown problem is encountered. If ever in doubt as to whether the patient requires oxygen, administer oxygen. If the patient is hypoxic, maximize the FiO_2 by providing high concentrations via nonrebreather mask. This will result in a high concentration of oxygen-saturated hemoglobin and, then, delivery of oxygen at the cellular level.

Clinical Insight

If ever in doubt as to whether a patient requires oxygen, administer oxygen.

If the breathing is inadequate due to an abnormal rate of less than 8 breaths per minute or greater than 30 breaths per minute with evidence of respiratory distress or failure or poor tidal volume, you must provide positive-pressure ventilation. *Apnea, inadequate tidal volume, and a respiratory rate of less than 8 or greater than 30 breaths per minute are indicators of physiological instability.*

When performing positive-pressure ventilation with a bag-valve-mask device, the adult tidal volume to achieve is 500 to 600 ml (8–10 ml/kg). The key to delivering an effective ventilatory volume is to produce visible chest rise with each ventilation. The ventilation should be delivered over a 1-second period, regardless of whether a mask is being used or the ventilation is being done in conjunction with an advanced airway. A 1- or 2-liter adult bag-valve-mask device can be used to provide positive-pressure ventilation. If a 1-liter bag is used, squeeze the bag so one-half to two-thirds of its volume is delivered with the ventilation. If a 2-liter bag is used, deliver one-third of the bag volume. A reservoir should be connected to the bag-valve mask and oxygen delivered at 10 to 12 lpm. Adult patients should be ventilated at a rate of 10 to 12 ventilations per minute. If the patient is in cardiac arrest, ventilation is delivered at a rate of 8 to 10 ventilations per minute. If ventilation is being provided to a patient with severe obstructive pulmonary disease or a condition that causes an increase in resistance to exhalation, a lower respiratory rate (6–8 per minute) should be used to allow for complete exhalation and prevention of "auto-PEEP."

Assess Circulation

Assessing circulation does not mean just checking the patient's pulse. The pulse is only one component in the circulation assessment. You are attempting to determine the patient's perfusion status. Thus, you need to assess the following components of circulation:

Clinical Insight

Assessing circulation is not just checking the pulse. You are attempting to determine the patient's perfusion status.

- Pulse
- Skin color, temperature, and condition
- Capillary refill

Also, you should identify any major bleeding during this phase, such as esophageal, vaginal, or gastrointestinal bleeding.

Assess Pulse

The purposes of pulse assessment during the initial assessment are to estimate the rate and determine the quality. You will obtain a more accurate pulse later, when you take a set of baseline vital signs.

First, palpate the radial pulse to determine if it is present. If it is not palpable, feel for the carotid pulse (Figure 1-10). Determine if the pulse is present, the

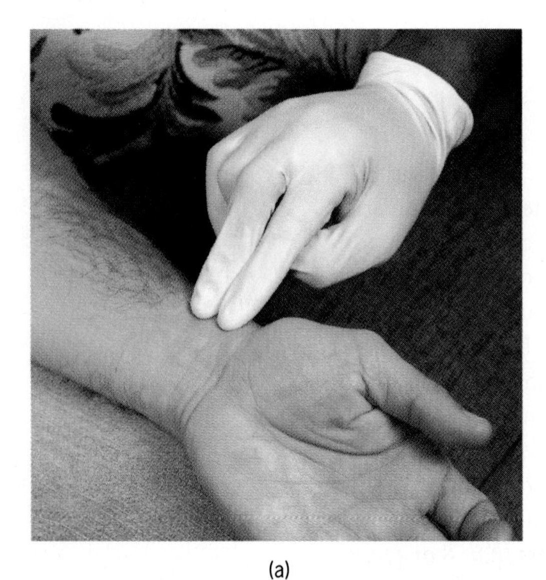

(a)

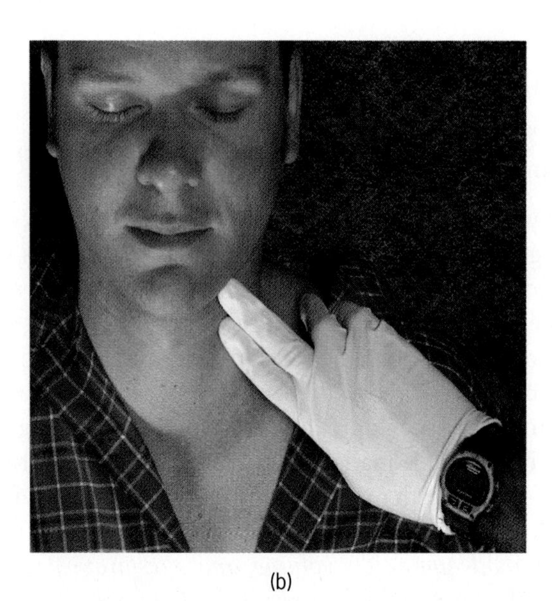

(b)

FIGURE 1-10
(a) Palpate the radial pulse. If it is not palpable, (b) feel for the carotid pulse.

approximate rate, and the regularity and strength. If a carotid pulse is not present, you must then manage the patient as a cardiac arrest and focus on resuscitation.

Once the pulse has been palpated, assess the approximate rate. You want to categorize the pulse as being fast (greater than 100 beats per minute), normal (between 60 and 100 beats per minute), or slow (less than 60 beats per minute). Tachycardia may indicate a cardiac dysrhythmia, poor perfusion, hypoxia, drug overdose or poisoning, fever, endocrine disturbances, heat emergency, anxiety, pain, or nervousness. Bradycardia may indicate a cardiac dysrhythmia, severe hypoxia, normal response to certain medications such as beta-blockers, drug overdose or poisoning, intense vagal stimulation, increase in intracranial pressure, or failure of an internal pacemaker.

The pulse rate must not be considered alone as a reason for intervention; it must be viewed as one of a series of signs and symptoms necessary to develop a field diagnosis. Do not treat the heart rate; treat the patient.

Cardiac dysrhythmias are the etiology of irregular pulses. The pulse may be regularly irregular, as in a normal sinus rhythm with bigeminy, or irregularly irregular, as in atrial fibrillation. Regardless, an irregular pulse or any indication of a potential dysrhythmia is definitely an indication that the patient requires application of a continuous cardiac monitor.

When assessing the pulse, determine if it is weak or strong. Weak pulses are typically correlated with hypotension and inadequate perfusion, which may be related to a multitude of conditions. A weak pulse may be associated with tachycardia, bradycardia, or a normal rate. Strong pulses are usually an indication of adequate cardiac output and blood pressure.

The location of the palpated pulse correlates with the perfusion status; however, it does not correlate well with the systolic blood pressure. It was once speculated that the presence of a radial, femoral, brachial, or carotid pulse could provide an estimate of the systolic blood pressure. More recently, it has been determined that this method of estimating a systolic blood pressure is not accurate and should not be employed in the clinical setting.

A study conducted by Deakin and Low found that patients who retained a radial pulse had an average systolic blood pressure of 72.5 mmHg. Of the subjects who had radial pulses, 83 percent of them had a systolic blood pressure of less than 80 mmHg. Eighty-three percent of the subjects who had palpable femoral and carotid pulses had a systolic blood pressure less than 70 mmHg and a mean systolic blood pressure of 66.4 mmHg. However, in support of the previous guidelines, none of the subjects who had only a carotid pulse had a systolic blood pressure greater than 60 mmHg. Thus, when assessing pulses based on location, it is more important to recognize that a pulse exists with perfusion and realize that the relationship between estimated systolic blood pressure and pulse location is not accurate.

A systolic blood pressure of 60 mmHg is required to perfuse the brain in most patients. Thus, if a carotid pulse is not palpated, you must begin chest compressions and aggressive resuscitation. *Indicators of physiological instability are weak or absent peripheral or central pulses, rates less than 60 or greater than 100, or irregular pulses.*

Identify Major Bleeding

Most often, it is the trauma patient who presents with major bleeding. In the medical patient, major bleeding is not usually the chief complaint. However, you might find a medical patient who has had recent surgery in which his incision has torn open, severe epistaxis (nosebleed) in an elderly patient with a history of hypertension, vaginal bleeding associated with spontaneous abortion, significant rectal bleeding associated with a gastrointestinal bleed, or massive hematemesis from ruptured esophageal varices. (See Chapter 9, Gastrointestinal Bleeding.) These and many other conditions may lead to massive blood loss, poor perfusion, and severe hypovolemic shock.

A patient with suspected internal bleeding requires expeditious transport.

The main difference between the medical patient and the trauma patient, typically, is the mechanism of injury and the source of bleeding. The management is usually the same, except that the trauma patient may present more often with external hemorrhage that can be controlled with direct pressure. The medical patient's bleeding is usually internal and not easily controlled. Most medical patients with internal bleeding require interventions not available in the prehospital setting; thus, expeditious transport is important.

Assess Perfusion

Perfusion can be assessed by checking the patient's skin color, temperature, and condition. Capillary refill can also predict perfusion status; however, it is not as reliable an indicator in the adult patient, as is discussed later.

Check the skin color by simple inspection. In dark-skinned patients, you can inspect the palms of the hands, mucous membranes inside the mouth and under the tongue (Figure 1-11), the conjunctiva (Figure 1-12), or the nail beds. Nail bed color is the least reliable indicator because nail polish, the environment, some chronic illnesses, and other conditions may affect color, providing an erroneous indication or making it impossible to check.

Abnormal skin colors are cyanotic, pale, red or flushed, mottled, and jaundiced. Cyanosis typically indicates hypoxia; however, it is a late sign. An early sign of hypoxia is pale, cool, clammy skin that results from sympathetic nervous system stimulation. Poor perfusion of the peripheral microcirculation produces a pale skin color. This usually results from the blood being shunted away from the periphery to the core circulation when there is loss of circulating intravascular volume, poor myocardial function, or severe vasoconstriction. Be aware that a cold environment also causes vasoconstriction as a thermoregulatory response and will produce pale skin. This is a normal response in a healthy individual, not a sign of shock. *Other than in a cold environment, pale or cyanotic nail, skin, or palm color is a sign of physiological instability.*

Red or flushed skin (erythema) results from vasodilation of the peripheral vessels and an increase in cutaneous blood flow. This can be associated with conditions

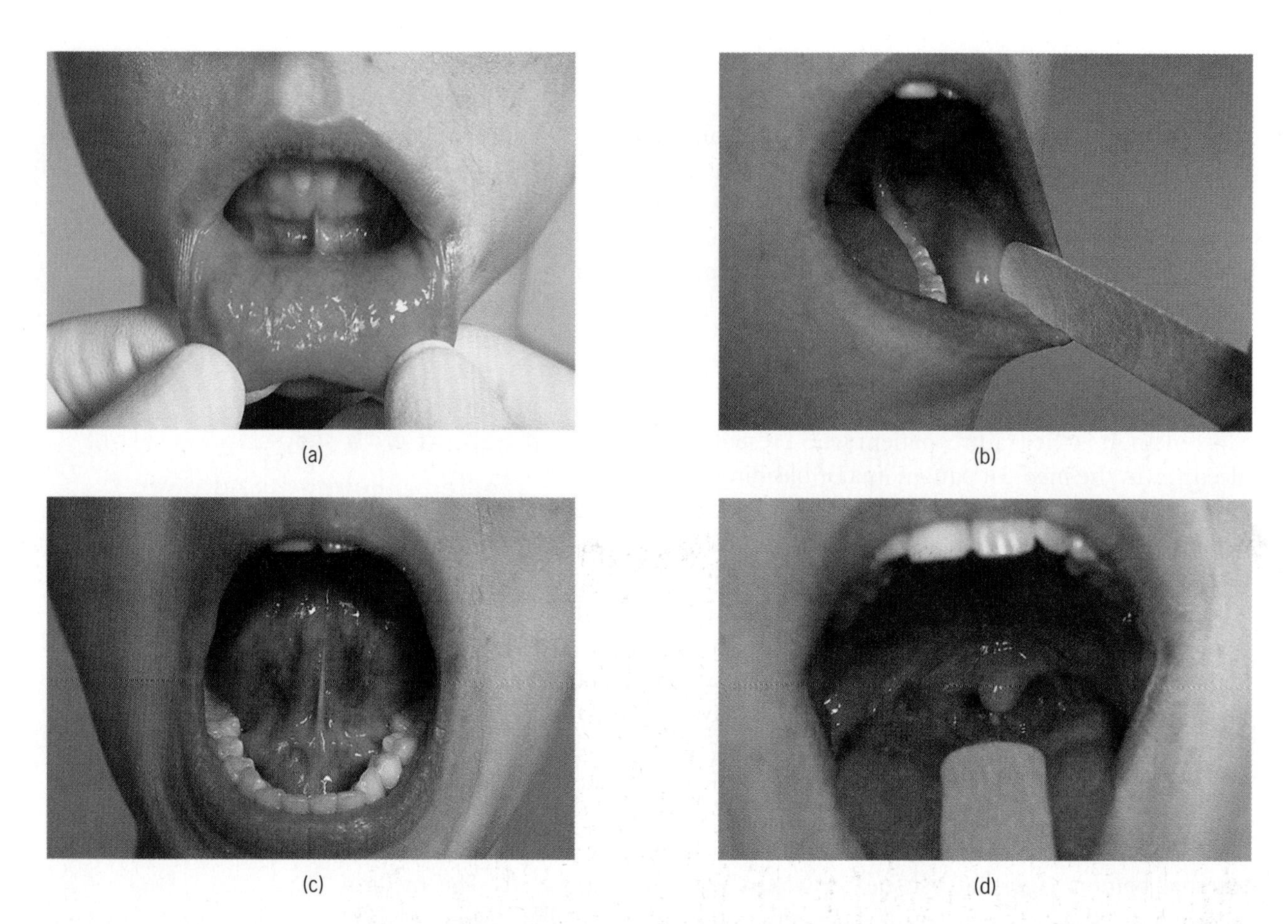

FIGURE 1-11
Inspect the mucosa (a) on the undersurfaces of the lips, (b) inside the cheek, and (c) under the tongue. (d) Have the patient say "aaahhh" while you examine the soft palate and uvula.

such as anaphylactic shock, drug overdose, poisoning, neurogenic shock associated with spine injury, inflammation, diabetic ketoacidosis, extreme heat emergencies, and fever. Red skin may also result from an increase in intravascular red blood cell volume known as polycythemia. Mottled (blotchy) skin is common with cardiovascular compromise or poor perfusion. Liver dysfunction usually produces a yellow, orange, or bronze skin tone from increased bile pigmentation known as jaundice. It is typically seen in patients with acute or chronic liver disease, chronic alcoholism, or with some endocrine disturbances.

Assess the skin temperature by partially removing your glove and placing the back of your hand or fingers on the patient's abdomen, neck, or face (Figure 1-13). The abdomen is the ideal location because it is the least influenced by environmental conditions when the patient is clothed. Determine if the skin is normal, hot, cool, or cold. Normal skin temperature is usually around 90 degrees Fahrenheit, which

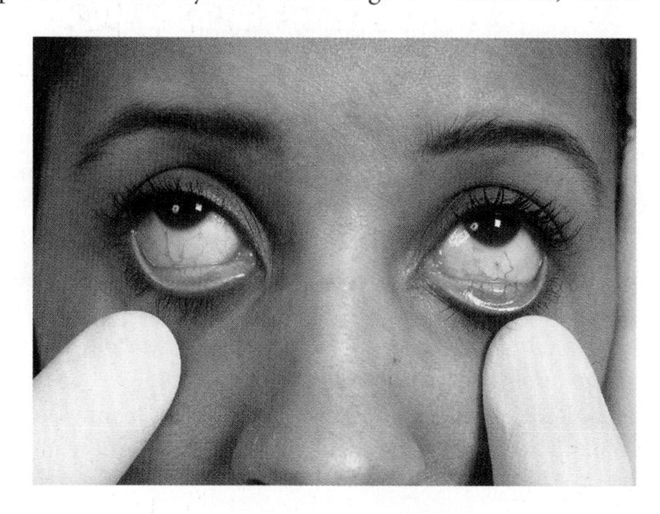

FIGURE 1-12
Skin color may be assessed by inspectingthe conjunctiva.

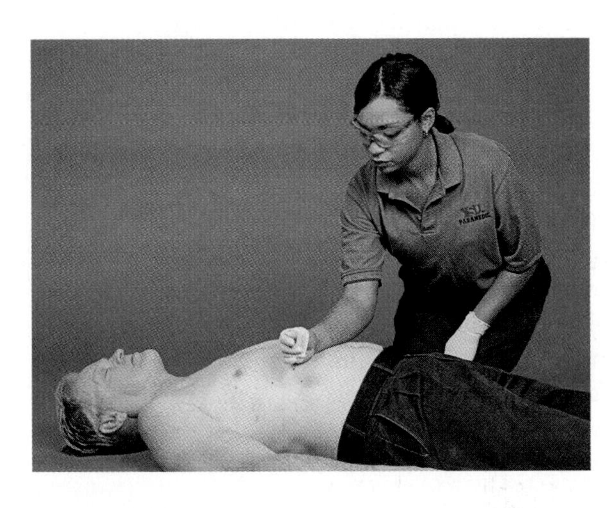

FIGURE 1-13
Assess skin temperature by partially removing your glove and placing the back of your hand or fingers on the patient's abdomen, neck, or face.

feels slightly warm to most people. Hot skin is typically associated with the elevated body core temperatures seen in severe fever and heat stroke. Poor perfusion and other conditions that cause vasoconstriction produce cool skin because the blood is being shunted to the core circulation, leaving little warm blood in the peripheral vessels. Cold skin is usually an indication of shock, cold exposure, or hypothermia.

Incidentally, an elderly patient with limited mobility can become hypothermic in his home during the cold months. He may turn down the thermostat to save on heating costs and inadvertently produce an environment cold enough to make him hypothermic. Thus, do not be surprised if an elderly patient found sitting in his recliner at home is hypothermic. This is commonly termed "urban hypothermia." Also, it does not take temperature extremes to produce hypothermia. You could find an intoxicated patient who has fallen asleep on a park bench on a night in which the temperature is 65 degrees Fahrenheit. A 65-degree night feels fairly warm to you and your partner, but the patient may have succumbed to hypothermia. The ingestion of alcohol results in accelerating heat loss and an increased susceptibility to hypothermia.

The condition of the skin refers to the amount of moisture in it. Extremely dry skin is usually an indication of severe dehydration, some drug overdoses, or poisoning. Moist skin may be found in patients with poor perfusion, fever, heat emergencies, cardiovascular compromise, exercise, exertion, drug overdose, or poisoning. Skin condition is best correlated with color and temperature to indicate the medical condition. For example, a classic sign of shock is pale, cool, moist skin.

Capillary refill is a quick method of assessing peripheral perfusion (Figure 1-14). However, it is not as accurate a measure as once believed. The problem with capillary

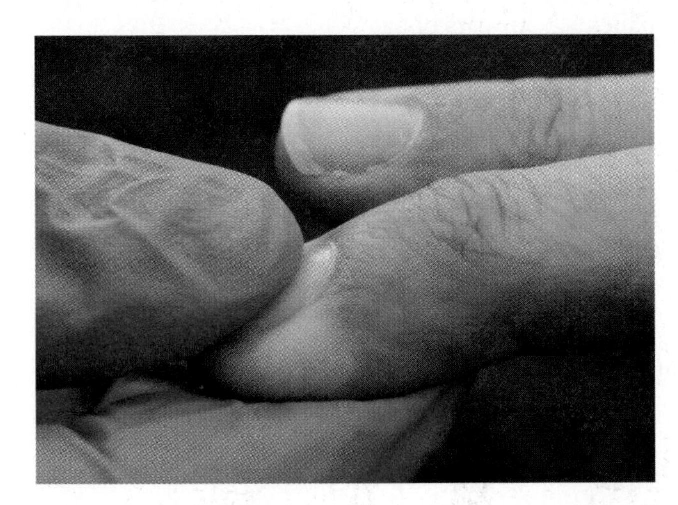

FIGURE 1-14
Capillary refill, a quick method of assessing peripheral perfusion, is not always a reliable measure.

Clinical Insight

The upper limits of normal capillary refill times at room temperature are 2 seconds for children and adult males, 3 seconds for adult females, and 4 seconds for the elderly.

refill in the adult patient is that it can be influenced by smoking, medications, environmental conditions, chronic medical conditions, and other conditions that impair peripheral circulation. (Capillary refill is a more accurate indicator of peripheral perfusion in infants and young children.) Also, it has been found that a normal capillary refill in some patients is longer than 2 seconds. Some people have normal capillary refill times of up to 4 seconds.

You should still assess capillary refill in all patients, but realize the limitations to interpreting the results. You must always consider other causes for a poor capillary refill test, one in which it takes longer than 2 to 3 seconds for color to return after the nail is pressed. For example, if the patient is found outside in a cold environment, you would expect the capillary refill to be delayed. Again, it is important to consider capillary refill as just one sign that should be viewed as only a component of the entire clinical picture. Treat the patient and not a sign.

Establish Patient Priorities

During the course of the initial assessment, you should have identified and managed any immediately life-threatening condition related to the airway, breathing, or circulation. The airway should be opened and kept open, high-flow, high-concentration oxygen applied or positive-pressure ventilation initiated as appropriate, and resuscitation begun for a pulseless patient. Based on your assessment findings and interventions, you can begin to determine your patient's priority status. Serious aberrations in the airway, breathing, or circulation findings will typically prompt you to consider the patient physiologically unstable. (Review Table 1-1.) These patients may have underlying conditions that will require aggressive assessment and management and expedited transport.

In addition to abnormalities in the initial assessment findings, the following could be considered high-risk findings or conditions that may warrant priority status. As you continue through the focused history and physical exam, detailed physical exam, if any, and ongoing assessment, the following should prompt you to recognize a priority medical patient and consider aggressive intervention:

- Abdominal finding of pain, tenderness, distention, or guarding
- Acute back or flank pain that is nonmusculoskeletal in a patient > age 60
- Gastrointestinal bleeding
- Profuse hematuria (blood in the urine)
- Major hemoptysis (bloody sputum)
- Wheezing
- Crackles (rales)
- Acute chest pain in a patient > 35 years of age
- Inappropriate diaphoresis
- Dizziness in a patient > 65 years of age
- Acute and severe headache
- Acute onset of motor deficit such as dysphagia (difficulty swallowing), dysphasia (difficulty speaking), facial or extremity paralysis or paresis
- Seizures
- Syncope
- Immersion accident
- Electrocution or lightning strike
- Caustic ingestion
- Poisoning

- Drug excess
- Pulseless extremity
- Clinically apparent jaundice
- Acute and severe edema to the lower extremities
- Acute neck stiffness with meningeal signs
- Labor and imminent delivery
- Complicated pregnancy
- Profuse vaginal bleeding
- Acute scrotal pain
- Hematemesis

Priority status may be determined at any time throughout the assessment. Also, you may categorize your patient as a priority, then, after further assessment, determine that the condition does not warrant a priority status. Bear in mind that the assessment approach is ongoing and that the patient's condition is dynamic; it can change at any point. An example of a drastic change would be a patient who is only complaining of nausea and weakness and appears not to have any physiological instability who then suddenly becomes pulseless and apneic. This is an extreme example. You must be prepared to recognize and manage changes in every patient, no matter how severe or how subtle.

FOCUSED HISTORY AND PHYSICAL EXAM

Once you have completed the scene size-up and initial assessment, the next step is to conduct a focused history and physical exam. This assessment is conducted to identify all other life-threatening conditions. The three main components of the focused history and physical exam are

- Gathering a history
- Performing a physical exam
- Assessing baseline vital signs

The order in which these steps will be performed is determined by the patient's mental status. In the responsive patient, the history will be the first step, followed by the physical exam and baseline vital signs. In the unresponsive patient or one with an altered mental status, the physical exam will be conducted first, followed by baseline vital signs and, finally, history gathering. In the medical patient, the chief complaint and medical history provide vital information for identifying the possible condition. Physical assessment findings are used to assist in making a differential diagnosis, to verify the condition, and to gauge its severity.

In the responsive patient, the history will be the first step, followed by the physical exam and baseline vital signs. In the unresponsive patient or one with an altered mental status, the physical exam will be conducted first.

In the responsive medical patient, the physical exam that will be conducted is a *focused medical assessment*—an exam that is focused more on the patient's chief complaint, signs, and symptoms and related body systems. For the unresponsive or altered mental status patient, a *rapid medical assessment* will be performed—a quick head-to-toe assessment similar to the rapid trauma assessment. You will be inspecting, palpating, auscultating, and percussing for evidence of abnormal findings associated with medical conditions. The unresponsive or altered mental status medical patient is already considered physiologically unstable and a priority patient by virtue of the chief complaint: unresponsiveness or altered mental status. The rapid medical assessment

Focused History and Physical Exam

Responsive Patient

1. History
2. Focused medical assessment
3. Baseline vital signs

Unresponsive or Altered Mental Status Patient

1. Rapid medical assessment
2. Baseline vital signs
3. History

will hopefully provide some clues, in the form of abnormal physical findings, as to why the patient is unresponsive or has an altered mental status.

The goal of the assessment is to move along the following continuum:

> Manage any life-threatening conditions found during the initial assessment and the focused history and physical examination → Begin emergency care → Continue assessment to attempt to establish a differential field diagnosis of the condition → Move from possibilities to probabilities of the suspected patient condition in order to → Provide continued and more precisely focused emergency care.

For example, consider the following scenario:

> You arrive on the scene of a call for shortness of breath. During the initial assessment, you concentrate on determining the extent of respiratory distress or respiratory failure and the level of hypoxia associated with the condition. You need to intervene immediately to provide airway management, positive-pressure ventilation, and oxygen therapy, without knowing the exact cause of the respiratory embarrassment. During the initial assessment and the focused history and physical exam, you gather information about the severity of the condition.
>
> After you have effectively managed the airway and breathing, you seek the cause of the respiratory distress or failure through further assessment. In this case, you determine the cause to be asthma, and you focus your continued management on treating the asthma through pharmacologic intervention with beta 2-specific medications and steroids. If you had identified a different cause, such as pneumonia, you would have managed the patient differently.

The idea is to manage all life threats and then continue to home in on the exact cause of the condition so more focused and appropriate pharmacologic and nonpharmacologic interventions can be undertaken. Incidentally, in some situations, it may be necessary to move to pharmacologic intervention early to establish an airway and breathing, such as in the anaphylactic patient. In that particular case, administration of intramuscular epinephrine may be required very early in the assessment process so an airway can be maintained and ventilation can be performed.

Clinical Insight

In the responsive medical patient, the information you gather in the history will then help to direct the focused medical assessment.

Responsive Patient

In the responsive medical patient, you must first gather the history, including the chief complaint, history of the present illness, past medical history, and current health status. The information you gather in the history will then help you direct the focused medical assessment.

For example, if the patient is complaining of retrosternal chest pain and dyspnea, you are not going to need to spend a lot of time evaluating the head. However, you will focus on areas of the body and body systems that may provide clues to the potential condition that is causing the chest pain and its severity. For example, you would assess the pupils for size and reactivity, the conjunctiva for pallor, cyanosis, or inflammation, and the oral mucosa for cyanosis. These may seem only remotely related to chest pain but may be an indication of hypoxia and the perfusion status and are worth checking in the chest pain patient, along with any other areas that may suggest signs of cardiac failure or hypoxia. Following the focused medical assessment, you would gather a set of baseline vital signs, which may also provide significant clues to the condition and its severity.

Based on the information gathered in the history, it may be necessary to provide interventions such as intravenous therapy and blood draw before you have completed the physical examination. Most often, these interventions are performed concurrently with the examination.

The following sections describe in more detail these elements of the focused history and physical exam for a responsive medical patient.

Assess Patient Complaints and Medical History

History may be gained through both verbal communication and nonverbal sources. Verbal communication would involve questioning the patient about his complaint, medical history, and so forth. The patient would be the primary historian, the person who provides the information. Nonverbal information consists mostly of clues in the environment, many of which you will have noted during your scene size-up. These would include such things as medication containers, a medical alert bracelet, or a wheelchair.

For example, an oxygen concentrator at the scene of a patient complaining of shortness of breath should make you suspect a chronic respiratory disease. Similarly, a patient who is in a hospital bed is probably a person with a long-term medical condition that limits his mobility. The shortness of breath may be a result of a pulmonary embolus related to the patient's immobility.

In the medical patient, you have to rely heavily on symptoms, because they are the most common reason a medical patient calls for EMS.

Keep in mind that physical assessment findings are objective, the observable signs of illness or injury. However, in the medical patient, you have to rely heavily on symptoms because they are the most common reason why a medical patient calls for EMS. Symptoms can only be described by the patient. We have to realize that we cannot see everything. For example, we cannot see chest pain, nausea, or dizziness. Also, we cannot see how badly it actually hurts. This is subjective information that must be gained from the patient through history taking and patient interviewing. Sometimes, however, a physical finding or posture may be a better indication of severity. As an example, a patient who is complaining of chest pain who presents with his fist clenched over his chest would have more severe chest pain than the patient who just points to the pain.

It is also important to realize that the patient may be responsive and able to answer your questions when you arrive at the scene, but later the patient may deteriorate and become confused, disoriented, or unresponsive. You may be the only person who had the opportunity to gain pertinent information about the chief complaint, present illness, and past medical history. A good example would be a patient suffering from a subarachnoid hemorrhage. When you arrive at the scene, the patient may be complaining of an excruciating headache. As you proceed with your assessment, the patient's condition continues to deteriorate. By the time you arrive at the emergency department, the patient is no longer responding to any stimuli. You may be the only health care provider who can deliver the history of the progression of events related to the aneurysm, and this may be a vital link in the continuum of care for this patient.

Clinical Insight

The best historian is usually the patient.

The best historian is usually the patient. Gather all the information you can from the patient. If you are asking questions, direct them to the patient and not the family. If the patient is in severe distress or is not able to answer the questions because of his mental status, then it is appropriate to direct the questions to the family members. Bystanders who are not family members can also be a source of information, but it is important to realize that bystanders are the most unreliable sources of information, so be cautious when reporting such information. It is a good idea always to identify the source of any information you report.

You can ask two types of questions to gather a history: open-ended (indirect) and closed (direct) questions. An open-ended question is a general question that does not suggest a specific answer and can help facilitate the flow of information. With open-ended questions, you can gather a large amount of information from the patient in a short period of time. An example of an open-ended question is "Can you describe your chest pain?" Direct or closed questions are very specific and suggest short responses, typically yes or no. An example of a direct question would be "Is the chest pain dull?"

It is appropriate to alternate between the two types of questions. The history taking usually begins with open-ended questions and moves to more specific closed or direct questions once you feel you have an idea of the chief complaint and present illness. Also, if the patient is having severe difficulty in breathing or terrible pain and is unable to answer with long sentences, you must use direct questions to gather the information because open-ended questions may exhaust your patient even further. Do not worsen the patient's condition with your patient interviewing techniques!

When gathering a history, employ some simple techniques. Introduce yourself and use the patient's name, if possible. For example, "Hi. My name is Mary Booth and I'm a paramedic. What is your name, sir? Okay, Mr. Edwards, I need to ask you some questions about why you called EMS." If the patient responds with a complaint of chest pain, probe further with "I need to ask you some questions about the pain you are experiencing."

Use compassion in your voice, yet be confident and firm. Do not be condescending or you will get little information from your patient. Avoid medical terminology because most patients do not understand it. For example, do not ask, "So is the pain radiating to the lumbar or sacral region?" The patient may respond simply no, not because the pain is not radiating there, but because he does not have a clue to what you are talking about and is embarrassed. Likewise, avoid treating the patient as if he is in kindergarten and using very simplistic terms unless it is appropriate for that particular patient.

Other good communication skills involve nonverbal techniques such as positioning, touch, tone, and eye contact. Do not position yourself authoritatively, that is, hovering above the patient. Get down to his level, if possible (Figure 1-15). Touch provides a great deal of reassurance and comfort. Use it appropriately with patients. The tone of your voice can portray empathy and a caring attitude or it can project just the opposite. Use eye contact when speaking with your patient. Also, patience is important. In situations that are not critical, allow the patient to answer at his pace, especially when the patient is elderly. A common problem with EMS personnel in history taking is a true lack of listening. Actually, they "listen" but do not really "hear" what the patient is telling them. You must be a good listener in order to be a good interviewer.

Chief Complaint The chief complaint is typically the reason why you are at the scene. It is usually one of the first pieces of verbal information gained from the

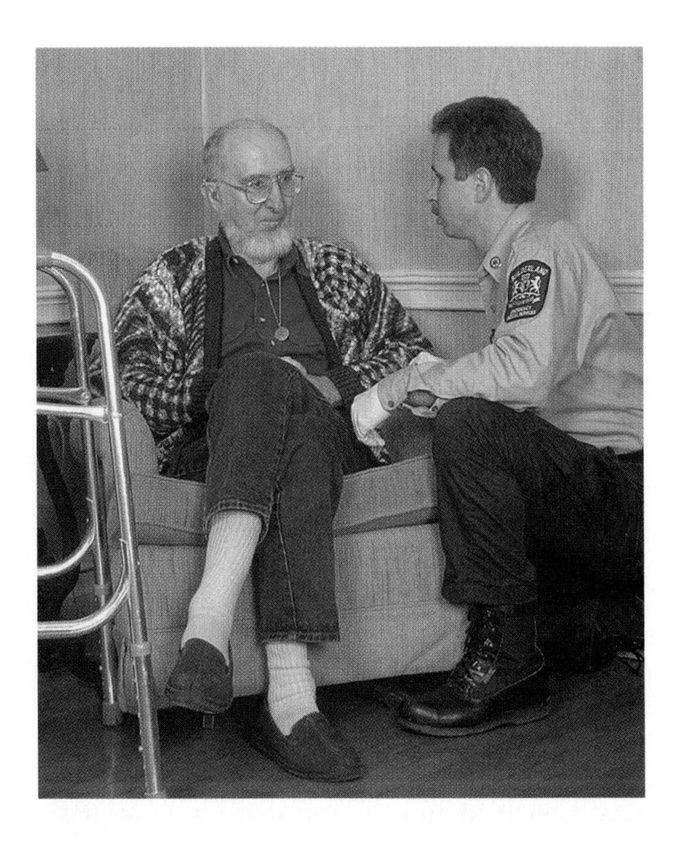

FIGURE 1-15
Position yourself at the patient's level, if possible.

patient ("Why did you call the ambulance?"). However, the complaint the patient describes at first is not necessarily the primary reason you were called. For example, you might be called for a complaint of abdominal pain. When you arrive on the scene, the patient states that he has had the abdominal pain for the last 3 weeks. You need to ascertain at this point what has changed that prompted the call to EMS ("So why did you call us *today*?"). The patient may have experienced an acute onset of bloody vomiting or dark tarry stools, or the pain may have become worse or changed in some other manner. This additional, refined information becomes as significant as the initial chief complaint.

The chief complaint is usually characterized by pain, dysfunction, discomfort, or an abnormal observation. When you describe the chief complaint in your report, use the patient's own words, if possible, such as "My chest hurts in the middle." You can further clarify the chief complaint in the history of the present illness and your report on the physical assessment findings. Avoid using diagnostic terms. Do not report "Patient complains of lung cancer." That is not the reason why you were called to the scene today. It should be an associated complaint, sign, or symptom, perhaps the fact that the patient's usual dyspnea has gotten worse. Remember that you may need to ask, "Why did you call us today?" to clarify the real complaint.

When ascertaining the chief complaint, do not develop tunnel vision. You need to remain aware of other possible complaints, signs, and symptoms that may initially appear subtle but are more important than the original complaint. Also, as emphasized earlier, do not let someone else at the scene provide you with the chief complaint unless the patient is unresponsive or has an altered mental status and does not respond appropriately. Attempt to gather the information from the patient; however, keep in mind that family members can sometimes provide a more complete and objective history (e.g., a history of alcohol use).

History of the Present Illness The history of the present illness is where the chief complaint is explored in much greater detail. The mnemonic OPQRST can help you remember the questions to ask:

- ***Onset/Setting.*** Determine the time of the onset. Ask for the date, day, and time. Determine if the onset was gradual or sudden. This alone may help rule out certain types of conditions.

  As already mentioned, you also want to know what the patient was doing at the time of onset. Was there a specific event associated with the onset of the symptom? For example you ask, "What were you doing when the chest pain came on?" The patient may respond, "Sitting in my recliner watching the news" or "Out playing basketball with my son." Either would have significant meaning.

  Establish whether this symptom is a single acute attack or whether there were previous occurrences. Determine whether the previous occurrences were daily, periodic, or chronic. Also, ask whether the previous occurrences were diagnosed. If the symptom is still present, ask about the progression. Is the symptom worse, better, or unchanged?
- ***Palliation/Provocation* (also called *Alleviation/Aggravation*).** Establish what provides relief and what makes the symptom worse. A patient with a complaint of dyspnea may indicate that sitting up makes breathing a lot easier, whereas lying flat makes the dyspnea much worse. Determine if the patient complaining of abdominal pain tried an over-the-counter antacid. If so, establish whether the pain was relieved, made better, or not changed. This information is useful when attempting to rule out certain conditions.
- ***Quality.*** Quality is the patient's perception of the pain. Some common descriptions are crushing, tearing, crampy, knifelike, dull, sharp, achy, and tight. Attempt to get the patient to describe the quality, and report it in the patient's own words.
- ***Radiation/Location.*** When evaluating location, determine whether the pain radiates or is stationary. Ask the patient to point to the pain with one finger. The patient may complain of referred pain—pain that occurs in another area of the body not directly associated with the body system that is affected by the condition. For example, when the diaphragm is irritated, the patient may complain of shoulder pain on the same side as the diaphragmatic irritation. Splenic injury or disease may cause left shoulder pain, and liver disease may produce right shoulder pain. Another example of referred pain is knee pain associated with a hip injury.

  The term "pain" is used if the sensation exists without being elicited by movement or palpation. The term "tenderness" is typically used when palpation is required to stimulate or evoke a pain response. You might ask, "Does the pain occur when you move or when you are lying still?"

Clinical Insight

Pain is a symptom that exists without pressure or palpation. _Tenderness_ is pain elicited on pressure, such as palpation.

OPQRST Questions

Onset
Palliation/Provocation
Quality
Radiation
Severity
Time

- ***Severity/Intensity.*** Intensity refers to the severity, or how badly the pain really hurts. Use a scale of 1 to 10 with 10 being the worst. Have the patient rate the intensity on the scale. If the patient has had this same pain before, have him compare it to the previous episode. Determine what intervention (e.g., hospitalization, surgery) was necessary following the previous episode.

  Assessing the severity of pain in a patient remains very subjective. The traditional 0 to 10 numeric pain scale was originally developed for assessing only chest pain. Currently, it is being used to assess any pain complaint. The report of the degree of severity differs widely from patient to patient.

  In an attempt to determine more accurately and objectively the severity of pain, it may be more helpful to use physical signs indicating discomfort or pain in addition to the patient's self-reporting of the intensity. For example, a patient complaining of chest pain who presents with a clenched fist over his chest should be considered to have much more severe pain than the patient who runs his hand in a general manner over his chest when questioned about the pain. The clenched fist would be more likely correlated with a severity close to 8 to 10 on the severity scale, whereas the general open hand over the chest would be more likely a 1 to 4 on the scale. If the patient points directly to the pain with one finger, it may be correlated with a severity of 5 to 7 on the scale.

  Look for other objective indicators of intensity such as sighs, moans, grimacing, slow movements, irritable demeanor, and limping. A patient who rubs or supports an affected area, shifts his posture frequently, or sits in a rigid posture is likely suffering from pain.

  Several pain assessment scales are used to attempt to quantify the amount of pain the patient is experiencing. The Wong-Baker FACES scale uses a variety of faces with varying degrees from smiles to visible discomfort by grimacing and crying to elicit a descriptive response from the patient. The scale is primarily used for children, more specifically children who are older than 3 years; however, it can be used for adults and elderly or those who are having difficulty communicating (Figure 1-16). Another pain scale, the FLACC behavioral scale, assesses the patient's face, legs, activity, cry, and consolability. This scale was designed to assess pain in children younger than 5 years. Again, however, the parameters assessed may be somewhat adapted to older children and adults.

  Note the patient's facial expression. A smiling, conversing person may have little pain, whereas the patient who sits with his jaw and teeth clenched would be experiencing more severe pain. Assess the patient's activity level and posture. A patient lying still may have little pain, whereas the patient who is shifting his posture and squirming or is rigid and tense may be having more severe pain.

  Elderly patients especially have a difficult time with the traditional 0 to 10 numerical pain rating scale. You can use the verbal descriptor scale as an alternative for the elderly or other adults who cannot rate the pain using the 0 to 10 scale. Carry a card with these descriptors: no pain, mild, discomforting, distressing, horrible, and excruciating. Show the card to the patient and have the patient select the best description of his pain. You would then document the pain from 0 to 5 with 0 being no pain and 5 representing excruciating pain.

  The traditional 0 to 10 numerical pain rating scale is a fast and easy method to assess and describe the severity of pain. However, it is subjective and varies widely from patient to patient.
- ***Time/Duration.*** Duration refers to the length of time the symptom has been present. You want to ask, "How long have you had the pain?" "When did it start?"

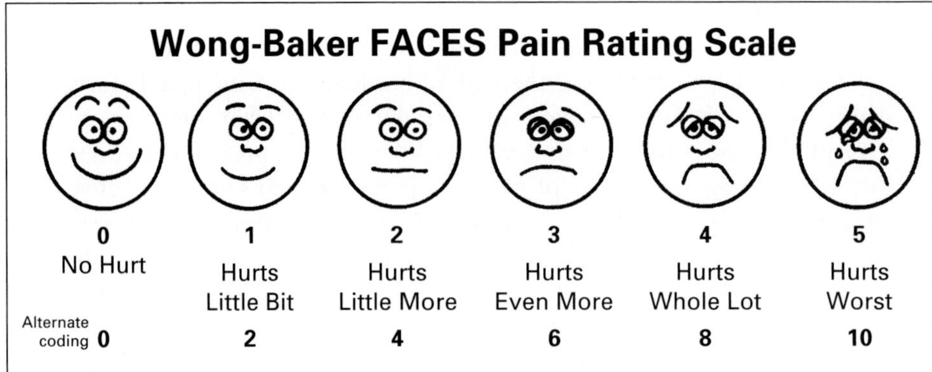

Brief word instructions: Point to each face using the words to describe the pain intensity. Ask the child to choose face that best describes own pain and record the appropriate number.

Original instructions: Explain to the person that each face is for a person who feels happy because he has no pain (hurt) or sad because he has some or a lot of pain. **Face 0** is very happy because he doesn't hurt at all. **Face 1** hurts just a little bit. **Face 2** hurts a little more. **Face 3** hurts even more. **Face 4** hurts a whole lot. **Face 5** hurts as much as you can imagine, although you don't have to be crying to feel this bad. Ask the person to choose the face that best desribes how he is feeling.

Rating scale is recommended for persons age 3 years and older.

FIGURE 1-16 The Wong-Baker FACES scale.

From Hockenberry, M.J., Wilson, D., Winkelstein, M.L.: *Wong's Essentials of Pediatric Nursing,* 7th ed., St. Louis, Mosby: 2005, p. 1259. Used with permission.

and "How long does it last when you get it?" Also, it is important to determine if the pain is constant (it does not go away) or intermittent (it comes and goes).

Another area it is often important to ask about, in conjunction with the OPQRST questions, is the following:

- *Associated Complaints.* Associated complaints are usually derived through direct questions. You want to attempt to determine what other complaints the patient has that may be directly related to this particular condition. For the patient complaining of chest pain, you would want to know about associated complaints such as dyspnea, nausea, lightheadedness, weakness, and palpitations. If the patient denies the symptom, you may want to document that as a pertinent negative, reported as "The patient denies associated dyspnea and nausea."

Past Medical History You also need to gain information about the patient's past medical history. Seek and document information that is pertinent to the current condition. You can use the mnemonic SAMPLE to help you remember questions that pertain to the past medical history:

- *Signs and Symptoms.* Ask about any signs or symptoms that the patient is now experiencing or noted before 911 was called. (The OPQRST questions can help elicit a description.)
- *Allergies.* Inquire about any allergies the patient may have, especially allergies to medications.
- *Medications.* Determine both prescription and nonprescription medications that the patient is taking. Ask whether the patient takes herbal supplements. Also, attempt to ascertain the patient's compliance in taking the medications. For example, you may be treating a patient who is actively seizing and who

SAMPLE Questions

Signs and symptoms
Allergies
Medications
Past medical history
Last oral intake
Events prior to illness

has a prescription for Dilantin. It is important to find out whether the patient takes the Dilantin as prescribed. If not, this may be the etiology of the acute seizure. The medication itself, or its interaction with another medication, may be the cause of the condition. You should either document all medications and their respective doses or take the medications to the emergency department with you. Either way, it is vital that the emergency department staff be made aware of the medications that the patient is currently taking.

- ***Past Medical History.*** This category can include the following:
  - ***Preexisting medical problems or surgeries.*** Ask the patient about any current or past medical illnesses such as heart disease, hypertension, respiratory conditions, diabetes mellitus, or stroke. Also, it is important to identify any major surgeries that the patient may have undergone. This may provide pertinent information about the severity of the past medical problems.
  - ***Physician.*** Attempt to identify the patient's physician. It may be helpful to ascertain if the patient is regularly seen by a physician for the current complaint. This may aid in establishing changes in the condition or severity.
  - ***Family History.*** A detailed family history is seldom relevant in the prehospital setting, except in the case of infectious disease transmission, when it becomes extremely important. When you are dealing with conditions such as TB or bacterial meningitis, the family history is also relevant to the patient's current status. The family cardiac history may be important when a young individual complains of typical cardiac-type chest pain. The family history may suggest the degree of cardiac risk. Also, conditions that are hereditary may be evaluated further through family history. In African Americans, ask about a history of sickle cell disease.
  - ***Social History.*** The patient's social history may help explain the etiology of the condition. Things you want to consider are the patient's housing environment, economic status, occupation, high-risk behaviors, and travel history. An elderly patient may succumb to heat stroke because of the lack of air conditioning in his living environment. You might find a patient who is malnourished, hypoglycemic, and thiamine deficient due to inadequate income. Occupational exposure to chemicals, heat, cold, and smoke may provide clues as to the etiology of the condition. Recent travel may have exposed the patient to infectious diseases, insects, animals, or other environmental conditions that may have triggered a specific disease process.
- ***Last Oral Intake.*** Knowing what the patient has eaten or drunk may help explain the present problem, such as in a diabetic patient who has forgotten to eat after taking insulin. Also, the association between the blood glucose

reading and the last oral intake is important to consider. If the patient reports eating a candy bar and having a bottle of sport drink a half hour prior to your arrival, you would expect the blood glucose reading to be elevated (120 to 140 mg/dl). However, if the patient indicates that he has not eaten anything for the last 13 hours and his blood glucose is 136 mg/dl, this would be reason for concern because you would expect to find a fasting blood glucose reading of 80 to 90 mg/dl. The hospital staff will also need last oral intake information if surgery is necessary.

- *Events Prior to the Illness.* Ask about what the patient was doing or experiencing just before becoming ill, such as whether the patient suffered a sudden severe headache or was actively exercising.

Current Health Status The current health status takes into account the patient's personal habits and is closely related to the past medical history. Components to consider in assessing the current health status of the patient are

- Tobacco use
- Use of alcohol or drugs—medicinal, recreational, or illicit
- Sexual/gynecological history
- Diet
- Screening tests
- Immunizations
- Exercise and leisure activity
- Patient's outlook

Perform a Focused Medical Assessment

In the responsive medical patient, the next step after the history would be the focused medical assessment, also known as the focused physical exam.

The focused exam is based on the information gathered from the history.

The focused exam is based on the information gathered from the history. If the patient's chief complaint is abdominal pain, you need to focus your attention on identifying signs of an acute abdomen or other medical conditions that may be related to the pain. This does not mean that you should develop tunnel vision and assess only the abdomen. You must also assess the other related body systems. As an example, there are cardiac and respiratory conditions that may present as abdominal pain. Thus, it would also be necessary to evaluate the cardiac and respiratory systems.

Techniques that you would use during a focused exam are the same as those you would use during a rapid medical assessment—the complete head-to-toe exam for an unresponsive or altered mental status patient, which is described later in this chapter. However, only certain components of the exam will be used—those that are relevant to the patient's complaint.

Clinical Insight

The "blink test," suddenly and rapidly flicking your fingers in front of the patient's face, is often used to differentiate a psychogenic coma from one that is truly metabolic or structural. Interpret the results cautiously because a truly comatose patient with open eyes may blink as the cornea is stimulated by the sudden air movement.

Perform a Neurologic Exam if Indicated When presented with a patient with a suspected neurologic insult, whether the patient is responsive, has an altered mental status, or is unresponsive, it is necessary to perform a more comprehensive neurologic examination. Isolate the exam to gathering information that will help you determine whether an injury or insult has occurred to the central nervous system. For the seasoned EMS practitioner, the assessment should take no longer than 60 seconds.

Determine the patient's mental status by using the AVPU scale and obtaining a Glasgow Coma score. (The Glasgow Coma Scale is discussed and illustrated in

Chapter 7, Altered Mental Status.) It is also important to assess the patient's orientation, short-term memory, attention, language capability, and ability to perform calculations. However, because it is usually not practical to do all of this in the prehospital environment, assess the following parameters to obtain key information about the patient's mental status:

- Is the patient oriented to place and time?
- Can the patient comprehend why EMS was called?
- Does the patient understand your concerns about his medical condition?
- Can the patient explain the risks if he refuses treatment?
- Does the patient exhibit the necessary decision-making ability to call EMS if he has refused care but changes his mind later?

Having the patient answer or demonstrate an understanding of these questions will provide information about gross mental status and identify potential deficits. Higher cerebral function is required to exercise reason, insight, and judgment. Getting these answers will also ensure the patient has consented to care. While the patient is answering, evaluate his speech for slurring, grammar, and vocabulary. Speech indicates cerebrum and cranial nerve function.

In the ambulatory patient, assess motor function by having the patient stand and take a few steps. Evaluate the gait to determine if it is smooth. Look for halting, a limp, or loss of balance (ataxic gait), which may indicate an insult to the cerebellum. Assess upper extremity function by testing grip strength and having the patient lift his arms above his head. Lower motor strength is tested through gait assessment.

Obviously, if you have any concerns about causing or aggravating a spinal cord injury, you should assess motor function while the patient is immobilized or while manual stabilization is being performed. To assess motor function in a nonambulatory patient, have him lift his thigh while flexing at the hip and then have him push down on your hands with his feet (plantar flexion).

Motor function is simply documented as adequate or near-normal, barely able to move, or absent. Be sure to compare the left and right extremities and the upper and lower extremities.

Assess pupillary function for size and reactivity. This, however, may provide limited information. Unequal pupils in a patient with an altered mental status are a serious sign of intracranial pathology, whereas unequal pupils in an awake patient with no neurologic deficit may be a normal finding or the result of direct cranial nerve damage. Assess the pupils for a sluggish response, which may indicate brain insult in the patient with an altered mental status. In the awake and alert patient, sluggish pupils are a nonsignificant finding.

This is an adequate neurologic examination to perform. However, if you have more time, you can do a more thorough assessment of cranial nerve function. This may be helpful when you are evaluating a patient with suspected brain injury, such as a stroke. Evaluate nerves II, III, IV, and VI by assessing the pupillary reaction to light and extraocular eye movements such as looking up, down, left, and then right. Normal speech tests nerves IX, X, and XII. To evaluate nerve VII, have the patient make a smile and raise both eyebrows. Clenching the teeth will assess a portion of the motor function of nerve V, while feeling facial sensations will test the sensory function of nerve V. Nerve VIII is checked by having the patient cover one ear with his hand and attempting to detect a whisper. Nerve XI is assessed by having the patient shrug his shoulders.

Note any nonpurposeful movements such as decorticate or decerebrate posturing. Evaluate the plantar (Babinski's) reflex by running a pen, your thumb, or

Clinical Insight

Elderly patients may exhibit a pattern of confusion that has an onset late in the day. Drugs that may cause a state of confusion in the elderly are histamine blockers, antidiarrheals, analgesics, antipsychotics, tricyclic antidepressants, antidysrhythmics, incontinence agents, sedatives, and hyponotics. A significant change in cerebral function and cognitive impairment in an elderly patient may be due to depression.

Clinical Insight

Pupil reactivity is one of the best ways to differentiate a structural from a metabolic etiology of coma. Pupil reactivity is usually preserved with metabolic causes of coma.

Clinical Insight

Babinski's reflex, dorsiflexion of the great toe with fanning and extension of the other toes, may be a normal presentation in an epileptic postictal patient.

Clinical Insight

Todd's paralysis, a transient focal weakness or paralysis of an arm or leg, may normally occur after an epileptic seizure and may indicate a focal cerebral lesion as the etiology.

other blunt object up the lateral edge of the sole of the foot from the heel to the toes. Dorsiflexion (upward movement, toward the body) of the great toe and fanning of the other toes is an abnormal response. The plantar reflex may indicate dysfunction to the cerebrum or spinal cord. The normal response is when the toes move downward (plantar flexion). Note that an abnormal Babinski's sign is a normal finding in a postictal patient. Also, some postictal patients suffer Todd's paralysis, a temporary hemiparesis or hemiplegia that resolves over a period of time.

Test all four extremities for both light touch and pain, as well as for motor function. Light touch and pain are carried by different afferent (sensory) nerve tracts in the spinal cord. Light touch is carried in the posterior columns of the spinal cord, whereas pain sensation is carried in the more anterior spinothalamic tracts. Moreover, pain tracts travel on the opposite side of the spinal cord from pain perception. For example, pain that the patient perceives from a pinch to the right hand is carried to the cerebrum by the spinothalamic tracts on the left side of the spinal cord. Conversely, the sensation of light touch is carried on the same side of the spinal cord as the perception of light touch. The sensation of light touch to the patient's right hand is carried to the cerebrum along the right side of the spinal cord. Therefore, by testing both light touch and pain in all extremities, you are testing sets of spinal tracts on both sides of the spinal cord. If only light touch or only pain were tested, you would be testing spinal tracts on only one side, and an incomplete spinal cord injury could be missed if either the posterior columns or the spinothalamic tracts were not injured and are still intact. Light touch is carried by a larger number of nerve tracts; thus, it is less specific and poorly localized in spinal cord injuries. Motor function is carried by corticospinal tracts in the spinal cord. These efferent (motor) nerve tracts carry the motor response from the cerebral cortex to the muscle group on the same side of the spinal cord as the muscle movement. Thus, movement of the right hand is carried by corticospinal tracts on the right side of the spinal cord.

To reemphasize: It is imperative in your neurologic assessment of the patient to test light touch, pain, and motor function in all four extremities. To test for light touch and pain, take a Q-tip with a wooden stick and break it. Use the cotton end of the Q-tip to test for light touch and the broken wooden part to check for pain response. Note carefully responses to both light touch and pain in all four extremities.

When performing a neurologic examination on a noncomatose patient who presents with any suspected signs or symptoms of stroke or on a patient who presents with an acute nontraumatic neurologic complaint, you should use one of the validated stroke screening evaluation tools, either the Cincinnati Prehospital Stroke Scale (CPSS) or the Los Angeles Prehospital Stroke Screen (LAPSS), to identify a potential stroke.

The CPSS (Figure 1-17) tests for 1) facial droop by having the patient show his teeth or make a smile, 2) arm drift by having the patient close his eyes and hold both arms straight out in front of him for 10 seconds, and 3) abnormal speech pattern and muscle palsies by having the patient say "you can't teach an old dog new tricks."

The LAPSS (Figure 1-18) takes into consideration other causes of altered mental status, such as hypoglycemia, hyperglycemia, or seizures, and also requires a physical test of asymmetry of strength. The information ascertained in the LAPSS is 1) age older than 45 years, 2) history of seizures or epilepsy, 3) duration of symptoms, 4) wheelchair or bedridden status of patient, and 5) blood glucose level. Asymmetry of strength is assessed by testing facial smile or grimace, grip, and arm strength.

Both screening tools are highly sensitive and specific. Any one abnormality in the physical tests of either the CPSS or the LAPSS is highly suggestive of stroke. According to the *2005 American Heart Association Guidelines for Cardiopulmonary Resuscitation and Emergency Cardiovascular Care*, if any one of the three CPSS

Cincinnati Prehospital Stroke Scale

Sign of Stroke	Patient Activity	Interpretation
Facial Droop	Have patient look up at you, smile, and show his teeth.	*Normal*: Symmetry to both sides. *Abnormal*: One side of the face droops or does not move symmetrically.
Arm Drift	Have patient lift arms up and hold them out with eyes closed for 10 seconds.	*Normal*: Symmetrical movement in both arms. *Abnormal*: One arm drifts down or asymmetrical movement of the arms.
Abnormal Speech	Have the patient say "you can't teach an old dog new tricks."	*Normal*: The correct words are used and no slurring of words is noted. *Abnormal*: The words are slurred, the wrong words are used, or the patient is aphasic.

Kothari, R.U., Pancioli, A., Liu, T., Broderick, J. "Cincinnati Prehospital Stroke Scale: reproducibility and validity." *Annals of Emergency Medicine.* 1999;33:373-378.

FIGURE 1-17 Cincinnati Prehospital Stroke Scale.

findings is abnormal, there is a 72 percent probability of stroke. Likewise, 93 percent of the patients who have suffered an acute stroke will respond *yes* or *unknown* with positive findings on the LAPSS, and 97 percent of the patients who present with positive findings on the LAPSS will have suffered an acute stroke. It is important that one of these evaluations is performed on any patient with suspicion of stroke.

Los Angeles Prehospital Stroke Screen (LAPSS)

Considerations	Yes	Unknown	No
Age **greater than** 45 years			
No history of seizures or epilepsy			
Duration of symptoms is **less** than 24 hours			
Patient is **not** wheelchair bound or bedridden			
Blood gluscose level **between 60 and 400 mg/dl**			
Physical exam to determine unilateral asymmetry	**Equal**	**R Weakness**	**L Weakness**
A. Have patient look up, smile, and show teeth		Droop	Droop
B. Compare grip strength of upper extremities		Weak grip No grip	Weak grip No grip
C. Assess arm strength for drift or weakness		Drifts down Falls rapidly	Drifts down Falls rapidly

Kidwell, C.S., Saver, J.L., Schubert, G.B., Eckstein, M., Starkman, S., "Design and retrospective analysis of the Los Angeles Prehospital Stroke Screen (LAPSS)." *Prehospital Emergency Care.* 1998;2:267-273.

Kidwell, C.S., Starkman, S., Eckstein, M., Weems, K., Saver, J.L., "Identifying stroke in the field: prospective validation of the Los Angeles Prehospital Stroke Screen (LAPSS)." *Stroke.* 2000;31:71-76.

FIGURE 1-18 Los Angeles Prehospital Stroke Screen (LAPSS).

This is a more comprehensive neurologic examination that may provide more information when subtle findings are necessary to form a differential field diagnosis. Remember: The neurologic exam should be accomplished in about 60 seconds.

Assess Baseline Vital Signs

The vital signs will be assessed following the focused physical exam. These preliminary measurements provide a baseline to which later readings can be compared, indicating improvement or deterioration in the patient's condition. Vital signs measurements are discussed later in the chapter.

Provide Emergency Care

Based on information you gather from the chief complaint, the history, the physical exam, and baseline vital signs, you will intervene and provide emergency care to your patient. This may include both pharmacologic and nonpharmacologic therapy. Intervening at the appropriate point depends on your ability to establish priorities and recognize conditions that warrant such treatment. Remember, you will begin with an assessment-based approach to identify and treat immediate life threats, and then you will move to developing a differential field diagnosis so you may provide advanced emergency care to the patient.

Unresponsive or Altered Mental Status Patient

Clinical Insight

Any unresponsive patient is considered to be unstable by nature of the presenting complaint: unresponsiveness.

Clinical Insight

Syncope with sudden onset or related to effort often has a cardiac etiology, usually due to a dysrhythmia. Dizziness, nausea, sweating, and yawning often precede vasovagal syncope.

The patient with an altered mental status or who is unresponsive should be considered to be physiologically unstable by nature of the presenting complaint: altered mental status or unresponsiveness. A rapid medical assessment, which is a systematic head-to-toe physical examination, is performed to identify signs potentially related to the etiology of the altered mental status or unresponsiveness. You will have already assessed and managed any life threats to the airway, breathing, and circulation during the initial assessment. As you perform the rapid assessment, you will be able to further assess the airway, breathing, and circulation, in addition to other signs of distress or illness.

For the unresponsive or altered mental status patient, the physical examination precedes vital signs measurements and history gathering.

Perform a Rapid Medical Assessment

The rapid medical assessment should be conducted systematically, beginning at the head and covering all major body cavities and body systems. The rapid medical assessment is designed to identify the more significant signs of medical illnesses or conditions. Four techniques (Figure 1-19)—inspection, palpation, auscultation, and percussion—are employed to gather information from the examination and to identify any abnormality or dysfunction.

Assess the Head Because the patient has an altered mental status or is unresponsive, and even though it is a medical call, it is important to inspect and palpate for any evidence of trauma (Figure 1-20). You may not expect to find any if you have not identified a mechanism of injury. Inspect and palpate for contusions, lacerations, depressions, abrasions, hematomas (swellings), ecchymosis (bruising), and punctures, keeping in mind that signs and symptoms of a subdural hematoma may occur up to 2 weeks or more after the initial injury, and findings may not be evident.

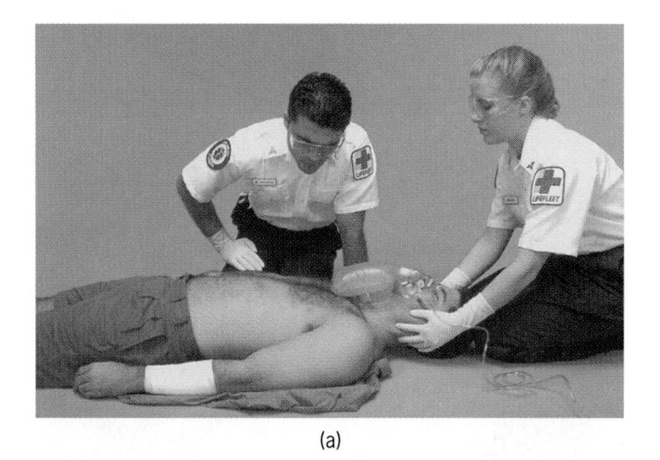

(a)

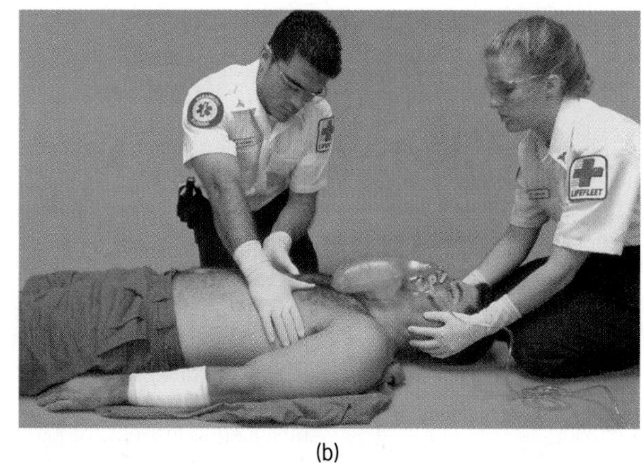

(b)

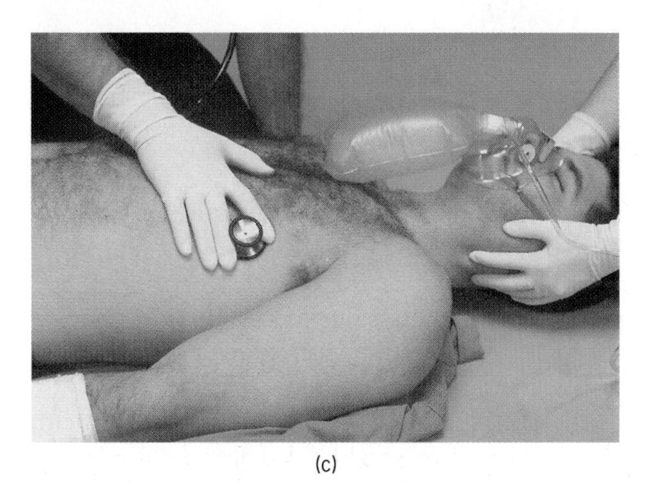

(c)

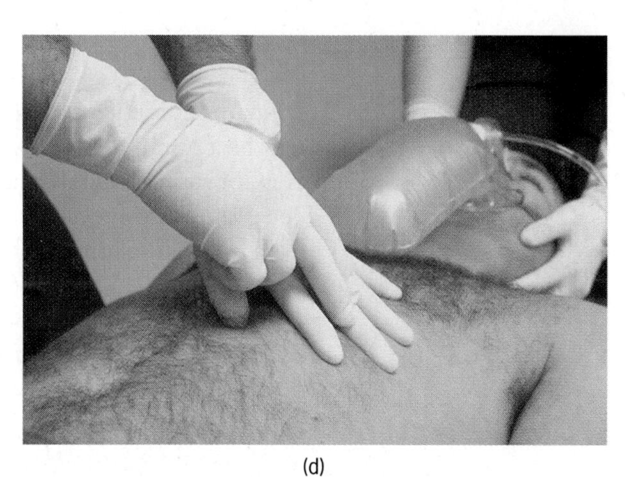

(d)

FIGURE 1-19
Four techniques of physical examination are (a) inspection, (b) palpation, (c) auscultation, and (d) percussion.

Inspect the face for symmetry. Look particularly at the corners of the mouth and the eyelids for asymmetry, which will appear as a droop. This may indicate stroke or a condition such as Bell's palsy. Also look for excessive swelling, erythema (redness), and urticaria (hives), indicating possible anaphylactic reaction.

Inspect the pupils for equality in size and reactivity. Unequal pupils indicate intracranial pathology, such as stroke. Cataracts may make the pupils appear cloudy, whereas glaucoma usually distorts the shape and size of the pupil, especially following surgical repair. The pupils may be dilated in response to drugs, poisoning,

Clinical Insight

If you suspect psychogenic coma in a patient, open the eyelids and assess eye deviation. If the eyes deviate upward with only the sclera showing (Bell's phenomenon), suspect psychogenic coma.

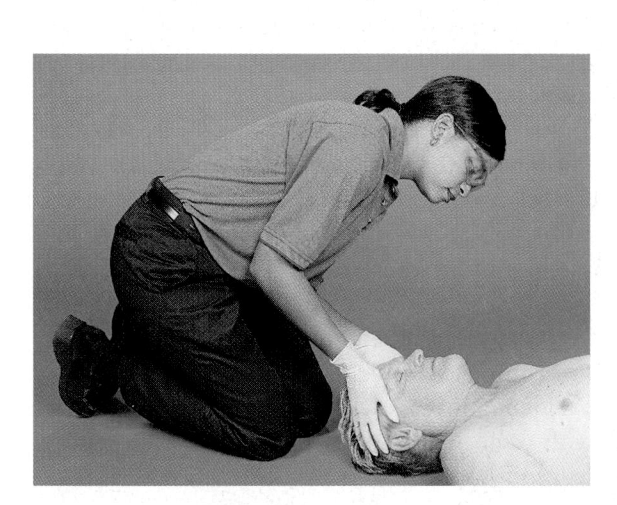

FIGURE 1-20
Inspect and palpate the head for contusions, lacerations, depressions, abrasions, hematomas, ecchymosis, and punctures.

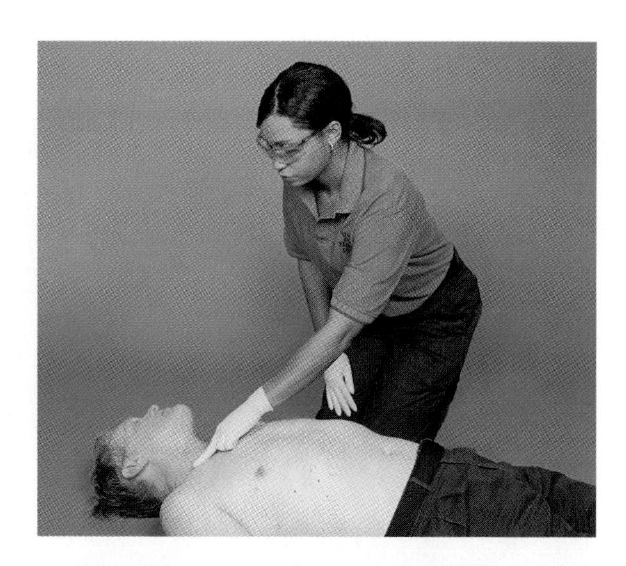

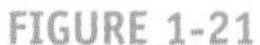

FIGURE 1-21
Inspect the neck for use of accessory muscles or retraction of the suprasternal notch, pendulum movements of the trachea, a tracheostomy tube, or a medical identification necklace. Inspect and palpate for subcutaneous emphysema. Inspect for jugular vein distention (JVD) with the patient's head and torso elevated to a 45-degree angle.

sympathomimetic medications, neurologic disorders, or injury. Constricted pupils may be a result of narcotic drug use or specific lesions in the pons. Also, note if the eyes appear to be sunken and dry, potentially indicating dehydration. Quickly pull down the bottom eyelid and inspect the conjunctiva. The conjunctiva may be pale from hypoperfusion, red from irritation or excessive hypertension, or cyanotic from hypoxia. Yellowed sclerae (icterus) indicate possible liver disease.

Open the mouth and quickly inspect the mucous membranes for cyanosis and pallor. Also, reassess for any evidence of bleeding, secretions, or vomitus that needs to be suctioned.

Assess the Neck Inspect the neck (Figure 1-21). In the medical patient, jugular venous distention (JVD) usually indicates right-sided heart failure. If possible, JVD should be inspected with the patient's head and torso elevated to a 45-degree angle. If the jugular vein is engorged more than two-thirds the distance from the base of the neck, it is considered to be significant. (It is important to note that a certain amount of jugular venous engorgement would be normal when a patient is lying flat.) Also, note if the jugular veins have a tendency to engorge during inspiration. This is termed Kussmaul's sign. If present, it may indicate increased intrathoracic pressure related to conditions such as severe acute asthma, tension pneumothorax, or pericardial tamponade.

Look for a medical identification necklace or tag containing pertinent information about the patient's condition or past medical history.

Inspect the neck for evidence of accessory muscle use and retraction in the suprasternal notch. If the muscles bulge and become prominent and the suprasternal notch retracts during inspiration, this suggests respiratory distress. (You may need to quickly reassess the breathing status.) Also, look for a medical identification necklace or tag containing pertinent information about the patient's condition or past medical history. Inspect and palpate the neck for subcutaneous emphysema, which appears as puffy skin and feels like bubble packaging. This commonly results from pneumomediastinum, where air dissects into the subcutaneous tissues from a ruptured bleb.

While inspecting the base of the neck, check for a tracheostomy tube or stoma. Secretions may build up, partially or completely obstructing the tube or stoma.

Palpate the trachea for movement during each ventilation. If the trachea moves in a pendulum motion with each breath, it may indicate an obstructed bronchus. Typically, the trachea will shift to the side of the obstruction.

In the nontrauma patient, flex the head and attempt to touch the patient's chin to his chest. If the neck is stiff or not supple and the patient presents with fever and an altered mental status, consider meningitis. If meningitis is suspected, flex the neck by moving the chin to the patient's chest. If the hips and knees then flex involuntarily, a response known as Brudzinski's sign, suspect meningitis.

Clinical Insight

Brudzinski's sign is the involuntary flexion of the hips and knees when the neck is flexed while the patient is supine. It is an indication of meningitis. This sign may be absent in the elderly.

Assess the Chest Expose the chest and inspect and palpate for symmetry, retractions of the intercostal muscles, and adequate rise and fall. Retractions of the intercostal muscles usually indicate significant respiratory distress. If you note retractions, quickly reevaluate the minute volume to determine the need for positive-pressure ventilation. This also may be an indication to expedite pharmacologic management of certain conditions associated with increased airway resistance, such as acute asthma. A barrel chest (increased anterior-posterior diameter from chronic air trapping) would likely indicate a patient with emphysema. Look for scars from open heart surgery. An implanted defibrillator or pacer is typically found as a bulge in the anterior chest wall. Place your hands with fingers spread apart on both sides of the chest wall. As the patient inhales, feel for symmetric rise and fall.

Clinical Insight

Approximately 5 to 10% of patients with ischemic heart disease will have reproducible chest pain on palpation of the thorax.

Auscultate the lungs (Figure 1-22) over the midclavicular line at the second intercostal space, at the fourth intercostal space midaxillary, and at the lower border of the thorax. If possible, have the patient sit up and auscultate over the posterior thorax at about the 8th to 10th thoracic vertebrae midscapular. This is especially important in the congestive heart failure patient to assess the basal areas of the lungs for crackles. When assessing the breath sounds, compare the right hemithorax to the left hemithorax. Assess for abnormal, or adventitious, breath sounds, including crackles, rhonchi, or wheezing.

Crackles, also known as rales, are heard more often during inspiration and are discontinuous sounds, each lasting only a few milliseconds. Crackles can be characterized as fine, high-pitched, and short in duration or coarse, low-pitched, and longer in duration. High-pitched crackles are referred to as sibilant, low-pitched crackles as sonorous. Crackles are caused by a disruption of airflow in the smaller airways. Crackles may be produced as a result of the terminal bronchioles and alveoli popping open during inspiration. Crackles are most often associated with fluid or exudate in or around the alveoli and terminal bronchioles. Conditions such as pneumonia and pulmonary edema produce crackles.

Rhonchi, also known as sonorous wheezes, are a much rougher, more rumbling sound and are much easier to hear. Rhonchi are more pronounced during expiration and produce a prolonged continuous sound. High-pitched rhonchi are

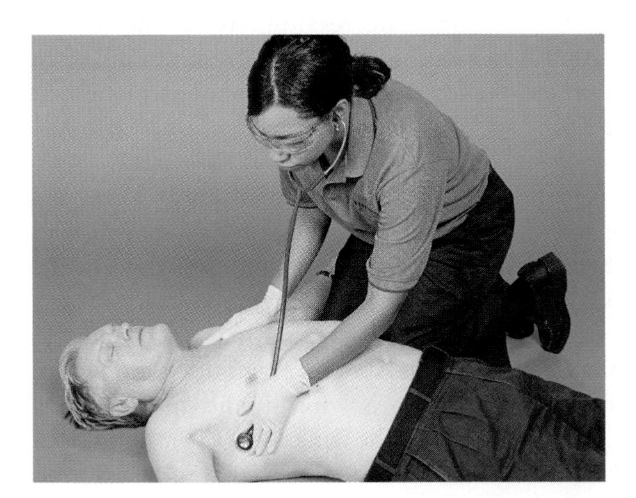

FIGURE 1-22
Inspect and palpate the chest for symmetry, retractions of the intercostal muscles, and adequate rise and fall. Look for barrel chest, scars from surgery, or an implanted defibrillator or pacer. Auscultate the breath sounds.

more sibilant and are associated with airflow obstruction in the smaller bronchi, such as in asthma. The low-pitched rhonchi are more sonorous and are produced in the larger bronchi. Rhonchi are produced by airflow through an airway obstructed with mucus or thick secretions, muscle spasm, growths, or external pressure. Coughing may clear the rhonchi, indicating mucus in the trachea or large bronchi. Rhonchi are often heard in chronic bronchitis, emphysema, and pneumonia.

Wheezes, also known as sibilant wheezes, are continuous, high-pitched musical sounds that are heard during both inspiration and expiration. Wheezes are caused by air flowing through a narrowed bronchiole. Bilateral wheezes are associated with bronchospasm commonly seen in asthma and bronchitis. Wheezes that are unilateral or localized to one area are more often associated with a foreign body. A tumor causing compression of the bronchial tree may produce wheezes that are consistent at the site of the lesion.

Clinical Insight

When a patient is wheezing, consider these conditions: asthma, emphysema, chronic bronchitis, congestive heart failure, anaphylaxis, foreign body obstruction at the bronchial level, and tracheobronchitis.

A friction rub is not associated with the respiratory tract; if present, however, it is discovered during auscultation. A rub is a dry, grating, crackling, low-pitched sound heard during inspiration and expiration. It is caused by inflammation and dried surfaces that become rough and rub over each other. If heard over the pericardium, it suggests pericarditis. When heard over the lungs, it usually indicates pleurisy. The pleural friction rub will be abolished when the breath is held, whereas the cardiac friction rub will continue during the breath holding.

Hamman's sign, or a mediastinal crunch, is indicative of mediastinal emphysema or air trapped in the mediastinum. The sounds heard may be crackling, clicking, or gurgling. The sounds are more synchronized with the heartbeat and less with respiration. A mediastinal crunch may be easier to hear during expiration and when the patient is leaning to the left or in a left lateral recumbent position.

You can percuss the chest to listen for abnormal sounds. Dullness, or hyporesonance, usually indicates fluid-filled lungs, as in pneumonia or pulmonary edema. A pleural effusion may produce localized dullness on percussion. Hyperresonance typically indicates air trapping associated with a pneumothorax or severe asthma attack or emphysema. Findings during percussion may be difficult to appreciate in the prehospital environment.

Note any abnormal respiratory pattern (see Chapter 5). Hyperpnea (deep breathing) and tachypnea (rapid breathing), such as Kussmaul's respirations associated with diabetic ketoacidosis, typically indicate a metabolic condition. Respirations that are rapid and shallow (central neurogenic hyperventilation) usually indicate brain injury, increased intracranial pressure, or metabolic problems. Cheyne-Stokes respirations are exhibited as a crescendo-decrescendo-apnea pattern that continuously repeats itself. Biot's, or ataxic, respirations have no coordinated pattern. Cheyne-Stokes, central neurogenic, and Biot's respirations often indicate central nervous system problems such as head injury, brain herniation, or increased intracranial pressure.

Assess the Abdomen Inspect the abdomen for evidence of any previous surgeries, distention, discoloration, and pulsating masses. The abdomen may distend due to air or fluid. Ascites, which is an abnormal accumulation of fluid in the intraperitoneal cavity, is usually related to cirrhosis, congestive heart failure, nephritic syndrome, peritonitis, or other disease. Distention may also be due to accumulation of blood from internal hemorrhage. It takes a significant amount of blood to distend the abdomen in a patient who is lying supine. In the supine patient, the blood has a tendency to accumulate in the flank area. The resulting discoloration is known as Grey Turner's sign and is due to collection of blood from

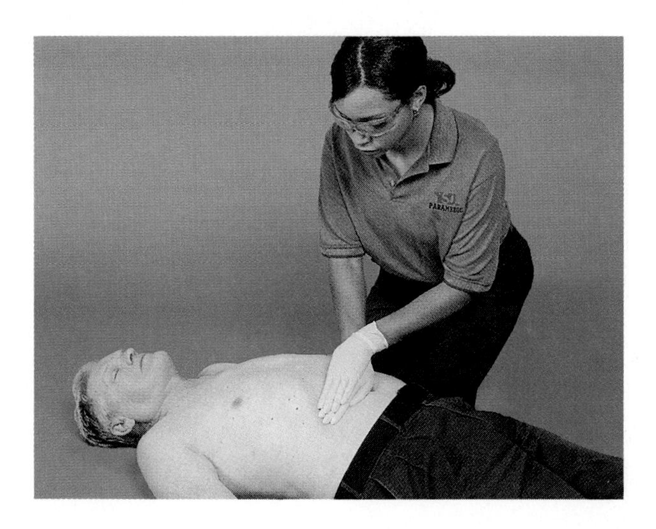

FIGURE 1-23
Inspect the abdomen for evidence of previous surgeries, distention, discoloration, or pulsating masses. Palpate for tenderness, rebound tenderness, guarding, rigidity, distention, or pulsating masses.

intraabdominal bleeding. Distention or discoloration may not develop for several hours, and therefore should be considered late signs of internal hemorrhage.

Palpate each quadrant of the abdomen for tenderness, rebound tenderness, guarding, and rigidity (Figure 1-23). You should start with the quadrant farthest away from the pain, leaving the painful quadrant for last. Rebound tenderness can be tested by quickly letting up on palpation pressure. Pain that is worse during abdominal wall recoil is suggestive of rebound. Guarding is a voluntary response where the patient tenses his abdominal muscles in response to your palpation. Rigidity is an involuntary muscular tension that the patient cannot control. Abdominal tenderness, pain, rebound tenderness, guarding, and rigidity are all signs of peritonitis. Also, palpate for any masses and distention. A pulsating mass found in the midline of the abdomen is likely from an aortic aneurysm. Ascites will feel spongy and distended.

Assess the Pelvis Inspect and palpate the pelvis for any evidence of bleeding or trauma (Figure 1-24). Also, inspect quickly for evidence of bowel or bladder incontinence or obvious rectal bleeding. In the pregnant patient who is in labor, inspect the vaginal area and perineum for crowning. Also assess for vaginal bleeding and any abnormal discharge.

Assess the Extremities Inspect the extremities for any evidence of trauma, ecchymosis (bruising), unusual erythema (redness), cyanosis, or mottling

Clinical Insight

A patient in diabetic ketoacidosis (DKA) may present with abdominal tenderness and guarding that could progress to abdominal rigidity with rebound tenderness. It is believed that the abdominal signs are due to dehydration, hypotension, and potassium deficit.

Clinical Insight

A positive Rovsing sign is an increase in right lower quadrant pain that intensifies when the left lower quadrant is palpated. This is an indication of peritoneal irritation due to appendicitis.

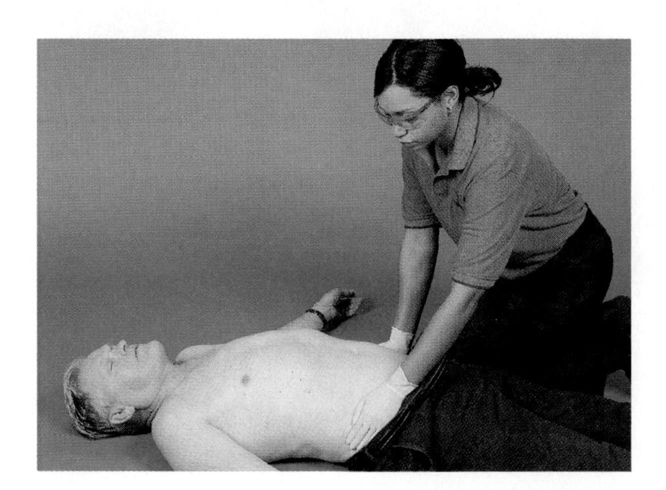

FIGURE 1-24
Inspect and palpate the pelvis for evidence of bleeding or trauma. Quickly inspect for evidence of bowel or bladder incontinence or for crowning in a patient in labor.

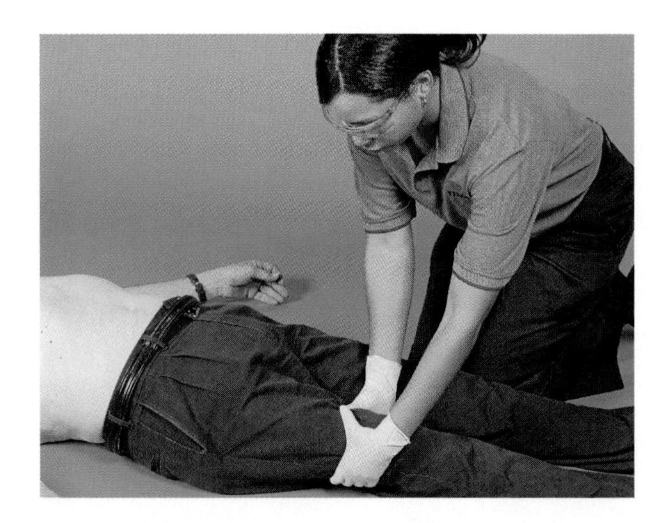

FIGURE 1-25
Inspect the extremities for evidence of trauma, ecchymosis, erythema, cyanosis, or mottling. Assess distal pulses and motor and sensory function.

Clinical Insight

Only 50% of patients with deep vein thrombosis complain of pain and swelling to the leg and have a positive Homan's sign (pain in the affected calf on dorsiflexion of the foot). Greater than 90% of pulmonary emboli originate from a lower extremity deep vein thrombosis.

(Figure 1-25). Erythema to an extremity that is warm and dry to touch may indicate a venous embolus. A pale, cool, cyanotic, and mottled extremity usually indicates an arterial thrombus. In dark-skinned patients, check for cyanosis by inspecting the nail beds, palms of the hands, oral mucosa, and conjunctiva.

Assess distal pulses and motor and sensory function in each extremity. The radial pulses should be assessed in the upper extremities, and the dorsalis pedis or posterior tibial pulses should be assessed in the lower extremities. Check the sensory function by painful stimulation and by light touch in the responsive patient. Watch for motor movement with the application of a painful stimulus in the patient with an altered mental status who cannot obey commands or who is responding only to painful stimuli. If the patient is responsive and able to obey your commands, ask the patient to identify which finger or toe is being touched on each hand or foot to assess sensory function. To assess motor function, ask the patient to grasp your fingers and squeeze as hard as possible. For the lower extremities, have the patient pull up and then push down with his foot against your hands. With both the upper and lower extremities, compare the strength of the right and left side. (Also review "Perform a Neurologic Exam if Indicated" earlier in this chapter.)

Assess for peripheral or dependent edema in the lower extremities (Figure 1-26). This may be a sign of right-sided heart failure, volume overload, or venous

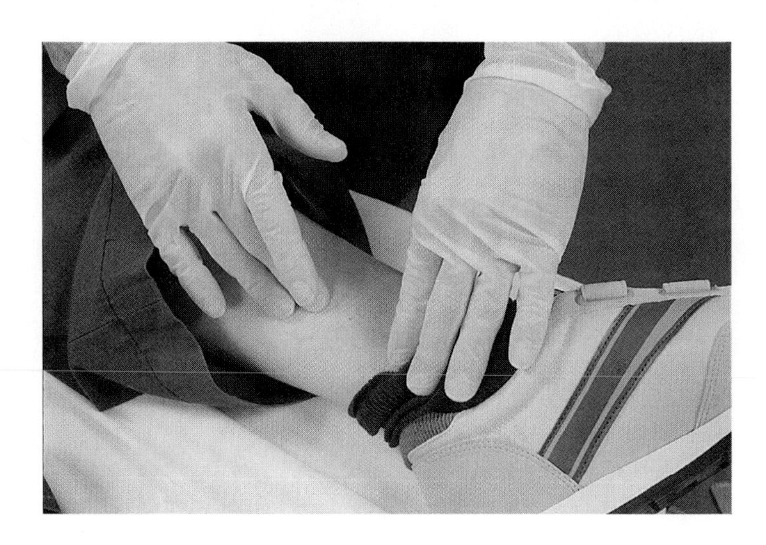

FIGURE 1-26
Assess for peripheral or dependent edema in the lower extremities.

hypertension. Compress the area over the tibia or medial malleolus for about 5 seconds to test for dependent edema. If an impression is left in the skin after you remove your finger or thumb, pitting edema is present.

Also look for a medical identification tag. These are commonly worn as bracelets, anklets, or necklaces.

Assess the Posterior Body Inspect and quickly palpate the posterior body. Look for discoloration to the flank areas, which may indicate intraabdominal hemorrhage. Palpate the small of the back for evidence of edema or fluid collection. This is termed presacral edema. Presacral edema is usually associated with conditions in which lymphatic fluid builds up, such as congestive heart failure.

Use Other Adjunctive Equipment as Needed

Other equipment can be used in conjunction with inspection, palpation, auscultation, and percussion to reveal additional information about the cause of the condition or to provide monitoring of vital functions. The following should be considered for the medical patient:

- *Continuous Cardiac Monitoring.* Application of the cardiac monitor (Figure 1-27) should be done no later than the focused history and physical exam. The electrocardiogram (ECG) may provide evidence as to the etiology of the condition. It is vital to identify life-threatening dysrhythmias and manage them, both pharmacologically and nonpharmacologically. Cardiac dysrhythmias may lead to complaints of chest pain, weakness, syncope, dyspnea, altered mental status, and other signs and symptoms of poor perfusion. Changes in the rhythm may indicate improvement or deterioration in the patient's condition. Also, a dysrhythmia may identify electrolyte disturbances. Continuous cardiac monitoring is imperative with any physiological instability or suspected cardiovascular, respiratory, or central nervous system problem. Continuous cardiac monitoring also provides a minute-to-minute read-out of heart rate. A 12-lead ECG should be performed whenever a myocardial infarction is suspected.
- *Pulse Oximetry.* A pulse oximeter (Figure 1-28) is an excellent piece of equipment to monitor oxygenation. Studies have shown that early detection of occult hypoxia is possible through pulse oximetry. A normal pulse oximeter

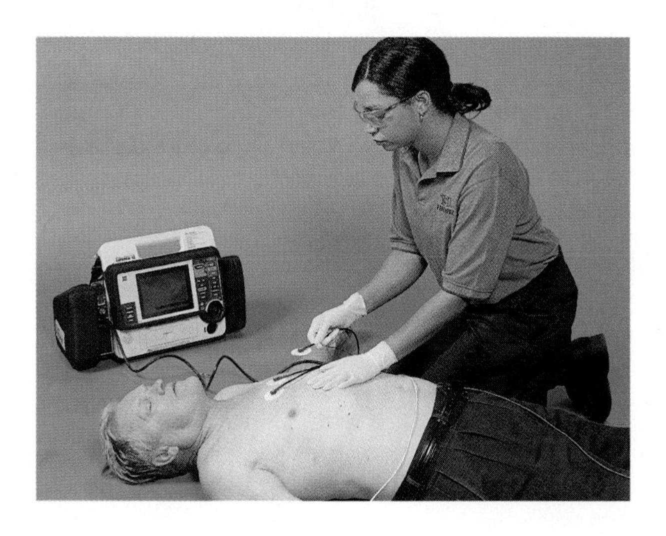

FIGURE 1-27
Apply the cardiac monitor for continuous cardiac monitoring no later than the focused history and physical exam.

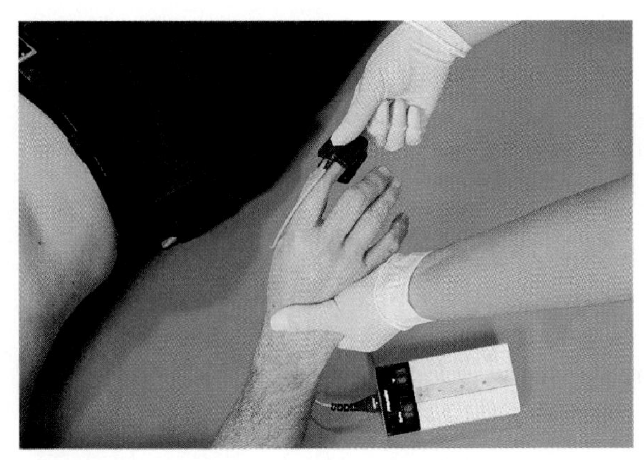

FIGURE 1-28
Use a pulse oximeter to monitor oxygenation.

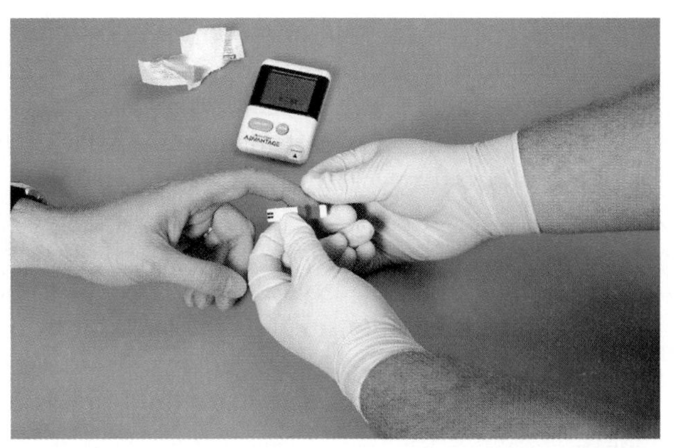

FIGURE 1-29
Use an electronic glucometer to measure blood glucose levels.

reading should be at or above 95 percent. An SpO_2 reading less than 95 percent typically warrants oxygen therapy. An SpO_2 reading of 90 percent correlates with an arterial blood gas oxygen level (PaO_2) of approximately 60 mmHg. You should consider positive-pressure ventilation and supplemental oxygen in this patient.

Be aware of the limitations of the pulse oximeter. (See Chapter 5, Dyspnea, Respiratory Distress, or Respiratory Failure.) Poor perfusion and hypothermia are two conditions that will produce erroneous readings. Also, fingernail polish, dried blood, and peripheral vascular disease will interfere with accurate readings. Be sure to look at the patient as a whole in response to the SpO_2 reading. It is only one piece of the puzzle in determining the patient's condition and directing emergency care. Remember to treat the patient and not the pulse oximeter reading

- ***Blood Glucose Level.*** If hypoglycemia is suspected, the patient presents with an altered mental status, or the cause of unresponsiveness is unknown, it is important to establish a baseline blood glucose level. This is achieved with an electronic glucometer (Figure 1-29). When assessing the glucose level using a capillary whole-blood glucometer, be sure to use a sample from a capillary stick obtained with a lancet. Do not use venous whole blood from an IV start or blood draw as the sample. A 15 percent difference in blood glucose values exists between venous and capillary blood, with the capillary sample providing a higher reading. Using a venous sample may provide an erroneously low blood glucose level.

If the blood glucose level is less than 60 mg/dl with symptoms, or less than 50 mg/dl with or without symptoms, treat for possible hypoglycemia. The glucometer is also useful in measuring excessively high blood glucose

Baseline Vital Signs
Respirations
Pulse
Skin
Blood pressure
Pupils

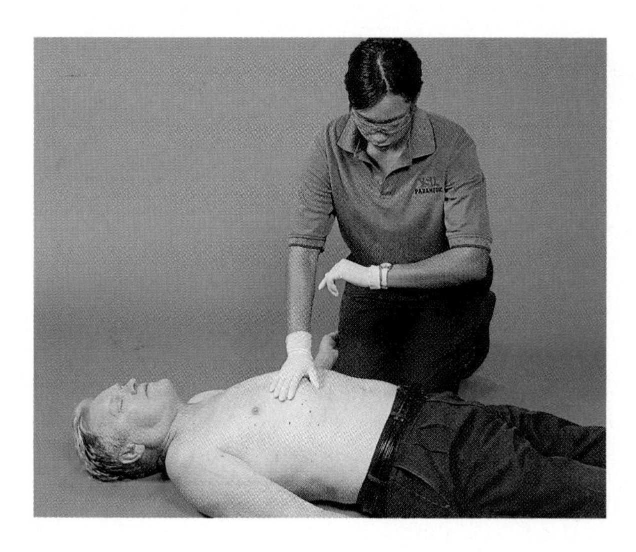

FIGURE 1-30
Assess the quality and rate of respiration.

levels that are found in diabetic ketoacidosis and hyperglycemic hyperosmolar nonketotic syndrome, which are also associated with altered mental status.

Assess Baseline Vital Signs

The basic vital signs that need to be assessed following the rapid medical assessment or the focused exam are

- Respirations
- Pulse
- Skin
- Blood pressure
- Pupils

If the patient is stable, assess the baseline vital signs every 15 minutes. In the unstable patient, the vital signs should be assessed every 5 minutes.

Respirations Assess the quality and rate of respirations (Figure 1-30). The quality is associated more with adequacy of tidal volume and workload of breathing. Look for evidence of labored breathing such as retractions, nasal flaring, or accessory muscle use. Inspect the chest for adequate rise and fall.

The respiration rate is typically between 8 and 24 per minute in the adult patient. Elderly patients typically have elevated respiratory rates and decreased tidal volumes. Thus, an increased resting respiratory rate in an elderly patient may not be a concern. However, it is important to closely monitor the tidal volume because a decrease may lead to poorer alveolar ventilation and a faster onset of hypoxia.

Elderly patients typically have elevated respiratory rates and decreased tidal volumes.

Tachypnea usually indicates hypoxia, acidosis, or other causes of ventilatory compromise, such as pulmonary edema, pneumonia, and pulmonary emboli, or other conditions or drugs that excite the respiratory center. Bradypnea may be an ominous sign of respiratory failure or the result of drug overdose, poisoning, or brain injury from stroke or other conditions that depress the respiratory center. Pay particular attention to abnormal respiratory patterns discussed earlier: Cheyne-Stokes, Biot's, central neurogenic hyperventilation, and Kussmaul's.

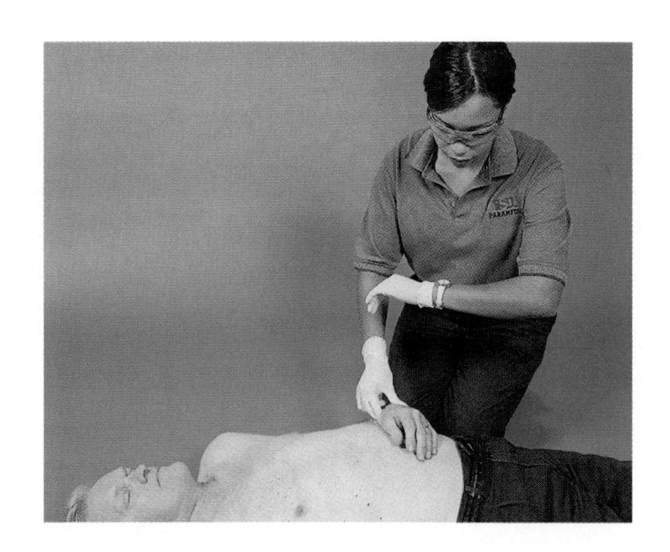

FIGURE 1-31
Assess the rate and quality of the pulse.

These may indicate various levels of brain injury or other medical conditions. (Abnormal respiratory patterns are discussed in more detail in Chapters 5 and 7.)

Pulse Determine the rate and quality of the pulse (Figure 1-31). The heart rate may be influenced by a wide range of factors, including cardiac disease, medications, drug overdose, poisoning, nervousness or anxiety, hypoxia, brain injury, and metabolic disturbances. Both tachycardia and bradycardia must be evaluated in relationship to other clinical signs and symptoms. One critical point is to determine if the heart rate is the etiology of a poor perfusion status. If so, you must focus a portion of your emergency management on stabilizing the rate in order to increase cardiac output and perfusion.

Clinical Insight

The heart rate typically increases by about 10 beats per minute for each increase of 0.6°C or 1°F in body core temperature.

The heart rate also reflects the health status of the individual. An extremely healthy individual may have a resting heart rate of 40 beats per minute. A heart rate of 90 beats per minute in this particular patient is significant. However, you may also find a 48-year-old who is not physically fit who has a resting heart rate of 86. A heart rate of 90 beats per minute in this patient does not represent a significant finding. Also, keep in mind that elderly persons have higher resting heart rates; a resting heart rate of 90 beats per minute in an elderly patient is normal.

Clinical Insight

A patient who suddenly stops taking beta-blockers may suffer an acute hypertensive emergency.

Be aware of the effects of certain medications on heart rate. If a patient is taking a beta-blocker, you would not expect tachycardia or high normal heart rates. Therefore, if you encounter a patient on a beta-blocker who is hypovolemic from a gastrointestinal bleed, a heart rate of 98 beats per minute would be a significant indicator of shock. Likewise, you would expect the patient on a beta-blocker to have lower resting heart rates. Also, a lower heart rate may increase your suspicion of the possibility of a digitalis drug overdose.

Clinical Insight

A pulse that has a regular rate and rhythm but alternates between strong and weak volume is typical of congestive heart failure. It is termed *pulsus alternans*.

The presence of the pulse in certain locations is also important in assessing perfusion. Central sites, such as the carotid and femoral, require less arterial pressure to generate a pulse. Peripheral sites, such as the radial and brachial, need higher arterial pressures to produce pulses. Therefore, loss of peripheral pulses is a potential indicator of a reduced cardiac output, decreased arterial pressure, and poor perfusion status.

The quality of the pulse may also provide information about the perfusion status. A weak pulse, whether it is peripheral or central, may indicate poor cardiac output and perfusion. Remember, it is important to view this as only one sign in your evaluation of the whole patient. A patient may be suffering

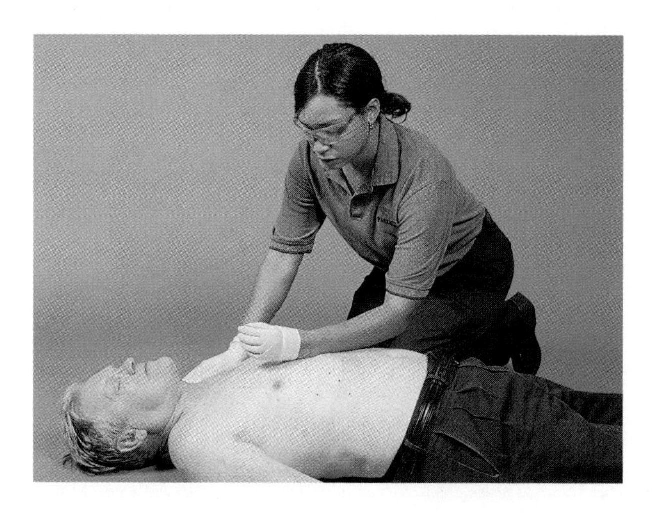

FIGURE 1-32
Assess relative skin temperature.

from an arterial embolus or some other vascular disease in the specific extremity in which the distal pulses are weak. Assess more than one pulse location. A strong and bounding pulse usually indicates adequate cardiac output and good perfusion.

When assessing the pulse, feel for a difference in amplitude during the inspiratory phase of respiration, especially in patients with respiratory complaints. If the pulse becomes weak or absent during inspiration, it may be an indication of an increased intrathoracic pressure, cardiac tamponade, adhesive pericarditis, advanced congestive heart failure, hypovolemia, or other conditions. This reduction or obliteration in the pulse is referred to as pulsus paradoxus. Pulsus paradoxus is a very subtle finding and hard to detect in the field.

Clinical Insight

Pulsus paradoxus is seen almost uniformly in patients with acute pericardial tamponade. Status asthmaticus and obstructive lung diseases also produce pulsus paradoxus.

Skin Assess the skin color, temperature (Figure 1-32), and condition. Abnormal skin colors include cyanosis, redness or flushing, pallor, mottling, or jaundice. It is possible to see a combination of skin colors in one patient. The patient with hypovolemic shock may present with pallor and cyanosis, whereas the patient with anaphylactic shock may exhibit flushing and cyanosis.

Abnormal skin temperatures may be hot, cool, or cold. Be sure you take into consideration the effect of the ambient temperature on the skin temperature. If it is extremely cold outside and you find the patient outdoors, you would expect the forehead to feel cold. The abdomen is the best area of the body to assess skin temperature because it is generally covered and less affected by environmental factors.

The condition of the skin refers to the level of moisture or dryness. The skin is normally dry to touch. However, a patient suffering from severe dehydration may present with extremely dry skin that tents when pinched. Turgor refers to the normal elastic recoil that occurs when the skin is pinched.The best place to assess for turgor of the skin is on the chest over the sternum. If you suspect dehydration, inspect the mucous membranes of the oral cavity for dryness and the eyes for lack of tear formation.

Clinical Insight

The skin is less elastic in older patients due to a change in the elastin in their skin. Thus, checking for skin turgor by examining for "tenting" has little value in older adults. It is an appropriate test in children.

Capillary refill also provides some indication of peripheral perfusion. However, as mentioned earlier, capillary refill can be greatly influenced by the environment, smoking, and disease states, medical conditions, or age or gender of the patient. Thus, a capillary refill of greater than 2 to 4 seconds, which may be considered to be abnormal, may not be a completely reliable indicator of poor perfusion. Consider capillary refill as one element in conjunction with other signs.

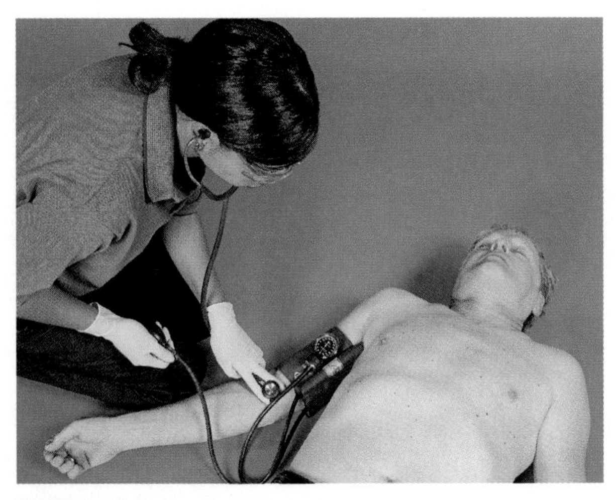

FIGURE 1-33
Assess the blood pressure by auscultation.

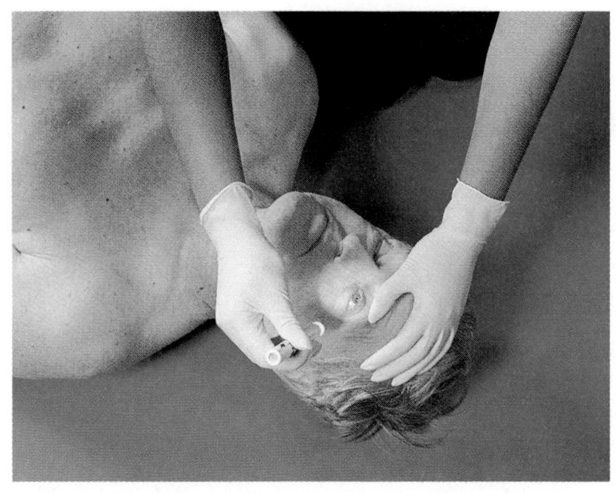

FIGURE 1-34
Assess the pupils for equality, size, and reactivity.

Blood Pressure Assess the blood pressure by auscultation (Figure 1-33) to obtain both a systolic and a diastolic reading. The normal ranges are systolic 100 to 140 mmHg and diastolic 60 to 90 mmHg. A diastolic blood pressure reading above 140 mmHg is usually considered a hypertensive emergency.

The difference between systolic and diastolic is the pulse pressure. A pulse pressure less than 25 percent of the systolic is considered to be narrow; one greater than 50 percent of the systolic is considered to be wide. A narrow pulse pressure is typically seen with vasoconstriction, increased peripheral vascular resistance, and potentially decreased cardiac output, as in hemorrhagic shock. A wide pulse pressure may be seen in brain herniation when Cushing's reflex increases the systolic but not the diastolic pressure.

Clinical Insight

Hypotension that occurs while standing is hard to interpret because approximately 10% of persons younger than 65 years and 11% to 30% of those older than 65 who are normovolemic will have a decrease in the systolic blood pressure of 20 mmHg or greater when standing.

When fluid or blood loss is suspected, test for orthostatic hypotension (also called postural hypotension). Place the patient supine for 2 minutes and assess his blood pressure and pulse. Then move him to a standing position for 1 to 2 minutes, and reassess the blood pressure and pulse. This allows about 7 to 8 ml/kg of blood to transfer to the lower extremities, decreasing preload, stroke volume, and cardiac output. A heart rate increase of more than 20 to 30 beats per minute is considered positive for orthostatic hypotension. The heart rate has been found to be the most sensitive indicator of volume depletion. A decrease in the systolic blood pressure of more than 200 mmHg is also significant. Orthostatic hypotension usually indicates significant intravascular blood or fluid loss, although many other conditions, including central nervous system disease and medications, have been implicated. Always support the patient during the test because an orthostatic drop in blood pressure may cause syncope.

Additional notes regarding blood pressure assessment: When assessing the blood pressure, look for pulsus paradoxus (the reduction or vanishing of the pulse or a drop in systolic pressure by greater than 10 mmHg when the patient inhales with no further drop after inhalation). A difference in the systolic blood pressure of 10–20 mmHg from one arm to the other may be an indication of an aortic dissection. A patient in shock may have extensive peripheral arterial vasoconstriction that impairs the Korotkoff sounds normally heard with auscultation, causing ineffective measurement and underestimation of systolic and diastolic pressures.

Pupils Assess the pupils for equality, size, and reactivity (Figure 1-34). When assessing pupils, in the absence of any suspected cervical spine injury, you may perform the oculocephalic test (Doll's eyes) in the comatose patient. Rotate the head quickly from one side to the other, watching the eyes. In a patient with an intact brainstem, the eyes will move conjugately in a direction opposite of the head turning and maintain focus on a distant point. If the eyes move in the direction of the head turning, it indicates brainstem dysfunction.

Also, assess for conjugate gaze, in which both eyes are positioned alike, to one side. It may indicate a pontine lesion on the same side as the gaze or frontal hemispheric infarction on the opposite side of the direction of the gaze. A dysconjugate gaze, where the eyes are deviated, focusing in different directions, usually indicates a brainstem lesion.

A dysconjugate gaze, where the eyes are deviated, focusing in different directions, usually indicates a brainstem lesion.

The pupils have a consensual reflex, meaning that if a light is shined into the right eye, the left pupil will react and constrict. If one pupil is dilated and fixed with no consensual reflex, it is most likely a result of herniation of the brain, a supratentorial lesion, or an aneurysm. If both pupils are midposition and fixed, suspect a midbrain lesion or brain herniation.

Check the extraocular eye muscles by having the patient follow your finger in different directions. Look for jerky movement or one eye that lags behind the other. If the patient is awake, ask about double vision.

Clinical Insight

Methanol, quinine, ergot preparations, and salicylates are four substances that may cause sudden painless loss of vision.

Obtain a History

In the unresponsive patient, the history should be obtained after the physical exam and vital signs have been assessed. Refer to the section "Assess Patient Complaints and Medical History" earlier in this chapter, which describes the history that should be gathered for the altered mental status or responsive patient. For the unresponsive patient, gather as much of this information as possible from family members or other bystanders.

Perform Interventions

The key with providing emergency care is to manage the immediate life threats as quickly as possible during the initial assessment and focused history and physical exam without forming a conclusive field diagnosis of the problem. If the patient is in respiratory distress, it is more important initially to determine the severity and begin managing the condition by oxygen therapy or positive-pressure ventilation than to determine the exact underlying condition. If the patient is in respiratory failure, he needs to be ventilated immediately, regardless of whether the condition is due to asthma, emphysema, or pulmonary edema.

Nevertheless, during the assessment, you must begin to formulate a field diagnosis because the asthma patient and the pulmonary edema patient are treated differently and can benefit significantly from specific pharmacologic therapy. Once life threats are under control, the management is truly patient and condition related. Some conditions require much more immediate pharmacologic intervention in order to reduce or abolish immediate life threats to the airway and breathing such as anaphylaxis or status asthmaticus.

By the conclusion of the focused history and physical exam, you should have managed all immediately life-threatening conditions. During the initial assessment, you would have established a patent airway and provided positive-pressure ventilation or supplemental oxygen. In addition, you should have recognized signs and symptoms of a physiologically unstable condition and begun to develop an emergency care plan. Typical interventions that may be performed during the initial assessment and the focused history and physical exam would include airway management, tracheal intubation, oxygen therapy, positive-pressure ventilation, intravenous therapy, and administration of medications to reverse immediately life-threatening conditions.

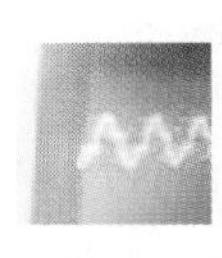

POSSIBILITIES TO PROBABILITIES: FORMING A DIFFERENTIAL FIELD DIAGNOSIS

Forming a differential field diagnosis requires close attention to all aspects of the patient assessment and the processing of complaints, signs, symptoms, and other diagnostic information. As the practitioner, you must stay focused and consider all information being fed to you through the assessment process, especially the subtle signs and symptoms. Through a critical thinking process, you must then associate the information and develop a mental list of possible conditions the patient may be suffering from. This list is completely dynamic and changes in every step in the assessment.

You start out in the process with a very broad list of possible conditions, or "possibilities" that the patient may be suffering from, based on the initial information typically provided to you by the dispatcher. As you gain more information from the initial scene characteristics and the patient's chief complaint, you revise your mental list by using a "rule-out" and "rule-in" system.

It must be understood that, during this time, you are providing patient care and continuing the assessment without any interruption. Also, what was "ruled in" as a possibility may be "ruled out" as quickly in the next step or phase of assessment. Thus, this becomes a mental process that is highly integrated with the information you are continuously collecting from the patient history and the physical examination. As you continue with the assessment and treatment, you are revising your mental "possibilities" list.

As you continue with the assessment and treatment, you are revising your mental "possibilities" list.

What you are working toward is ideally narrowing down your "possibilities" to one, two, or three "probabilities," that is, what the patient is likely suffering from. This is your differential field diagnosis. You then typically provide additional emergency care based on that probability or field diagnosis. Until you are at the probability phase, your emergency management of the patient is likely to be general and not as involved. When moving through the assessment process, your approach should always proceed from the most critical diagnoses to the less critical conditions.

When responding to an emergency scene, the EMS professional must process the information provided by the dispatcher, such as a report of a "56-year-old male complaining of chest pain." No matter how much or little information is provided, you take that information, process it, and begin to attempt to categorize the patient as a medical or trauma patient. However, as evident as it may seem, do not develop tunnel vision and miss critical and often subtle indicators of a condition simply because you were focused in one direction.

As an example, you may be called to a scene for a "fall with a possible hip fracture." As you enter the residence, you note the patient lying supine on the living room floor with internal rotation of the left lower extremity, obvious ecchymosis to the left hip, and complaints of pain to the left lateral thigh and left knee. Based on the dispatch information, patient complaint, and scene characteristics, you would categorize the patient as a trauma patient with a possible hip fracture or dislocation. (As a note of interest, the knee and hip are innervated by the obturator nerve. Therefore, any patient who has fallen and is complaining of pain only to the knee, typically at the distal anterior thigh and medial aspect of the knee, and does not complain of hip pain, should be thoroughly assessed for a possible hip dislocation or fracture. The knee pain may be the only indicator of the fracture or dislocation to the hip.)

It would be easy at this point to focus on the possible fracture or dislocation and provide emergency care only for that injury. You may arrive at the emergency department with a nicely and neatly immobilized hip but with a patient who is in critical condition from another cause that you missed due to your failure to consider all "possibilities" and perform a thorough assessment. The key question to ask this patient is "How did you fall?" It is vital to distinguish whether the patient "tripped and fell," "got dizzy," or "passed out" and fell. If the latter is true, the patient could be suffering from a much more serious problem than a hip injury.

The patient may be experiencing episodes of a potentially lethal dysrhythmia such as ventricular tachycardia, have suffered a stroke, have an electrolyte imbalance, or be hypoxic from a pulmonary embolism. There are myriad conditions or "possibilities" that could have caused the patient's dizziness or caused him to suffer a syncopal episode. You must consider all possibilities and conduct your investigation through your assessment, looking for evidence to support or invalidate the possibilities. If a possibility is becoming more evident, search harder both to support your finding and to identify other possibilities.

The first step in this critical thinking process is to take the dispatch information and develop a broad list of possibilities. This prevents you from developing tunnel vision and sets the pace of your assessment. Next, you collect the information from the scene size-up, begin to develop a mental picture of the potential mechanism of injury, and "rule in" or "rule out" possibilities. For example, if you are called to the scene for a patient complaining of a "very tender left calf," you may include in your possibilities an arterial embolism, deep venous thrombosis, tibia or fibula fracture, muscle injury, or tendon rupture as just a few of the possibilities on your mental list.

The first step in the critical thinking process is to take the dispatch information and develop a broad list of possibilities.

When arriving at the scene, you find a patient lying in a hospital bed. The family states the patient is nonambulatory and confined to the bed. The family denies any falls or stress placed on the patient's lower extremities and indicates that she has been bedridden for the last several months. Based on this information, you are beginning to "rule out" traumatic injury from your list of possibilities; however, it will not be completely "ruled out" until the physical examination confirms no evidence of trauma or objective signs of injury. Then, the fracture and muscle and tendon injury possibilities will be effectively "ruled out."

In contrast, in a patient with a tender calf after a long period of immobility, the possibility of a deep vein thrombosis is "ruled in" and becomes a much stronger possibility. During the physical examination of the extremity, if the calf is found to be warmer and slightly larger than the opposite calf and tender to touch, a deep vein thrombosis moves from a "possibility" to a "probability."

In summary, differential field diagnosis is a dynamic mental process that requires input and integration of information discovered from every aspect of the scene size-up, history, and physical exam. The process flows as shown in the "Differential Field Diagnosis Process" flowchart that follows. An example of how you would proceed with the "possibilities" to "probabilities" critical thinking process for the previously mentioned 56-year-old male patient complaining of chest pain is featured in the chart titled "Possibilities-to-Probabilities Critical Thinking."

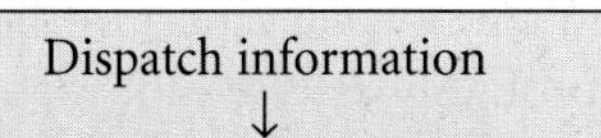

Differential Field Diagnosis Process

Dispatch information

↓

Develop mental list of possibilities proceeding from most critical to least critical

↓

Collect and process scene size-up information

↓

POSSIBILITIES

↓

Determine patient's chief complaint → Rule out (R/O) possibilities

↓

POSSIBILITIES

↓

How does the general impression correlate with conditions? → R/O possibilities
(Posture, appearance, age, gender, race)

↓

POSSIBILITIES

↓

Information obtained from the initial assessment → R/O possibilities
(Mental, airway, breathing, and circulatory status)

↓

POSSIBILITIES

↓

SAMPLE History
(OPQRST, pertinent negatives, and relevant symptoms) → R/O possibilities

↓

POSSIBILITIES

↓

Focused physical exam or rapid medical assessment findings
(Relevant signs, pertinent negatives, subtle signs, elicited responses) → R/O possibilities

↓

POSSIBILITIES

↓

Other pertinent tests and monitoring device results
(Blood glucose level, SpO_2, 12-lead ECG, I-Stat) → R/O possibilities

↓

POSSIBILITIES

↓

Response to initial treatment
(Oxygen therapy, IV fluids, positioning) → R/O possibilities

↓

PROBABILITIES
(Differential diagnosis)

↓

CONTINUED EMERGENCY CARE
(Medication administration, advanced assessment, notification)

Possibilities-to-Probabilities Critical Thinking

Example: 56-Year-Old Male Complaining of Chest Pain

An example of how you would proceed with the possibilities-to-probabilities critical thinking process.
Follow the information input, listing of possibilities, and rule-out reasoning as you work your way through the assessment.

<table>
<tr><th colspan="2">DISPATCH</th></tr>
<tr><td colspan="2">Information Input: 56-year-old male with chest pain</td></tr>
<tr><td>Possibilities: Myocardial infarction
Unstable angina
Aortic dissection
Pulmonary embolism
Pneumothorax
Tension pneumothorax
Acute pericarditis
Esophageal rupture
Stable angina
Pneumonia
Esophageal reflux
Esophageal spasm
Musculoskeletal injury
Peptic ulcer disease
Cholecystitis
Herpes zoster
Anxiety or panic disorder
Hyperventilation
Sickle cell disease
Cocaine use
Rib fracture</td><td>Rule-Out Reasoning: Not enough information yet to rule out any of the possibilities</td></tr>
<tr><th colspan="2">SCENE SIZE-UP</th></tr>
<tr><td colspan="2">Information Input: Find patient in residence lying in semi-Fowler's position on living room couch. No evidence of trauma to patient, no oxygen equipment, bottles, drug paraphernalia. Patient covered with blanket.</td></tr>
<tr><td>Possibilities: No additional possibilities</td><td>Rule-Out Reasoning: Not enough information</td></tr>
</table>

INITIAL ASSESSMENT

Information Input: General impression: white male patient in his mid-50s lying with head propped up on pillows, dressed in pajamas at 2:00 P.M., looks ill, note accessory neck muscle use and rapid respiratory rate

Patient is alert and responding, talking in short sentences with gasps for breath in between, RR approximately 22/minute and a decreased tidal volume, radial pulse strong with an approximate HR of 110/minute, skin very warm and slightly moist to touch, capillary refill less than 2 seconds

Treatment: Support patient's semi-Fowler's position, apply a nonrebreather at 15 lpm. Apply pulse oximeter and ECG monitor. Start an intravenous line of normal saline at TKO rate.

Possibilities:	**Rule-Out Reasoning:**
Sickle cell crisis	Sickle cell disease usually affects African Americans; patient is a white male.
Hyperventilation	Patient's respirations are only 22/minute with a less-than-normal tidal volume.

HISTORY

Information Input: Chief complaint: chest pain

- O gradual onset over last 3 days
- P made worse by cough and deep breaths; no relief with positioning
- Q sharp stabbing pain
- R none, pain located over left lateral chest and costal chondral margin
- S 5 on a 1-to-10 scale
- T short duration after cough or when breathing deep, intermittent

Associated complaints:

Dyspnea:	Began more than week ago and progressively got worse; worse when lying flat
Cough:	Thick sputum, green-yellow in color
Weak and dizzy:	Worsens with standing
Fever:	Hot alternating with chills
Cold:	Patient complains of a head cold that has persisted for last 2 weeks
Allergies:	None known
Medications:	Lipitor; aspirin 325 mg
Past medical history:	Hyperlipidemia
Last oral intake:	45 minutes prior to EMS arrival, cup of soup
Events:	Lying in bed, pain occurs with cough and deep breathing over past few days; denies any injury
ECG monitor:	Sinus tachycardia; Rate: 114/minute; 12-lead ECG normal
SpO_2	89 percent on room air; 93 percent on NRB 15 lpm

Possibilities:	**Rule-Out Reasoning:**
Esophageal rupture	Pain of esophageal rupture is acute, severe, pleuritic, usually preceded by vomiting, abdominal or back pain typical, and dysphagia. This patient's onset of pain was gradual and no other signs/symptoms typical of esophageal rupture.
Esophageal reflux	Pain of esophageal reflux is typically substernal, and burning in nature, dysphagia, radiation interscapular, occurs after large meal, no relation to exertion, comes when lying down. This patient's pain located over left lateral chest and no other signs/symptoms typical of esophageal reflux.
Anxiety or panic disorder	This patient not emotionally upset; appears ill, not apprehensive. Does not have typical findings associated with anxiety/panic such as sighing respirations, chest wall tenderness on palpation, pain usually located over precordium, or history of panic disorder.
Aortic dissection	Pain of aortic dissection is typically sudden onset, constant, and interscapular, amplitude difference of pulses, BP variance. This patient's pain was gradual in onset, intermittent, not interscapular, and has no other findings associated with aortic dissection.
Pulmonary embolism	With pulmonary embolism, dyspnea and pain are sudden onset, chest pain is constant, dyspnea greater complaint than pain. Although this patient does have dyspnea, the onset was gradual and the pain intermittent.
Peptic ulcer	Peptic ulcer pain is aching and burning, epigastric, relieved with food or antacid. This patient's symptoms are different, not related to ingestion of food.
Cholecystitis	Pain of cholecystitis is epigastric and RUQ, referred pain to right scapula, check for RUQ pain on palpation of abdomen. This patient's pain is located over the left lateral chest and costal chondrial margin.
Musculoskeletal	Typical findings with musculoskeletal chest pain is aggravated by movement, history of injury or muscle exertion, has related tenderness on palpation of chest, increases with exertion. This patient has no history of injury, pain worsens with cough and deep breaths rather than exertion.
Rib fracture	Patient has no history of trauma; pain was gradual in onset, which is not typical of rib fracture.
Esophageal spasm	Pain of esophageal spasm is usually interscapular, and dysphagia is common. This patient's pain is left lateral and costal chondrial. No dyspnea is noted.

HISTORY *(continued)*	
Stable angina	This patient's chest pain not typical of stable angina; he has no increase with exertion or increased myocardial workload, no relief from oxygen, and duration of pain longer than the 15 minutes typical of stable angina.
Unstable angina/myocardial infarction	Again, this patient has pain atypical of unstable angina or MI and does not have these typical characteristics of unstable angina/MI: sudden onset, radiation, skin that is cool as well as diaphorectic, nausea, constant pain. This patient has a normal 12-lead ECG.
Pericarditis	Pain of pericarditis typically radiates to the back, arm, and shoulder, is constant, and is aggravated in a supine position. This patient's pain does not radiate, is intermittent, and is aggravated by cough or deep breathing rather than position.

FOCUSED PHYSICAL EXAM

Information Input:

Pupils:	Midsize, rapid response
Conjunctiva:	Slight cyanosis
Oral mucosa:	Slight cyanosis
	Dry
Neck:	No JVD in Fowler's position
	No subcutaneous emphysema
	No tracheal deviation
	No evidence of trauma
	Sternocleidomastoid muscle use on inspiration
Chest:	No signs of trauma on inspection
	No increase in anterior-posterior chest diameter
	Scalene muscle use
	Pectoralis muscle use
	No scars
	Symmetric chest rise
	No tenderness on palpation
	Breath sounds present all lobes
	Crackles (rales) in all left lung fields
	Crackles (rales) in right lower lobe
	Tactile fremitus indicates increased vibration
	Dull on percussion

FOCUSED PHYSICAL EXAM *(continued)*	
Abdomen:	Soft, nontender No scars No evidence of trauma No RUQ tenderness No pulsating masses
Extremities:	Strong pulses in all extremities Good neurologic function Good motor function No discoloration or edema Slightly diaphoretic Normal color, warm
Posterior:	No presacral edema No discoloration No tenderness on palpation
Vital Signs:	BP 114/88 mmHg HR 118/minute Sinus tachycardia R 22/minute, labored SpO_2 93 percent on NRB Temperature 101.4°F

FIELD DIAGNOSIS	
Field Diagnosis:	Pneumonia
Key Indicators:	Gradual onset, history of recent cold, sputum production, patient in pajamas at 2:00 P.M. indicates not feeling well for a period of time, labored breathing with accessory muscle use, skin is warm to touch, pain aggravated by coughing and deep breathing, sharp stabbing pain, dyspnea that was gradual in onset, green-yellow sputum, sinus tachycardia, normal 12-lead ECG, poor SpO_2 reading, crackles on auscultation, tactile fremitus indicating consolidation, fever of 101.4°F.
Management:	Place patient in position of comfort, continue oxygen therapy, run IV line at TKO, continue to monitor ECG and SpO_2.

DETAILED PHYSICAL EXAM

A detailed physical exam is a much more comprehensive examination that is typically conducted after the focused history and physical exam, and only after all life-threatening conditions have been effectively managed. The purpose is to identify all other non-life-threatening conditions or injuries and manage them. Many of the same steps that were performed in the focused exam or the rapid medical assessment are repeated in the detailed physical exam. This exam is more detailed than the focused exam or the rapid medical exam, and it allows you to truly focus on findings that will contribute to developing a differential diagnosis.

However, because most medical patients' assessments are based on the chief complaint and history and not on the presenting signs of illness, a detailed physical exam in the medical patient is of limited usefulness. In the trauma patient, where most of the information needed to form a field diagnosis and manage the patient is gathered from the physical examination, a detailed physical exam is much more important to perform. Thus, it is usually performed in the trauma patient and not in the medical patient. In any case, a detailed exam should be conducted only when available time and the patient's condition allow it.

ONGOING ASSESSMENT

The ongoing assessment is performed after the focused history and physical exam. This exam could be performed in the back of the ambulance while en route to the emergency department or while you are still at the scene. Or you may begin the ongoing assessment at the scene and continue it in the back of the ambulance.

The purposes of the ongoing assessment are to determine any changes in the patient's condition and to assess the effectiveness of your interventions. You should continually reassess all patients, regardless of the level of criticality and responsiveness. This will identify whether the management that you have provided is effective or not and will provide evidence of deterioration or improvement in the patient's overall condition.

Clinical Insight

The ongoing assessment should be performed on all patients regardless of the level of criticality and responsiveness—every 15 minutes in the stable patient, and every 5 minutes in the unstable patient.

The key to managing the medical patient is to assess, intervene, reassess, intervene, reassess, intervene, reassess, and so forth. Your interventions should be followed by a reassessment, which is the ongoing assessment. In the stable patient, it should be performed every 15 minutes, whereas in the unstable patient it should be performed every 5 minutes.

The steps in the ongoing assessment are

- Repeat the initial assessment.
- Reassess and record vital signs.
- Repeat the focused assessment for additional complaints.

Ongoing Assessment

Repeat the initial assessment.
Reassess and record vital signs.
Repeat the focused assessment for additional complaints.
Check interventions.
Note trends in the patient's condition.

- Check interventions.
- Note trends in the patient's condition.

Repeat the Initial Assessment

The first step in the ongoing assessment is to repeat the initial assessment. This is to identify any changes and new life threats to the airway, breathing, or circulation. An example would be a patient who has now developed secretions in the oral cavity. You would immediately suction the secretions to prevent aspiration. Or, during your reassessment, you may note that the patient's minute ventilation is poor and immediately elect to provide positive-pressure ventilation. The reassessment is conducted no differently than the first time the initial assessment is performed.

The steps are as follows:

- Reassess the mental status
- Reassess the airway
- Reassess circulation including pulse, bleeding, and perfusion status (skin color, temperature, and condition and capillary refill)
- Reestablish patient priorities

Reassess and Record Vital Signs

During the ongoing assessment, reassess the respiratory rate and quality, breath sounds, pulse rate and quality, skin, pupils, and blood pressure. Also, record the rhythm on the ECG monitor, the pulse oximeter reading, the blood glucose level, the end-tidal CO_2 reading, or other assessment tool findings. Record each of the vital signs and readings, as well as the time that they were taken.

Repeat the Focused Assessment for Other Complaints

If the patient begins to complain of another symptom or a change in the original symptom, repeat the history, using OPQRST questions related to the particular complaint. Conduct a focused exam on that particular area or related body system. For example, if the patient now begins to complain of breathing difficulty, go back and assess the mouth, neck, chest, abdomen, and extremities, looking for additional evidence as to the severity and cause of the breathing difficulty.

Check Interventions

Determine if your emergency care is effective and has changed the patient's condition. Ensure that all the equipment is in proper working order and that the interventions are still appropriate. For example, reassess the tracheal tube placement by reassessing breath sounds, absence of sounds over the epigastrium, end-tidal CO_2 monitor reading, pulse oximeter reading, centimeter marking level of the tube at the patient's lip line, security of the tracheal tube holder, and the pilot balloon to ensure the cuff is still inflated. It is important to assess equipment that is used for airway management, ventilation, intravenous therapy, drug administration such as an intravenous infusion, infusion pumps, oximeter, capnograph, continuous ECG monitor, and other devices that are used to either continuously monitor the patient's condition or manage the patient's condition.

Note Trends in the Patient's Condition

Changes in the patient's condition will be the basis for further intervention and reassessment. Also, these changes can provide information as to whether your patient is improving or deteriorating. Any trends in the patient's condition are imperative to note and document for establishing a continuum of care.

SUMMARY

Information gathered from assessment of the patient is pivotal in providing accurate and effective emergency care. In the medical patient, information gained from the chief complaint and history are generally more useful in guiding patient care than information from the physical exam.

Your goal in the assessment is to identify and manage all immediately life-threatening conditions during the initial assessment and focused history and physical exam, regardless of the exact cause of the problem, looking for indicators of physiological instability. You should also be gathering additional information to make judgments about the etiology of the condition as a basis for more advanced emergency care. So you move from an assessment-based format focused on identification and management of immediate life threats to a more diagnostic-based approach focused on making a differential field diagnosis that may allow you to provide specific interventions for that particular condition.

Reassessment that is performed in the ongoing assessment is also vital and involves continuously monitoring for changes in the patient's condition, identifying any developing life threats, and monitoring interventions and equipment used in management of the patient. Also during reassessment, trends in the patient's condition, seen as either improvement or deterioration, are determined and recorded.

SCENARIO FOLLOW-UP

You arrive on the scene and find an 86-year-old male patient who is lying supine on the couch. His daughter states that the patient has been complaining of shortness of breath over the last few days.

Scene Size-Up

While entering the house, you scan the scene and do not notice any potential hazards. An oxygen tank is located in the corner of the room with a large roll of tubing. No other scene characteristics are pertinent.

Initial Assessment

You approach the patient and call out his name. He is not alert and does not respond with any eye opening or motor movement. In your general impression, you note severe cyanosis to his upper chest, neck, and face. He is a thin and frail elderly gentleman who has an obviously increased anterior-posterior chest diameter—the barrel chest characteristic of emphysema. He has a nasal cannula applied with 2 lpm of oxygen being administered. You instruct your partner to prepare the bag-valve mask for positive-pressure ventilation with supplemental oxygen.

Again, you yell, "Sir, can you open your eyes?" The patient does not respond, so you perform an earlobe pinch. There is no response. You insert an oropharyngeal airway and note no gag reflex. You instruct your partner to begin bag-valve-mask ventilation at a rate of 8 ventilations per minute with a tidal volume that produces visible chest rise, with each ventilation being delivered for a 1-second period. Initially, you instruct him to hyperventilate for approximately 1 minute, then decrease the rate to 14 breaths per minute. You ensure the reservoir is attached to the bag valve and the oxygen is flowing at 10 to 12 lpm.

Next you assess the patient's radial pulse, which is weak and rapid. You note that his skin has a slightly pink tone with cyanosis to the upper body and is hot and moist. Based on the initial assessment findings of cyanosis and inadequate breathing, you categorize him as being physiologically unstable and a priority patient.

Focused History and Physical Exam

Because the patient is unresponsive, you perform a rapid medical assessment. You assess the pupils, which are equal and react sluggishly to light. The conjunctiva is pale and cyanotic. You inspect the mucosa inside the mouth and find diffuse cyanosis. The patient's jugular veins are flat, and there is no evidence of subcutaneous emphysema. You quickly inspect the chest and confirm your earlier impression of a significantly increased anterior-posterior diameter. You note it as a barrel chest. You quickly ask the daughter if the patient has a history of emphysema. She responds, "Oh, my yes. He's had emphysema for over 15 years now. It's gotten much worse this past year, though." At this point, you instruct your partner to reduce the ventilatory rate to 8 ventilations per minute to reduce the incidence of auto-PEEP.

You place your hands on the patient's chest, spreading your fingers out with your thumbs on the sternum, and feel the chest rise and fall. There is minimal spontaneous movement. You note retraction of the intercostal muscles, suprasternal notch, and supraclavicular spaces. You auscultate the chest and find coarse crackles and rhonchi in both apices, bases, and lateral lobes. Percussion reveals a duller resonance than that which is associated with emphysema.

The abdomen is soft and not distended. You inspect and palpate the extremities, noting no peripheral edema. Pulses are present in all four extremities, but the patient does not respond to a pinch to any of the extremities. You log roll the patient and quickly inspect and palpate the posterior body, noting no pertinent findings.

You place the patient on the cardiac monitor and find a sinus tachycardia at a rate of 126 beats per minute. An occasional PVC is noted. The spontaneous respiratory rate is 42 and extremely shallow. His radial pulse is weak, mostly regular, and is obliterated during inspiration. The blood pressure is 102/84 mmHg. His skin is warm to hot, slightly moist, and showing slight cyanosis to the upper body. However, the cyanosis is beginning to improve with positive-pressure ventilation. You attach a pulse oximeter, which reveals an SpO_2 of 80 percent.

As you prepare the equipment to perform tracheal intubation, you begin to gather the SAMPLE history. The daughter is the primary historian. You ask about symptoms of which the patient has been complaining. She states that he was seen by a physician last week for an extremely bad chest cold. He has not been taking the medications that the physician prescribed. He developed a bad productive cough and began to complain about being much more short of breath than usual. He felt a lot weaker than usual, too. She states that, "When he lies flat or lower than normal, he gets real bad." You ask if anything makes the breathing easier, and she states, "Just bed rest and no activity."

You ask the daughter to attempt to rate the patient's description of the severity on a scale of 1 to 10, with 10 being the most severe. She guesses a 9. He is allergic to penicillin and contrast dye. He is taking Theodur, uses an inhaler, and is on 2 lpm of oxygen continuously. He has had no significant past medical history except for the diagnosis of emphysema approximately 15 years ago. His last oral intake was yesterday evening at about 10 P.M. when he had a cup of hot tea. She states, "I thought he was just sleeping on the couch until I tried to wake him. I thought it was unusual that he was lying without his pillows. He was just watching television when I last saw him."

You perform the orotracheal intubation, assess tube placement, and secure the tracheal tube. Lung compliance is fairly poor. You initiate an intravenous line of normal saline with an 18-gauge angiocath and draw blood. You quickly test the blood glucose level, because of his altered mental status, and find it normal at 92 mg/dl. You continue to monitor his cardiac rhythm, which remains a sinus tachycardia. You prepare the patient for transport and move him to the ambulance.

Ongoing Assessment

En route you reassess the airway by reassessing tracheal tube placement. No epigastric sounds are heard, and breath sounds are heard bilaterally. Diffuse crackles and rhonchi are also heard over all lung fields. The radial pulse is still present, and the skin has "pinked up" from the cyanotic tone. It remains warm and slightly moist. The blood pressure is now 108/82 mmHg. The pulse oximeter reading has increased to 90 percent. The cardiac monitor shows sinus tachycardia with fewer PVCs. You check the intravenous line to ensure it is still patent and running well. You switch the oxygen from the portable tank to the onboard oxygen outlet.

You suspect the patient is suffering from pneumonia, which is worsening his emphysema. Therefore, you do not consider drug therapy at this time. You contact medical direction and provide a report. No further orders are given. You continue to perform an ongoing assessment every 5 minutes until you arrive at the hospital emergency department.

The patient is admitted with diffuse bilateral pneumonia. He is placed on a ventilator in the medical intensive care unit.

FURTHER READING

1. Bickley, L.S., R.A. Hoekelman, and B. Bates. *Bates' Guide to Physical Examination and History Taking.* 7th ed. Philadelphia: Lippincott-Raven, 1999.
2. Bledsoe, B.E., R.S. Porter, and R.A. Cherry. *Paramedic Care: Principles and Practice—Volume 2, Patient Assessment.* Upper Saddle River, NJ: Pearson/Prentice Hall, 2006.
3. Brady, W. "Missing the diagnosis of acute MI: challenging presentations, electrocardiographic pearls, and outcome-effective management strategies," *Emergency Medicine Reports,* 1997;18(10):91-101.
4. Cummins, R.O., ECC Senior Editor. *ACLS Provider Manual.* Dallas: American Heart Association, 2001.
5. Davis, M., S. Votey, and G. Greenough. *Signs and Symptoms in Emergency Medicine.* St. Louis: Mosby, 1999.
6. Deakin, C. and L. Low. "Accuracy of the advanced life support guidelines for predicting systolic blood pressure using carotid, femoral, and radial pulses: observational study," *BMJ,* 2000;321:673-764.
7. DeLorenzo, R.A. "Demystifying the neuro exam," *JEMS,* 1997;22(9):68-88.
8. Ferri, F. *Clinical Advisor: Instant Diagnosis and Treatment.* St. Louis: Mosby, 2002.
9. Fordyce, W. *Behavioral Methods for Chronic Pain and Illness.* St. Louis: Mosby, 1976.
10. American Heart Association. *Guidelines 2000 for Cardiopulmonary Resuscitation and Emergency Cardiovascular Care. Circulation,* 2000;102(suppl)(8).
11 Hamilton, G.C., A.B. Sanders, G.R. Strange, and A.T. Trott. *Emergency Medicine: An Approach to Clinical Problem Solving.* 2nd ed. Philadelphia: W.B. Saunders, 2003.
12. Kalarickal, O. "Neurological history and physical exam," *eMedicine Journal,* 2001;2(12). http://www.emedicine.com.
13. Kidwell, C.S., J.L. Saver, G.B. Schubert, M. Eckstein, and S. Starkman. "Design and retrospective analysis of the Los Angeles Prehospital Stroke Screen (LAPSS)," *Prehospital Emergency Care,* 1998;2:267-273.
14. Kidwell, C.S., S. Starkman, M. Eckstein, K. Weems, and J.L. Saver. "Identifying stroke in the field: prospective validation of the Los Angeles Prehospital Stroke Screen (LAPSS)," *Stroke,* 2000;31:71-76.
15. Markovchick, V. and P. Pons. *Emergency Medicine Secrets.* 2nd ed. Philadelphia: Hanley & Belfus, 1999.
16. Marx, J.A., R.S. Hockberger, and R.M. Walls. *Rosen's Emergency Medicine: Concepts and Clinical Practice.* 5th ed. St. Louis: Mosby, 2002.
17. May, H.L., ed. *Emergency Medicine.* 2nd ed. Boston: Little Brown and Company, 1992.
18. McCaffery, M. and C. Pasero. *Pain: Clinical Manual.* 2nd ed. St. Louis: Mosby, 1999.
19. Mistovich, J.J., B. Hafen, and K. Karren. *Prehospital Emergency Care.* 6th ed. Upper Saddle River, NJ: Pearson/Prentice Hall, 2000.
20. Pons, P. and D. Cason, eds. *Paramedic Field Care: A Complaint-Based Approach.* St. Louis: American College of Emergency Physicians, Mosby–Year Book, 1997.
21. Porth, C.M. *Pathophysiology: Concepts of Altered Health States.* 5th ed. Philadelphia: Lippincott-Raven, 1998.
22. Rund, D., R. Barkin, P. Rosen, and G. Sternbach. *Essentials of Emergency Medicine.* 2nd ed. St. Louis: Mosby, 1997.
23. Russell, I., Z. Baig, G. Quin, G. McCarthy, and C. Deakin. "Accuracy of ATLS guidelines for predicting systolic blood pressure," *BMJ,* 2001;322:552.
24. Schneider, S. "Nonmyocardial infarction chest pain: differential diagnosis, clinical clues, and initial emergency management," *Emergency Medicine Reports,* 1995;16(25):247-254.
25. Seidel, H., J. Ball, J. Dains, and G. Benedict. *Mosby's Guide to Physical Examination.* 4th ed. St. Louis: Mosby, 1999.
26. Spurlock, P. "An emergency nurse's pain management initiative: Mercy Hospital's experience," *Journal of Emergency Nursing,* 1999;25:383-385.
27. Sucholeiki, R. "Syncope and related paroxysmal spells," *eMedicine Journal,* 2001;2(7). http://www.emedicine.com.
28. Swartz, M. *Textbook of Physical Diagnosis: History and Examination.* 4th ed. Philadelphia: W.B. Saunders, 2002.
29. Victor, K. "Properly assessing pain in the elderly," *RN,* 2001;64(5):45-49.

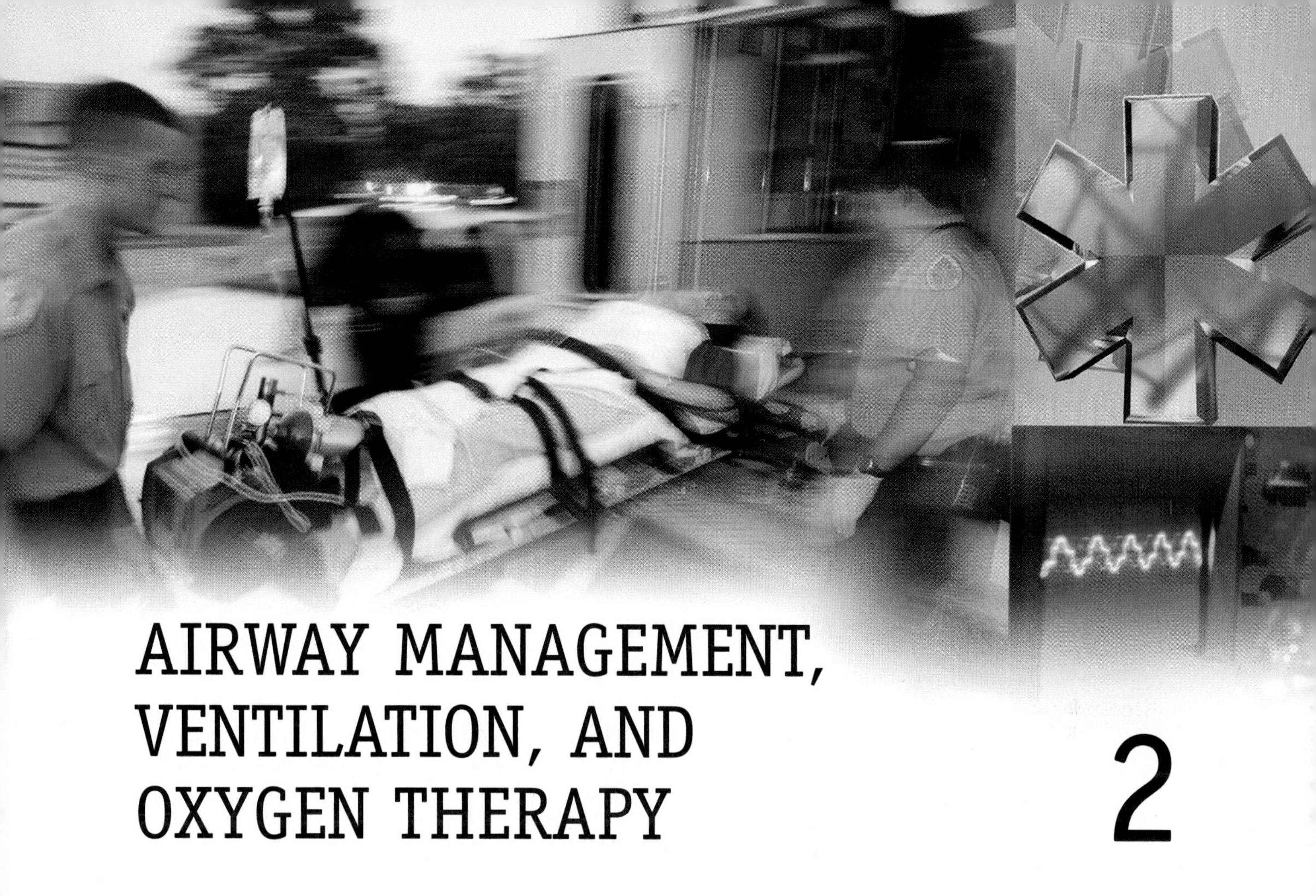

AIRWAY MANAGEMENT, VENTILATION, AND OXYGEN THERAPY

2

The airway is the portal of entry for oxygen into the human body. Establishing an airway is the first priority of resuscitation because, without an adequate airway, all other medical treatments are futile. Despite the fact that the A (airway) of the ABCs is emphasized so commonly, the airway is often overlooked in the actual treatment of patients with acute medical conditions. In this chapter, we review some principles of basic airway management and the tracheal intubation procedure. We then discuss other advanced measures of airway control, including rapid sequence intubation. The chapter also stresses appropriate methods of patient monitoring after the airway has been secured.

Topics that are covered in this chapter are

- Anatomy and Physiology
- Oxygen Supplementation
- Airway Management
- Ventilation Equipment and Techniques
- Tracheal Intubation
- Alternative Methods of Intubation
- Alternative Airway Devices
- Surgical Techniques of Airway Control
- Rapid Sequence Intubation
- Guidelines for Airway and Ventilation Support

SCENARIO

You are dispatched on an emergency call for an "unconscious unknown." As you reach the dispatched location, you are met by a man who frantically explains that he found his wife unconscious beside an open bottle of sleeping pills and a fifth of Scotch. You quickly survey the area for any obvious hazards and move in to evaluate the patient.

You find a middle-age female breathing eight times per minute with shallow, snoring respirations and a pool of fresh vomit beside her.

How would you proceed with the immediate resuscitation of this patient?

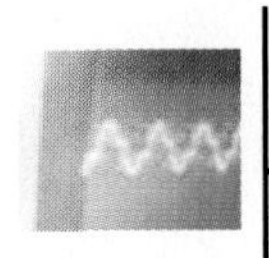

ANATOMY AND PHYSIOLOGY

Upper Airway Anatomy

The upper airway begins at the openings of the nose and mouth and ends in the trachea at the bottom of the larynx.

Air enters the body through the nose and mouth. Here, the air is warmed, humidified, and filtered before passing into a larger cavity called the pharynx. The posterior portion of the nose is the nasopharynx, and the large cavity in the back of the mouth is the oropharynx. The pharynx represents the common beginning for both the respiratory and digestive systems. Distally, the pharynx divides into two channels: The esophagus leads to the digestive tract; the trachea leads to the lungs. With vomiting, gastric contents enter the pharynx, where they may gain access to the tracheobronchial tree if airway protective mechanisms fail.

The muscular tongue is the largest structure to occupy the oral cavity. As a result of its size, the tongue is the most common source of airway obstruction, particularly in patients with an altered level of consciousness. The tongue has significant muscular attachment to the mandible, or jaw bone, which explains why anterior movement of the mandible (as in a chin lift) moves the tongue forward and relieves airway obstruction.

A large cartilaginous structure, the epiglottis, protects the trachea from blood, secretions, vomitus, and material intended for the digestive system (Figure 2-1). Most tracheal intubation techniques require manipulation of the epiglottis. In front of the epiglottis is a recess that forms at the base of the tongue called the vallecula. Ligaments attach the base of the tongue to the epiglottis so that pulling the deep portions of the tongue forward, as with a curved laryngoscope blade, also elevates the epiglottis. The aryepiglottic folds, along with the epiglottis, define the glottic opening. The upper portion of the epiglottis is innervated by the ninth cranial nerve (glossopharyngeal nerve), whereas the lower portions of the epiglottis and vocal cords are innervated by the tenth cranial nerve (vagus nerve). Stimulation of the lower portions of the epiglottis may produce *laryngospasm.* Injury to the branches of the vagus nerve (superior laryngeal nerve and recurrent laryngeal nerve) may result in permanent hoarseness.

laryngospasm forceful contraction of the laryngeal muscles.

Beneath the epiglottis is the larynx, the upper portion of the trachea, which contains the vocal cords. This structure is located in front of the fourth and fifth cervical vertebrae anatomically. The false vocal cords lie above the true vocal cords. The larynx is defined externally by the thyroid cartilage, or Adam's apple. Just below this area is the cricoid cartilage or cricoid ring. This is the only completely circular support in the tracheobronchial tree. Direct pressure on the anterior

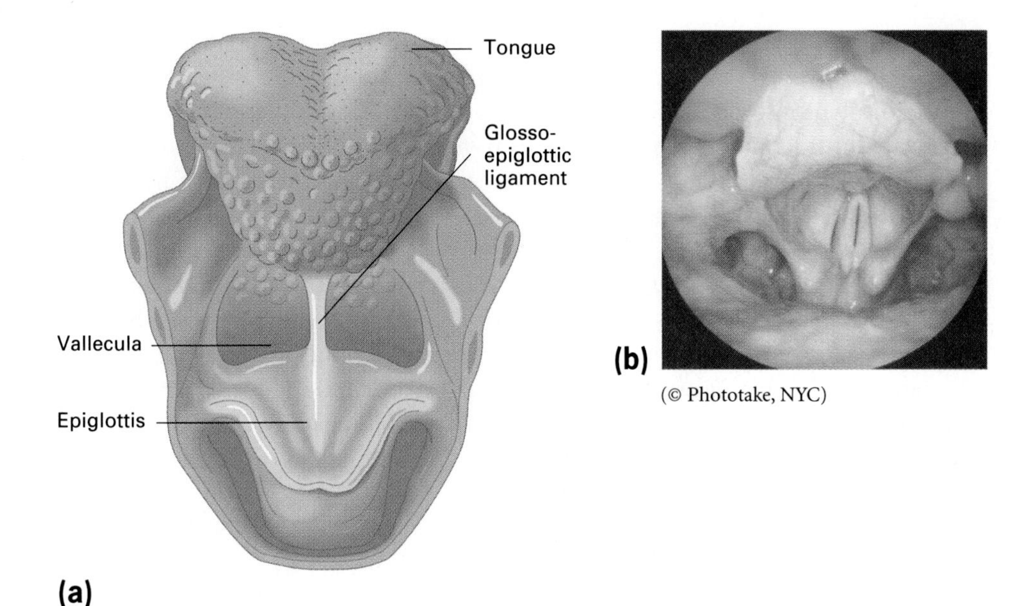

(© Phototake, NYC)

FIGURE 2-1
(a) The epiglottis. (b) Laryngoscopic view of the glottis, closed during the act of swallowing.

surface occludes the esophagus, which lies posteriorly, and prevents aspiration. There is a small diamond-shaped membrane between the thyroid cartilage and cricoid ring called the cricothyroid membrane. This is an important landmark for establishing a surgical airway. As the larynx projects into the pharynx, it defines deep posterior recesses called the pyriform fossa. This is a site where a tracheal tube tip may commonly become lodged, particularly during blind insertion procedures.

An obstruction of the airway is often characterized by its location. Supraglottic obstruction occurs above the larynx, whereas subglottic obstruction occurs at the level of the larynx or below.

Below the cricoid ring, the trachea is characterized by a series of cartilaginous rings that support this portion of the airway. Each of these tracheal rings is C-shaped. The trachealis muscle completes the circular support of each ring. The trachea proceeds distally until it divides at the carina into the right and left mainstem bronchi.

Upper Airway Physiology

A major function of the larynx is protection of the upper airway, which is in continuity with the alimentary system. During swallowing or coughing, contraction of the laryngeal muscles leads to tight closure of the glottic opening and downward movement of the epiglottis. These movements serve to protect the tracheobronchial tree. Laryngospasm is an exaggerated form of this protective mechanism.

In defining whether a patient is in need of airway protection, it is difficult clinically to determine whether these mechanisms remain intact. The testing of a gag reflex is not a reliable indicator of these airway protection mechanisms. Therefore, it should be assumed that any patient who is unable to maintain a patent airway without assistance requires aggressive airway management.

Testing the gag reflex is not a reliable indicator of airway protection. Assume that any patient who is unable to maintain a patent airway without assistance requires aggressive airway management.

Manipulation of the upper airway produces characteristic physiological responses. For example, manipulation of the upper airway as occurs during intubation typically results in the release of systemic catecholamines (epinephrine and norepinephrine). Clinically, this results in an elevation in blood pressure and heart rate during the intubation process. Generally, this is well tolerated unless the patient has an elevated intracranial pressure (e.g., from intracerebral hemorrhage) or underlying cardiac disorder (e.g., cardiogenic shock). Opioid drugs such as morphine sulfate and beta-blocking agents have been used successfully to protect against these effects.

A separate reflex independently produces a rise in intracranial pressure during intubation attempts. This can be particularly harmful if not addressed because brain blood flow is determined by the difference between mean arterial blood pressure and intracranial pressure. If the mean arterial blood pressure remains unchanged, then the intubation attempt can produce a significant reduction in brain blood flow during the procedure. Lidocaine, administered intravenously or by local spray, can blunt this airway response.

Lower Airway Anatomy

The lower airway begins at the point where the larynx branches into right and left mainstem bronchi. This point is known as the carina. The right mainstem bronchus branches off at a lesser angle than the left mainstem bronchus. For this reason, aspirated foreign matter is more likely to enter the right lung. For the same reason, a tracheal tube, if advanced too far, will usually come to rest in the right mainstem bronchus rather than the left.

The bronchi subdivide into smaller and smaller bronchioles that terminate at the sac-like alveoli. The exchange of oxygen and carbon dioxide takes place between the alveoli and the pulmonary capillaries (Figure 2-2).

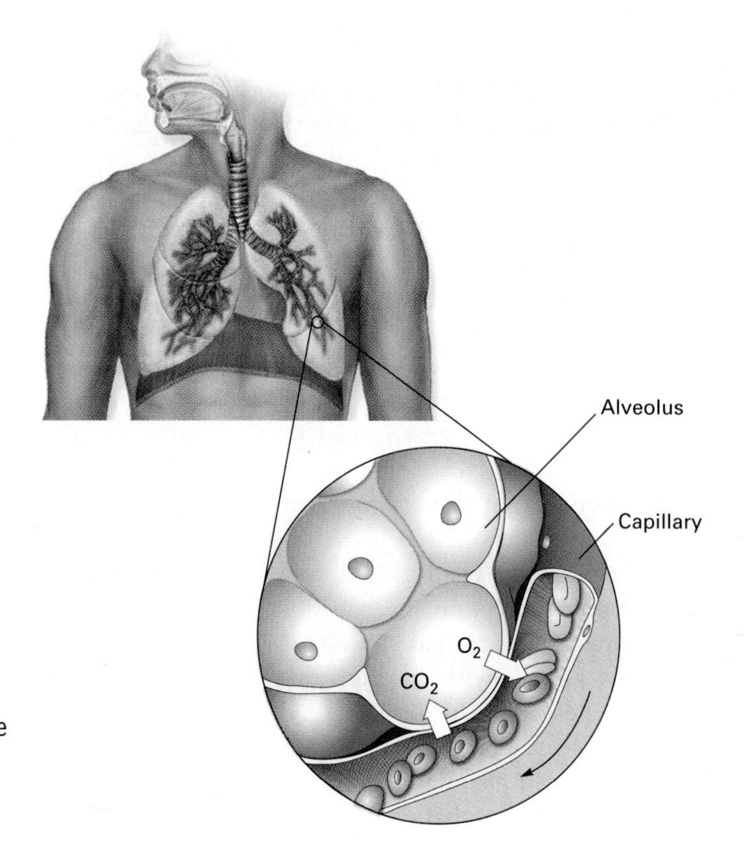

FIGURE 2-2
The exchange of oxygen and carbon dioxide occurs between the alveoli and the pulmonary capillaries across the alveolar/capillary membrane.

Respiratory Physiology

The major functions of respiration are to provide oxygen for cellular metabolism and to eliminate carbon dioxide produced by metabolic processes of the body. In addition, because of the relationship of carbon dioxide to acid–base balance, the lungs provide the most rapid physiological response to pH changes in the body.

Oxygen is derived from our external environment and is drawn into the lungs during the inspiratory phase of respiration (Figure 2-3a). During this phase, the chest wall expands as the intercostal and neck muscles contract and the diaphragm flattens. This creates negative pressure (a vacuum) within the lungs, drawing oxygen and other gases from the environment through the trachea into the respiratory tree. Inspiration is an active process that requires the expenditure of significant energy.

The major determinants of the alveolar content of oxygen include the inspired fraction of oxygen (generally 21 percent of room air) and the ventilatory rate as reflected in the measured concentration of arterial carbon dioxide.

During expiration (Figure 2-3b), the diaphragm and ribs return to their normal resting state. Positive pressure is created within the chest cavity, which forces gases (particularly carbon dioxide) out of the chest. In most cases, expiration is a passive process and requires no energy consumption. However, in asthmatic patients and those with chronic obstructive pulmonary disease (COPD), there may be obstruction of air flow along with reduced elasticity of the lungs, and exhalation becomes an active process, also expending energy.

In patients with respiratory failure, ventilation is performed by emergency care personnel using manual or mechanical techniques (e.g., bag-valve-mask ventilation or portable transport ventilation). In this case, inhalation is based on positive pressure forcing oxygen and other gases into the lungs with passive exhalation of carbon dioxide by the patient.

Two factors affect the ability to ventilate a patient adequately: resistance and compliance. *Resistance* refers to the ease with which gases flow into an open space (airway or alveolus). The major factor that determines airway resistance

Two factors affect the ability to ventilate a patient adequately: resistance and compliance.

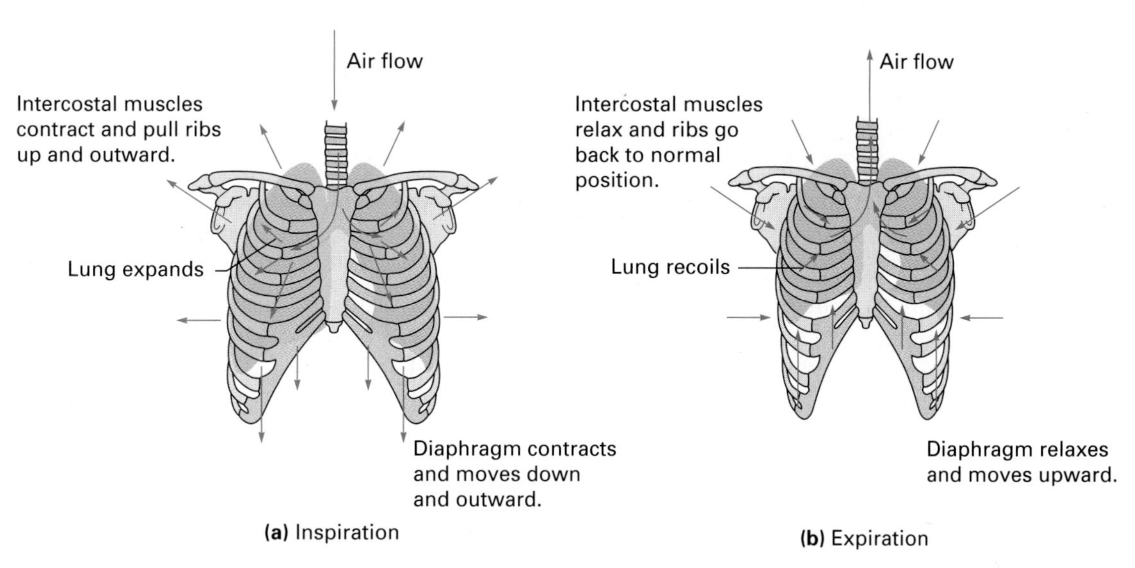

FIGURE 2-3
The phases of respiration: (a) inspiration and (b) expiration.

resistance the opposition of the body to the passage of gases into an open space (e.g., airway resistance to ventilation).

compliance the elasticity of the lungs; the change in lung volume in response to a change in pressure.

is the cross-sectional diameter of the trachea and upper airway structures. The change in resistance is proportional to the fourth power of any change in the cross-sectional diameter of the airway. Thus, any decrease in the diameter by a factor of 2 (e.g., with tracheal edema from an inhalation injury) results in a 16-fold increase in airway resistance. *Compliance* is the mathematical description of the elasticity of the lungs and is defined as the change in lung volume produced by a change in pressure. A decrease in compliance can be appreciated as an increase in the effort needed to "bag" a patient. Greater pressure is needed to achieve the same lung volume in patients with decreased lung compliance, such as patients with COPD.

Greater pressure is needed to achieve the same lung volume in patients with poor lung compliance, such as patients with COPD.

Once oxygen reaches the alveoli, it must then pass into the small capillaries that are found in the distal portions of the lungs. This process is known as *diffusion*. This is usually a very efficient process, owing in part to the tremendous surface area of the alveoli and the small distance between the alveolar and capillary membranes.

diffusion movement of a gas from an area of higher concentration to an area of lower concentration, as in the passage of oxygen and carbon dioxide across alveolar and capillary membranes.

ventilation process of getting air or oxygen to the alveoli of the lungs.

perfusion adequate supply of blood to the tissues.

pulmonary shunting the mixture of unoxygenated blood with oxygenated blood leaving the lungs caused by a mismatch between ventilation and perfusion of lung segments—either insufficient air reaching the alveoli or insufficient blood reaching the capillaries—as occurs with atelectasis.

atelectasis a collapsed or airless lung or lung segment.

hypoxemia insufficient oxygenation of the blood; an arterial oxygen level less than 80 torr.

hypoxia inadequate oxygen delivery to the tissues.

For diffusion to occur most efficiently, all of the oxygenated alveoli must come in contact with unoxygenated blood from the pulmonary arterial system. In other words, all ventilated segments of the lung (V) are equally matched by capillary perfusion from the pulmonary circulation (Q). Normally, there is some physiological mismatch of *ventilation* (V) of alveoli and blood flow (Q) through the alveolar capillaries, or *perfusion*. For example, when the patient is upright, there is better ventilation of the upper segments of the lung, but less blood flow through the same segments because of the effects of gravity. This physiological mismatch accounts for the fact that the measured difference between alveolar and arterial oxygen concentration is approximately 5 to 15 torr.

Any further mismatch of ventilation and perfusion of lung segments will cause unoxygenated blood to mix with oxygen-enriched blood leaving the lungs, creating a condition known as *pulmonary shunting* (Figure 2-4). This can occur when a segment of lung is collapsed (*atelectasis*), when pneumonia is present, or when the patient experiences a pulmonary embolism. In each condition, the alveolar arterial difference will be greater than 15 torr. Damage to the alveoli (e.g., from cigarette smoking, asbestos inhalation, or fluid accumulation from pulmonary edema) will also prevent effective diffusion and increase the difference between alveolar and arterial oxygen. In addition, any process that increases the interstitial space between the alveolus and the pulmonary capillary, such as pulmonary edema, may reduce the efficiency of oxygen diffusion.

Ultimately, oxygen that enters the bloodstream must be transported to the tissues. Although some oxygen (less than 1 percent) can be dissolved in the plasma (the noncellular portion of the blood), most oxygen is transported to the tissues bound to hemoglobin, a protein found on the outside of red blood cells. The normal level of hemoglobin is between 12 and 14 g of protein per dl of blood. Patients with anemia (especially less than 7 g/dl), therefore, are less able to provide adequate oxygen delivery to tissues.

Under normal conditions, the measured arterial concentration of dissolved oxygen is 80 to 100 torr. Measured oxygen levels below 80 torr are known as *hypoxemia*. This condition is contrasted with *hypoxia*, which is the inadequate delivery of oxygen to the tissues. It should be remembered that oxygen delivery depends on both an adequate arterial oxygen content and an adequate cardiac output.

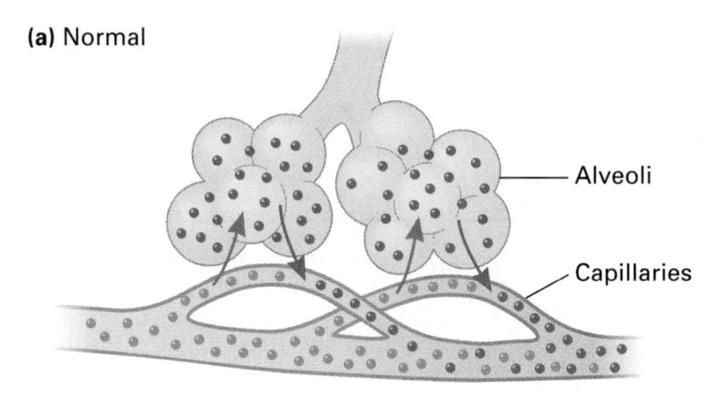

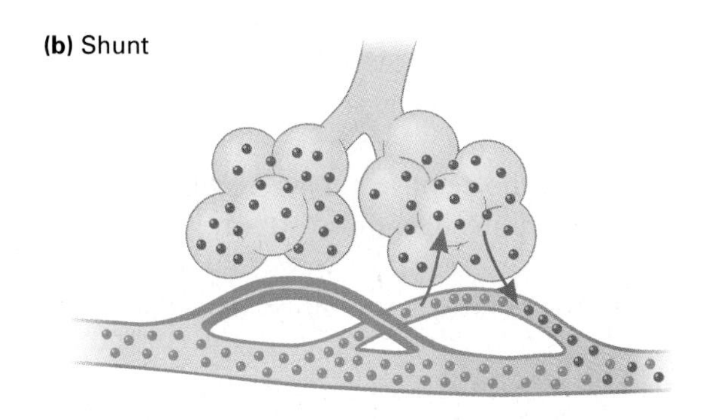

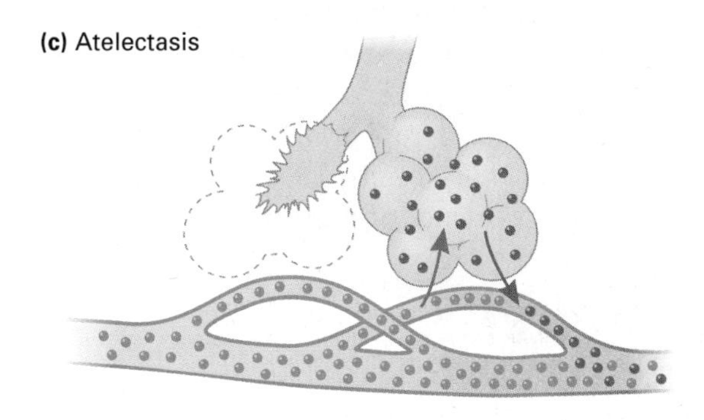

FIGURE 2-4
Diffusion of oxygen from alveoli to capillaries: (a) normal, (b) shunting, (c) atelactasis.

OXYGEN SUPPLEMENTATION

Many patients with medical illness will have greater oxygen requirements than in the normal healthy state. As a result, higher oxygen concentrations must be made available to the patient above the normal 21 percent that is present in the air we breathe. A variety of methods are available to increase the amount of inspired oxygen, including nasal cannula, nonrebreather mask, simple face mask, partial rebreather mask, and the Venturi mask.

A few points are worthy of emphasis here. Any patient with a medical illness that requires greater concentrations of oxygen should not have oxygen withheld for any reason. This is particularly true of patients with underlying COPD. (See Chapter 5, Dyspnea, Respiratory Distress, or Respiratory Failure.) In these patients, there has been an undue fear that providing higher oxygen concentrations will depress respiration; however, the damaging effects of oxygen deprivation far outweigh any potential for respiratory depression, especially during the relatively short duration of prehospital care.

Also, remember that blood oxygen saturation as measured by pulse oximetry is not a true reflection of tissue oxygen concentration. Therefore, you should not

Clinical Insight

Patients who require oxygen because of an underlying disease process should never have supplemental oxygen withheld because of chronic underlying lung disease. The patient's need for oxygen should supersede any concern about depressing the patient's respiratory drive by administering high concentrations of oxygen.

assume that because the patient has an acceptable oxygen saturation reading, adequate concentrations of oxygen are reaching the tissues.

AIRWAY MANAGEMENT

All patients who are unable to protect their airway adequately should be considered candidates for definitive airway management.

The most common reason for airway management is the inability to maintain airway patency, usually as the result of a depressed level of consciousness. This generally occurs in patients with drug or alcohol intoxication, head injury, stroke, seizure, or other metabolic disease. Patients who have an alteration in mental status should be closely assessed for their ability to maintain an open airway. If this fails, definitive airway control must be established. Patients who maintain a gag reflex may still require tracheal intubation if other indications for airway management are present.

Clinical Insight

Testing a patient's gag reflex is an inadequate method of determining the patient's ability to maintain airway patency. The presence of a gag reflex does not guarantee that a patient is able to adequately maintain an open airway nor does it guarantee that the patient will not aspirate secretions, blood, or vomit.

Another important group of patients who require airway management are those with signs of hypoxia or respiratory failure. The most extreme example of this would be the patient with cardiorespiratory arrest. However, any respiratory ailment (see Chapter 5) may progress to the point where ventilatory support and acute airway management are indicated.

Finally, any patient who presents with a medical condition that may ultimately result in airway compromise should have the airway addressed before airway compromise actually develops. For example, an anaphylactic reaction may result in *angioedema* involving the upper airway and may require early airway intervention. Infections such as Ludwig's angina (infection involving the soft tissues of the anterior portion of the neck) and retropharyngeal abscesses (see Chapter 5) may also eventually lead to airway compromise. Here again, you must carefully monitor the patient's airway for any evidence of deterioration.

angioedema an immunologically produced swelling of the skin, mucous membranes, or internal organs.

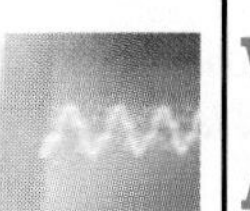

VENTILATION EQUIPMENT AND TECHNIQUES

Many patients are not capable of supporting their own ventilatory needs. This is common in patients with conditions that cause central nervous system depression (e.g., drug overdose, alcohol intoxication, metabolic diseases, stroke) or in patients with respiratory failure. Ventilatory failure must be addressed promptly. A variety of alternative ventilatory support methods are available. Selection depends on the equipment available and the perceived advantages of each technique. These methods include mouth-to-mask ventilation, two-person bag-valve-mask ventilation, and flow-restricted, oxygen-powered ventilation. The single-person bag-valve-mask technique is believed to be the least effective method of ventilation.

Indications for Airway Management

Patients requiring airway management are those who have

- An altered mental status or depressed level of consciousness (as with drug or alcohol intoxication, head injury, cerebral vascular accident, seizure, metabolic disease)
- Signs of hypoxia or respiratory failure
- A medical condition that may ultimately result in airway compromise (as with anaphylaxis or epiglottitis)

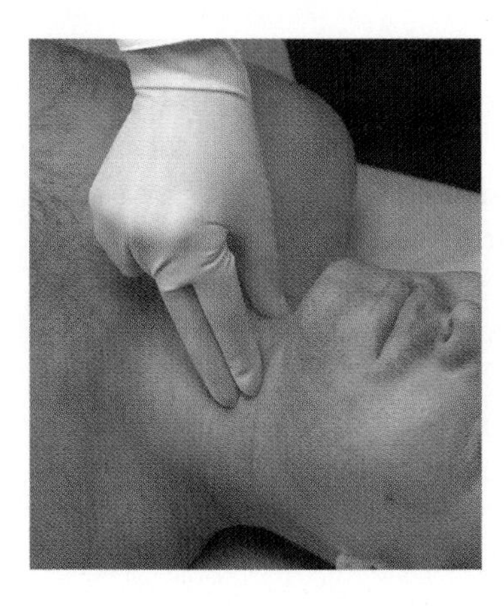

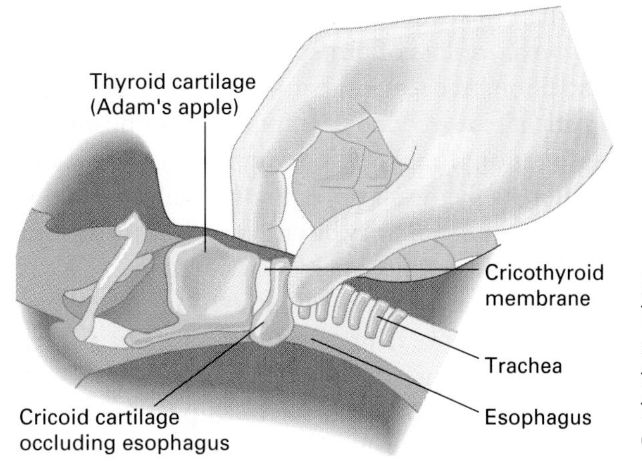

FIGURE 2-5
To perform cricoid pressure, use the thumb and the index finger to apply firm posterior pressure on the cricoid ring.

With each technique, the rescuer provides positive-pressure ventilation. This means that, instead of air being drawn into the lungs as the result of negative pressure created by an expanding thorax, the rescuer forces air into the lungs. In addition to providing assistance to ventilation, this reduces the patient's oxygen requirements by reducing the energy requirements during respiration.

Take care to avoid injuring the patient by ventilating too aggressively. Aggressive ventilation can lead to complications, including pneumothorax, as well as air in the mediastinal and subcutaneous tissues. Additionally, overly aggressive ventilation can cause gastric distention and increased risk of aspiration. Insufflation of air into the stomach raises the pressure in the stomach above that which can be occluded by the normal muscular tension in the lower esophageal sphincter muscle (10 torr). To avoid this complication, make sure that *cricoid pressure* is applied with any form of positive-pressure ventilation.

cricoid pressure application of pressure on the cricoid cartilage to prevent gastric insufflation, regurgitation, and aspiration and to aid in visualization of the vocal cords; also known as the **Sellick maneuver.**

To apply cricoid pressure (Figure 2-5), first locate the cricoid ring. This is identified as the first cartilaginous ring beneath the thyroid cartilage. Use your thumb and index finger to apply firm pressure on the anterior portion of the cricoid ring in order to occlude the esophagus. Do not perform this maneuver if the patient is actively vomiting, because esophageal rupture may result.

Cricoid pressure prevents air from being forced into the stomach by resisting a pressure gradient of up to 100 torr. This reduces the risk of gastric distention and aspiration. Additionally, during attempts at tracheal intubation, this procedure forces the glottic opening posteriorly into the intubator's field of vision. Finally, if the intubation is performed properly, the tracheal tube can be felt to pass beneath the thumb and index finger of the person applying cricoid pressure, which provides an additional method of confirming proper tube placement.

TRACHEAL INTUBATION

Successful placement of a tracheal tube is the definitive method of securing an airway. In essence, the length of the trachea is extended to the end of the tracheal tube, which is under your control. You can deliver oxygen directly to the lungs and can manipulate the patient's tidal volume. Meanwhile, the tracheal tube protects the tracheobronchial tree from contamination by vomit, blood, or secretions.

Successful placement of a tracheal tube is the definitive method of securing an airway.

Tracheal intubation is indicated in any situation in which the patient cannot support his own airway. As noted earlier, this would include any patient who has an altered mental status, severe hypoxia, or loss of protective reflexes due to a medical condition (e.g., a stroke). In addition, tracheal intubation should be undertaken if there is a need to control the patient's oxygenation because of significant obstruction to the airway or risk of aspiration from bleeding, vomiting, or secretions or to support the patient's ventilation as the result of respiratory failure. Finally, it should be mentioned that tracheal intubation may be employed for therapeutic reasons (e.g., as a means of drug delivery in certain emergency situations).

One aid to tracheal intubation should be mentioned at this point: the gum elastic bougie. It has been used to assist in tracheal intubation when there is inadequate visualization of the vocal cords. The gum elastic bougie is a long tube-like device with a flexible tip that can be inserted behind the epiglottis and passed blindly through the vocal cords. The tracheal tube is slid over the proximal end of the device and advanced into the trachea using the gum elastic bougie as a guide (Figure 2-6).

The orotracheal method of tracheal intubation is reviewed in Figures 2-7a–f. (Also see "Nasotracheal Intubation" later in this chapter.)

It should be remembered that tracheal intubation can be performed without the aid of sedating medications only in patients who are profoundly obtunded or who are in cardiac arrest. In most cases, the procedure is performed either by using sedative agents as adjuncts to produce a profound state of sedation (see "Rapid Sequence Intubation" later in this chapter) or by using a combination of sedating medication in low doses and local tracheal anesthesia to depress protective reflexes.

Patient monitoring equipment that should be available during the procedure includes

- Cardiac monitor
- Pulse oximeter

If possible, place a cardiac monitor and pulse oximetry on the patient before initiating a tracheal intubation.

The cardiac monitor and pulse oximetry should be placed on the patient before beginning the intubation procedure unless the intubation is being performed for a truly emergent condition such as apnea. The ECG tracing and oxygen saturation should be monitored continuously during the intubation procedure.

FIGURE 2-6
The gum elastic bougie.
(Photo courtesy of Roy Alson, M.D.)

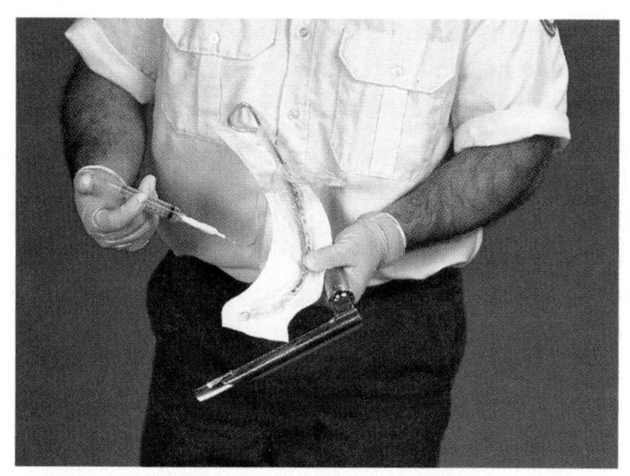

FIGURE 2-7a Make sure the equipment has been assembled and tested.

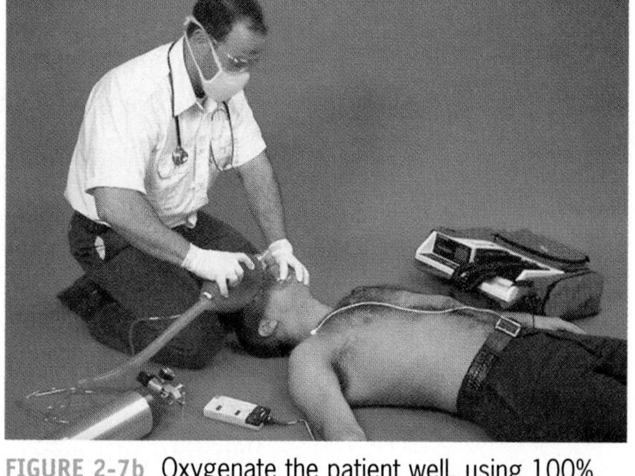

FIGURE 2-7b Oxygenate the patient well, using 100% oxygen.

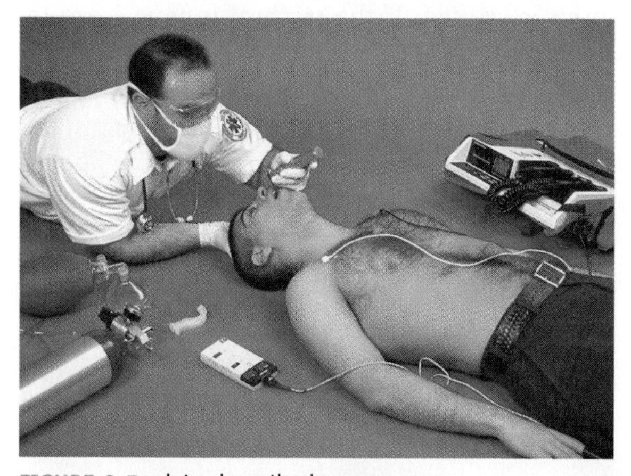

FIGURE 2-7c Introduce the laryngoscope.

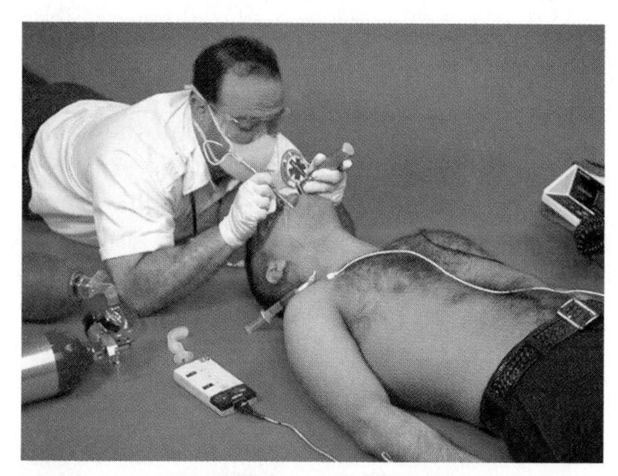

FIGURE 2-7d Visualize the end of the tube as you pass it between the vocal cords.

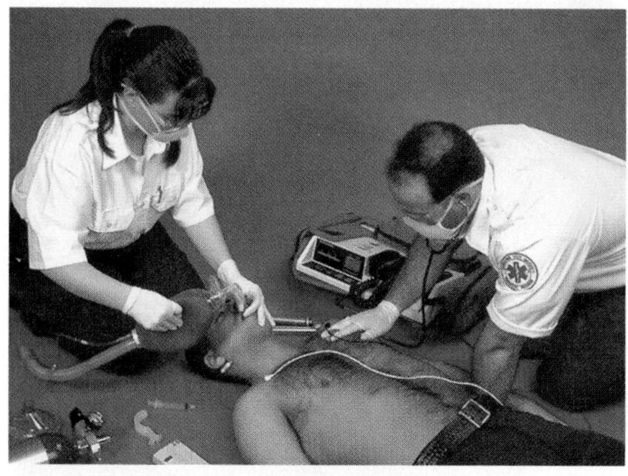

FIGURE 2-7e Confirm tube placement.

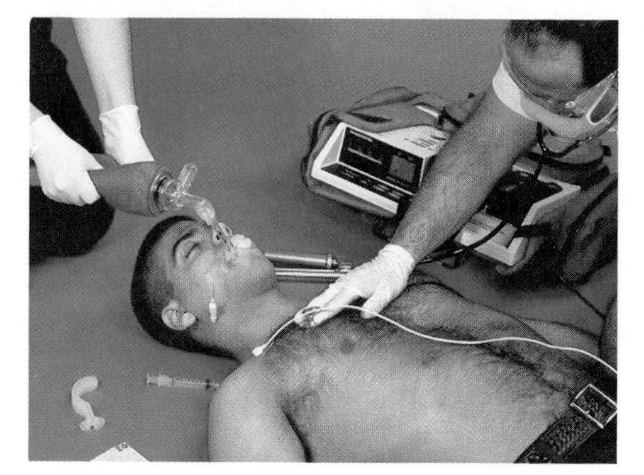

FIGURE 2-7f Secure the tube and reconfirm tube placement.

It is also strongly recommended that a method of assessing appropriate tube placement be available. This could be either of the following (Figures 2-8a–c):

- End-tidal CO_2 detection device
- Esophageal detection device

These devices supplement clinical protocols used to determine correct placement of the tracheal tube in the trachea. Evidence suggests that using clinical methods alone may incorrectly identify improper tube placement in a significant percent of cases where a tracheal tube is placed.

End-tidal CO_2 detection devices are placed in the ventilation circuit. They indicate the presence of exhaled carbon dioxide by demonstrating a color change, wave form, or partial pressure reading. The continued detection of carbon dioxide indicates appropriate tube placement in the trachea. This device is less useful in cases of cardiac arrest, where carbon dioxide production and elimination by the lungs may be limited.

The continued detection of carbon dioxide indicates appropriate tube placement in the trachea.

Esophageal detection devices operate on the principle that the esophagus is a collapsible tube, whereas the trachea, with its cartilaginous circular support, is not collapsible. The detection device is inserted onto the end of the tracheal tube, and a bulb is compressed or a syringe plunger is pushed in. When the bulb is released or the plunger withdrawn, a vacuum is created. If the tracheal tube is correctly placed in the trachea, the trachea will remain open, air will rush through it from the lungs, and the bulb will distend or plunger withdrawal will not be impeded. However, if the tracheal tube has been improperly inserted in the esophagus, the vacuum that has been created will collapse the esophagus, and the bulb will only partially refill or you will feel resistance as you try to withdraw the plunger. These devices can also be used to verify placement of the pharyngotracheal lumen (PtL) and Combitube airways in either the trachea or esophagus.

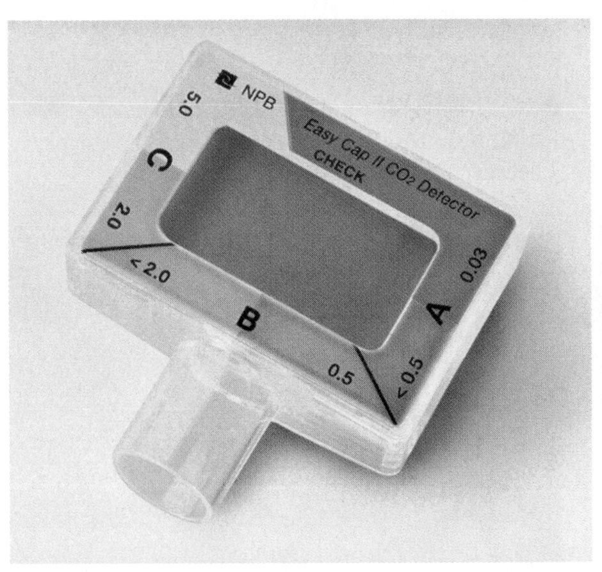

(a)

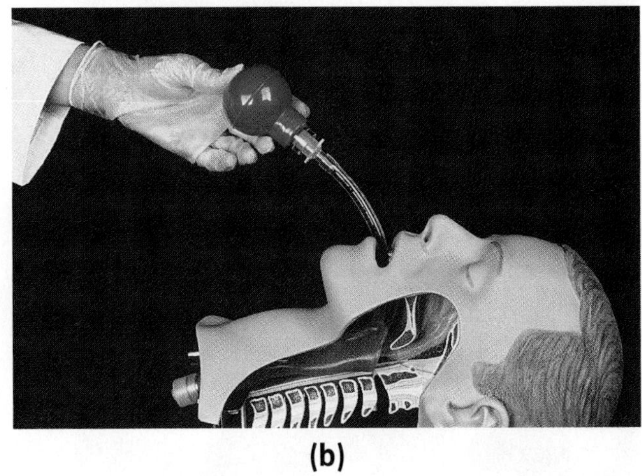

(b)

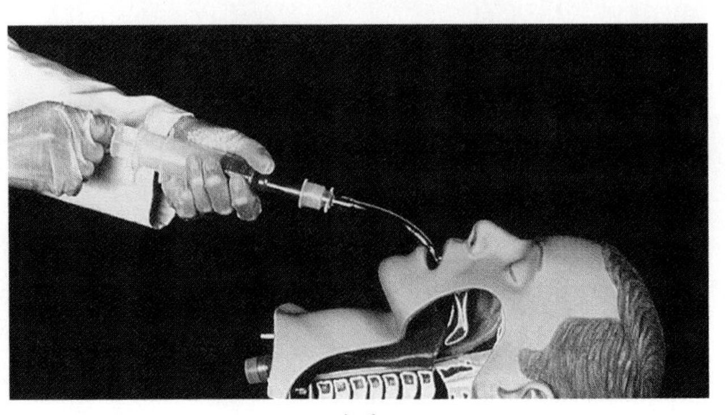

(c)

FIGURE 2-8
(a) End-tidal CO_2 detector.
(© Nellcor Puritan Bennett, Inc.)
(b) Bulb-type esophageal detection device.
(© Ambu, Inc.)
(c) Syringe-type esophageal detection device.
(© Ambu, Inc.)

Confirmation of Tracheal Tube Placement

To confirm tracheal tube placement

- Listen for absence of sounds in the epigastrium.
- Listen for equal bilateral breath sounds.
- Visualize the tube for appearance of mist.
- Use an end-tidal CO_2 detection device or an esophageal detection device.

To summarize, confirm tube placement in the following manner:

1. Listen first for sounds in the epigastrium. Presume that any air heard rushing into the stomach with ventilation is from an esophageal positioning of the tracheal tube. If this happens, remove the tube immediately and repeat the procedure. Be prepared for regurgitation of stomach contents.
2. Listen for breath sounds over each side of the chest. You should hear breath sounds in both the apices of each lung and the lateral intercostal spaces. At the same time, observe for symmetric rise and fall of the chest wall with ventilation. A decrease in breath sounds on one side of the chest may indicate that the tube has been advanced too far, with the tip resting in one of the mainstem bronchi. Typically, a right mainstem intubation is seen. Should this occur, deflate the balloon and pull the tube out 1 to 2 cm, based on auscultation of the chest to confirm the presence of bilateral breath sounds.
3. Visualize the tube for the appearance of mist, which suggests tracheal positioning.
4. Finally, confirm placement using an end-tidal CO_2 detection device or an esophageal detector (as explained earlier).

Clinical Insight

A confirmatory device such as an end-tidal CO_2 detector or a mechanical device such as an esophageal detection device must be used to confirm proper intubation. A significant portion of tracheal tubes believed to be in the trachea by clinical measures alone are later found to be placed in the esophagus.

Secure the tube using an appropriate method. In addition to adhesive tape or intravenous tubing, a variety of commercially available tube-securing devices are available. Make a note of where the centimeter marking on the tracheal tube rests against the corner of the mouth. As a general guideline, the tube should be positioned at 21 cm in an adult female and 23 cm in an adult male. Reconfirm this marking and tube placement after any patient movement or transfer. Additionally, the intubated patient may be secured on a long backboard with a cervical collar in place to prevent movement of the neck and potential dislodgement of the tracheal tube.

One final point must be emphasized. Prior to any procedure where exposure to blood or body secretions is possible, those performing the procedure should take proper body substance isolation precautions, including protective gloves, mask, and eye shield.

Take appropriate body substance isolation precautions, including gloves, mask, and eye shield, before performing an intubation.

There are several possible complications associated with intubation. As already mentioned, esophageal intubation is perhaps the most significant because it can lead to a disastrous outcome. Anoxic brain injury and death can result from unrecognized esophageal intubation. Placement in one of the mainstem bronchi is another significant complication. A patient suffering this complication will present with absent or decreased breath sounds on the unventilated side. Occasionally, these patients may be difficult to ventilate, leading emergency care personnel to suspect the development of a tension pneumothorax. Patients with mainstem intubation have mistakenly undergone needle decompression of the chest under these circumstances. Other complications include mucus plugging, soft tissue injury, placement of the tracheal tip at the glottic opening, and bleeding.

The intubation procedure itself can also lead to unrecognized hypoxia, particularly if attempts at intubation are prolonged and pulse oximetry is not routinely used during the procedure. Alterations in the patient's vital signs, including hypertension, bradycardia, or tachycardia, can also occur. In addition, a variety of cardiac dysrhythmias have been reported during intubation attempts.

Soft tissue damage to the mouth, lips, teeth, pharynx, tongue, epiglottis, and vocal cords may result. Stimulation of the epiglottis and vocal cords has led to laryngospasm in some cases, resulting in difficulty ventilating and oxygenating the patient. Finally, stimulation of the posterior oropharynx and loss of the protective epiglottic reflexes may lead to vomiting and aspiration of gastric contents during the procedure.

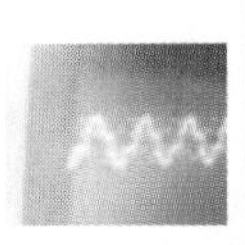

ALTERNATIVE METHODS OF INTUBATION

Nasotracheal Intubation

Nasotracheal intubation is a commonly employed alternative to orotracheal intubation. This blind approach is commonly used in the out-of-hospital environment because of a number of advantages it offers over the orotracheal approach. The technique can be successfully performed with the patient in a variety of positions. Unlike orotracheal intubation, it can be easily accomplished when the patient is in an upright or semi-upright position. Also, the nasotracheal route is better tolerated in the patient who is lethargic but not unconscious. Finally, it is an alternative approach in patients where an orotracheal approach is not possible because of difficulties in the oropharynx. Patients with seizures and a clenched jaw, patients with significant swelling in the oropharynx, or patients with *trismus* (contraction of the muscles of mastication) as the result of infectious processes may be intubated using a nasotracheal approach.

trismus muscle spasm resulting in clenching of the jaw.

There are also disadvantages with the nasotracheal approach. Blind nasotracheal intubation requires some skill and persistence when compared to the orotracheal approach. The success rate for the procedure is significantly lower than for tracheal intubation, and soft tissue injury is more common with this technique. In addition, the patient must have some spontaneous ventilatory effort for the procedure to be performed successfully. The technique cannot be performed on a completely apneic patient.

Finally, there are some delayed consequences of nasotracheal intubation that must be considered. As a rule, tracheal tubes inserted nasotracheally have a smaller lumen then those inserted using the orotracheal route. Smaller tracheal tubes increase airway resistance, which may increase the work of spontaneous ventilation, and this may create some difficulty in getting the patient off a mechanical ventilator. In addition, some hospital procedures, such as bronchoscopy, can only be performed on a size 8.0-mm tracheal tube or larger. Such tubes are typically too

Indications for Nasotracheal Intubation

Nasotracheal intubation is appropriate as an alternative to orotracheal intubation when the patient

- Cannot be placed in a supine position
- Is lethargic but not unconscious
- Has difficulties with the oropharynx, such as swelling or copious secretions that inhibit visualization of the vocal cords
- Has a clenched jaw

large to be used for nasotracheal intubation. Finally, nasotracheal intubation has a higher incidence of complications, including sinusitis and soft tissue injury.

The following equipment is needed for nasotracheal intubation:

Oxygen source
Bag-valve mask
Tracheal tube
Water-soluble lubricant
Syringe
Suctioning equipment
Method to secure the tracheal tube (tape, intravenous tubing, or commercially available device)
Stethoscope

Nasotracheal intubation should be undertaken in the following manner (Figures 2-9a–f):

1. The patient should be well oxygenated with 100 percent oxygen, using a full face mask in the case of a spontaneously breathing patient or a bag-valve mask in the case of a patient with decreased ventilatory effort. Administer high-flow, high-concentration oxygen for approximately 3 to 5 minutes. Lubricate a nasopharyngeal airway, and place it in the nostril in which the insertion will be attempted. A water-soluble lubricant should be used, preferably lidocaine jelly. A vasoconstricting agent such as 0.25 percent phenylephrine (Neosynephrine) should also be administered prior to an attempt.
2. Pass a lubricated 6.5- to 7.5-mm tracheal tube directly posterior through the nare. You may feel some resistance. You can overcome this by gently rotating the tube, but do not use significant force. "Curl" the tube prior to the procedure to allow a significant anterior displacement of the tip of the tube during insertion. Alternatively, an Endotrol tube can be used. This tube has a cable that is used to curl the tip of the tube more anteriorly when the ring attached to the cable is pulled during the procedure.
3. Gently and slowly push the tube through the pharynx to the point at which breath sounds are heard loudest. At this point, the tube is resting just above the glottic opening. Advancing the tube beyond this point results in a marked decrease in sounds heard. You can aid auscultation by removing the bell of the stethoscope and placing the open tubing into the adapter end of the tracheal tube. Alternatively, a whistle-like device called a BAAM is available that can be placed over the tracheal tube adapter to augment the breath sounds.
4. Observe the patient for each inspiration. During a deep inspiration, quickly advance the tube. This should result in the tube passing through the vocal cords when they are wide open. Typically, the patient will buck and cough after successful intubation. A prominence noted on either side of the larynx suggests that the tube has come to rest in the pyriform fossa. If this happens, pull the tube back and rotate it laterally during subsequent attempts.
5. Confirm tube placement. Do this after inflating the balloon cuff with 5 to 10 ml of air.
6. Secure the tube, using an appropriate method. Make a note of the centimeter marking of the tracheal tube as it rests against the opening of the nare. As a general guideline, the tracheal tube adapter should be within a few centimeters of the nares. Reconfirm this marking and tube placement after any patient movement or transfer.

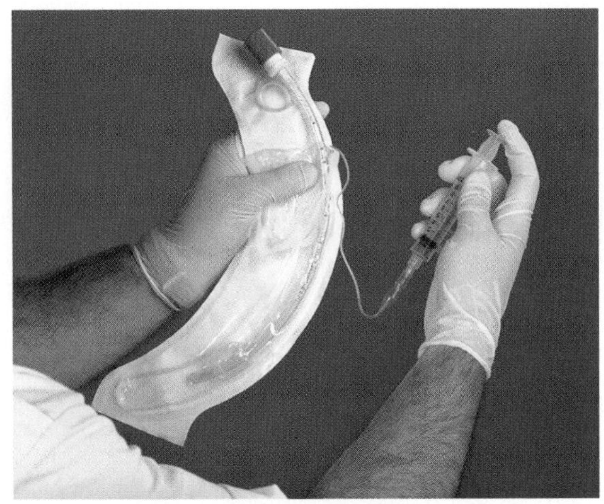

FIGURE 2-9a Make sure the equipment has been assembled and tested.

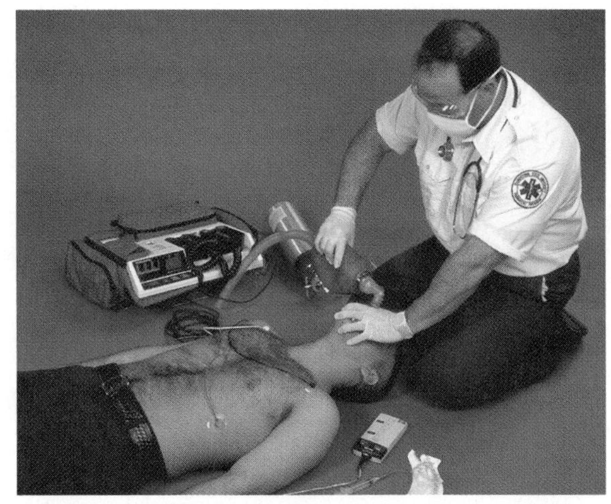

FIGURE 2-9b Oxygenate the patient well, using 100% oxygen.

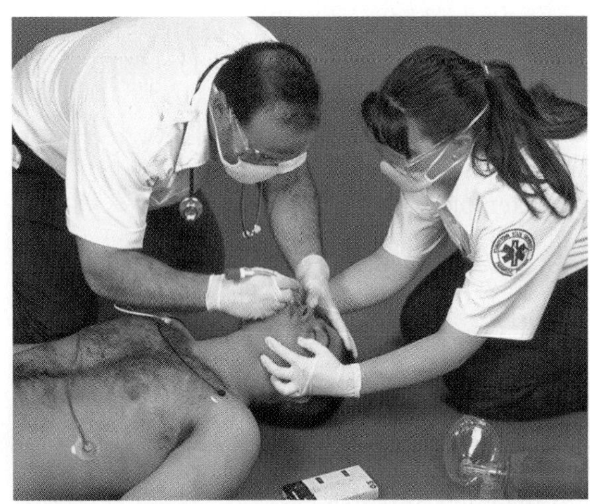

FIGURE 2-9c Position head and insert lubricated tube into the nare.

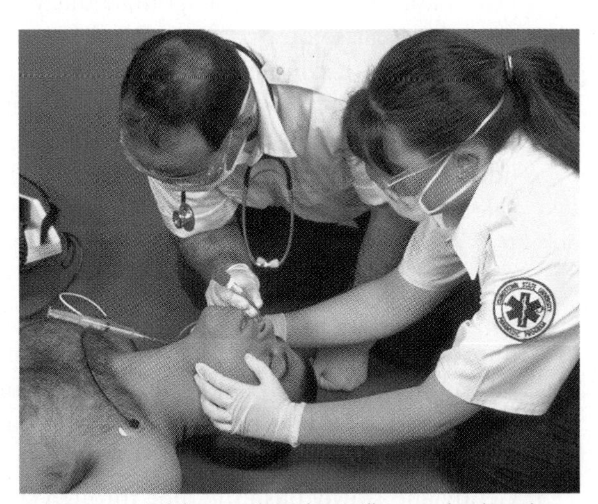

FIGURE 2-9d Advance the tube until properly placed.

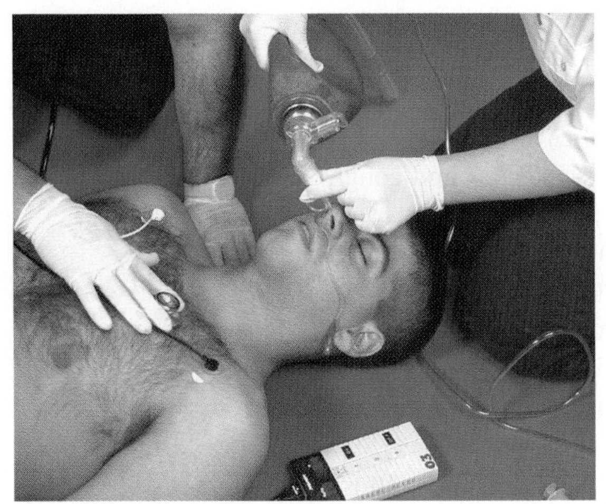

FIGURE 2-9e Confirm tube placement.

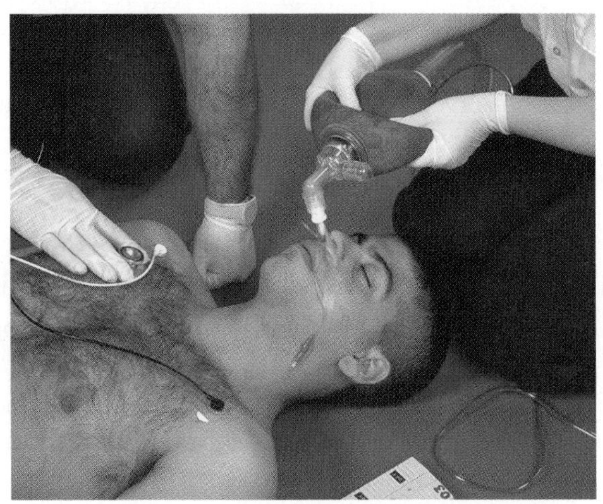

FIGURE 2-9f Secure the tube and reconfirm tube placement.

Complications of nasotracheal intubation are similar to those for orotracheal intubation. As already mentioned, infectious complications and soft tissue injury are more common with the nasotracheal technique. It should also be mentioned that, once the nasotracheal tube has been advanced into the pharynx, a laryngoscope blade can be used to locate the tube tip. Using Magill forceps, the tube can be advanced past the vocal cords using a technique similar to that used for orotracheal intubation, if necessary.

Digital Intubation

Digital intubation is a blind intubation technique that enables emergency care personnel to pass a tracheal tube when the patient is in a position that is not conducive to oral or nasal intubation and is unresponsive. In addition, this is an alternative approach to consider when other methods of intubation have already been attempted unsuccessfully in the unconscious patient. The digital technique is particularly useful when secretions prevent adequate visualization of the cords or when equipment failure precludes appropriate visualization. This technique requires minimum equipment because the care provider guides the tube into the larynx using his fingers only. The major risk of this procedure is injury to the care provider from the patient's teeth, causing direct exposure to oral secretions. The technique should be reserved for those patients who have a severely depressed level of consciousness, are unresponsive, or are paralyzed.

The following equipment is needed for digital intubation:

Oxygen source
Bag-valve mask
Tracheal tube
Stylet
Water-soluble lubricant
Syringe
Suctioning equipment
Method to secure the tracheal tube (tape, intravenous tubing, or commercially available device)
Stethoscope

Digital intubation should be performed in the following manner (Figures 2-10a and b):

1. The patient should be well oxygenated with 100 percent oxygen, using a full face mask in the case of a spontaneously breathing patient or a bag-valve mask in the case of a patient with decreased ventilatory effort. Administer high-flow, high-concentration oxygen for approximately 3 to 5 minutes.

Indications for Digital or Lighted-Stylet Intubation

Digital intubation or lighted-stylet intubation is appropriate as an alternative to orotracheal or nasotracheal intubation when the patient

- Has a severely depressed level of consciousness, is unresponsive, or is paralyzed
- Is in a position not conducive to orotracheal or nasotracheal intubation
- Has copious secretions that inhibit visualization
- Has already had an unsuccessful intubation attempt with orotracheal or nasotracheal intubation

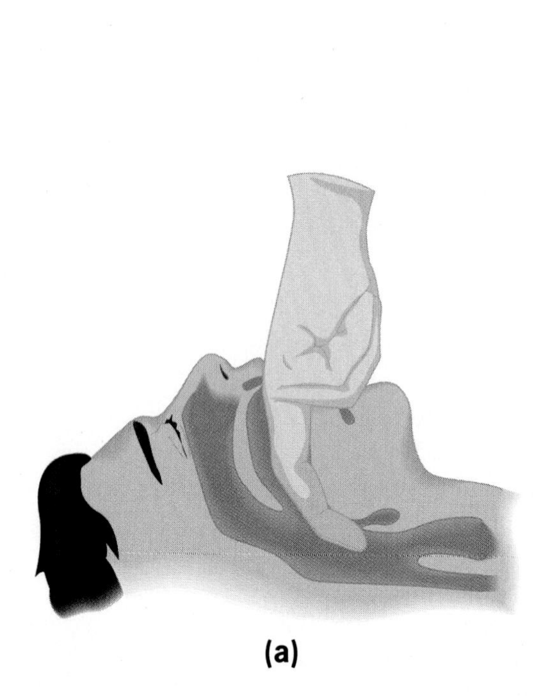

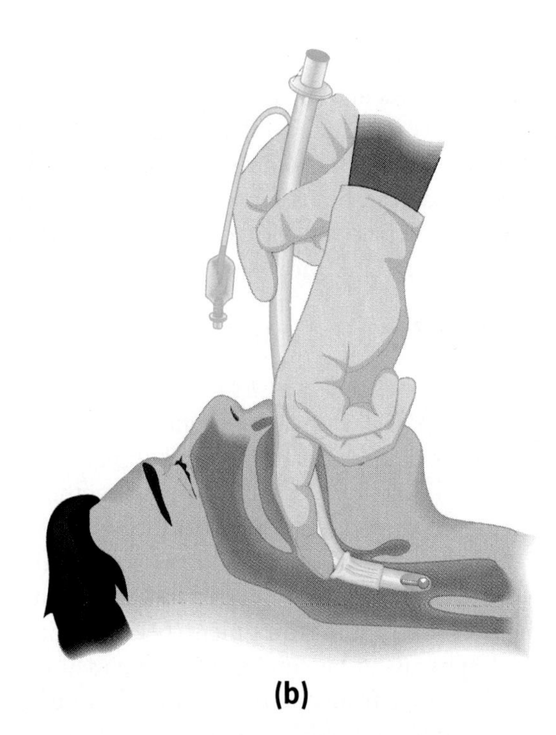

FIGURE 2-10
(a) To perform digital intubation, insert the index finger and the middle finger of your dominant hand into the patient's mouth and pull the base of the tongue forward. Locate the epiglottis and pull it forward, using your middle finger. (b) Use your other hand to advance the lubricated tube and stylet through the mouth, past the vocal cords, and into the trachea.

2. Insert the index and middle finger of your dominant hand into the mouth and use them to pull the base of the tongue forward. You can insert a bite block to prevent the patient from injuring you. Locate the epiglottis and pull it forward, using your middle finger.
3. Use your other hand to advance the lubricated tube through the mouth. (The lubricated stylet will have been placed into the lumen of the tube and molded into a J shape.) Then, slide the tube past the vocal cords into the trachea, using your index and middle finger to guide the tube.
4. Remove the stylet and inflate the balloon cuff with 5 to 10 ml of air.
5. Confirm tube placement using the methods described earlier for orotracheal intubation.
6. Secure the tube using an appropriate method. Make a note of the centimeter marking of the tracheal tube as it rests against the corner of the mouth. Reconfirm this marking and tube placement after any patient movement or transfer.

Lighted-Stylet Intubation

Lighted-stylet intubation takes advantage of the fact that a high-intensity light at the end of a stylet can be seen through the soft tissues of the neck when the stylet is properly placed in the trachea. In this technique, the tracheal tube and lighted stylet are advanced blindly into the mouth, guided toward the larynx, and then slid into the trachea.

The indications for this technique are similar to those for other blind methods; it should be considered when orotracheal intubation is not practical because of the patient's position, copious secretions, or equipment failure. The procedure is somewhat limited by the fact that it is difficult to appreciate the light emitted from the stylet in the presence of bright ambient lighting, such as direct sunlight. However, lighted-stylet intubation is better tolerated than digital intubation and puts the care provider at less risk.

Lighted-stylet intubation is better tolerated than digital intubation and puts the care provider at less risk.

The following equipment is needed for lighted-stylet intubation:

Oxygen source
Bag-valve mask
Tracheal tube
Special high-intensity lighted stylet
Water-soluble lubricant
Syringe
Suctioning equipment
Method to secure the tracheal tube (tape, intravenous tubing, or commercially available device)

Lighted-stylet intubation should be performed in the following manner (Figures 2-11a and b):

1. The patient should be well oxygenated with 100 percent oxygen, using a full face mask in the case of a spontaneously breathing patient or a bag-valve mask in the case of a patient with decreased ventilatory effort. Administer high-flow, high-concentration oxygen for approximately 3 to 5 minutes.

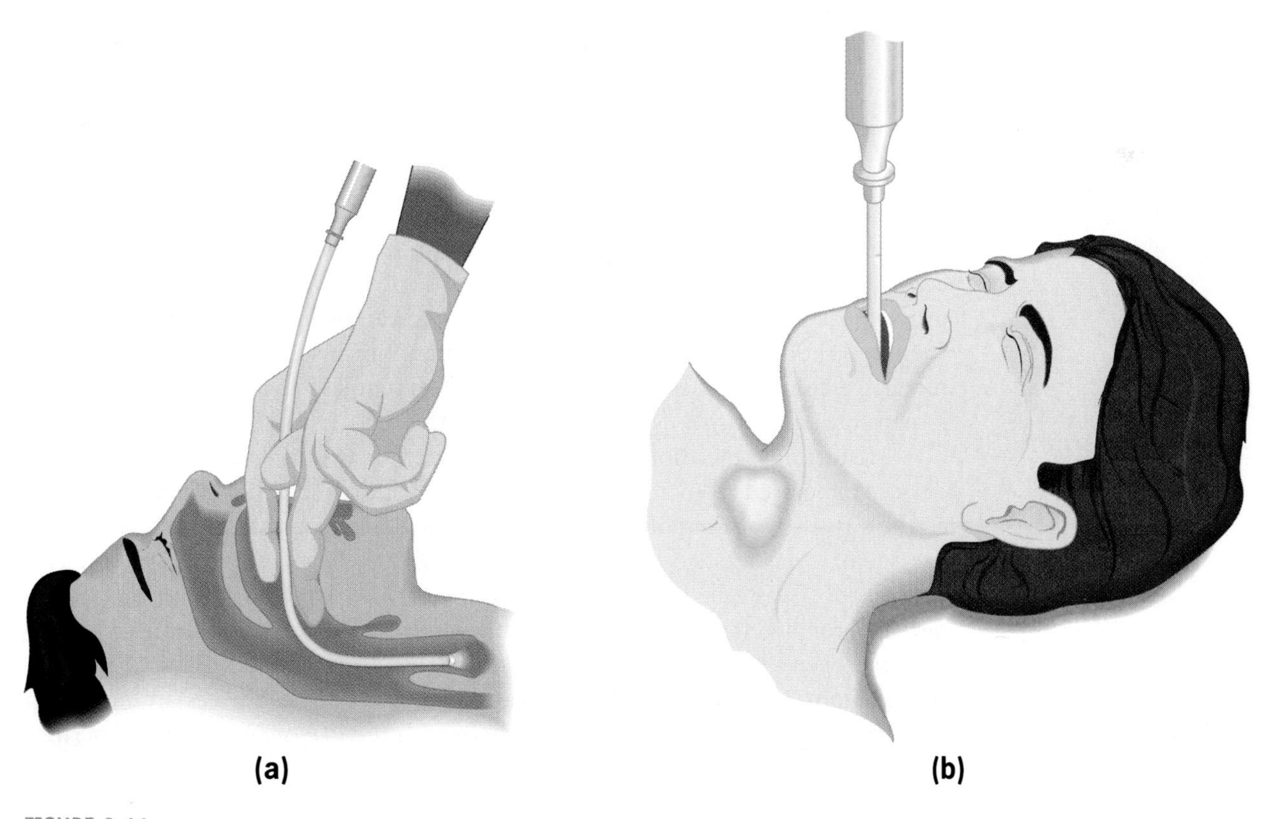

FIGURE 2-11
(a) To perform lighted-stylet intubation, insert the index finger and the middle finger of your dominant hand into the patient's mouth, depressing the base of the tongue. Advance the tube and stylet deep into the pharynx and past the epiglottis.
(b) The tip of the stylet is correctly placed in the trachea if you can see a distinct, bright light in the middle portion of the neck.

2. Thread the tube over the distal portion of the lighted stylet and fit the adapter to the end of the tube. Bend the stylet to a curved J or hockey stick configuration just beyond the end of the tracheal tube.
3. Advance your index and middle fingers into the patient's mouth, depressing the base of the tongue. Use your thumb to stabilize the chin. Alternatively, the laryngoscope can be used to elevate the tongue. Advance the tube and stylet deep into the pharynx, along the midline, so the tip passes the epiglottis.
4. The tip of the stylet is in the correct position if you can see a distinct, bright light in the middle portion of the neck after the stylet has been advanced. After confirming that the light is distinctly visible, advance the tube 1 to 2 cm and withdraw the stylet.
   a. If the light you see across the neck is faint or diffuse, the tube is in the esophagus. Remove the tube and the stylet, and bend the distal portion of the stylet into a more pronounced curve before reattempting intubation.
   b. If you see a distinct, bright light lateral to the thyroid cartilage, the tip of the stylet has been advanced into the pyriform fossa. Withdraw the tube and the stylet, and redirect them toward the midline.
5. After inflating the balloon cuff with 5 to 10 ml of air, confirm tube placement using the methods described earlier for orotracheal intubation.
6. Secure the tube, using an appropriate method. Make a note of where the centimeter marking of the tracheal tube rests against the corner of the mouth. Reconfirm this marking and tube placement after any patient movement or transfer.

ALTERNATIVE AIRWAY DEVICES

Although tracheal tube placement by direct visualization is the definitive way to manage the patient's airway, a high degree of manual skill and frequent practice are required to remain proficient. Alternative devices have been developed that can provide adequate ventilation for the patient and can be inserted by those with less training. The devices discussed in this segment are inserted using a blind technique, which requires less skill. However, skill is required to assess the appropriate lumen through which to ventilate the patient.

Historically, the esophageal obturator airway (EOA) was the first of these devices to be used as an alternative method of ventilation. The obturator protected the airway by sealing off the esophagus. The device was later modified to allow passage of a nasogastric tube into the stomach to relieve gastric distention. This modification was called an esophageal gastric tube airway (EGTA). Although both devices provide effective ventilation when used properly, a significant complication had been the unrecognized insertion of the obturator into the trachea, leading to hypoxia and death in many cases. As a result, these devices are no longer used, and most services have replaced them with the PtL or Combitube described in the following sections.

The PtL airway and the esophageal-tracheal Combitube were refinements on the concept of the EOA/EGTA that offered the additional safety factor and benefit of being able to ventilate the trachea if the device came to rest in that position. However, each device also allows occlusion of the pharynx and indirect ventilation of the trachea using an alternative port.

Pharyngotracheal Lumen Airway

The PtL airway is designed as a longer tube passing through a shorter, wider tube, each with its own distal balloon (Figure 2-12). A stylet is placed in the lumen of the longer tube, which is designed to rest in either the trachea or the esophagus. The shorter tube has a larger balloon that, when inflated, occludes the pharynx.

During insertion, if the longer tube is inserted into the trachea, then the stylet is removed and the trachea is directly ventilated through the ventilation port. If, however, the esophagus is intubated, the distal balloon is inflated to occlude the esophagus, and ventilation is performed using the port attached to the shorter tube. In this case, ventilation of the trachea occurs indirectly because the pharynx and esophagus are occluded and the ventilations are directed into the trachea. One unique feature of this airway device is the fact that the balloon cuffs can be inflated separately or simultaneously. Because the pharyngeal balloon occludes the pharynx, it offers the advantage of preventing blood or secretions in the mouth or nose from entering the trachea.

The greatest limitation with the use of the PtL is that the care provider must determine whether the longer tube has been placed in the esophagus or the trachea. Studies have shown that this skill is difficult to master without a significant amount of training and supervision.

The device is used in patients who are unconscious, without a gag reflex, and in whom an orotracheal or nasotracheal intubation could not be accomplished or is not within the scope of practice of the emergency care provider. Approval by the service medical director is needed before the device is used.

The PtL is not used in patients younger than 16 years of age or shorter than 5 feet tall. It should not be used in patients with known esophageal disease or patients who may have ingested a caustic substance.

The following equipment is needed:

Oxygen source
Bag-valve mask
PtL
Water-soluble lubricant

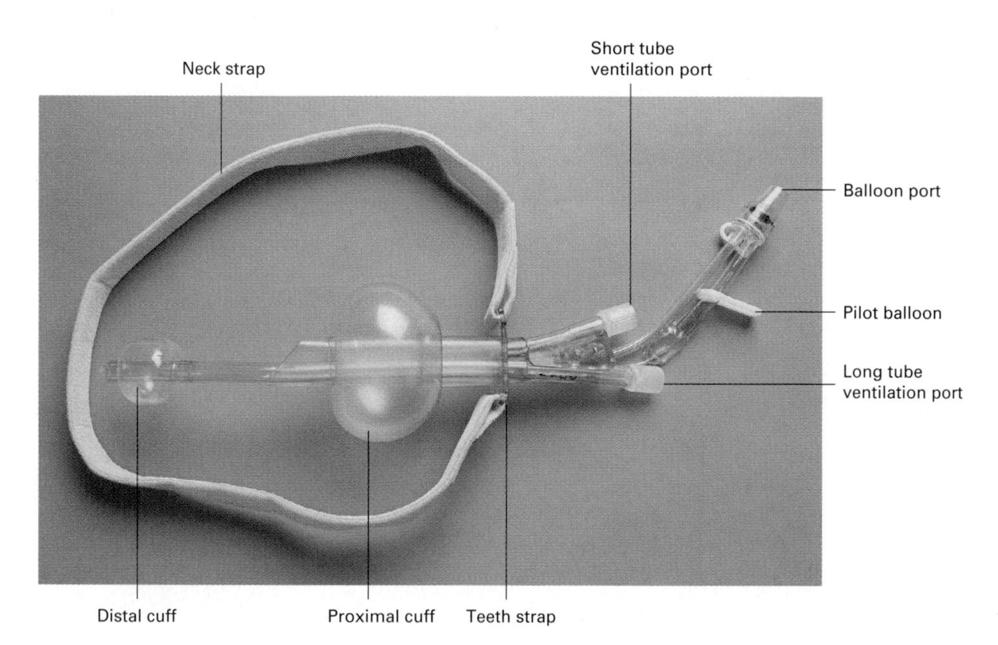

FIGURE 2-12
Pharyngotracheal lumen (PtL) airway.
(Photo courtesy of Michal Heron.)

Syringe
Suctioning equipment
Stethoscope

PtL insertion should be performed in the following manner (Figure 2-13):

1. The patient should be well oxygenated with 100 percent oxygen, using a full face mask in the case of a spontaneously breathing patient or a bag-valve mask in the case of a patient with decreased ventilatory effort. Administer high-flow, high-concentration oxygen for approximately 3 to 5 minutes.
2. The patient's head should be hyperextended slightly. Pull the jaw and tongue forward using your nondominant hand. Insert the PtL through the mouth along the natural curve of the pharynx. Continue to pass the tube until the teeth strap is at the level of the patient's teeth.
3. Fasten the neck strap around the patient's neck. Inflate both balloon cuffs simultaneously by breathing into the common balloon port with a sustained effort.
4. After cuff inflation, ventilate the shorter, wider tube. If no air is heard entering the epigastrium and the chest rises and falls symmetrically, then the longer balloon is occluding the esophagus. Air is being forced into the trachea as the result of esophageal and pharyngeal occlusion. Continue to ventilate using this port.
5. If air is heard entering the stomach and the chest is not rising with each breath, then the longer tube has been inserted into the trachea. Remove the stylet and use the bag-valve device to ventilate the 15-mm port attached to the longer tube. Reconfirm tube placement by listening to the lungs and epigastrium. An end-tidal CO_2 detector or esophageal detection device can be used to determine tube placement.

If the patient should regain consciousness or develop a gag reflex, remove the PtL as soon as possible. Turn the patient onto the left side in a slight Trendelenburg position. Deflate the balloons and quickly withdraw the airway. A nasogastric tube can be passed into the port that is not ventilated to allow for removal of stomach contents prior to airway removal. Suction equipment should be available because vomiting is common after removal.

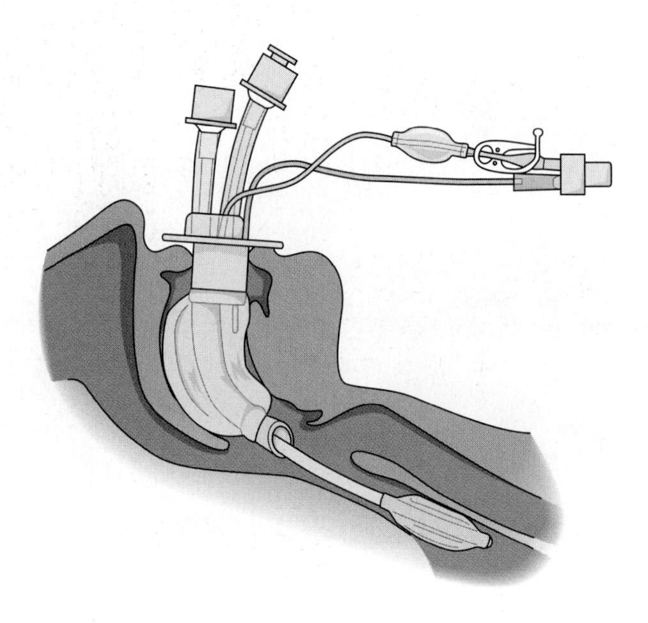

FIGURE 2-13
The PtL airway in place in the esophagus.

Esophageal-Tracheal Combitube Airway

The Combitube is similar in basic design to the PtL with some minor differences. Instead of having one tube inside the other, a partition separates the two lumens of the Combitube (Figure 2-14). There is a ventilation port for each lumen. The longer, blue tube (#1) is the proximal port; the shorter, clear tube (#2) is the distal port, which opens at the distal end of the tube. The Combitube has two inflatable cuffs—a 100-ml cuff just proximal to the distal port and a 15-ml cuff just distal to the proximal port.

Like the PtL, the Combitube is designed so it can be seated in either the esophagus or the trachea. Ventilation is first attempted through the longer, blue port (#1), which will be successful if the device has been placed in the esophagus and is most common. If ventilation through port #1 is not successful, the tube has been placed in the trachea, and ventilation through the shorter, clear port (#2) will be successful.

The Combitube has the same limitations as the PtL, in that appropriate use depends on the rescuer's ability to identify correct placement. Contraindications for use are similar to those for the PtL.

The following equipment is needed:

Oxygen source
Bag-valve mask
Combitube
Water-soluble lubricant
Syringe
Suctioning equipment
Stethoscope

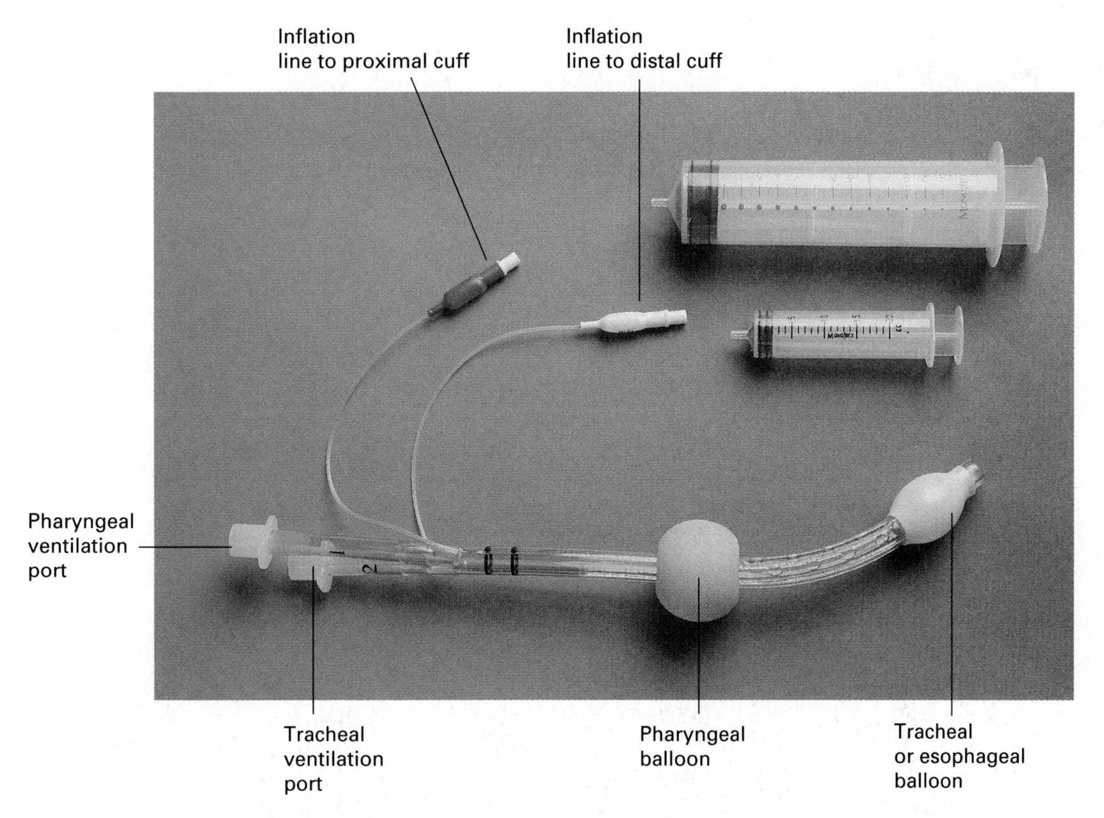

FIGURE 2-14
Esophageal-tracheal Combitube airway.
(Photo courtesy of Michal Heron.)

Combitube insertion is performed in the following manner:

1. The patient should be well oxygenated with 100 percent oxygen, using a full face mask in the case of a spontaneously breathing patient or a bag-valve mask in the case of a patient with decreased ventilatory effort. Administer high-flow, high-concentration oxygen for approximately 3 to 5 minutes.
2. The patient's head should be placed in a neutral position. Pull the jaw and tongue forward using your nondominant hand. Insert the Combitube through the mouth along the natural curve of the pharynx. Continue to pass the tube until the black rings on the device are at the level of the patient's teeth.
3. Inflate both cuffs, first the proximal cuff with 100 ml of air, then the distal cuff with 15 ml of air.
4. Use a bag-valve mask to ventilate through the longer, blue port (#1). If no air is heard entering the epigastrium and the chest rises and falls symmetrically, then ventilation is successful. Air is being forced out of openings along the tube and, because the esophagus and the pharynx are occluded by the inflated cuffs, the oxygen has nowhere to go but into the trachea (Figure 2-15a). Continue to ventilate using this port.
5. If air is heard entering the stomach and the chest is not rising with each breath, then assume that the tube has been inserted into the trachea. Use a bag-valve device to ventilate through the shorter, clear port (#2), which will force air into the trachea through the distal end of the tube (Figure 2-15b).
6. Confirm tube placement by listening to both the lungs and the epigastrium. An end-tidal CO_2 detector or esophageal detection device can be used to further confirm tube placement.

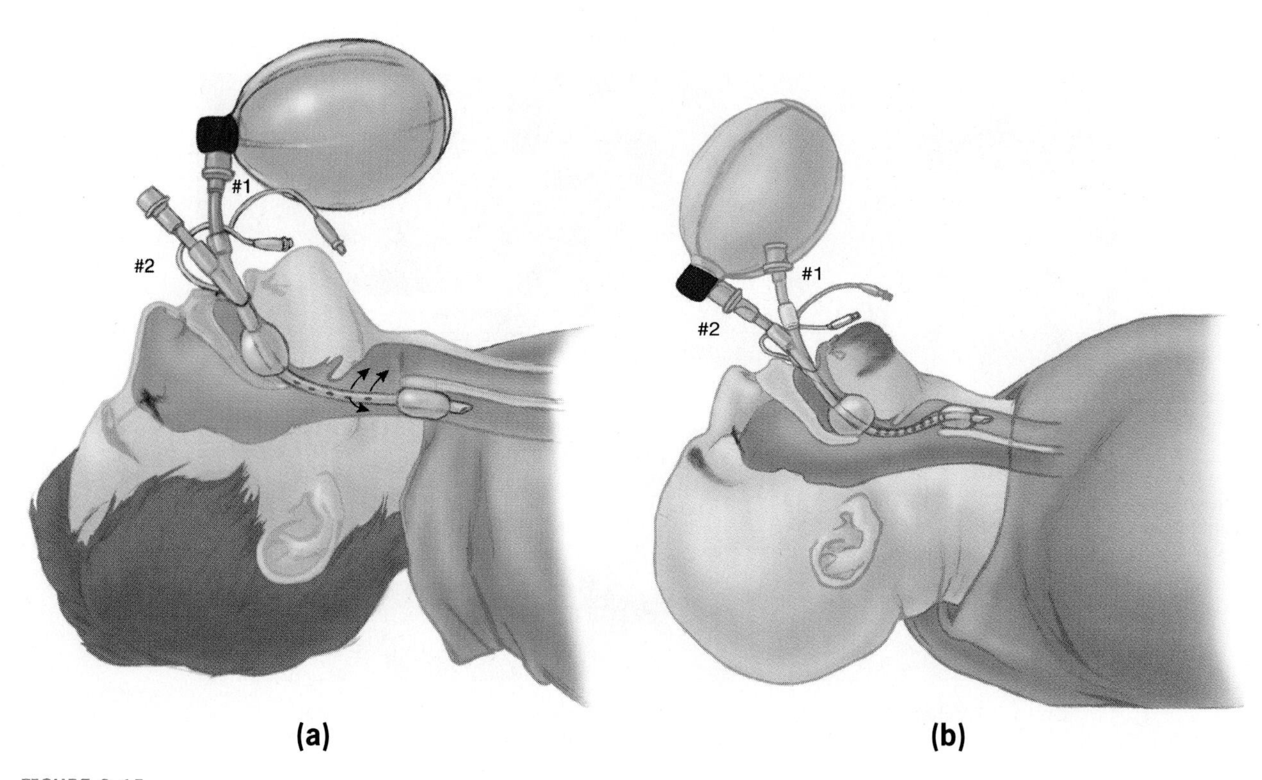

FIGURE 2-15
(a) With the Combitube, first ventilate through the longer, blue tube (#1). Ventilation will be successful if the tube has been placed in the esophagus, as is most common. (b) If ventilation through tube #1 is not successful, ventilate through the shorter, clear tube (#2). Ventilation will be successful if the tube has been placed in the trachea.

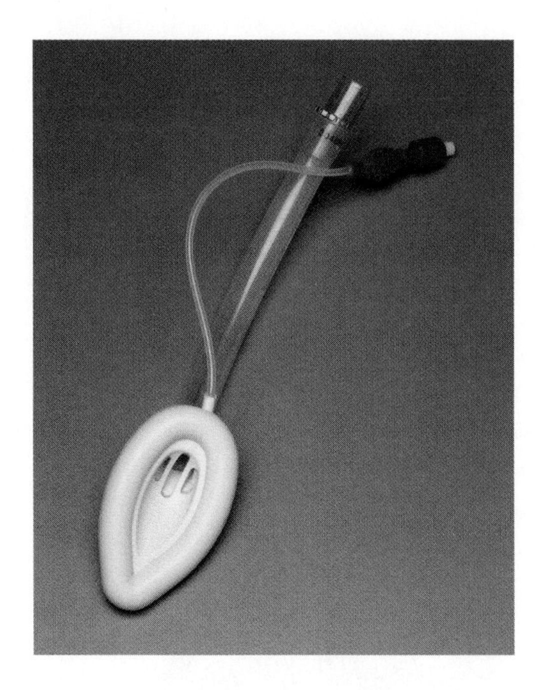

FIGURE 2-16
The standard laryngeal mask airway (LMA).
(© Gensia Automedics, Inc.)

If the patient should regain consciousness or develop a gag reflex, remove the Combitube as soon as possible. Turn the patient onto the left side in a slight Trendelenburg position. Deflate the balloons and quickly withdraw the airway. Suction equipment should be available because vomiting is common after removal.

Laryngeal Mask Airway

The laryngeal mask airway (LMA) is an alternative airway device that provides direct ventilation through the glottic opening. The airway is inserted without direct visualization of the glottis. The airway consists of three components: airway tube, mask, and inflation line (Figure 2-16). When properly inserted, the LMA lies just above the glottic opening. Two bars that sit over the mask aperture prevent the epiglottis from occluding the lumen. Ventilation is performed via a standard 15-mm adapter that can be connected to a ventilation bag. The device is most useful for patients who cannot be intubated using conventional methods and in whom bag-valve-mask ventilation is not possible. Studies have shown that the device can be used with only a minimal amount of training, and success rates are comparable to those with tracheal intubation.

The device comes in sizes ranging from 1 to 6. Sizes 2, 2 ½, and 3 are for children. Size 4 is typically used for women and size 5 for men.

To insert a standard LMA, the following equipment is needed:

Oxygen source
Bag-valve mask
Laryngeal mask airway
Water-soluble lubricant
Syringe
Suctioning equipment
Stethoscope

LMA insertion should be performed in the following manner (Figures 2-17a–f and Figure 2-18):

1. The patient should be well oxygenated with 100 percent oxygen, using a full face mask in the case of a spontaneously breathing patient or a bag-valve

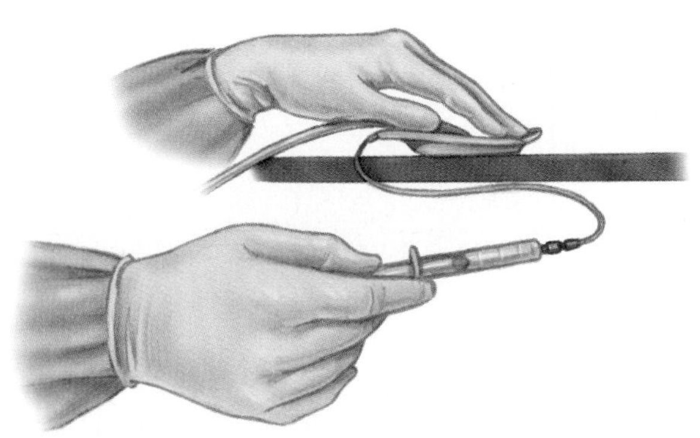

FIGURE 2-17a Tightly deflate the cuff so it forms a smooth "spoon shape." Lubricate the posterior surface of the mask with water-soluble lubricant.

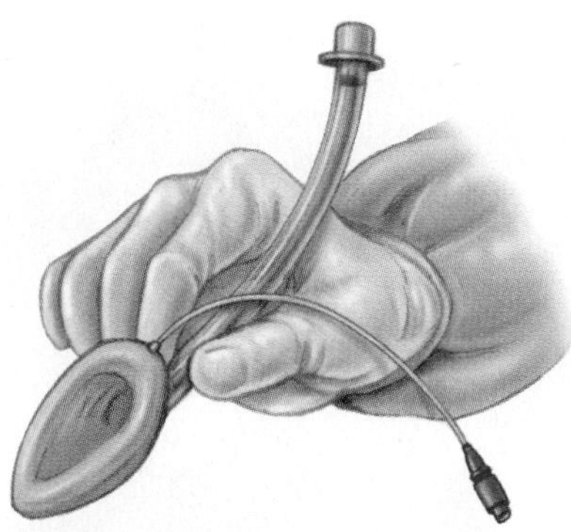

FIGURE 2-17b Hold the LMA like a pen, with the index finger at the junction of the cuff and the tube.

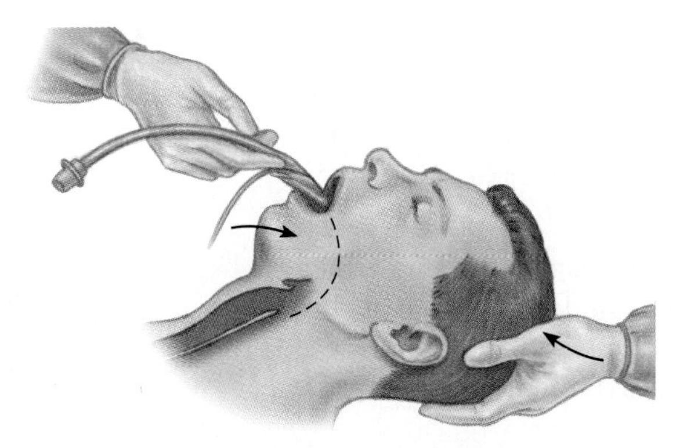

FIGURE 2-17c With the patient's head extended and the neck flexed, carefully flatten the LMA tip against the hard palate.

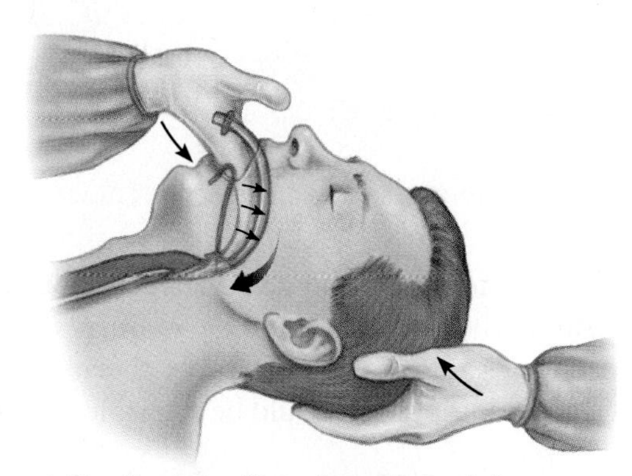

FIGURE 2-17d Use the index finger to push cranially, maintaining a pressure on the tube with the finger. Advance the mask until definite resistance is felt at the base of the hypopharynx.

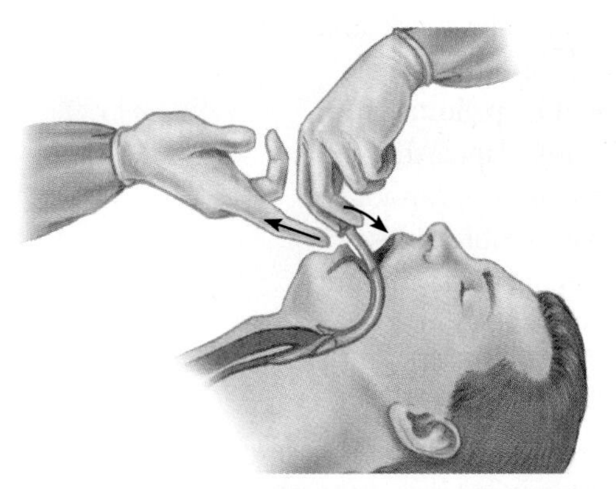

FIGURE 2-17e Gently maintain cranial pressure with the one hand while removing the index finger.

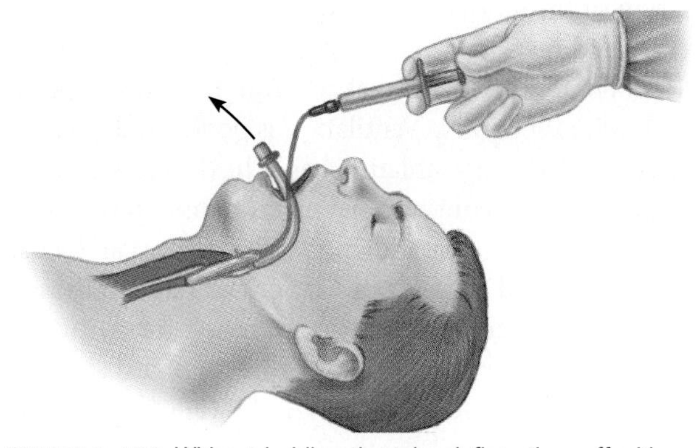

FIGURE 2-17f Without holding the tube, inflate the cuff with just enough air to obtain a seal (to a pressure of approximately 60 cm H_2O).

Maximum LMA Cuff Inflation Volumes

LMA Size	Cuff Volume (air)	LMA Size	Cuff Volume (air)
1	up to 4 ml	3	up to 20 ml
1½	up to 7 ml	4	up to 30 ml
2	up to 10 ml	5	up to 40 ml
2½	up to 14 ml	6	up to 50 ml

Source: LMA Instruction Manual, Table 5, p. 28

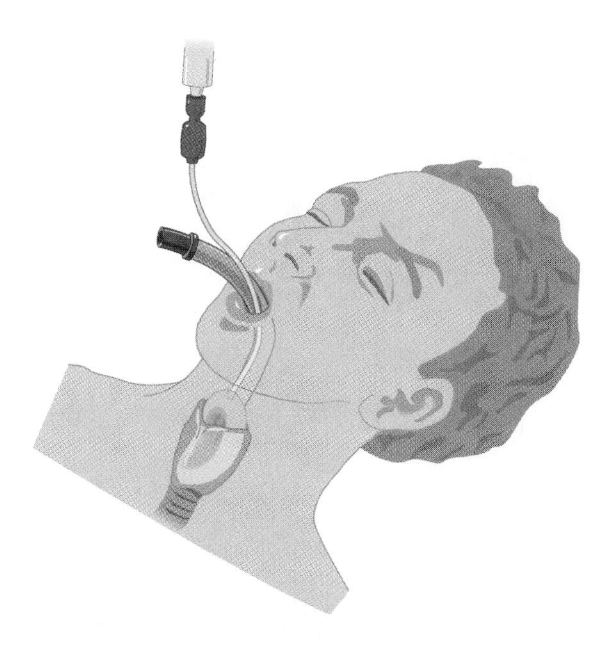

FIGURE 2-18
The laryngeal mask airway (LMA) in place.

mask in the case of a patient with decreased ventilatory effort. Administer high-flow, high-concentration oxygen for approximately 3 to 5 minutes.

2. The patient's head should be placed in the classic sniffing position. The cuff of the LMA should be completed deflated. Lubricate the posterior portion of the mask.
3. Pull the jaw and tongue forward, using your nondominant hand. Insert the LMA through the mouth along the natural curve of the pharynx, holding the device like a pencil at the junction of the tube and mask with the aperture facing forward. Continue to pass the tube until resistance is met.
4. The cuff should be inflated to approximately 60 cm H_2O once the device is properly seated. This is approximately 30 ml of air for a size 4 mask; a size 5 mask will require approximately 40 ml (see inflation volumes chart with Figures 2-17a–f). Failure to maintain a good seal above the glottic opening may indicate overinflation of the cuff.
5. Ventilate the patient using a ventilation bag with peak airway pressures not to exceed 20 cm H_2O. This reduces the amount of gastric insufflation. An end-tidal CO_2 detection device can be used to confirm placement.

A modification of the standard LMA, an intubating LMA (the LMA-Fastrach) is now commercially available. A tracheal tube can be passed through the LMA-Fastrach, allowing successful intubation of the patient. In this device, the standard LMA has been modified by adding a rigid steel shaft with a handle that lies over the ventilating tube. Additionally, there is a V-shaped ramp at the mask aperture that directs the tracheal tube toward the glottic opening. Finally, an epiglottic elevating bar replaces the two bars found on the standard LMA (Figure 2-19). Insertion of the LMA-Fastrach device requires more skill on the part of the operator, as does the subsequent passing of the tracheal tube through the device.

Insertion of the LMA-Fastrach (Figures 2-20a–f) is similar to insertion of the standard LMA, except that the handle is held as the LMA-Fastrach is advanced and seated against the glottis and the cuff inflated. A ventilation bag can then be connected to the adaptor at the end of the LMA-Fastrach handle to ventilate the

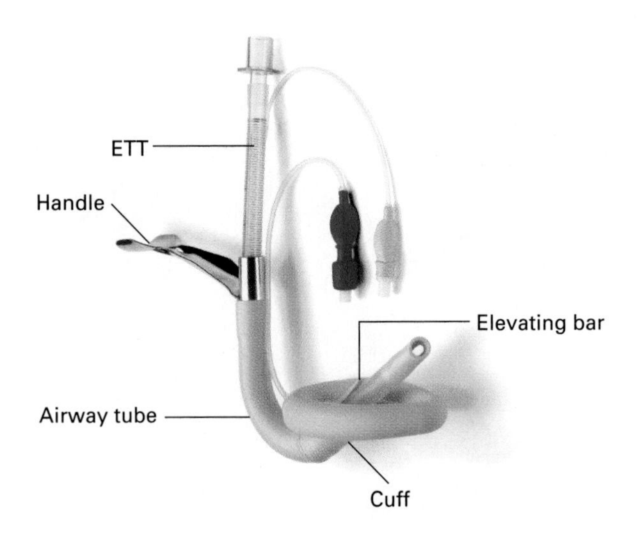

FIGURE 2-19
The intubating LMA.
(© LMA North America, Inc.)

patient. To insert a tracheal tube, the handle of the LMA-Fastrach is lifted upward as a lubricated ETT is advanced through the lumen of the LMA-Fastrach handle. Passage with minimal resistance indicates proper placement of the tracheal tube. Compatible tracheal tubes are available.

The LMA-Fastrach should be removed following successful intubation, and the patient should be well ventilated. The mask cuff is then inflated, and the 15-mm tracheal tube adapter is removed. While the LMA-Fastrach is removed using a curved motion on the handle, forward pressure is applied to the proximal end of the ETT. Once the end of the ETT is level with the end of the LMA-Fastrach handle, a stabilizing rod is inserted and the LMA-Fastrach is completely withdrawn.

Aspiration is the major complication with the use of an LMA. This is a particular concern among pregnant patients and those with gastric distention from bag-valve-mask ventilation. The device does not fully protect the glottic opening. Other complications include laryngospasm, airway trauma, and unsuccessful placement in less than 2 percent of patients. Specific complications with the LMA-Fastrach are posterior pharyngeal edema and posterior distracting force applied to the cervical spine with insertion of the device in patients with potential spinal cord injury.

Aspiration is the major complication with the use of an LMA. The device does not fully protect the glottic opening.

If the patient should regain consciousness or develop a gag reflex, remove the LMA as soon as possible. Turn the patient onto the left side in a slight Trendelenburg position. Deflate the cuff and quickly withdraw the airway. Suction equipment should be available because vomiting is common after removal.

Several newer devices designed to be placed into the upper airway using a blind technique are being used in some systems. These include the perilaryngeal airway (CobraPLA), laryngeal tube airway (King LT), oropharyngeal airway (PAxpress), and pharyngeal airways (SLIPA, COPA).

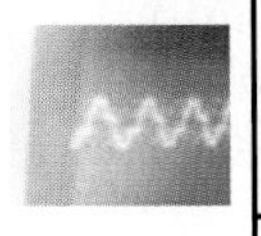

SURGICAL TECHNIQUES OF AIRWAY CONTROL

Placement of a tracheal tube using an orotracheal or nasotracheal approach is the ideal method of securing an airway in a patient who requires it. Unfortunately, all emergency care providers will encounter the rare patient who, either for technical reasons or because of medical contraindications, cannot be intubated by any of

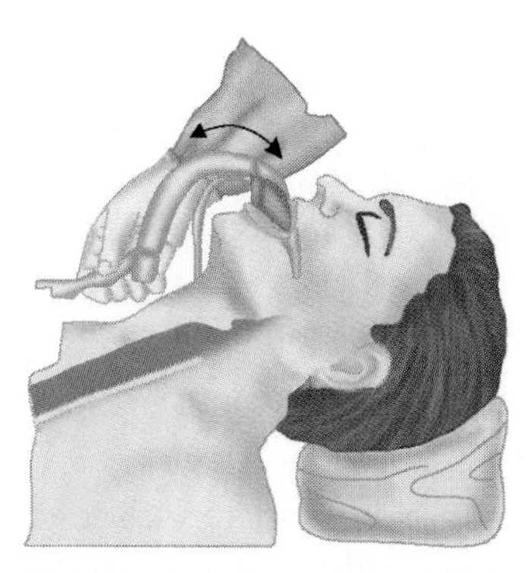

FIGURE 2-20a Hold the LMA-Fastrach handle parallel to the patient's chest. Position the mask tip so it is flat against the hard palate just posterior to the upper incisors.

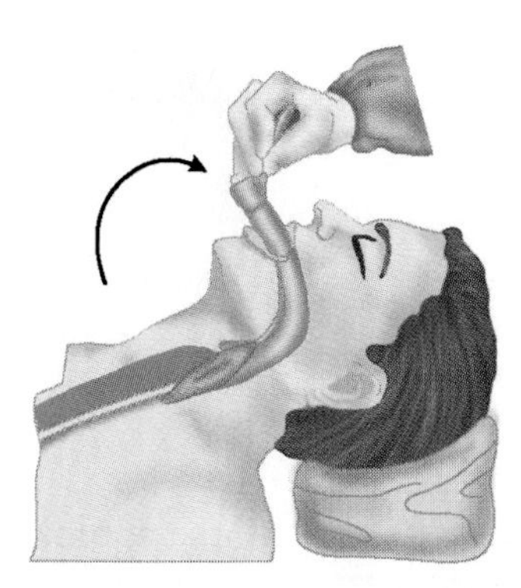

FIGURE 2-20b Swing the mask into place in a circular movement, maintaining pressure against the palate and posterior pharynx.

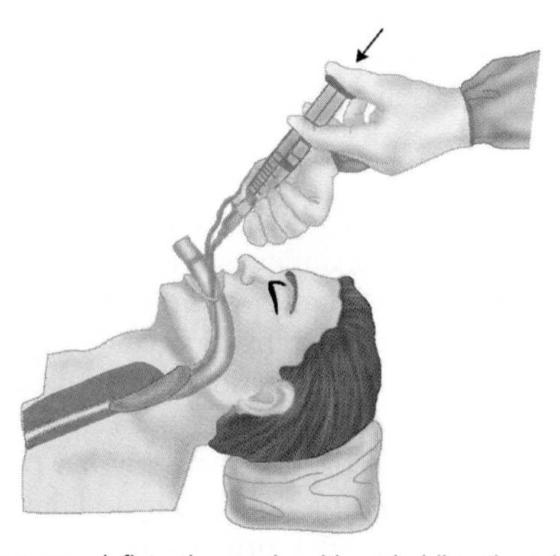

FIGURE 2-20c Inflate the mask, without holding the tube or handle, to a pressure of approximately 60 cm H_2O.

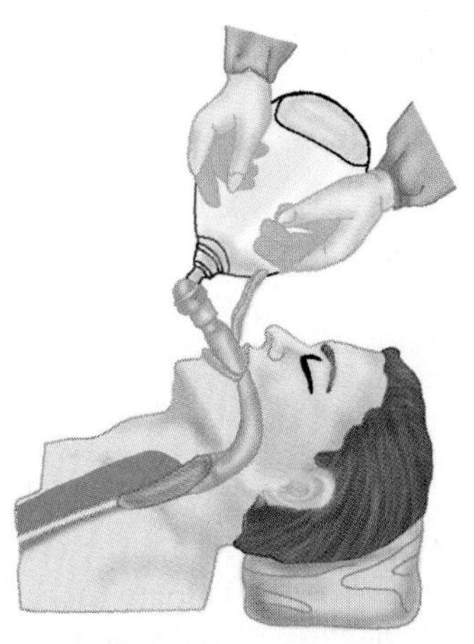

FIGURE 2-20d Connect the LMA-Fastrach to the bag-valve or other ventilation device and ventilate the patient before intubating.

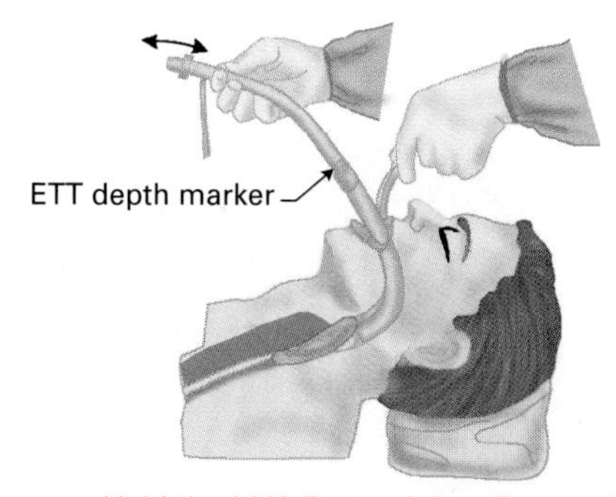

FIGURE 2-20e Hold the LMA-Fastrach handle steady while gently inserting a lubricated tracheal tube into the metal shaft.

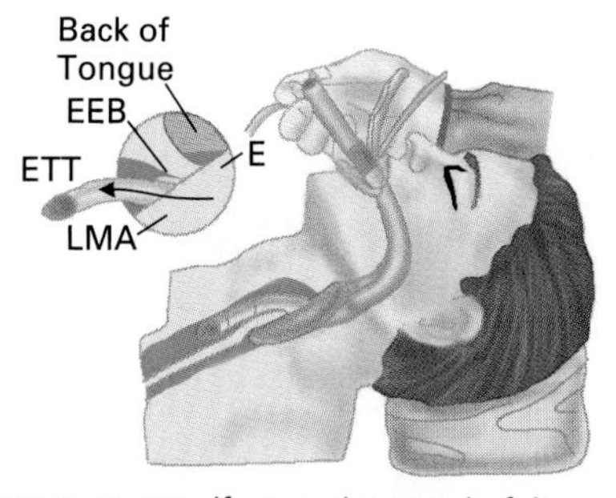

FIGURE 2-20f If no resistance is felt, continue to advance the tracheal tube, while holding the LMA-Fastrach steady, until intubation has been accomplished. Following successful intubation, remove the LMA-Fastrach and ventilate the patient well.

KEY
E Epiglottis
EEB Epiglottic Elevating Bar
LMA LMA-Fastrach™
ETT Endotracheal Tube

Indications for a Surgical Airway

A surgical technique is appropriate in patients in whom an emergency airway is indicated and tracheal intubation cannot be achieved, for example patients who

- Have anatomical distortion of the landmarks used for intubation (e.g., those with prior head or neck surgery)
- Have direct obstruction of upper airway structures (e.g., from infection or anaphylaxis)

Clinical Insight

Surgical approaches to airway management should be the method of last resort to secure an airway. When attempting a tracheal intubation, you should have at least one alternative method available to secure the airway if you are unsuccessful. If the patient has been adequately sedated or paralyzed, digital intubation or a lighted-stylet intubation are alternative methods for performing a tracheal intubation. In other cases, an LMA, PtL, or Combitube should be attempted before a surgical airway is used.

these approaches. Such patients include those with anatomical distortion of the landmarks used for intubation (e.g., patients with prior head and neck surgery) and those with direct obstruction of upper airway structures (e.g., from infection or anaphylaxis).

In those patients where an emergency airway is indicated and tracheal intubation cannot be achieved, a surgical approach to securing an airway should be considered. An important consideration prior to attempting a surgical airway in the field is to consider whether a less invasive procedure (e.g., a bag-valve mask, PtL, Combitube, or LMA) can be used to effectively ventilate the patient. In general, surgical approaches are most successful when they are attempted in a controlled environment.

Note that the inclusion of surgical techniques in this text does not authorize their use by local providers. To use surgical techniques, the emergency care provider must have prior authorization by the local medical director.

With all surgical techniques, location of the cricothyroid membrane is critical to successful insertion. This membrane is located anteriorly between the lower thyroid cartilage (Adam's apple) and the cricoid ring (Figure 2-21). You can best locate the cricothyroid membrane by identifying the broad, flat thyroid cartilage. Palpate the superior portion of this structure to appreciate the thyroid notch. The notch is the most common site for misplacement of a surgical airway. Then, slide your fingers along the thyroid cartilage toward the patient's feet until you feel the first ring-like structure, which is the cricoid ring. The diamond-shaped recess lying above the superior portion of the ring is the cricothyroid membrane. You will appreciate this as a soft depression in the cartilage.

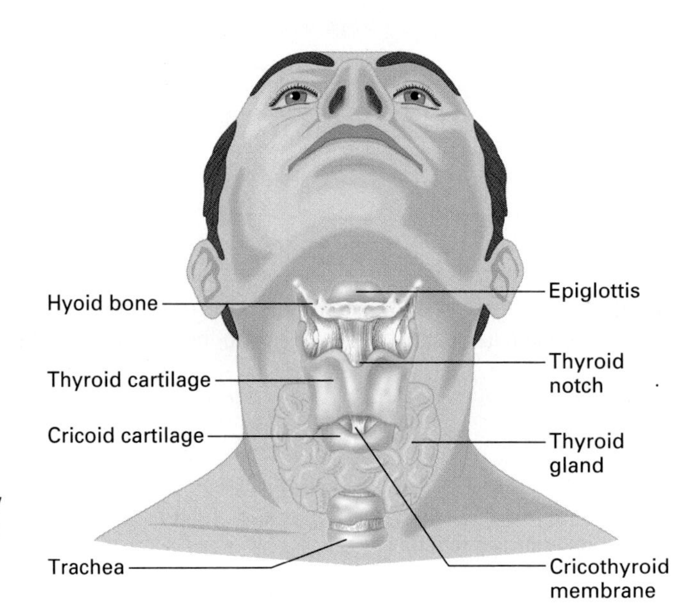

FIGURE 2-21
The cricothyroid membrane is located anteriorly between the lower thyroid cartilage (Adam's apple) and the cricoid ring.

Surgical Airway Techniques

Surgical techniques of airway control include

- Percutaneous transtracheal jet ventilation
- Retrograde intubation
- Surgical cricothyroidotomy

Percutaneous Transtracheal Jet Ventilation

Percutaneous transtracheal jet ventilation is a technique in which a catheter is inserted into the cricothyroid membrane and high-pressure oxygen is driven into the tracheobronchial tree. It should be remembered that this is only a temporary solution to airway management until a more definitive airway can be established. Although the patient can receive an adequate supply of oxygen with this technique, the success of percutaneous transtracheal ventilation is limited by the accumulation of carbon dioxide within the patient's body. Therefore, this method of ventilation may be used safely for only 30 to 45 minutes.

Oxygen is supplied to the patient with this technique via the 50-psi pressure port on the oxygen tank regulator. To allow this, the proximal end of a commercially manufactured jet ventilation tubing is threaded so it will securely attach to the threaded high-pressure port on the tank regulator. Additionally, the commercially manufacturerd oxygen tubing is reinforced so it is capable of handling the high pressure that is needed for this technique to work. Because of the high pressure required, it is recommended that the jet ventilation technique *not* be used if the commercially manufactured high-pressure ventilation equipment is not available. Only under an extreme emergency should an alternative to the commercial equipment be used to perform jet ventilation. This alternative is created by removing the BVM adapter from a 3.0-mm tracheal tube and using it as an interface between the IV catheter hub and the BVM. Ventilation could then be performed via the BVM, with oxygen flowing under slow but firm pressure. If exhalation difficulty is encountered, an additional 14- or 12-gauge needle can be placed beside the first one as an additional exhalation port.

It should be remembered that a patient younger than age 12 does not have complete circular support of the trachea. Consequently, a surgical cricothyroidotomy is not used in this age group; needle cricothyroidotomy is the emergency airway of choice in children younger than age 12.

The following equipment is needed for percutaneous transtracheal jet ventilation:

Antiseptic solution
14- or 12-gauge over-needle catheter
10-ml syringe
High-flow oxygen source
Oxygen tubing with connector and opening (Figure 2-22) or valve

Percutaneous transtracheal jet ventilation should be performed in the following manner (Figure 2-23).

1. Locate the cricothyroid membrane. Cleanse the skin on the neck overlying the cricothyroid membrane as much as practical.
2. Stabilize the skin using the thumb and the index finger of your nondominant hand. Advance the needle, with the syringe attached, into the lower half of the cricothyroid membrane at a 45-degree angle toward the feet.

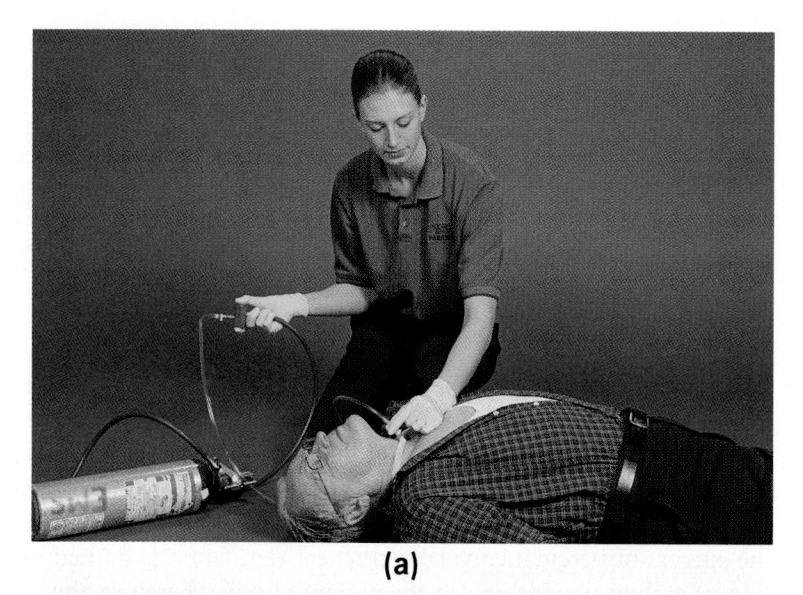

(a)

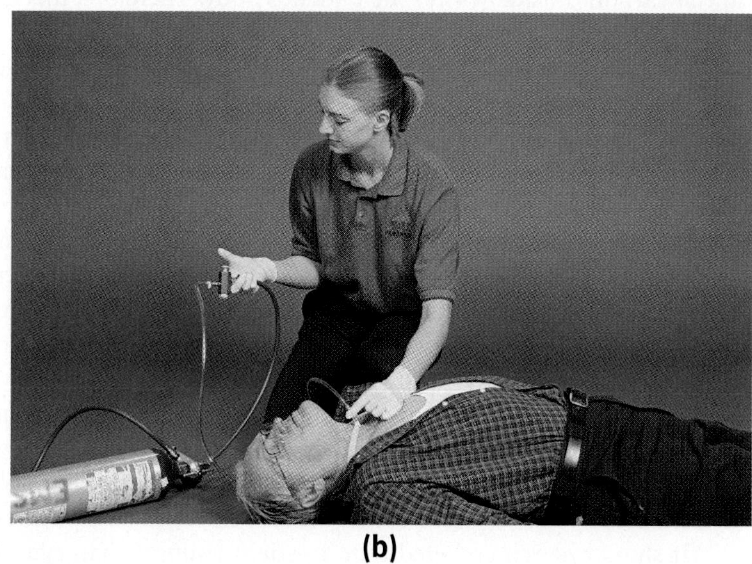

(b)

FIGURE 2-22
(a) Depress the trigger on the valve to allow insufflation. (b) Release the trigger to terminate insufflation.

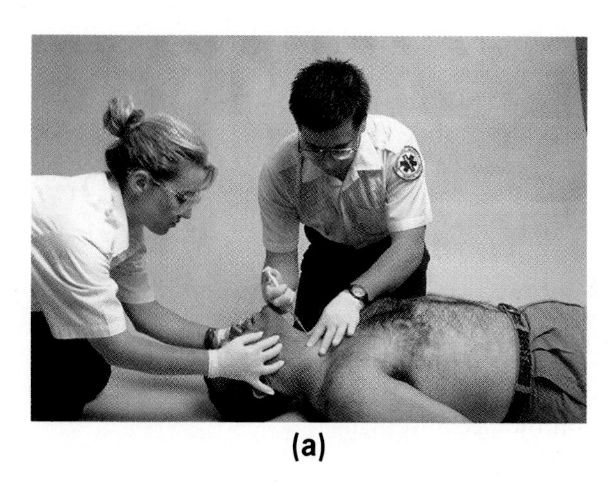

(a)

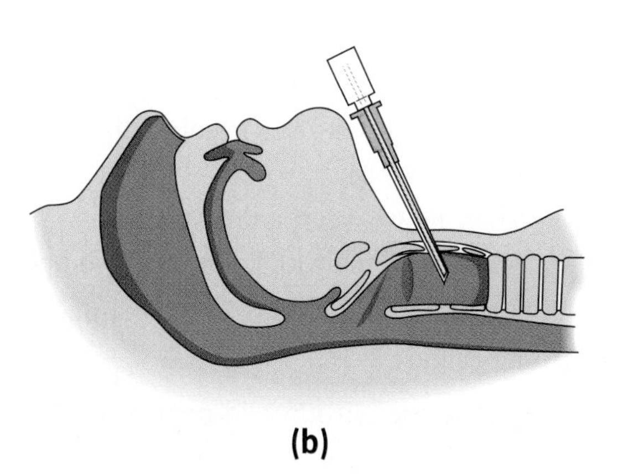

(b)

FIGURE 2-23 (a) To perform percutaneous transtracheal jet ventilation, insert the needle, with the syringe attached, into the lower half of the cricothyroid membrane at a 45° angle toward the feet. (b) The catheter properly placed through the cricothyroid membrane into the trachea.

3. Advance the catheter while applying negative pressure on the syringe. The drawing of air into the syringe signifies needle entry into the trachea.
4. Slide the catheter off the needle and advance it until the hub rests against the neck. Affix the catheter to the skin.
5. Attach the oxygen tubing to the hub. The other end of the tubing should be attached to a high-flow oxygen source.
6. Ventilate the patient by depressing the trigger on the valve of the jet ventilation tubing to direct oxygen into the trachea for 1 second. Release the trigger for a total of 2 seconds to allow exhalation. The chest wall should be seen to rise and fall symmetrically, and no swelling should be appreciated in the neck.

Complications of this technique include improper placement of the puncture, particularly into the thyroid notch. Puncturing the posterior wall of the trachea and extension into the esophagus have been reported. Although there are few major blood vessels in the area, severe hemorrhage and hematoma formation have been reported, occasionally leading to shock, infection, and airway compromise. The thyroid gland, which is just below the cricothyroid membrane, may be damaged during the procedure. Finally, air may be found in the soft tissues of the neck or in the mediastinum if the catheter tip is improperly placed in the subcutaneous tissues.

Retrograde Intubation

Retrograde intubation is a procedure in which a guidewire is passed, using a needle cricothyroidotomy, to direct an tracheal tube into proper position. This technique differs from a standard needle cricothyroidotomy in that the needle is directed toward the head, allowing the guidewire to pass from below the glottis into the mouth. The tracheal tube is then placed over the guidewire, guided into the trachea, and subsequently positioned. This technique is particularly useful in patients whose medical conditions result in a loss or distortion of the normal airway landmarks, such as patients with angioedema, severe burns, or surgical resection of the larynx.

The following equipment is needed for retrograde intubation:

Oxygen source
Bag-valve mask
Antiseptic solution
14- or 12-gauge over-needle catheter
10-ml syringe
Guidewire
Appropriately sized tracheal tube

Retrograde intubation should be performed in the following manner (Figures 2-24a–e):

1. Locate the cricothyroid membrane. Cleanse the skin on the neck overlying the cricothyroid membrane as much as practical.
2. Stabilize the skin using the thumb and the index finger of your nondominant hand. Advance the needle, with the syringe attached, into the lower half of the cricothyroid membrane at a 45-degree angle toward the head.
3. Advance the catheter while applying negative pressure on the syringe. The drawing of air into the syringe signifies needle entry into the trachea.
4. Slide the catheter off the needle and advance it until the hub rests against the neck.

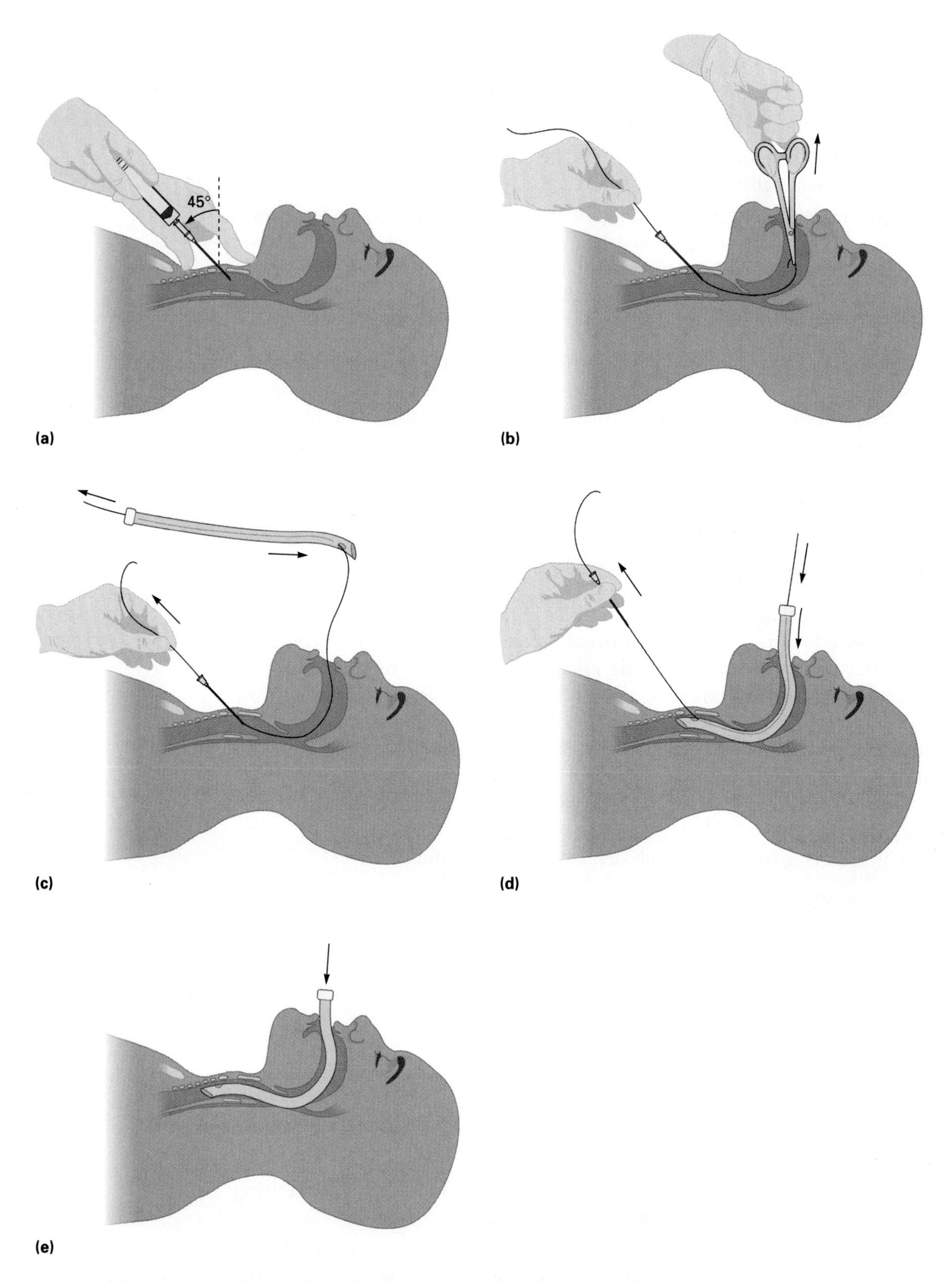

FIGURE 2-24 (a) Insert the needle, with the syringe attached, into the lower half of the cricothyroid membrane at a 45° angle toward the head. (b) Pass the wire through the needle into the oropharynx. Grasp the distal end of the wire and pull it out through the mouth. (c) Engage the wire with the end of the tracheal tube. (d) Pull the tracheal tube into position in the trachea. (e) Confirm proper tube placement.

5. Pass the wire through the catheter and continue to advance the wire, watching for it to appear in the patient's oropharynx. A J-wire should be used to prevent puncturing of soft tissues. It should measure at least 24 inches for ease of handling. Grasp the distal end of the wire (with a hemostat, if available), and pull it out through the mouth. Be sure to also hold the proximal end so the wire is not pulled completely through the catheter.
6. Then, place the distal end of the guidewire through the lumen of the tracheal tube or through the Murphy eye (small opening at the tip of the tracheal tube). While maintaining traction at both ends of the guidewire, slide the tube into the oropharynx along the guidewire until you meet resistance. At this point, the tip of the tracheal tube is resting below the glottis at the level of the cricothyroid membrane.
7. Withdraw the catheter and guidewire with one hand while applying slight downward pressure to the end of the tracheal tube. As you pull the guidewire beyond the end of the tracheal tube, there will be a decrease in resistance at the end of the tube, which will allow you to advance it into the trachea.
8. Confirm proper tube placement in a manner similar to that used for other methods of intubation.

Although there are no absolute contraindications to this technique, it requires a great deal of manual dexterity. The procedure may also be time consuming in inexperienced hands. It should be used only by those care providers who are trained in the technique and with approval of local medical direction.

The complications of this technique are similar to those listed for needle cricothyroidotomy. In addition, damage to the vocal cords and oropharynx are possible from the guidewire and tracheal tube.

Although there are no absolute contraindications to retrograde intubation, it requires a great deal of manual dexterity and may be time consuming in inexperienced hands.

Surgical Cricothyroidotomy

The technique of surgical cricothyroidotomy involves a direct incision of the cricothyroid membrane with subsequent passage of an appropriate airway. Although a tracheostomy tube can be used and several commercial cricothyroidotomy kits are available, placement of a standard tracheal tube through the incision is an acceptable method of securing an airway in the prehospital setting. Normally, the tube should be about one full size below the typical selection used for an orotracheal approach. This means that in an adult male, a size 7.0 is appropriate for placement through the cricothyroid incision, whereas a 6.0 or 6.5 should be used in an adult female.

Remember that a surgical incision in the neck is a very invasive solution to airway management that should be considered only after other measures have failed. The care provider should consider less invasive measures such as bag-valve-mask ventilation until a more controlled environment can be reached. However, if these measures do not succeed in providing appropriate ventilation, then a surgical cricothyroidotomy should be attempted, provided that this is within the provider's scope of practice as defined by local medical direction. A surgical airway should not be attempted in children younger than age 10 because the cricoid ring is the *only* circular support for pediatric patients.

The following equipment is needed for a surgical cricothyroidotomy:

Oxygen source
Bag-valve mask

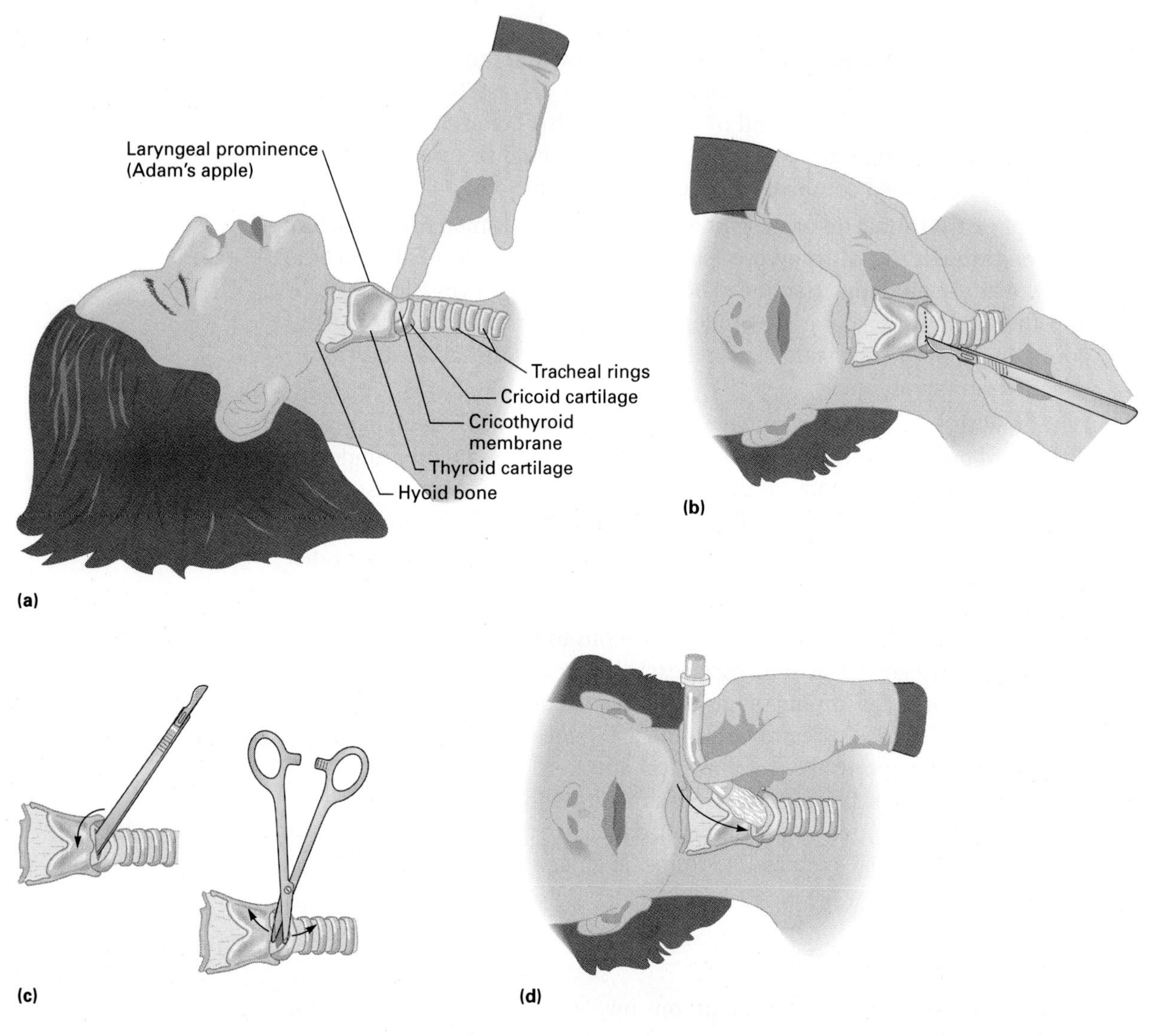

FIGURE 2-25
To perform a surgical cricothyroidotomy: (a) Locate the cricothyroid membrane. (b) Use a scalpel blade to puncture the cricothyroid membrane. (c) Use the scalpel handle or hemostat tips to open the incision. (d) Insert the tracheal tube through the incision into the trachea.

Antiseptic solution
Scalpel blade (#10 or #11)
Hemostats (optional)
Appropriately sized tracheal tube

A surgical cricothyroidotomy should be performed in the following manner (Figure 2-25):

1. Locate the cricothyroid membrane. Cleanse the skin on the neck overlying the cricothyroid membrane as much as practical.
2. Stabilize the skin using the thumb and the index finger of your nondominant hand. Make a 2-cm longitudinal incision through the skin over the cricothyroid membrane.
3. Use the scalpel blade to puncture directly through the cricothyroid membrane.

4. Use your little finger to maintain patency of the puncture. Insert the handle of the scalpel into the incision, and rotate the handle 90 degrees to open the incision. Alternatively, you can insert the tips of the hemostat into the incision and open them to provide access to the trachea.
5. Insert the tracheal tube into the trachea with the tip directed toward the feet. The tube should be inserted only 1 to 2 centimeters beyond the end of the balloon cuff. Alternatively, the tube may be shortened by cutting off the top few centimeters of the tube and reinserting the 15-mm adapter. This may make the tube easier to manage.
6. Inflate the cuff and stabilize the tube. Ventilate the patient using a standard ventilation bag.
7. Verify tube placement, using the methods described earlier.

Several commercially available kits use a needle cricothyroidotomy through which a guidewire and dilator are passed to expand the opening in the cricothyroid membrane. A tracheostomy tube is ultimately placed through this opening into the trachea.

The complications of surgical cricothyroidotomy are similar to those listed for needle cricothyroidotomy. Because a larger incision is made, hemorrhage and local infection can be significant problems with a surgical approach.

RAPID SEQUENCE INTUBATION

Emergency care providers must often secure a patent airway under the most difficult conditions. In the ideal situation, the intubation process would be undertaken in controlled conditions similar to those provided for patients undergoing elective surgery. Unfortunately, emergency patients have generally not been well prepared prior to intubation; specifically, it must be assumed that emergency patients have a full stomach prior to the procedure.

However, given these limitations, the intubation process can be somewhat controlled with the aid of drugs that produce a sedating and amnestic state (*induction*) and the addition of drugs that produce muscular paralysis (paralytic agents). This procedure is most commonly used when the patient has a clinical condition that requires emergent intubation (e.g., impending respiratory failure) but is too awake or combative to tolerate the procedure. This organized sequence of induction and paralysis is commonly referred to as a *rapid sequence intubation.*

induction the introduction of drugs that produce sedation and amnesia.

rapid sequence intubation an organized sequence of induction and paralysis used to aid and control an invasive procedure such as intubation.

It must be immediately noted that, in terms of prehospital airway control, this process is far from rapid. In fact, proper performance of the procedure requires precise timing and a deliberate attention to details. Often, this procedure takes significantly more time than standard intubation procedures.

Prior to undertaking a rapid sequence intubation, you should anticipate any difficulties. If possible, ask the patient about previous intubation procedures and complications with anesthetic or sedative agents. Physical findings that also suggest a difficult intubation include a short, thick neck, prominent central incisors, a small mandible, limited motion of the jaw or neck, or previous surgical or traumatic alteration of the anatomy.

You should be able to place three fingers between the prominence of the mandible and the hyoid bone (Figure 2-26). Ask the patient to open his mouth. Ideally, the entire posterior pharynx, tonsils, and uvula will be visible (Figure 2-27). Complete inability to see these structures predicts that the intubation will be

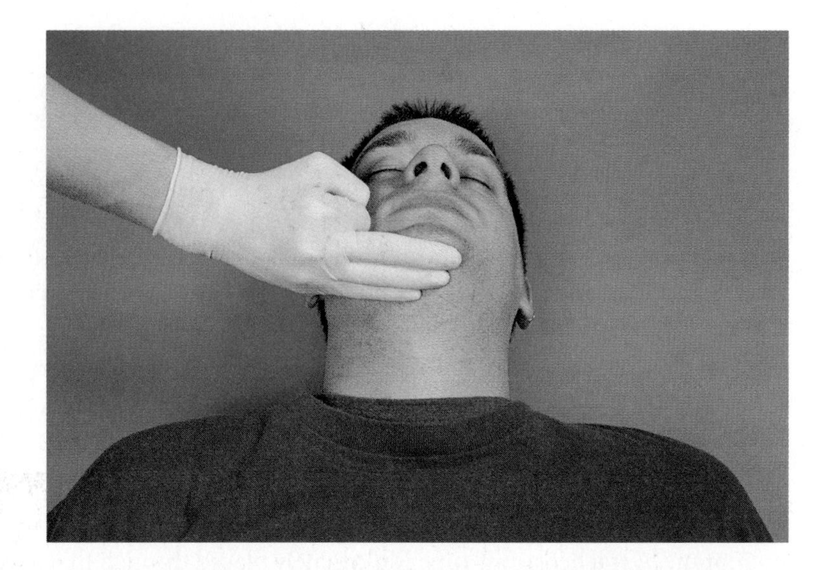

FIGURE 2-26
To perform a rapid sequence intubation without difficulty, you should be able to place three fingers between the prominence of the mandible and the hyoid bone.

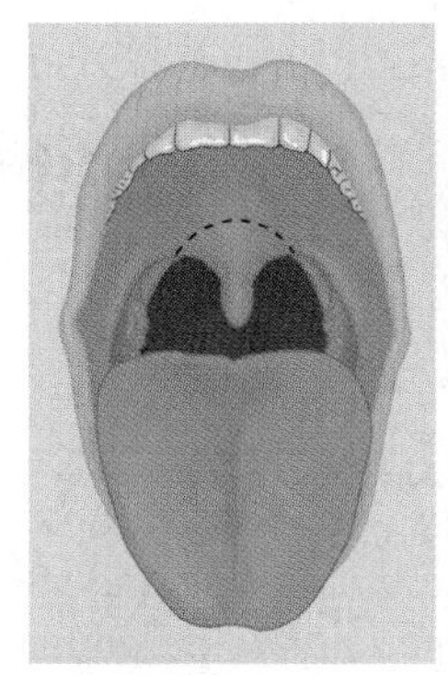

Soft palate, uvula, fauces, pillars visible

No difficulty

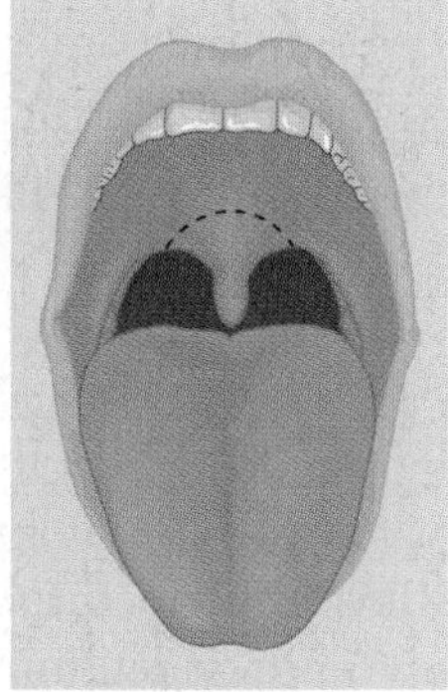

Soft palate, uvula, fauces visible

No difficulty

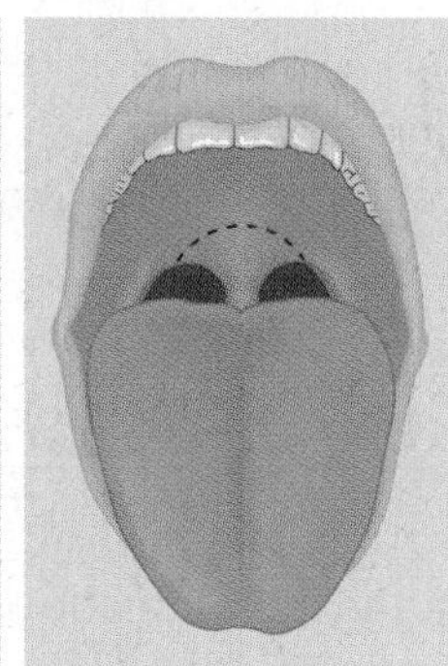

Soft palate, base of uvula visible

Moderate difficulty

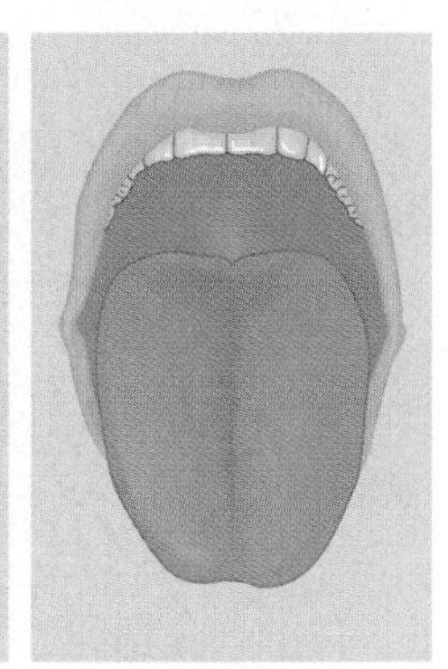

Hard palate only visible

Severe difficulty

FIGURE 2-27
Before performing a rapid sequence induction, ask the patient to open his mouth. Ideally, the entire posterior pharynx, tonsils, and uvula will be visible.

difficult, and an alternative method (e.g., blind nasotracheal or retrograde approach) should be considered.

Additionally, prehospital protocols for rapid sequence intubation including a trial of a few breaths using bag-valve-mask ventilation is imperative prior to attempting a rapid sequence intubation. Remember that if a paralytic agent is administered and the attempt should fail, assisted ventilation must be carried out until the effects of the paralytic agent are gone and spontaneous ventilatory effort returns.

General Procedure

An overall outline of rapid sequence intubation is presented in the following paragraphs. The specific medications used during the procedure will vary according to local protocol. It must again be emphasized that preparation prior to the procedure and adequate personnel are the keys to a successful rapid sequence intubation.

1. The procedure begins with early preparation of all materials. An appropriately sized tracheal tube with an intact balloon cuff should be available. A working laryngoscope and suction equipment should also be ready. Finally, any medications used in the procedure are drawn up and accessible for immediate administration.

2. Hyperoxygenate the patient for approximately 3 to 5 minutes. This will allow the patient to maintain an adequate oxygen saturation during the procedure without ventilatory assistance by filling the lungs with 100 percent oxygen. Place the spontaneously breathing patient on high-flow, high-concentration oxygen by nonrebreather mask. Do not attempt to assist the patient's breathing if ventilation is adequate because this increases the risk of gastric distention and subsequent aspiration. If, however, the patient does not have an adequate ventilatory effort, assist ventilations using a bag-valve-mask device with 100 percent oxygen. Cricoid pressure should be applied if bag-valve-mask ventilation is required. Once applied, cricoid pressure should not be removed until the airway is secured.
3. Closely monitor the patient throughout the procedure. At a minimum, perform cardiac monitoring. Closely observe the patient's level of consciousness and spontaneous movements throughout the procedure. Finally, obtain and document continuous pulse oximetry readings, if available.
4. There are several medications you may administer before initiating the procedure in order to protect against side effects that are associated with the rapid sequence intubation technique. These include the following:
   a. Atropine may be administered to prevent bradycardia that develops with the use of certain paralytic medications and is associated with the intubation procedure. This drug is particularly useful in pediatric patients where a dose of 0.02 mg/kg is given (minimum dose of 0.1 mg). The adult dose is 0.5 to 1.0 mg IV, which is administered 3 minutes before the procedure.
   b. Lidocaine may be administered to prevent the rise in intracranial pressure that is associated with the use of succinylcholine and the intubation procedure itself. A dose of 1.0 to 1.5 mg/kg IV is given several minutes before the procedure.
   c. A "defasciculating" dose of a nondepolarizing paralytic agent may be administered if succinylcholine is used. (Fasciculations are fine musucular movements that occur following administration of succinylcholine.) The dose is typically one-tenth of the normal intravenous dose of the chosen agent. As an example, a defasciculating dose of vecuronium is 1 mg; a normal paralyzing dose is approximately 10 mg IV push.
5. Then, administer a sedative/hypnotic agent in order to produce a state of sedation and facilitate the procedure. Ideally, this medication also results in a state of amnesia for the procedure. Several agents are available and should be chosen based on the training of the provider and clinical condition of the patient.
6. As the patient becomes sedated, cricoid pressure should be applied to prevent aspiration and to assist the intubation procedure. A few bag-valve ventilations should be given to assess ability to provide rescue ventilation. Further ventilations with a bag-valve mask should be administered only if oxygen saturation drops to less than 90 percent.
7. Next, administer a paralyzing agent until a state of complete muscular relaxation is achieved.
8. With cricoid pressure continued, carry out orotracheal intubation as quickly and carefully as possible. Confirm tube placement, using the standard methods described previously, and inflate the tracheal tube cuff. Only then should cricoid pressure be released. Finally, secure the tube in place.
9. Additional sedation and paralysis of the patient should be based on local protocol.

Sedative Agents

Several pharmacologic agents can be chosen to produce a state of sedation prior to paralyzing a patient for intubation. The agents vary in their ability to produce an appropriate level of sedation. Other properties of these medications include analgesia (pain relief) and amnesia (inability to recall the procedure). These agents should be used in conjunction with paralytic medications. Keep in mind that many of these agents have shorter duration of action than the paralytic agents. Therefore, multiple doses must be administered while the patient remains paralyzed. Some of the more common agents used to produce sedation are listed as follows.

Midazolam Midazolam is a short-acting benzodiazepine medication that produces both sedation and amnesia. In addition, the drug reduces anxiety associated with the procedure (anxiolysis). The drug has no analgesic properties. The usual induction dose of midazolam is 0.1 mg/kg IV, with a typical adult dose of 5 to 10 mg. Older patients are particularly sensitive to the drug. The drug has an onset of action of 60 to 90 seconds and a duration of action of approximately 30 minutes. In addition to significant respiratory depression, midazolam can cause significant hypotension. Diazepam (Valium) can be used in doses of 0.2 mg/kg, but it has both a longer onset and a longer duration of action. Other disadvantages of diazepam include pain on intravenous injection and prolongation of the effects of neuromuscular blocking agents.

Thiopental Thiopental is an ultra-short-acting barbiturate medication. These drugs produce sedation, but do not have analgesic or amnestic properties. The typical dose of thiopental is 3 to 5 mg/kg. The onset of action is within 30 seconds of administration, with a duration of action of 5 to 10 minutes as the drug is redistributed from the brain to other tissues. As with the benzodiazepines, thiopental can produce both respiratory depression and hypotension. The drug should be used with extreme caution in patients with decreased circulating volume and hypertension because it has a profound effect on blood pressure in these patients. In addition, the drug may cause laryngospasm. Finally, an exaggerated vagal response along with increased mucous secretions have been noted with this agent. As a result, the drug should be used cautiously in patients with airway obstruction, severe cardiac disease, and asthma.

Methohexital Methohexital is a rapid-acting barbiturate. It has similar actions to thiopental, and both drugs have the potential advantage of reducing intracranial pressure. The drug has no analgesic properties. The dose of methohexital is 0.75 to 1.5 mg/kg IV. Pain may be noted at the injection site. The onset of action is 30 to 45 seconds (approximately one arm-to-brain circulation) with a duration of action of 2 to 4 minutes, although there are some effects of the drug that last for hours after administration. The complications are similar to those of thiopental.

Propofol Propofol is a rapid-acting phenol that can be used to produce rapid anesthesia. Like methohexital, the onset of the drug is rapid (15 to 30 seconds). Recovery is rapid following intravenous injection. Disadvantages of the drug include pain on injection, profound cardiac depression (particularly in the elderly or in hypertensive patients in whom the drug is rapidly injected). The drug is given at a total dose of 2.0 to 2.5 mg/kg in adults, typically given 40 mg every 10 seconds to effect. The dose should be reduced by one-half in the elderly. A continuous infusion can be used for long-term sedation.

Fentanyl Fentanyl is an opioid narcotic that is 100 times more potent than morphine. The drug can produce a state of sedation and also has potent analgesic effects. A typical sedating dose is 3 to 5 μg/kg. This produces an effect within approximately 90 seconds that has a duration of action of 30 to 40 minutes. As with other sedating agents, hypotension can occur, although its cardiovascular effects are minimal. With fentanyl, hypotension is typically caused by parasympathetic-induced bradycardia. At higher doses, muscular rigidity (particularly of chest muscles) can be produced, especially with rapid administration. Fentanyl is not as useful as other agents in this setting because of the longer time to onset of action and the variable effect of the drug at the dose cited.

Fentanyl is not as useful as other agents in the prehospital setting because of the longer time to onset of action and the variable effect of the drug at the dose cited.

Ketamine Ketamine is a drug chemically related to PCP that produces a state called dissociative anesthesia. This drug has sedative, analgesic, and amnestic properties. The drug can cause an increase in heart rate and in myocardial oxygen demand, so it should be used cautiously in patients with severe coronary artery disease. Ketamine can also produce bizarre hallucinations, which can be prevented by administering a benzodiazepine along with this agent. However, the hemodynamic and respiratory effects of the drug are few. In particular, it can be administered safely to patients who are mildly hypotensive. Ketamine also causes bronchodilation, making it useful in intubating patients with reactive airway disease. The dose is 1 to 2 mg/kg IV, which produces an effect within 60 seconds. The duration of action is 10 to 15 minutes. Ketamine does not depress protective airway reflexes and, as a result, laryngospasm can occur with intubation attempts using this drug.

Etomidate Etomidate is a nonbarbiturate sedative/hypnotic agent. The drug is useful because of its rapid onset, duration of action, and limited side effects. The drug is administered at a dose of 0.3 to 0.6 mg/kg IV. There may be pain noted at the injection site. The drug has a peak duration of action at 2 to 4 minutes. Jerking of the muscles (myoclonus) may be noted after the drug has been given. The patient may also experience nausea and vomiting after use of the drug. Repeated doses of the drug may be given safely without evidence of cumulative effects.

Clinical Insight

Etomidate is an excellent choice as an induction agent for a rapid sequence intubation. It has a rapid onset and short duration of action. Additionally, it has neuroprotective effects and virtually no effect on the cardiovascular system, unlike the other induction agents listed. Finally, it does not depress the patient's respirations and may produce intubating conditions without the need for a paralyzing drug.

Neuromuscular Blockade

The major agent used to achieve a successful intubation with a rapid sequence technique is a paralyzing medication. To understand the various medications and their consequences, you must understand the basics of transmission at the *motor endplate* (Figure 2-28). The motor endplate is the point at which the nerve and muscle interact so the nerve impulse is converted into a muscular contraction.

For a muscular contraction to occur, an impulse must be conducted down the nerve to the motor endplate. When the impulse reaches the endplate, stored *acetylcholine* (a chemical messenger) is released and diffuses across to receptors on the muscle side of the motor endplate. The binding of acetylcholine to the appropriate receptors creates an electrical change along the muscle cell that, in turn, leads to chemical changes within the muscle cell that result in muscular contraction. It is important to note that acetylcholine acts as a chemical messenger for both the sympathetic and parasympathetic nervous systems.

motor endplate the point at which nerve and muscle interact.

acetylcholine chemical, released when a nerve impulse reaches the motor endplate, that binds to receptors on the muscle cells, creating electrical and chemical changes that result in muscle contraction.

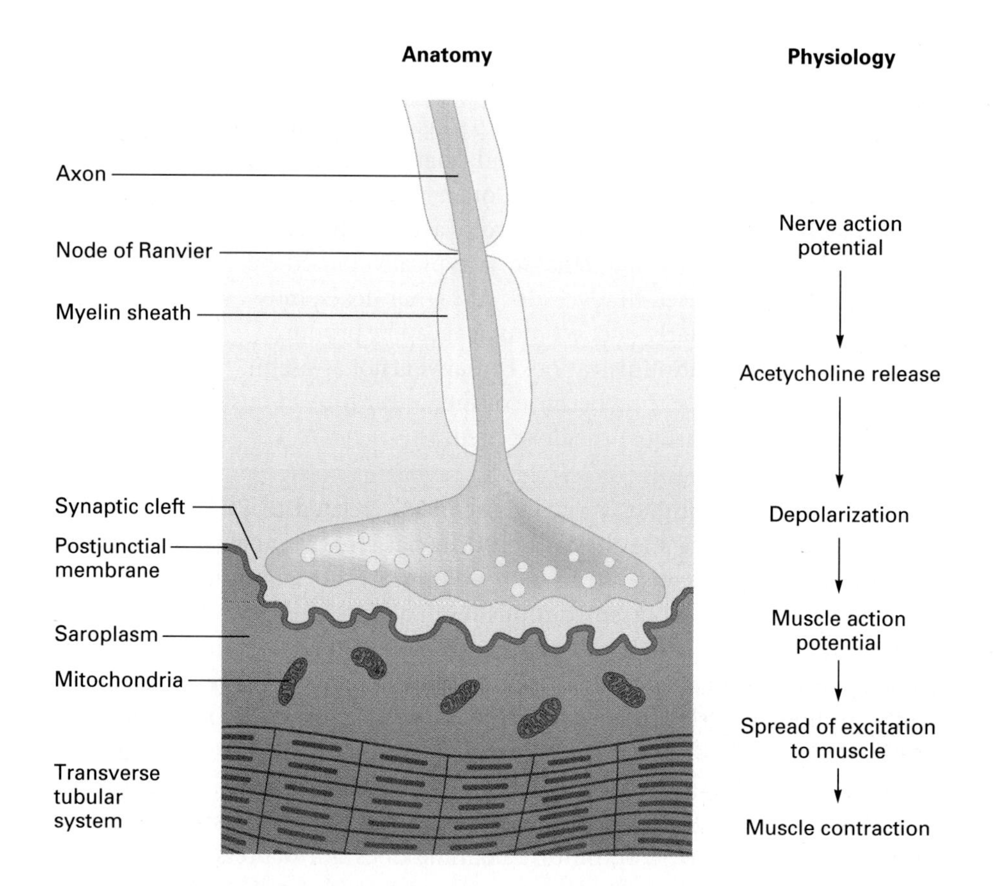

FIGURE 2-28
The motor endplate is the point at which the nerve and muscle interact.

depolarizing agents paralytic agents chemically similar to acetylcholine that bind to muscle receptor sites, cause muscle contraction, and then continue to occupy the receptor sites, preventing further contraction.

Paralytic agents produce their effects in one of two ways: as depolarizing agents or as nondepolarizing agents. *Depolarizing agents* are chemically similar to acetylcholine and act by binding to the receptor sites, causing a spontaneous contraction of all muscles. The receptor sites then remain occupied by the depolarizing agent and are thus unable to produce any further contractions. Succinylcholine, which is structurally two acetylcholine molecules bound together, is the only clinically available depolarizing agent.

Nondepolarizing agents also combine with the acetylcholine receptors on the muscle cells. However, no chemical changes occur at these sites and, as a result, no depolarization occurs. Instead, there is an inability to generate any muscular contractions because the receptor sites are now occupied by the nondepolarizing drug. There are many available nondepolarizing agents, which vary in their onset, duration of action, and associated side effects.

Depolarizing Agents

Succinylcholine As noted earlier, succinylcholine acts by causing widespread contractions of the muscles and remaining chemically bound to the motor endplate receptors. Clinically, these contractions are manifest by fasciculations, which are weak, disorganized contractions of various muscles. Bound succinylcholine makes the muscles unresponsive to acetylcholine released at the nerve ending until the drug is metabolized. The enzyme responsible for breakdown of succinylcholine is called pseudocholinesterase.

The standard adult dose of succinylcholine is 1.5 mg/kg IV push. It has an onset of action of 30 to 60 seconds. The duration of its effect is from 3 to 10 minutes. The rapid onset and short duration of action make succinylcholine nearly ideal for use in a rapid sequence intubation. If the patient cannot be successfully intubated, ventilation need only be supported for about 10 minutes before spontaneous respirations recover.

Succinylcholine has some important side effects that must be considered in patient selection. The drug can cause an elevation in the serum potassium level. This is a particular concern in patients with existing elevation in their potassium levels (e.g., chronic renal failure patients), as well as in patients with neuromuscular disorders (Guillain–Barré syndrome, stroke, myasthenia gravis) or extensive tissue injury (e.g., from major trauma, burns, muscular diseases, sepsis, and tetanus). In the latter group, potassium elevation is noted only after days of injury; therefore, succinylcholine can be used in early airway management of these patients.

Succinylcholine causes a rise in intracranial, intragastric, and intraocular pressure. In head-injured patients, pretreatment with lidocaine may prevent the unwanted rise in intracranial pressure. Cricoid pressure is used during the rapid sequence intubation to prevent any harmful effects of a rising intragastric pressure.

Finally, because acetylcholine acts at many sites in the sympathetic and parasympathetic nervous systems, a variety of effects can be seen, including bradycardia, tachycardia, hypertension, and cardiac dysrhythmias. Bradycardia can be prevented by pretreatment of the patient with atropine.

Nondepolarizing Agents

Vecuronium Vecuronium is an intermediate-acting nondepolarizing agent. At a dose of 0.1 mg/kg, vecuronium has an onset of action of approximately 1 minute with a peak effect in 3 to 5 minutes. Vecuronium has a duration of action of 30 to 45 minutes. The duration of action may be prolonged in hypothermic patients. In general, vecuronium is free of many side effects.

Pancuronium Pancuronium is a long-acting nondepolarizing agent. An administered dose of 0.04 to 0.1 mg/kg produces paralysis in 2 to 3 minutes, with a duration of effect of 60 to 75 minutes. Increases in heart rate and hypertension have been seen with the use of pancuronium. Histamine release, which is a significant problem with other nondepolarizing agents and is manifest by hypotension and flushed skin, is not prominent with the use of pancuronium. However, because of its long duration of action and relatively long onset of action, it is more commonly used in maintaining paralysis than as a primary paralyzing agent in a rapid sequence intubation.

Rocuronium Rocuronium is a short-acting nondepolarizing agent. At a dose of 0.6 to 1.2 mg/kg, rocuronium has an onset of action of approximately 1 minute with a peak effect in 2 to 3 minutes. Rocuronium has a duration of action of 20 to 30 minutes. Like vecuronium, rocuronium has few side effects. The drug should be used with caution in patients with liver disease and obesity.

It should be noted that this is not a conclusive list of all drugs used for rapid sequence intubation; new drugs are being introduced constantly. You should refer to emergency medicine or anesthesia texts for a more complete discussion of these medications.

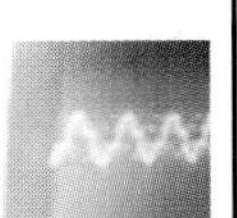

GUIDELINES FOR AIRWAY AND VENTILATION SUPPORT

Patient Assessment

To assess and manage a patient's airway and ventilation, you should always take an organized approach, working from the most basic to the more complex methods of airway and ventilatory support (Figure 2-29). Constant reassessment of the patient

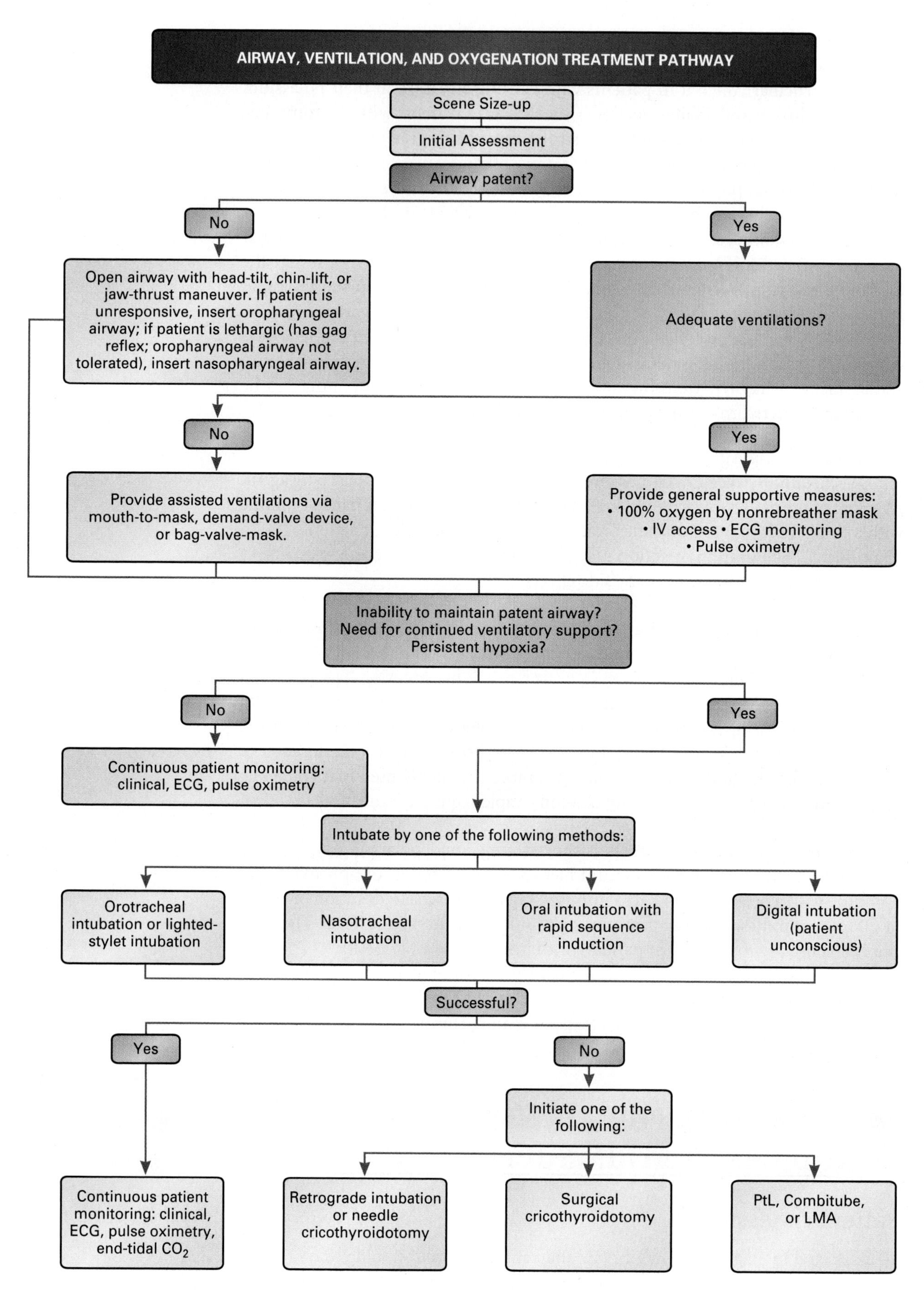

FIGURE 2-29
Airway, ventilation, and oxygenation treatment pathway.

is imperative because the airway needs and degree of ventilatory assistance required may vary based on a changing clinical condition. Finally, you must also consider any limitations placed on your scope of practice as defined by local medical direction.

Always take an organized approach to airway and ventilatory support, working from the most basic to the more complex methods.

The first question to be considered is: Does the patient have a patent airway? If there is any evidence of upper airway obstruction, the initial approach should involve either a head-tilt, chin-lift or a jaw-thrust maneuver (if trauma is suspected) to support the airway. If the patient is unconscious, then an oropharyngeal airway is used to provide continuing airway support; in the lethargic patient, a nasopharyngeal airway is better tolerated. Patients who require continued airway support are candidates for tracheal intubation.

The next consideration is: Does the patient have an adequate ventilatory effort? Is there evidence of respiratory failure? Patients who are unable to support their ventilatory needs will require assisted ventilation. Noninvasive methods of ventilation, such as continuous positive airway pressure (CPAP) ventilation, should be considered. (See Chapter 5, Dyspnea.) As stated earlier, the selection of the appropriate support will be based on the equipment available, the skills of the rescuer, and the needs of the patient. Mouth-to-mask, demand-valve ventilation, or bag-valve-mask ventilation should be considered. Here again, if the patient requires a prolonged period of assisted ventilation, tracheal intubation must be considered.

One final consideration is the need for oxygen supplementation. *Does the patient appear hypoxic or have a clinical condition such as shock or chest pain that will require oxygen supplementation?* Any patient who requires oxygen supplementation should receive as close to 100 percent inspired oxygen as possible. Spontaneously breathing patients should be placed on a nonrebreather mask. Patients who are being assisted with a bag-valve mask should have a reservoir attached to the ventilation device to assure near 100 percent inspired oxygen.

Continued patient assessment should be performed using clinical indicators, cardiac monitoring, and pulse oximetry. Any patient who requires continued airway support, who remains hypoxic, or who demonstrates persistent ventilatory failure should have a definitive airway established. Orotracheal intubation is the generally accepted standard for airway control. However, depending on the condition of the patient, the skills of the rescuer, and the scope of practice authorized by medical direction, nasotracheal intubation or orotracheal intubation using a rapid sequence intubation technique are appropriate alternatives. In the unconscious patient, lighted-stylet or digital intubation should be considered.

If difficulties are encountered, alternative airways such as the PtL or Combitube should be considered. Finally, if there are anatomical limitations, or if an airway cannot be established using any of the previously mentioned methods, a surgical approach (surgical cricothyroidotomy or needle cricothyroidotomy) should be considered if authorized by medical direction.

Patient Monitoring

In addressing a patient's airway and ventilation, we must remember that we are manipulating some of the body's most basic functions. This will often produce a response in the patient, usually involving the sympathetic and parasympathetic nervous system. As a result, it is important that the patient be closely monitored when any airway maneuver or ventilation technique is used.

The following parameters should be continuously monitored in any patient who is having interventions involving the airway or ventilation: patient condition,

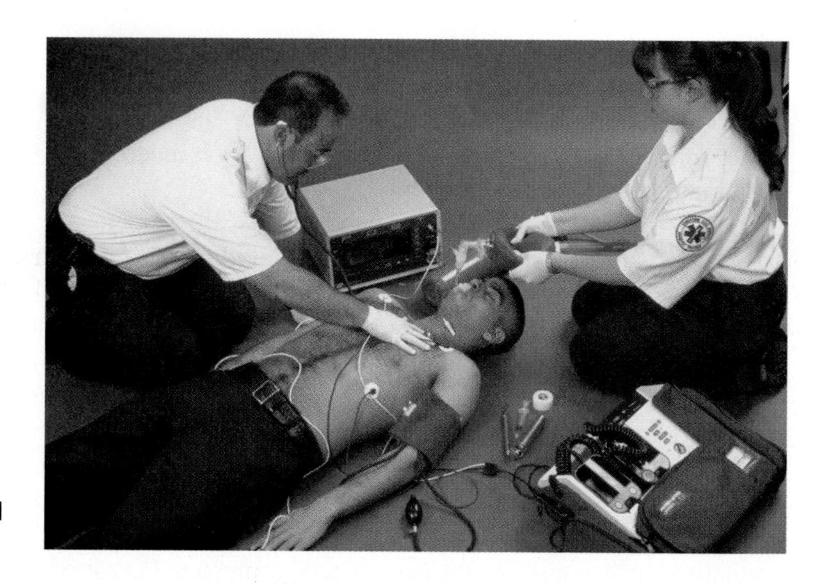

FIGURE 2-30
Intubated patient with cardiac monitor, oximetry, blood pressure measurement, and capnography.

cardiac monitoring, blood oxygenation, blood pressure evaluation, and, if the patient is intubated, capnometry or capnography (Figure 2-30).

Patient Observation

Clinical observation of the patient is extremely important. Often, emergency care personnel are guilty of using technology such as cardiac monitoring, pulse oximetry, and capnometry or capnography as a substitute for sound clinical skills.

For any patient who requires an airway intervention, frequently assess the level of consciousness, as well as the skin color and mucous membranes, for signs of hypoxia.

For any patient who requires an airway intervention, frequently assess the level of consciousness, as well as the skin color and mucous membranes, for signs of hypoxia. Patients should become more alert and calm after an airway intervention as oxygen is delivered to the brain. If, however, the patient becomes less responsive or more agitated with intervention, problems with the delivery of oxygen to the patient must be considered. The skin and mucous membranes should be carefully observed for signs of adequate oxygenation. The presence of cyanosis, particularly in the mucous membranes around the mouth, suggest inadequate oxygenation.

For patients who are receiving assisted ventilations, continually observe the chest wall for an adequate rise and fall with each ventilation. If a mask is used, assess the effectiveness of the seal and depth of ventilations. In addition, consider the ease of ventilation, which reflects both peak airway pressure and lung compliance. The patient should demonstrate the signs of appropriate oxygenation suggested previously.

Cardiac Monitoring

An additional component of patient assessment is continuous cardiac monitoring (Figure 2-31). Patients who require supplemental oxygen are at risk of developing hypoxia. Among the early signs of hypoxia are cardiac rhythm disturbances, including tachycardia and bradycardia, as well as premature atrial and ventricular beats. Ventricular tachycardia, ventricular fibrillation, pulseless electrical activity, and asystole are rhythms that develop with profound hypoxia.

Another important argument for continuous cardiac monitoring is the fact that any manipulation of the patient's airway produces strong autonomic (parasympathetic and sympathetic) responses from the body. Tachycardic rhythms and bradycardia can develop with instrumentation of the upper airway. In addition, the patient's blood pressure can show significant changes during the procedure.

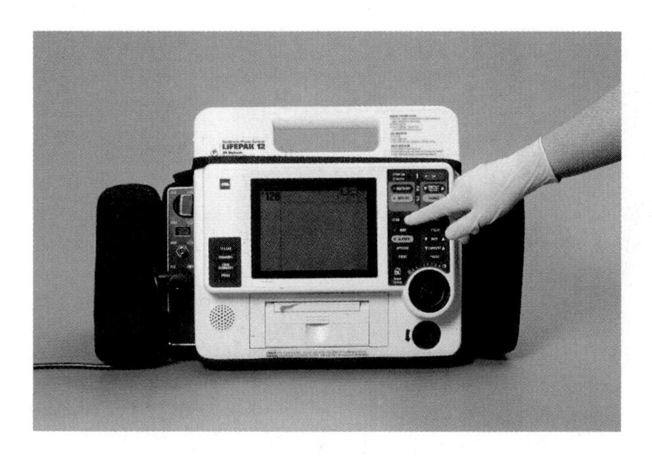

FIGURE 2-31
Cardiac monitor.

If a significant bradycardic response develops, consider administration of atropine 0.5 to 1.0 mg IV prior to further attempts at airway manipulation.

Pulse Oximetry

Pulse oximetry (Figure 2-32) is useful for providing a continuous measurement of blood oxygenation. Specifically, pulse oximetry measures the amount of bound hemoglobin. (Remember that hemoglobin is the blood protein responsible for oxygen transport.)

With pulse oximetry, the oxygen saturation is determined by evaluating the different absorption of oxygenated and deoxygenated arterial blood measured at two different wavelengths (red and infrared light). The difference in the absorption of light at these two wavelengths can be converted to a saturation reading. In addition to emitting the appropriate wavelength of light and detecting absorption, the oximetry probe also detects arterial pulsation. A properly functioning probe gives an instantaneous measurement of the patient's heart rate and can be compared to the cardiac monitor to determine if the probe is functioning accurately. Appropriate signal detection also gives an indication of adequate tissue perfusion.

A variety of pulse oximetry products are available. The probes can be mechanically attached to the fingers or toes or applied by adhesive to these areas. Additionally, the nose and earlobes have been used.

Keep in mind that pulse oximetry has several limitations. For example, a drop in the oxygen saturation will lag behind the withdrawal of oxygen by 30 to 60 seconds. Therefore, you must still carefully monitor the oxygen source while you are administering supplemental oxygen to a patient. Also, pulse oximetry readings are difficult to obtain in patients who are hypotensive, have poor peripheral perfusion, or who are cold. Finally, other gases, most notably carbon monoxide, have the same absorptive

Clinical Insight

Remember that hemoglobin containing bound carbon monoxide has similar absorptive properties as oxyhemoglobin. Therefore, a patient with significant carbon monoxide poisoning may appear to have normal oxygen saturations as measured by pulse oximetry. As a result, pulse oximetry is not useful in determining oxygen saturation or the response to oxygen therapy in carbon monoxide poisonings.

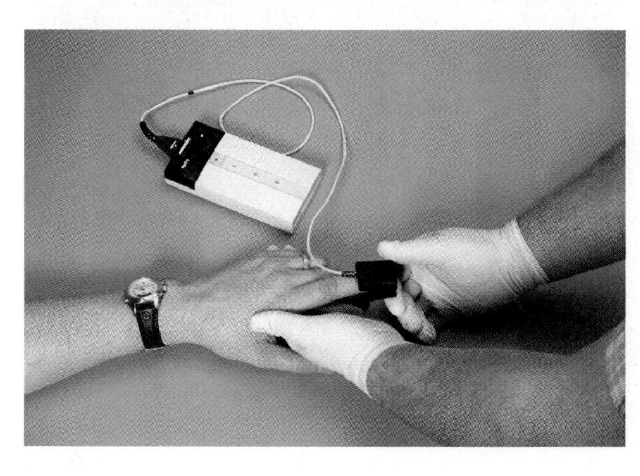

FIGURE 2-32
Pulse oximeter.

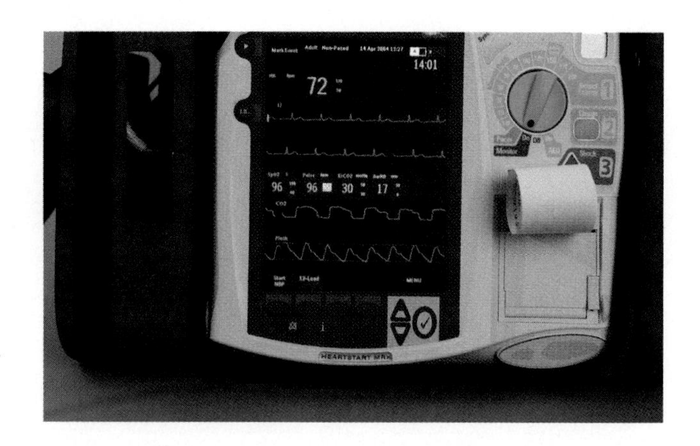

FIGURE 2-33
Quantitative electronic end-tidal CO_2 detector.
(Scott Metcalfe)

properties as oxygen when bound to hemoglobin. Therefore, patients with significant carbon monoxide poisoning will display falsely high oxygen saturation readings.

Also keep in mind that oxygen saturation readings give little information about the ventilatory status of the patient. Clinical evidence of hypoventilation, such as low respiratory rate, decreased tidal volume, and lethargy, should be evaluated. Other adjuncts such as capnography may be helpful.

Capnography/Capnometry

Capnography is the determination of carbon dioxide (CO_2) levels during the phases of ventilation. Although some products display a continual tracing of CO_2 levels (capnograph), the most commonly used units display only a numerical value (capnometry) of the CO_2 reading at the end of each breath (end-tidal CO_2) (Figure 2-33).

The level of CO_2 is determined by an adapter, placed in the ventilation circuit, which emits infrared light. CO_2 levels are determined by absorption of a specific wavelength of light. Alternatively, some disposable CO_2 detectors take advantage of a color change that is caused by expired CO_2. As a rule, the level of CO_2 measured by capnometry is approximately 2 to 5 torr lower than the level in arterial blood, but wide patient-to-patient variability exists.

Continuous end-tidal CO_2 measurements are useful as a measure of the adequacy of ventilation (Figure 2-34). This is particularly true in patients who have undergone tracheal intubation. In addition, the presence of end-tidal CO_2 reflects appropriate placement of the tracheal tube in the trachea. Many systems require a measurement of end-tidal CO_2 after tracheal tube placement as a method to confirm appropriate tube placement.

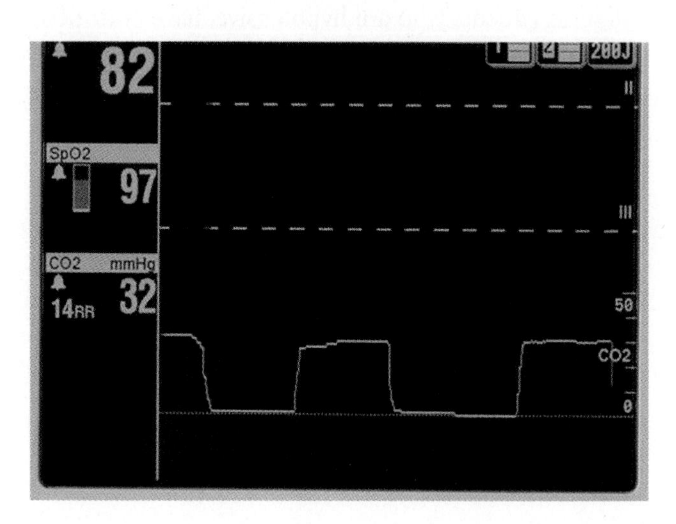

FIGURE 2-34
Continuous waveform capnography.
(Scott Metcalfe)

SUMMARY

Assuring adequate oxygenation and appropriate ventilation are the first priorities you must address in any patient with medical illness.

Patients with depressed mental status, structural airway problems, or inadequate ventilation will require support to maintain an open airway and appropriate ventilation. The methods available to assure an adequate airway and ventilation include manual airway maneuvers, mechanical airway adjuncts, and tracheal intubation.

Although orotracheal intubation remains the ideal method of providing definitive airway and ventilatory support, a variety of alternatives exist, including nasotracheal intubation, digital intubation, lighted-stylet intubation, and several surgical airway approaches. For those situations in which definitive intubation is not possible, options such as the PtL, Combitube, or LMA can assist in airway support.

Patients who require such support should be monitored carefully by using repeated clinical observation, cardiac monitoring, and continuous pulse oximetry. Capnometry or capnography is useful for patients who require tracheal intubation.

SCENARIO FOLLOW-UP

A man reports that he found his wife unconscious beside an open bottle of sleeping pills and a fifth of Scotch. As you approach this unresponsive patient, you continue to assess the area for any immediate hazards. You put on your gloves, mask, and eye shield because it is clear that the patient will require immediate airway intervention and ventilatory support. Noting that there does not appear to be any evidence of direct trauma, you perform an immediate head-tilt, chin-lift maneuver as you instruct your partner to bring the airway supplies and suction to the patient's side.

You quickly clear the oropharynx of larger food particles, sweeping with your fingers, then use a tonsil tip catheter to clear the upper airway. There is minimal response by the patient to these maneuvers, and the patient's skin color and respiratory rate fail to improve. After your partner returns with a bag-valve-mask device and an oxygen source, you begin two-person bag-valve-mask ventilation. A third rescuer applies a cardiac monitor and pulse oximeter. The patient's heart rate increases from 50 to 80 beats per minute with ventilation, and the pulse oximetry improves from 80 to 96 percent saturation. However, the patient's mental status and respiratory rate do not improve. You deduce that the patient will require prolonged ventilatory and airway support and decide that tracheal intubation is immediately indicated.

Although you believe that a standard orotracheal intubation would be best, the amount of vomitus and secretions in the oropharynx are likely to make this difficult. The patient does have some reflexive movement of the mouth; thus, a digital approach is not likely to be safe. Finally, you select a nasotracheal approach, realizing that it may be difficult to perform with the patient's shallow respirations. Fortunately, you are successful in this approach and, after suctioning the tracheal tube using a flexible catheter, you proceed with further stabilization of the patient.

You transport the patient to the hospital. Later, you receive a note from the patient's husband thanking you for helping his wife and letting you know that she has recovered from the incident and is seeking counseling for some personal problems.

FURTHER READING

1. ARBOUR, R. "Mastering neuromuscular blockade," *Dimensions of Critical Care Nursing: DCCN,* 2000; 19(5):4-16; quiz 17-20.
2. BLANDA, M. and U.E. GALLO. "Emergency airway management," *Emergency Medicine Clinics of North America,* 2003;21(1):1-26.
3. DEEM, S. and M.J. BISHOP. "Evaluation and management of the difficult airway," *Crit Care Clinics,* 1995;11(1):1–27.
4. FRAKES, M.A. "Rapid sequence induction medications: an update," *Journal of Emergency Nursing: JEN: Official Publication of the Emergency Department Nurses Association,* 2003;29(6):533-540.

5. GRINER, R.L. II. "The laryngeal mask airway: attributes and inadequacies," *AANA Journal,* 1996;64(5):485-496.
6. HASTINGS, D. "Airway management skills," in J.E. Campbell, ed., *Basic Trauma Life Support for Paramedics and Advanced EMS Providers.* 4th ed. Upper Saddle River, NJ: Pearson/Prentice Hall, 2000.
7. HASTINGS, D. "Optional skills," in J.E. Campbell, ed., *Basic Trauma Life Support for Paramedics and Advanced EMS Providers.* 4th ed. Upper Saddle River, NJ: Pearson/Prentice Hall, 2000.
8. JAGIM, M. "Emergency: airway management," *The American Journal of Nursing,* 2003;103(10):32-35.
9. OSSMAN, E.W., E.A. BARTKUS, and M.L. OLINGER. "Prehospital pearls, pitfalls and updates," *Emerg Med Clinics NA,* 1997;15(2):283–301.
10. REED, A.P. "Current concepts in airway management for cardiopulmonary resuscitation," *Mayo Clin Proc,* 1995;70(12):1172-1184.
11. RICH, J.M., A.M. MASON, T.A. BEY, P. KRAFFT, and M. FRASS. "The critical airway rescue ventilation, and the combitube: part 1," *AANA Journal,* 2004;72(1):17-27.
12. RICH, J.M., A.M. MASON, T.A. BEY, P. KRAFFT, and M. FRASS. "The critical airway, rescue ventilation, and the combitube: part 2," *AANA Journal* 2004;72(2):115-24.
13. RICH, J.M., A.M. MASON, and M.A.E. RAMSAY. "AANA Journal course: update for nurse anesthetists. The SLAM emergency airway flowchart: a new guide for advanced airway practitioners," *AANA Journal,* 2004;72(6):431-439.
14. STEWART, R.D. and J.E. CAMPBELL. "Initial airway management," in J.E. Campbell, ed., *Basic Trauma Life Support for Paramedics and Advanced EMS Providers.* 4th ed. Upper Saddle River, NJ: Pearson/Prentice Hall, 2000.
15. THOMAS, S.H., C.K. STONE, T. HARRISON, and S.K. WEDEL. "Airway management in the air medical setting," *Air Med J,* 1995;14(3):129-138.

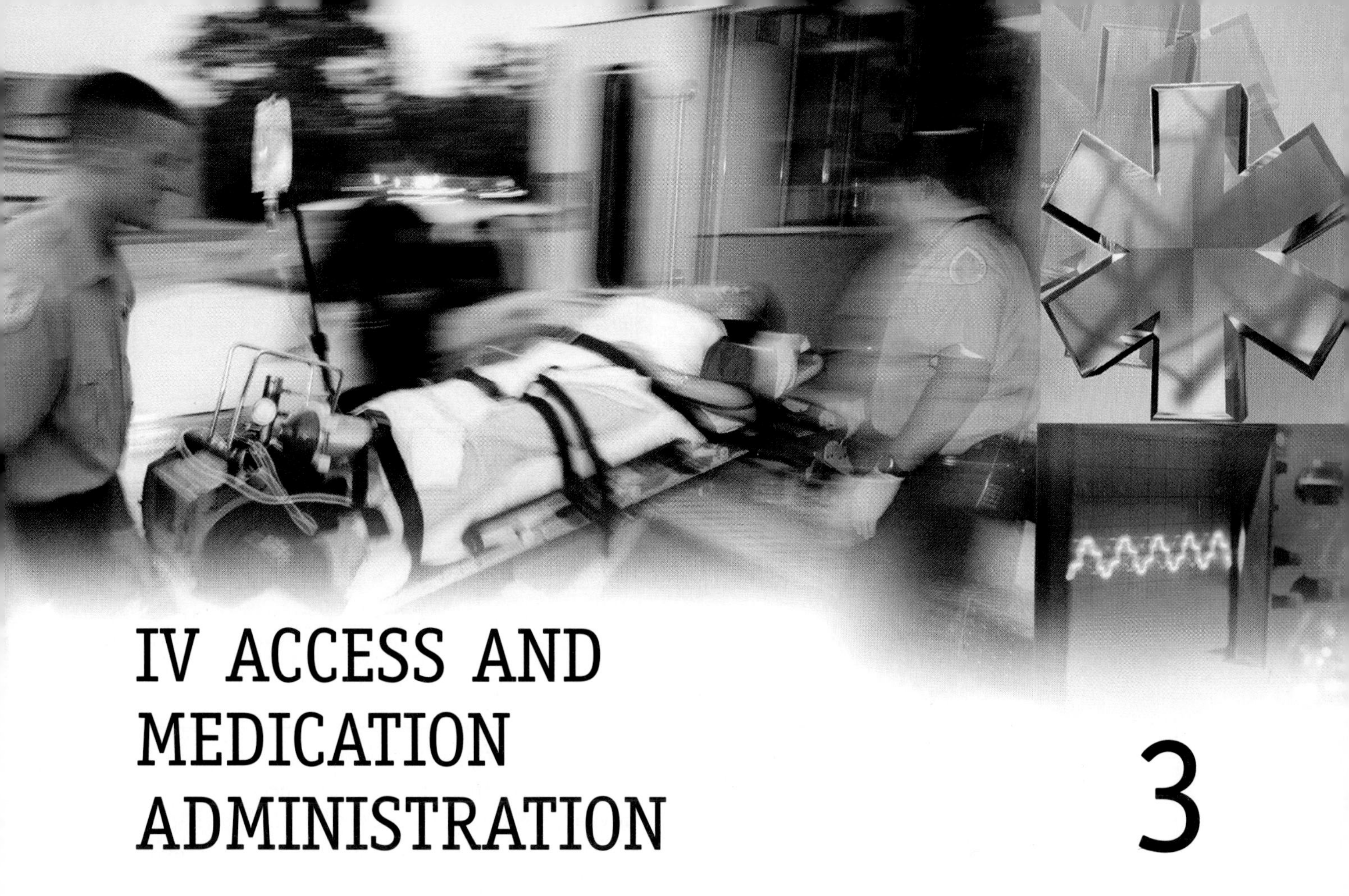

IV ACCESS AND MEDICATION ADMINISTRATION

3

One of the major differences between the care of the medical patient and that of the trauma patient is the ability to significantly impact the patient's condition through the use of medications. In the medical patient, medications are used to control cardiac dysrhythmias, correct shock, relieve pain, and more. Immediate correction of urgent traumatic conditions is largely surgical. The use of IV and other methods of medication administration is an important difference between basic and advanced field providers. Not only does the advanced training provide the skills necessary to gain IV access and administer medications, it should also provide the clinical decision-making skills to identify when vascular access and medications are necessary.

Topics that are covered in this chapter are

- Medication Administration
- Medication Administration Methods
- Venous Access
- Intraosseous Infusion
- Delivering Medication by Injection
- Other Methods of Medication Administration

SCENARIO

Your advanced life support unit is dispatched to a call for a "man down." Fire department EMTs are on the scene rapidly and radio you that the patient is in cardiac arrest.

On arrival at the scene, you and your partner gather your equipment, including cardiac monitor and defibrillator, drug box, and airway supplies. Because you already know you will be working a cardiac arrest, you put on gloves and protective eyewear.

The EMTs have defibrillated the patient with two sets of three shocks each. They report that the 59-year-old male patient had collapsed after dinner, without warning. The EMTs continue CPR while your partner prepares to defibrillate again. You prepare to intubate the patient. The patient's cardiac rhythm converts to asystole.

You intubate the patient. Your partner sets up a bag of normal saline and attempts an IV in the patient's left arm. The IV attempt is unsuccessful.

What should you and your partner do next for this patient?

INTRODUCTION

The two main purposes of this chapter are to review medication administration procedures and to discuss the decision-making process necessary when deciding whether to use these advanced skills. The information in this chapter, combined with the other procedural and clinical topics in other chapters, helps provide information for forming such clinical decisions.

MEDICATION ADMINISTRATION

Medication administration is a great responsibility. Although medications can correct life-threatening heart dysrhythmias, reverse diabetic conditions, and relieve pain, they can also cause serious complications or death if administered improperly or to a patient who has allergies to a medication. Some common rules are taught to any medical professional who has the responsibility for administering medications. These are often referred to as the "five rights":

- ***Right medication.*** Am I administering the correct/intended medication?
- ***Right dose.*** Am I administering the right amount of the medication? Is the medication's concentration correct? Is the rate of administration correct?
- ***Right route.*** Am I administering the medication via the right route? (Some medications, when delivered by the wrong route, have much different effects than intended.)
- ***Right patient.*** Am I administering the medication to the patient who needs it and for whom it is intended?

The Five Rights

Right medication
Right dose
Right route
Right patient
Right time

- ***Right time.*** Will the patient benefit from this medication at this particular place and time? Is this medication clinically indicated for the patient's current condition?

Most of the other chapters in this textbook deal with the last two items (right patient, right time). The first three items (right medication, right dose, right route) relate to the actual administration of a medication, the subject of this chapter. Administering a medication should always be taken seriously.

A final right, right documentation, has also been suggested. There are few situations where documentation is more important than medication administration. Remember to document the IV attempt(s), location, catheter gauge, fluid administered, amount of fluid administered, and type of administration set. For any medication administration, note the date, time, medication, amount, route, site, and effects of the medication. Always document any problems, errors, or complications noted during care and provide a verbal report of suspected problems to the receiving hospital staff.

MEDICATION ADMINISTRATION METHODS

There are many methods of administering medications. *Parenteral* routes (those not using the digestive system) are the most common in the emergency setting. The oral, sublingual, and rectal (*enteral*) routes are used for specific situations.

parenteral routes routes of medication other than by the digestive tract, including intravenous, intramuscular, subcutaneous, intraosseous, transdermal, tracheal, and inhalation.

enteral routes routes of medication through the digestive tract, including oral, sublingual, and rectal.

Medication administration routes with some of the pros and cons of each are:

- ***Intravenous.*** A mainstay of advanced emergency care, aseptically started peripheral IVs provide rapid, predictable absorption with minimal complications.
- ***Intraosseous.*** This route is used when IV access cannot be obtained. Formerly used largely in pediatric patients, some recent devices facilitate the use of intraosseous infusion in adults.
- ***Intramuscular.*** Used more frequently in routine medical care, IM injections provide a less predictable and slower absorption rate than IVs. IM injections may be used when IV access cannot be obtained (e.g., Glucagon).
- ***Subcutaneous.*** Subcutaneous injections are used to obtain intentionally slower absorption for prolonged effect. Epinephrine has been injected via this route for conditions such as anaphylaxis.
- ***Tracheal.*** This route provides rapid absorption of certain medications (epinephrine, lidocaine, atropine, and naloxone). Most sources recommend an increase in concentration and/or volume of any drug administered by the tracheal route.
- ***Inhalation.*** Drugs that affect the respiratory system act rapidly and efficiently when administered by this route. Inhaled drugs may be administered via aerosolized treatments and inhalers.
- ***Transdermal.*** Some medications, such as nitrates, are effectively absorbed through the skin. This route provides constant, prolonged administration of the medication.
- ***Oral.*** With the exception of activated charcoal and syrup of ipecac, most oral medications are not even considered for use in an unstable patient. Absorption from the digestive tract of an unstable patient ranges from

unpredictable to absent, as does the ability of the unstable patient to swallow or to protect the airway from aspiration.

- ***Sublingual.*** Some medications, such as nitroglycerin, are efficiently absorbed from under the tongue. Sublingual injection (injection into the vascular area under the tongue) may also be used for some medications.
- ***Rectal.*** Medications may be absorbed through the rectal mucosa. One indication for this route is Valium administration for a seizure patient when IV access is not possible.
- ***Intranasal.*** Medications (including naloxone) may be administered by syringe or "atomizer" and absorbed through the nasal mucosa.

As distance increases between the administration site and the target organ, the absorption time increases and the reliability of absorption decreases.

The main principle to remember when administering medications in the emergency setting is: Medications administered close to the central circulation are absorbed rapidly and reliably. As distance increases between the administration site and the target organ, the absorption time increases and the reliability of absorption decreases.

VENOUS ACCESS

Note: Always use appropriate body substance isolation techniques when performing any procedure that has the potential to expose you to a patient's blood or other body luids.

Clinical Insight

Clinical judgment includes when—and when not—to start an IV or give a medication. It is sometimes more difficult to decide that a patient does not need the IV or medication than that he does. Use the entire clinical picture for your decision. Err on the side of caution if in doubt.

Decision Making

There are many factors that influence the decision to initiate IV access and administer medications. The most obvious and important consideration is: What decision will benefit my patient the most?

Considerations for the use of (or decision not to use) IV or medication therapy include

- Standing orders
- The need to administer medications or deliver a fluid challenge
- Your perception of the patient's stability
- Benefit versus risk analysis
- Consultation with medical direction

A term for the combination of these considerations is "clinical judgment." It is a main purpose of this text to provide practical information on a variety of adult medical emergencies that will help you make appropriate decisions regarding patient care procedures such as IV therapy.

peripheral veins the veins of the arms and legs and the external jugular vein.

central veins veins that are part of the central circulation, including the internal jugular vein, the subclavian vein, and the femoral vein.

Peripheral and Central Lines

The two main types of venous access are peripheral and central. *Peripheral venous* access is widely practiced in the out-of-hospital setting. Medications and fluids are administered into veins of the arms and legs, as well as into the external jugular vein. Peripheral IV access is relatively safe, easy, and effective in the prehospital setting.

Central venous IVs are not common in the field. There is a higher risk of serious complications with central cannulation, and the technique is difficult to

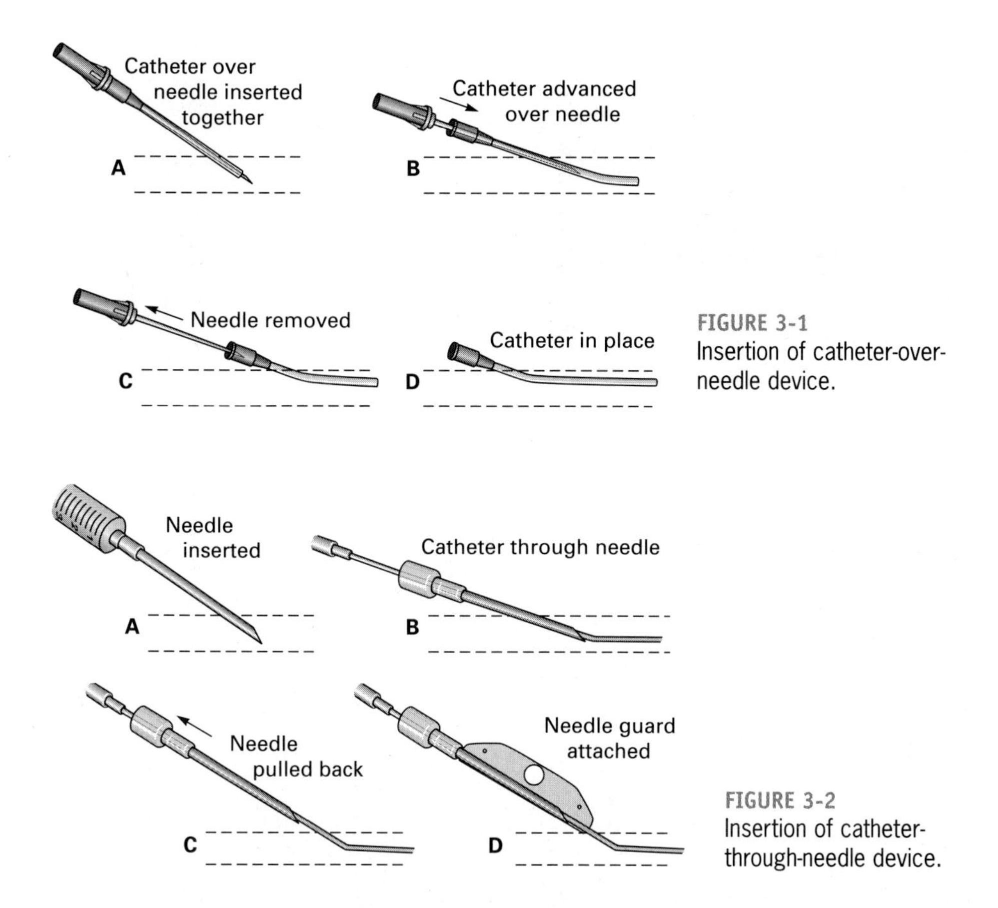

FIGURE 3-1
Insertion of catheter-over-needle device.

FIGURE 3-2
Insertion of catheter-through-needle device.

master, especially when not performed frequently. This text focuses on peripheral venous cannulation because of the predominance of this procedure in the field. If you are allowed or required to do central IVs, knowledge and practice are essential. Please refer to the many excellent sources of in-depth information available on this topic.

Three general types of intravenous needle or catheter are available:

- ***The catheter-over-needle device*** (Figure 3-1). This is by far the most common device used for peripheral venous cannulation. The catheter is placed over the needle, and the needle and the catheter are inserted simultaneously into the vein. The needle is removed, and the catheter remains in place.
- ***The catheter-through-needle device*** (Figure 3-2). A catheter is fed through a larger-bore needle into the vein. This method is used frequently for central venous cannulation.
- ***The hollow needle or "butterfly."*** This type is used primarily in pediatric patients. The metal needle remains inside the patient's vein. This leads to a higher rate of infiltration and damage to the vein.

Performing Venipuncture

Once a decision is made to initiate IV therapy, several other considerations exist:

- ***Where will I start the IV?*** For patients who require a medication or fluid bolus, veins closest to the central circulation are largest (larger-bore IVs may be used) and provide an efficient route for the medications to reach the central circulation (Figure 3-3a–c).

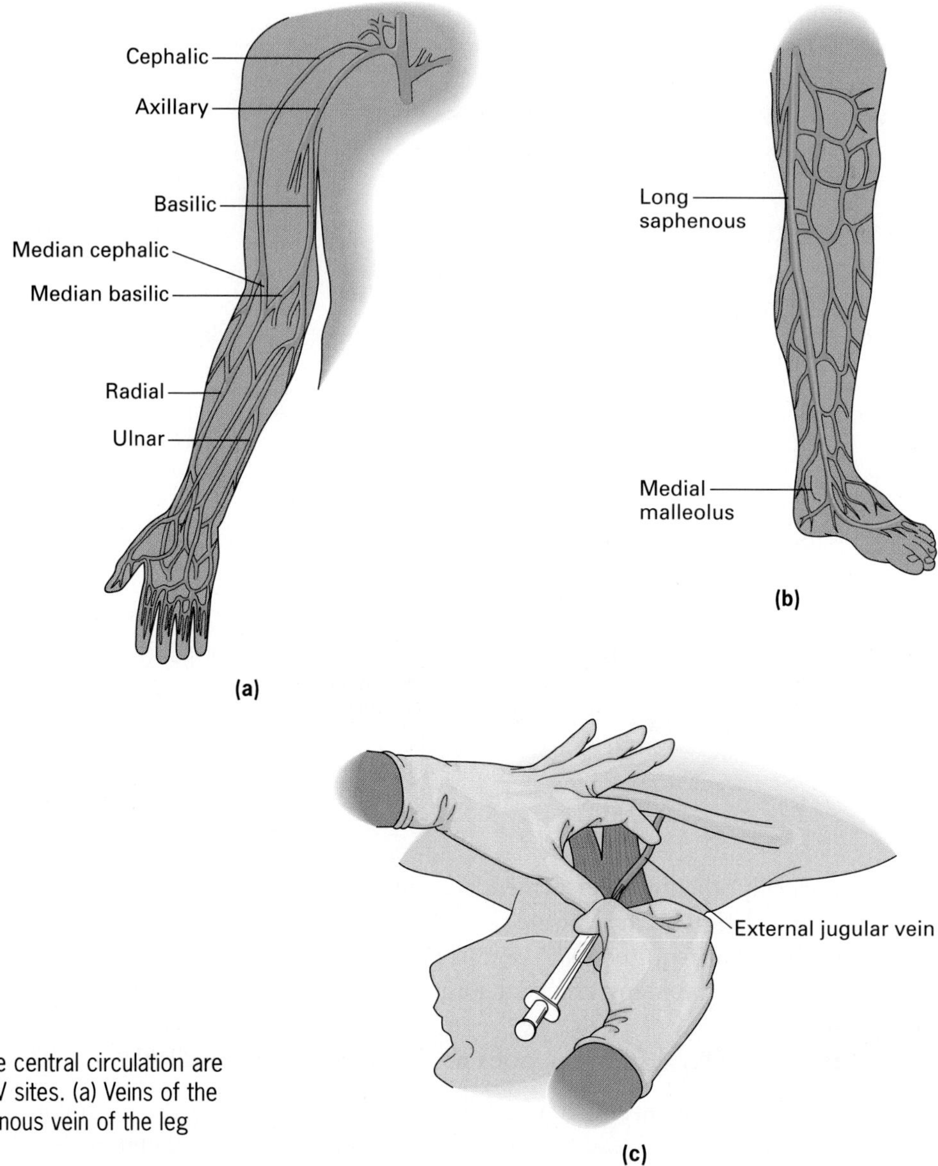

FIGURE 3-3
Peripheral veins closest to the central circulation are generally the most effective IV sites. (a) Veins of the hand and arm (b) Long saphenous vein of the leg (c) External jugular vein

- ***What catheter size and type will I use?*** Choose an IV catheter that will be functional in a worst-case scenario. Often, IVs are started as a "precaution" but are not large enough to handle the type of administration that turns out to be needed (e.g., a fluid challenge or large-volume injection such as D_{50}).
- ***Where should I perform the venipuncture?*** Examine the benefits and risks of starting the IV at the scene versus en route to the hospital. Although this is often a consideration in trauma, there are also medical applications. You will also find that getting the patient into a suitable position will improve your chances for success in starting an IV. If you are in a cramped space or have to reach across a patient, moving the patient to the stretcher or to a different position will be beneficial. Starting the IV in the ambulance may expedite transport and increase the equipment you have available. However, starting an IV in a moving ambulance can be challenging.
- ***If the first IV is unsuccessful, how many will I try?*** In this case, weigh the benefits versus the risks and delays in continued attempts to gain access. Criteria

for determining this include time, patient stability, alternative routes of medication administration available, and the patient's comfort and consent. Also, the more attempts that are made, the fewer the options that will be available for ED personnel to obtain peripheral venous access.

Patients who are candidates for fibrinolytic therapy should not receive multiple venipunctures unless necessary to stabilize a critical condition, because fibrinolytic drugs decrease clotting and increase the danger of serious bleeding from any wound.

Clinical Insight

We pride ourselves on the ability to start an IV in the worst of situations—and many consider missed IVs as the ultimate failure in patient care. It will happen. When it does, remember that there are many facets of patient care, including excellent basic life support, compassionate emotional care, and alternative methods of administering medications. Do not lose sight of the end goal because of problems along the way.

Procedure for Peripheral Venipuncture

To perform a peripheral venipuncture (Figure 3-4a–f),

1. Take body substance isolation precautions.
2. Choose an appropriate IV solution for the patient's condition.
3. Attach IV tubing to the bag and run fluid through the tubing.
4. Determine where you will be starting the IV. Choose a peripheral site to look for a vein.
5. Apply a venous tourniquet (the obvious exception is for the external jugular, where the proximal portion of the vein is occluded by pressing on it with a finger). This should not eliminate all blood flow, just impede the return of venous blood, which will engorge the veins.
6. Choose a vein. Vein choice is important. Choose a vein that appears to be anchored. Superficial veins may look large and tempting but may roll.
7. Cleanse the skin over and around the vein with an antiseptic wipe.
8. Insert the needle and catheter, bevel up. When you enter the vein, you will feel a "pop." You may also see a flash of blood in the hub of the catheter.
9. When you have felt the pop, advance the needle and catheter slightly to ensure that you are in the vein. You may attach a small syringe to the catheter and withdraw blood to verify placement in the vein.
10. While grasping the hub of the needle, advance the catheter over the needle and into the vein.
11. Completely remove the needle. Remove the tourniquet. Be sure that one hand is holding the hub of the catheter so it does not become dislodged from the vein.
12. Attach the tubing to the catheter and begin the flow of fluids. Observe for signs of infiltration.
13. Be sure to dispose of the contaminated sharp in an appropriate container. Do not recap needles.
14. Cover the site where the catheter enters the skin with a sterile dressing or sterile commercially available device. Secure the catheter and tubing to prevent accidental displacement.
15. Monitor the IV site, tubing, and any drip medications for complications.
16. Document IV location, catheter size, fluid, and time.

Procedure for External Jugular Cannulation

As has been mentioned throughout this chapter, peripheral IVs placed closest to the central circulation are the most effective. Although located in the neck (Figure 3-5a), the external jugular vein is considered a peripheral site. This site is used in cardiac arrest or when other peripheral sites cannot be obtained in critical situations.

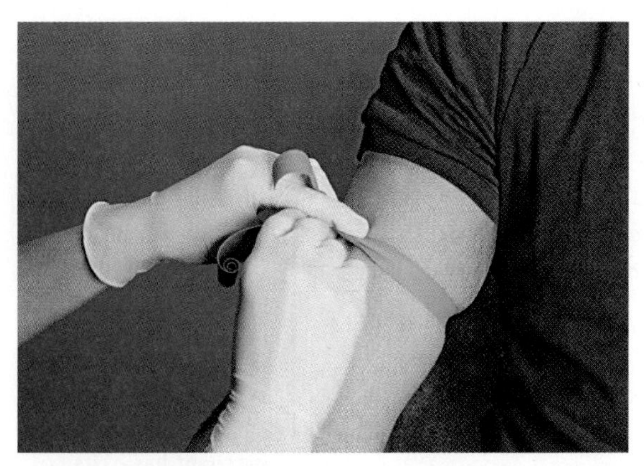

FIGURE 3-4a Apply a venous constricting band.

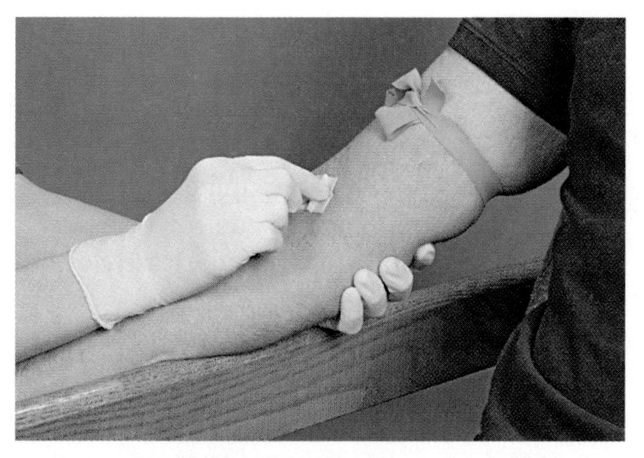

FIGURE 3-4b Cleanse the site with an antiseptic.

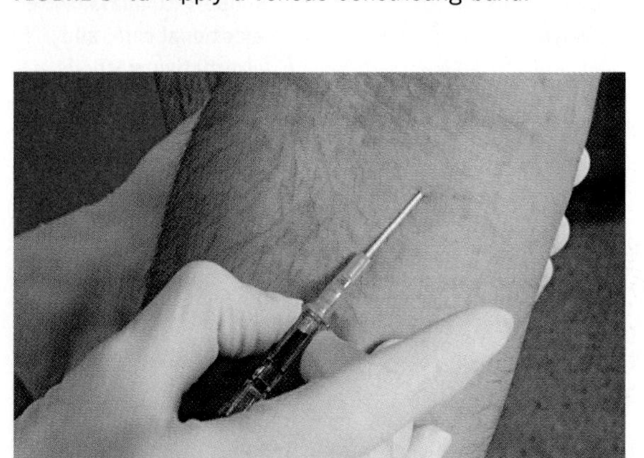

FIGURE 3-4c Insert the catheter and stylet into the lumen of the vein until flashback is noted. Advance the catheter and stylet another 1 to 2 mm and then thread the catheter off the stylet.

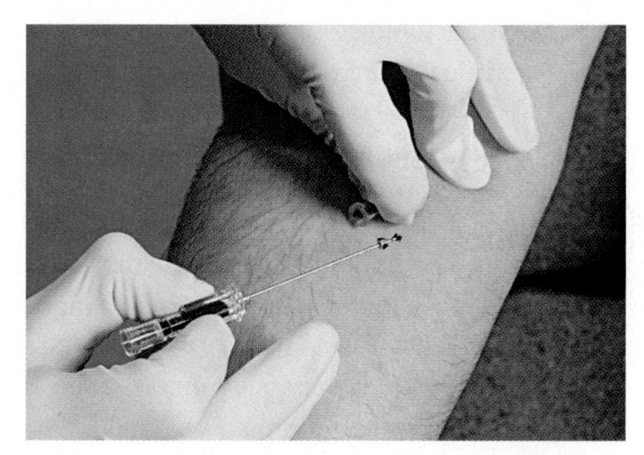

FIGURE 3-4d Tamponade the proximal portion of the vein with a finger and remove the stylet. Ensure that the safety device covers the needle, and dispose of the sharps properly.

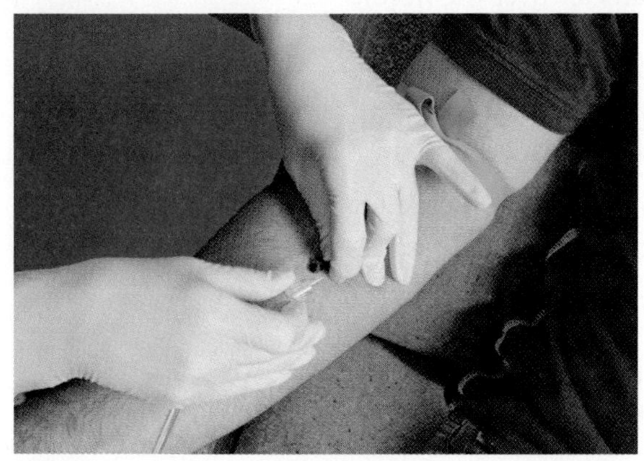

FIGURE 3-4e Attach IV tubing to the catheter hub. Remove the venous constricting band and initiate and adjust the fluid flow.

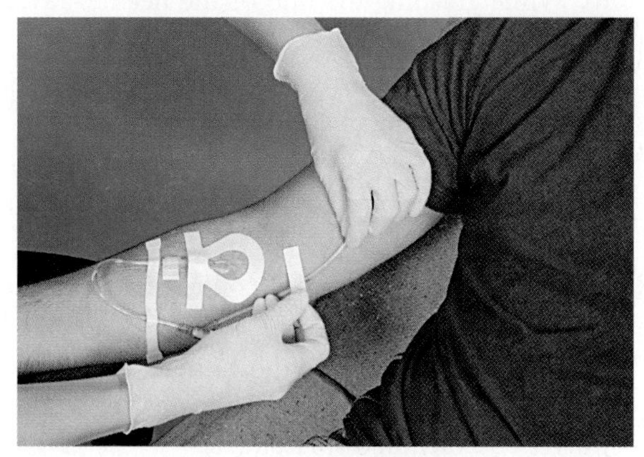

FIGURE 3-4f Apply a sterile protective cover over the insertion site and secure the tubing in place.

To perform an external jugular cannulation (Figure 3-5b),

1. Take body substance isolation precautions.
2. Place the patient in a Trendelenburg position. Turn the patient's head to the opposite side.
3. Cleanse the injection site with an antiseptic wipe.

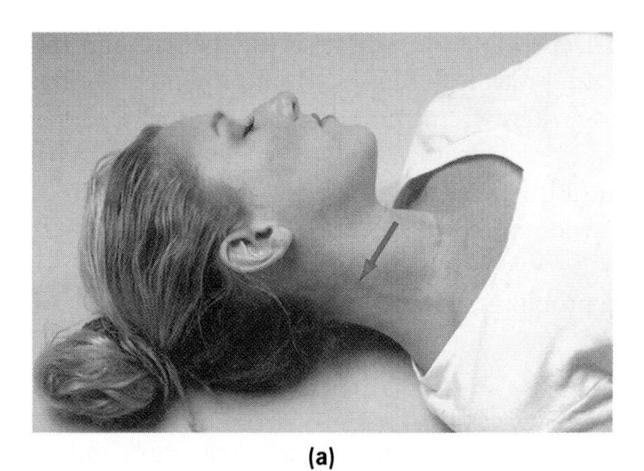

(a)

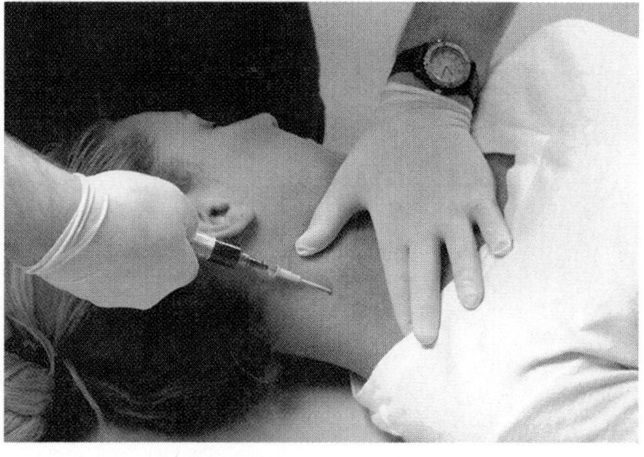

(b)

FIGURE 3-5
The external jugular vein is considered a peripheral IV site. (a) Location of the external jugular vein. (b) Cannulation of the external jugular vein.

4. Place one gloved finger on the proximal portion of the external jugular vein just above the clavicle to occlude blood flow and distend the vein.
5. Using a 14- or 16-gauge catheter, align the catheter with the vein. The catheter should be pointing in the direction of the shoulder. Puncture the vein midway between the angle of the jaw and your finger, which is acting as the tourniquet.
6. Continue the procedure as you would for any other peripheral IV. *Note:* Some recommend attaching a syringe to the needle so IV placement can be checked.

Heparin or Saline Locks

When continuous IV fluids are not necessary, but occasional medication drips or boluses may be needed, heparin or saline locks are used (Figure 3-6). These devices also decrease the risk of accidental fluid overload or electrolyte derangement. If seated in a suitable vein, and if protocols allow, blood may be withdrawn from the lock.

Complications of Intravenous Therapy

Complications associated with IV therapy are rare and include extravasation (infiltration) of IV fluids, hematoma, local infection, and phlebitis. More serious complications such as sepsis or embolization are possible.

Complications may include extravasation (infiltration), hematoma, local infection, phlebitis, sepsis, and embolization.

Extravasation is an occasional complication. The use of butterfly catheters and the use of catheters near a joint

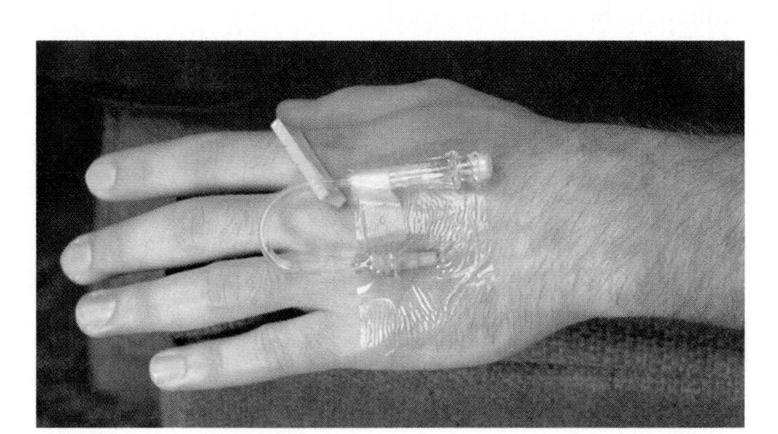

FIGURE 3-6
A heparin or saline lock regulates IV flow and decreases the risk of accidental fluid overload or electrolyte derangement.

increase the risk of extravasation. Depending on the size of the patient and the location of the IV, up to 1 liter of fluid may leak unnoticed into surrounding tissue. Hypertonic solutions and those with extreme deviations from the body's pH may cause pain and tissue damage or tissue death.

Complications may also occur if the IV bag and tubing are not monitored. A "runaway IV" (one that is flowing wide-open) may quickly overload the medical patient with fluid. Kinked tubing will prevent fluid and medications from reaching the patient. When troubleshooting problems, be sure to check the entire length of IV from the bag to the catheter.

Intravenous Solutions

IV solutions are classified in many ways. Some IV solutions are crystalloids, meaning they have small molecules and a low osmotic pressure. These solutions are typically used in the field. Normal saline and lactated Ringer's solution are crystalloid solutions commonly used for patients in shock.

Colloid solutions have large molecules and a higher osmotic pressure. These solutions will remain in the vascular space and are theoretically best in situations where fluid resuscitation is required. Unfortunately, most colloid solutions (whole blood or packed red blood cells, plasma, and plasma substitutes) are expensive, have strict requirements for temperature, and limited expiration dates, which make use in the field impractical.

Solutions are also classified by their tonicity (hypo-, hyper-, or isotonic):

- *Hypotonic solutions* have a lower solute concentration than the body's cells. One hypotonic solution, for example, is 0.45 saline (sodium chloride).
- *Hypertonic solutions* have a greater solute concentration. An example is hypertonic (3.0%) saline (sodium chloride).
- *Isotonic solutions* have a solute concentration equal to the body's cells. Lactated Ringer's solution and normal (0.9%) saline are examples of isotonic solutions.

The final method of classifying solutions is by their content (e.g., dextrose, saline, lactated Ringer's solution). This classification also helps determine an appropriate solution. For example, stroke and head injury patients are not given dextrose-containing solutions, whereas diabetic patients may benefit from the dextrose.

Flow Rates

microdrip set an intravenous administration set that delivers 1 milliliter with 60 drops of fluid.

macrodrip set an intravenous administration set that delivers 1 milliliter with 10 or 15 drops of fluid.

IV solutions are delivered through administration sets. These sets are either microdrip or macrodrip. With a *microdrip set,* 60 drops equal 1 milliliter. With a *macrodrip set,* 10 drops (or 15, depending on the set) equal 1 milliliter. It is essential to know the type of set you are using in order to calculate the flow rate of an IV and to accurately deliver any medications by IV drip or piggyback.

To calculate a flow rate in gtt (drops) per minute, use the following equation:

$$\text{gtt/min} = \text{volume to be infused} \times \text{gtt/ml of administration set} \div \text{time of infusion in minutes}$$

For example, if you were to deliver 100 ml per hour using a macrodrip set:

$$\text{gtt/min} = (100 \times 10) \div 60 \text{ Result: approximately 17 gtt/min}$$

IV Administration of Medications

The preferred route of medication administration is through an IV line. With the exception of central lines, peripheral IV lines are the most dependable and rapid way of administering medication to the critical or potentially unstable patient. Because this method of administration provides rapid access to the patient's circulation, the potential hazards are also greater. Errors in medication, dose or concentration, or undiscovered allergies may prove rapidly fatal. Caution must be taken in all parts of the preparation and actual administration of the medication.

IV administration provides rapid access to the circulation, so potential hazards are also greater. Caution must be taken in preparation and administration.

IV Bolus or "Push" Administration In this method, the given dosage of medication is administered all at once, as a *bolus.* The steps for IV *push* medication administration, listed here, assume that an IV line has already been established (Figure 3-7a–d). Remember: *Always take appropriate infection control precautions and use sterile technique.*

bolus a concentrated dose of medication given rapidly by intravenous injection.

push the method of administering a bolus of medication intravenously in one rapid dose.

1. Identify the drug to be administered. Verify the need for the drug, the route, concentration, dose, expiration date, and clarity of the liquid. Check for allergies and contraindications. Verify that the IV line is patent and running.
2. Draw up the correct amount of medication (or verify the amount in a preloaded syringe).
3. Choose a port in the IV tubing. The one closest to the point of entry into the patient is usually preferred. Cleanse the port with an antiseptic wipe.

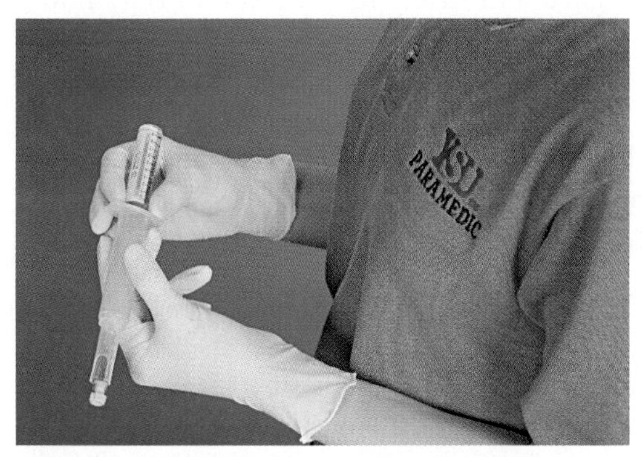

FIGURE 3-7a Draw up the correct amount of medication (or verify the amount in a preloaded syringe).

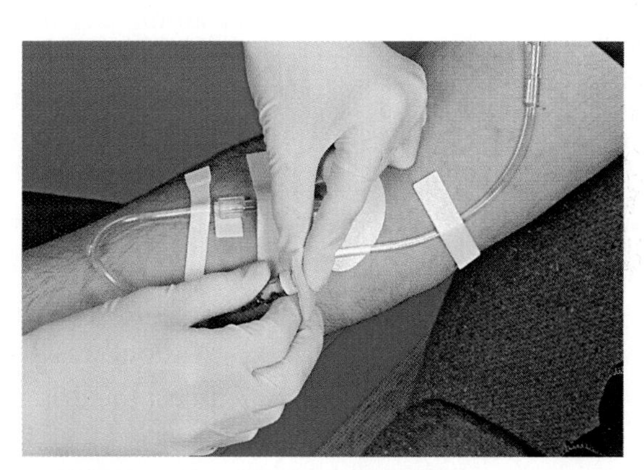

FIGURE 3-7b Cleanse the injection site.

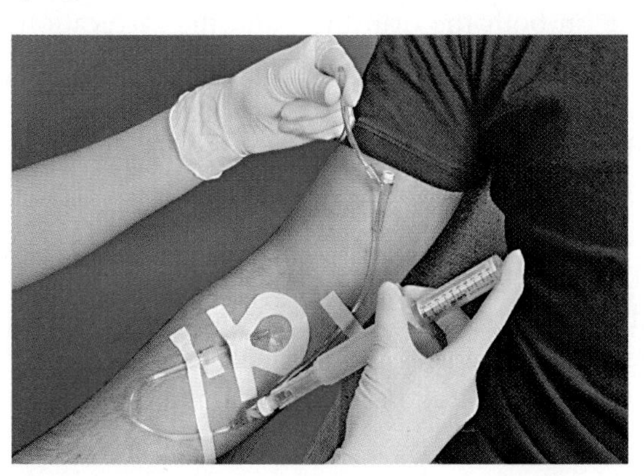

FIGURE 3-7c Insert the needle into the medication port. Pinch the tubing above the port.

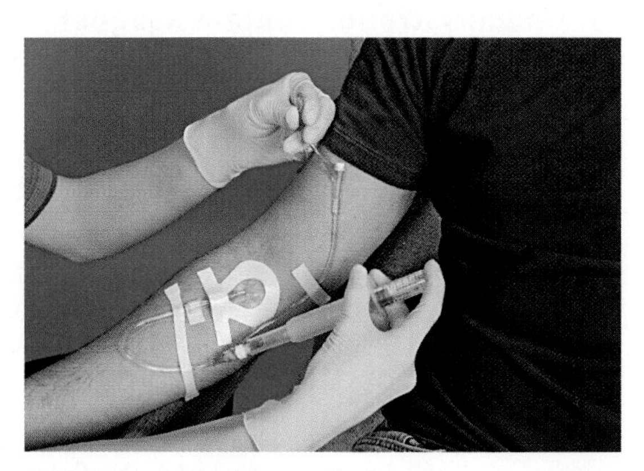

FIGURE 3-7d Inject the medication at an appropriate rate.

4. Carefully insert the needle of the syringe containing the medication into the center of the port. Pinch the tubing above the port to prevent backflow.
5. Inject the medication. Be sure to inject the medication at an appropriate rate. Some medications (e.g., adenosine) require very rapid administration, whereas others (e.g., morphine, verapamil) are administered slowly. Medications will be moved to the circulation faster if a saline flush (approximately 20 ml) is used after administration.
6. Discard the sharp in an appropriate container.
7. Monitor the patient, the IV and drip rate, and the patient's reaction to the medication frequently.
8. Record the time of administration and any reactions (or lack of reactions).

Note: Many medications are now administered using a needleless system. This has become an OSHA requirement.

drip slow intravenous administration of a medication, one drop at a time.

IV Drip or "Piggyback" Administration Medications that are beneficial to a patient as an IV bolus may be additionally beneficial when given as a *drip,* that is, in smaller amounts over time. A prime example is lidocaine, which is given by bolus and followed by a drip. Many other medications can also be given via drip, including epinephrine and nitrates, and it is the only route of administration for medications such as dobutamine and dopamine.

Because syringes or vials containing medications to mix for IV drip administration contain a higher concentration of medication than IV bolus medications, never administer a medication designed exclusively for drip use directly into a vein.

piggyback IV drip administration of a medication achieved by inserting the drip medication administration set into a port in the original intravenous line.

Remember as you read the following steps (Figure 3-8a–d) that an IV drip, or *piggyback,* requires two full IV setups (bags, tubing, alcohol wipes, etc.)—one being the original IV setup with fluid running at a TKO (to keep open) rate, the other being the medication infusion setup that will be "piggybacked" onto the first setup via a port in the tubing of the original IV setup:

1. Be sure the original IV line is patent, dependable, and flowing properly. Without this line, the piggyback drip will not be possible.
2. Inject the drip medication into the second IV bag. Be sure to use the proper amount and concentration of the medication to get the correct mg/ml in the drip bag. As with any medication administration, use sterile technique. Cleanse the port on the IV bag, and then insert the syringe with the medication. Verify the expiration date on both the drip fluid and the medication. Allow the medication to properly mix with the fluid.
3. Assemble the IV delivery tubing with the freshly mixed drip bag. Flow the fluid through the tubing to eliminate bubbles.
4. Place a sterile needle on the end of the tubing attached to the piggyback bag. Cleanse a port on the original IV tubing, and insert the needle attached to the drip tubing. Secure the tubings so the needle does not become dislodged. (Most agencies and hospitals use "needleless" systems for drips and medication administration. These systems are shown in figures included in this chapter.)
5. Open the flow on the drip tubing, and watch for IV flow in the drip chamber. Close the flow on the original IV. The only fluid being delivered to the patient is now from the piggybacked IV drip with medications added.

Syringes or vials containing medications to mix for IV drip administration contain a higher concentration of medication than IV bolus medications. Never administer a medication designed exclusively for drip use directly into a vein.

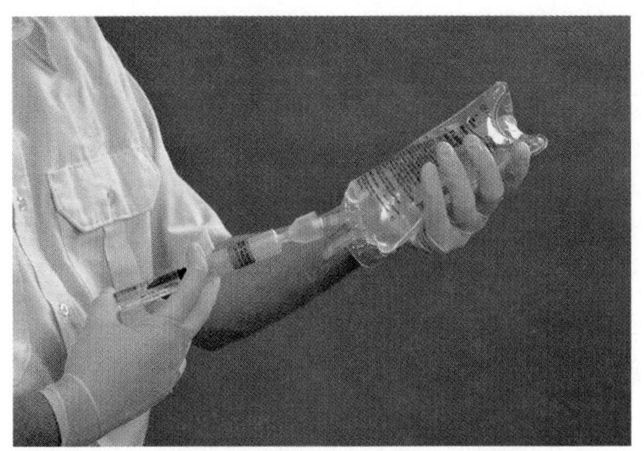

FIGURE 3-8a Inject the correct amount of the drug into the IV bag and allow the medication to mix with the fluid in the bag.

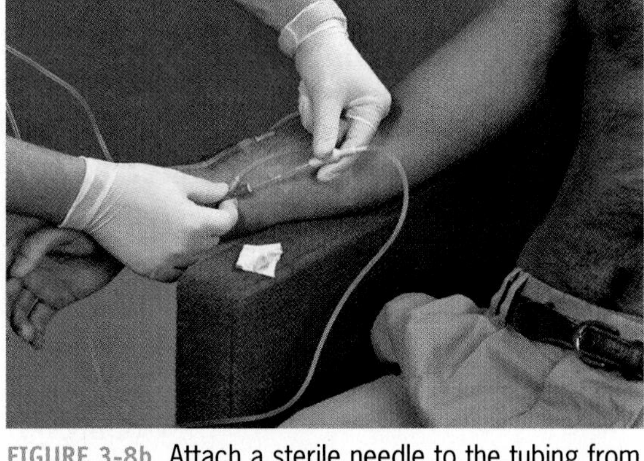

FIGURE 3-8b Attach a sterile needle to the tubing from the piggyback bag and insert it into a cleansed port on the original IV tubing.

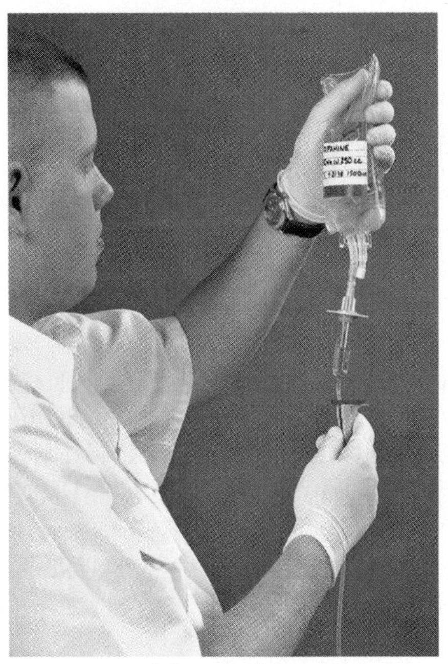

FIGURE 3-8c Adjust the flow rate.

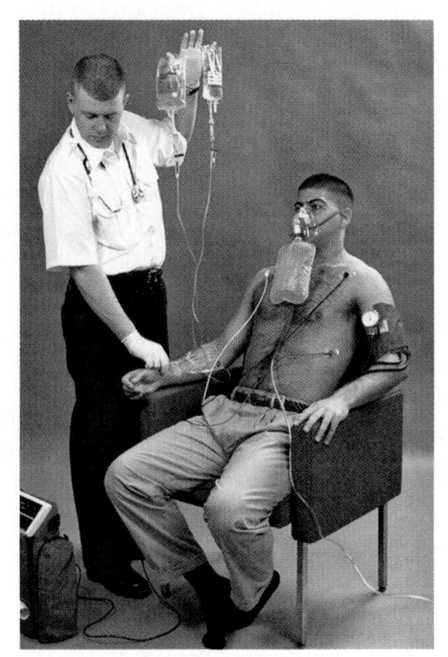

FIGURE 3-8d Monitor the patient.

6. Set the flow rate to deliver the medication amount you want to deliver over the appropriate time.
7. Carefully label the IV bag with the medication, concentration or amount of medication in the bag, the date and time started, and your initials. In patients where there are multiple lines and drips running, it may also be beneficial to use a small piece of tape to label the tubings near the patient because they are not always easily traced back to the bag. Not all medication boluses may be administered into IV solutions containing drip medications, because some medications have an adverse interaction.

Calculating Flow Rates for IV Drip Medications Complex IV drip calculations can bend even the best EMS minds under pressure. Fortunately, many IV drip solutions have been devised in round numbers and divisible figures to make these calculations easier. Moreover, a multitude of field guides, charts, and software provide precalculated information to providers administering drip medications. In

Medication dosage guides, charts, and software can prevent errors in calculation. They do not eliminate the need for careful selection, mixing, and administration.

reality, these practical charts can prevent errors in calculation. They do not eliminate the need for careful selection, mixing, and administration of the medication—potential areas for other human errors in this complex task.

Because practicing calculation will promote understanding and help prevent errors, it is reviewed here. The two essential determinations are as follows:

1. *How many mg/ml is my IV solution?*
   Using a popular example, 2 g of lidocaine (2,000 mg) is injected into a 500-ml bag of D_5W. This provides a concentration of 4 mg of lidocaine per ml of D_5W (4 mg/ml).
2. *How much fluid will I have to run at this concentration to get the desired dose?*
   Using a 60 gtt/ml microdrip set, 60 gtt/min (1 ml/min) would deliver 4 mg of lidocaine to the patient per minute.

Therefore: 15 gtt/min = 1 mg/min lidocaine
30 gtt/min = 2 mg/min lidocaine
45 gtt/min = 3 mg/min lidocaine

Dopamine is a more challenging example, where the medication dose must be calculated based on μg/kg/min. Using 400 mg of dopamine (400,000 μg) in a 500-ml bag of D_5W, we obtain a concentration of 800 μg/ml. If we are looking to administer 5 μg/kg/min to a patient who weighs 75 kg, our calculation would be as follows:

To determine the amount of dopamine that would be administered per minute we would multiply 5 × 75 = 375. This is the number of μg × the weight of the patient in kg to determine how many μg per minute we will administer to this patient. (Be sure to use the patient's weight in kg: 1 kg = 2.2 lb.)

The further math may be done in a number of ways. A simple proportion comparing μg and drops will develop an answer rapidly:

375:800 as X:60

This statement says that 375 μg is to 800 μg as *X* gtt are to 60 gtt (1 ml). To work this out, set it up as an equation:

$$\frac{375}{800} = \frac{X}{60} \quad \text{(cross multiply to get)} = 800X = 22{,}500$$

$$\text{Then, } \frac{22{,}500}{800} = 28.125$$

So, you would administer 28 gtt/min to this patient.

If you used your practical senses even before going to the math, you would have realized that 375 μg/min is almost half of 800 μg/min. This means that if you delivered 30 gtt/min (half of 60 gtt, which would equal 400 μg) you would have been mighty close. Unfortunately, "mighty close" is not always acceptable in medicine. This does, however, give you a way to check and see if your answer is in the ballpark.

None of the mathematical formulas for figuring dosages are known for accuracy when sirens are wailing and calculations are being performed in a moving ambulance. Use the math calculations you have learned and your common sense to check the reasonableness of the dosages you will administer . . . but experienced care providers and emergency department personnel frequently use the charts!

INTRAOSSEOUS INFUSION

Intraosseous (IO) infusions have been recommended in pediatric patients for many years. For adults, the relative ease of IV cannulation and numerous accessible sites available when compared to pediatric patients has traditionally left the option of IO infusions in adults a distant second in prehospital medicine. With the advent of newer intraosseous devices for adults, however, intraosseous infusion has become an option in the critically ill adult patient.

The infusion of significant quantities of fluid and administration of medication is clearly possible via the IO route. Additionally, there has been increased marketing of and interest in use of these devices in adults, so the concept is reviewed here. Always follow local protocols for infusion methods and acceptable devices.

IO devices currently available for adults are most commonly inserted into the tibia or sternum. For this discussion, we use the tibia in describing the placement and function of the IO needle and infusion (Figure 3-9). The tibia has a diaphysis, or shaft, and an epiphysis at each end of the bone. The diaphysis contains two types of bone: compact bone, which is the rigid and relatively solid bone found on the outside, and spongy bone, which is found in the center or cortex of the bone. The spongy bone resembles a net with marrow filling in the spaces of the net.

Bones are very vascular. Haversian canals (also known as central canals) within bone each contain one or more blood vessels. Canals of Volkman (also known as perforating canals) link the bone marrow with the Haversian canals and, therefore, with the entire circulatory system. Thus, fluids and medications introduced into the IO space are rapidly absorbed into circulation.

The IO needle (also called a bone marrow needle because of its placement in the marrow space) is placed in the anterior tibia. In pediatric patients, the needle is placed 1 to 3 cm distal to the tibial tuberosity. In an adult, the needle is inserted approximately two finger-widths (3–4 cm) below the tibial tuberosity. The needle must come to rest in the IO (marrow) space.

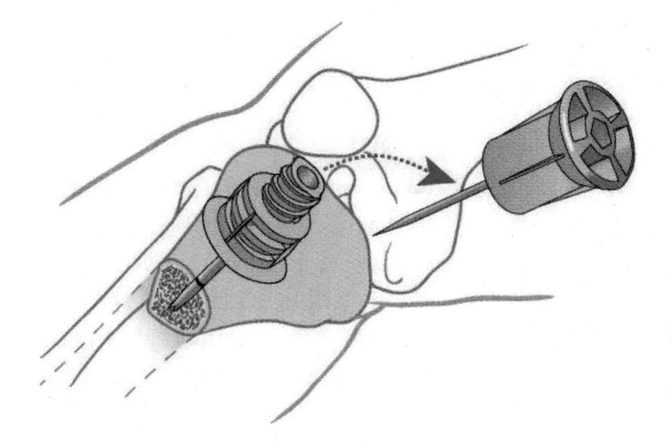

FIGURE 3-9
Intraosseous device inserted into the tibia.
(© Vidacare)

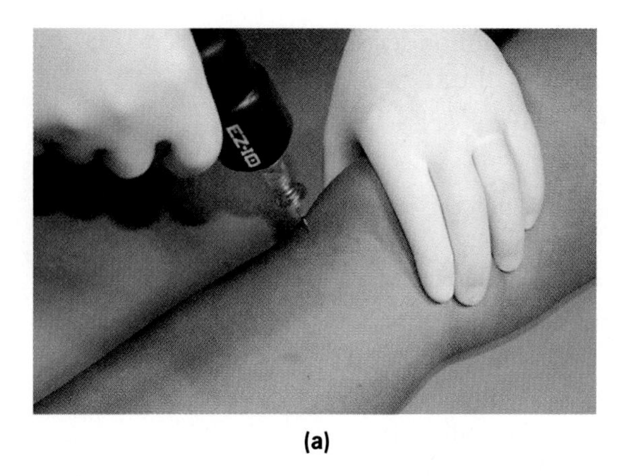

(a)

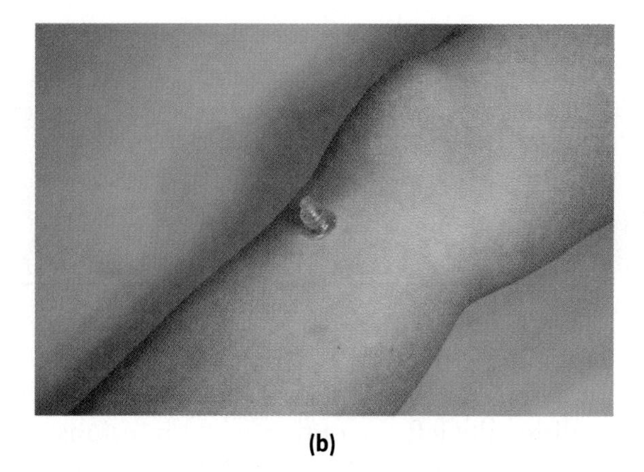

(b)

FIGURE 3-10
(a) The EZ-IO intraosseous device inserting a needle into the anterior tibia. (b) The EZ-IO needle in place in the tibia.
(© Vidacare)

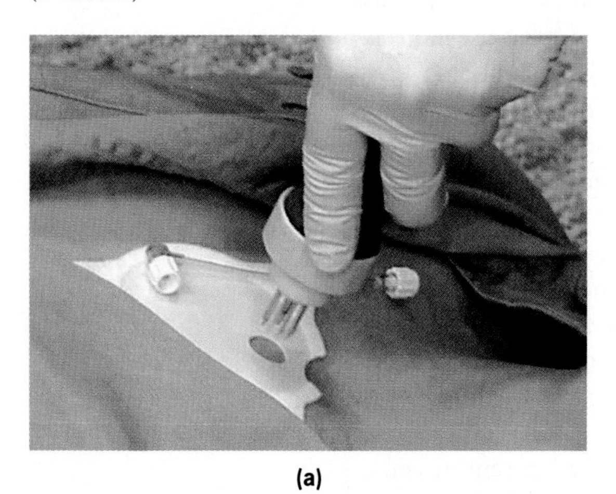

(a)

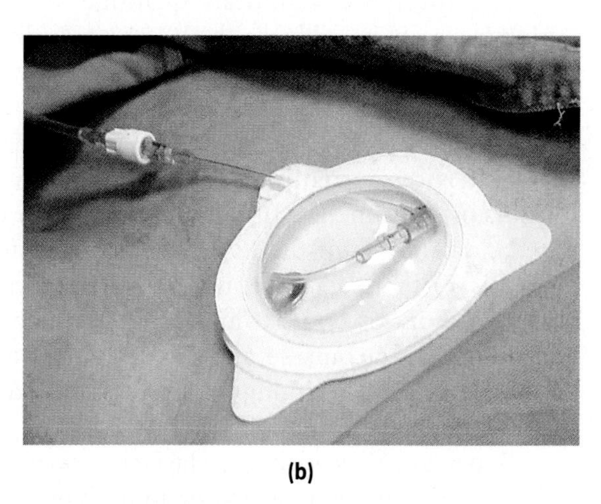

(b)

FIGURE 3-11
(a) The F.A.S.T.-1 intraosseous device inserting a needle into the sternum. (b) The F.A.S.T.-1 needle in place in the sternum.
(© Pyng Medical Corporation)

Unlike techniques of peripheral intravenous insertion, IO infusion procedures vary widely depending on the device and insertion location chosen. Refer to the manufacturer's recommendations for these procedures. Figures 3-10 and 3-11 show two IO devices and placements.

DELIVERING MEDICATION BY INJECTION

Although intramuscular, subcutaneous, and other forms of injection are frequently given in the nonemergent health care setting, field use of these injections is usually limited to occasions where an IV cannot be obtained or for specific medications that cannot be administered intravenously.

In a patient suffering shock or another medical or traumatic emergency, intramuscular or subcutaneous absorption may become slowed, unpredictable, or even nonexistent.

Injections into muscle and subcutaneous tissue have benefits such as relatively predictable absorption and longer duration of action. These attributes generally apply to the healthy patient. When patients are suffering shock or where other medical conditions exist, however, the absorption may become slowed, unpredictable, or even nonexistent.

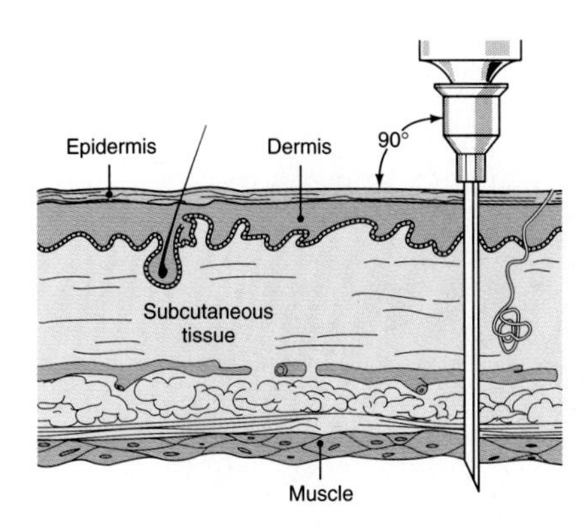

FIGURE 3-12
Intramuscular injection is made at a 90° angle into the muscle. Draw back the plunger slightly to ensure that the needle is not in a blood vessel.

Intramuscular Injection

Intramuscular (IM) injections are delivered into muscle, using a 1½-inch, 21-gauge or similar needle (Figure 3-12). The needle must be long enough to ensure the medication is delivered into the deep muscle tissue. The length and gauge of the needle may vary. If a viscous material such as an oil is to be injected, a larger-gauge needle may be used. The size of the patient and the amount of subcutaneous tissue varies from patient to patient. This will affect the choice of needle length and technique.

IM injections, depending on the site chosen, may be used to deliver 1 to 5 ml of medication.

The deltoid (arm) injection site is isolated by locating the acromial process on the lateral side of the arm. Choose a location 1 to 2 inches (2–3 finger-widths) below the acromial process. Visualize an inverted triangle with the wide base below the acromial process and the point one-third of the way down the humerus (Figure 3-13). Only about 1 ml of medication may be injected into this site. Beware of the radial nerve when injecting into the deltoid muscle.

Injection into the buttocks is most frequently into the gluteal muscles. There are two methods of isolating this injection site. The first is to draw an imaginary line from the posterior superior iliac spine to the greater trochanter of the femur (Figure 3-14a). The injection would then be given in the area on the lateral side

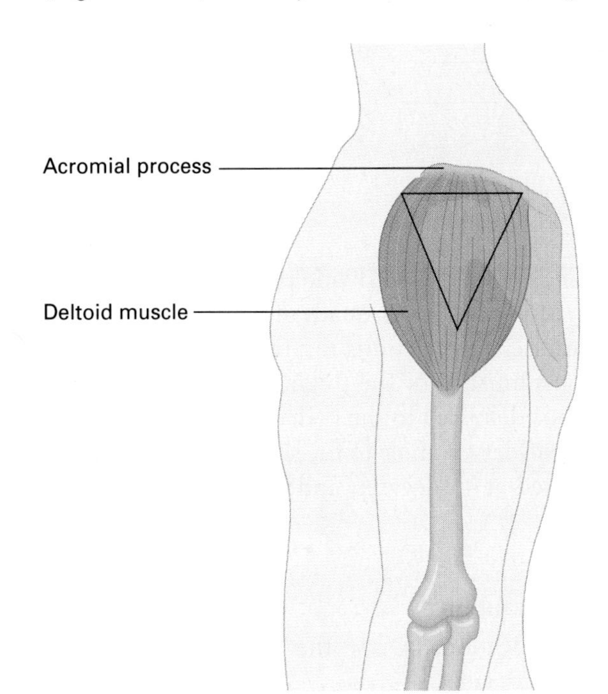

FIGURE 3-13
The deltoid injection site is 1 to 2 inches (2–3 finger-widths) below the acromial process. It can also be located by visualizing an inverted triangle with the wide base below the acromial process and the injection site about one-third of the way down the humerus.

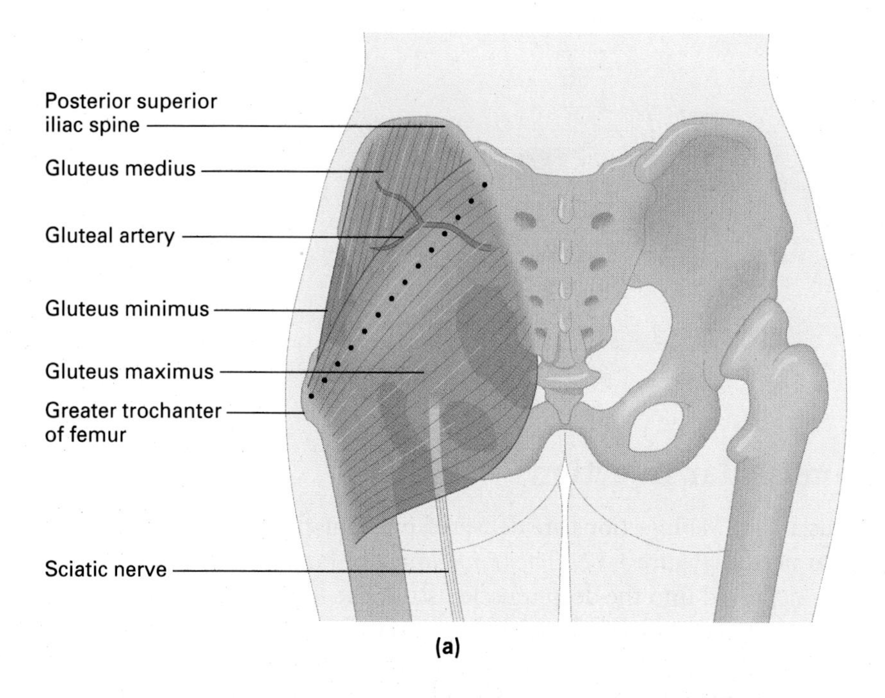

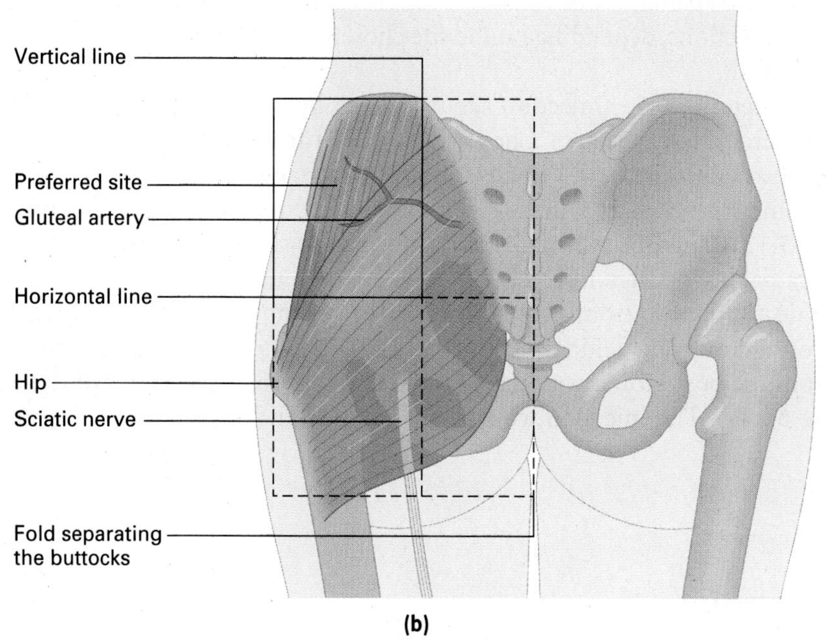

FIGURE 3-14
Locate the gluteal injection site by either of two methods: (a) Draw an imaginary line from the posterior superior iliac spine to the greater trochanter of the femur, and inject on the lateral (up and out) side of that line. (b) Divide the buttocks into quadrants and inject in the upper, outer quadrant 2 to 3 inches below the iliac crest.

(up and out) of that line. The second method is to divide the buttocks into four quadrants. The injection is given in the upper, outer quadrant 2 to 3 inches below the iliac crest (Figure 3-14b). Intramuscular injections may also be performed in the rectus femoris and vastus lateralis muscles of the thigh. These sites are often used for self-injection or for injections delivered to the pediatric patient.

IM injections are delivered at a 90-degree angle to the skin. This is in contrast to the subcutaneous, which is delivered at 45 degrees, and the intradermal at 15 degrees (Figure 3-15).

To perform an IM injection (Figure 3-16a–f),

1. Take body substance isolation precautions.
2. Gather the equipment and medications. Draw the medication into the syringe (or prepare the preloaded device).

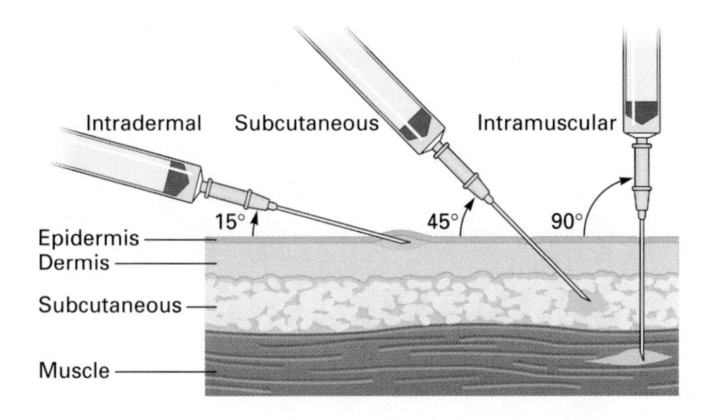

FIGURE 3-15 Intramuscular injections are delivered at a 90° angle to the skin, subcutaneous injections at a 45° angle, and intradermal injections at a 15° angle.

3. Prep the site of injection with an antiseptic wipe.
4. Insert the needle at a 90-degree angle into the muscle tissue beneath the skin.
5. Draw back slightly on the plunger of the syringe to ensure that you are not in a blood vessel. If you see blood flow into the syringe, remove the needle—do not inject the medication. Choose another site.

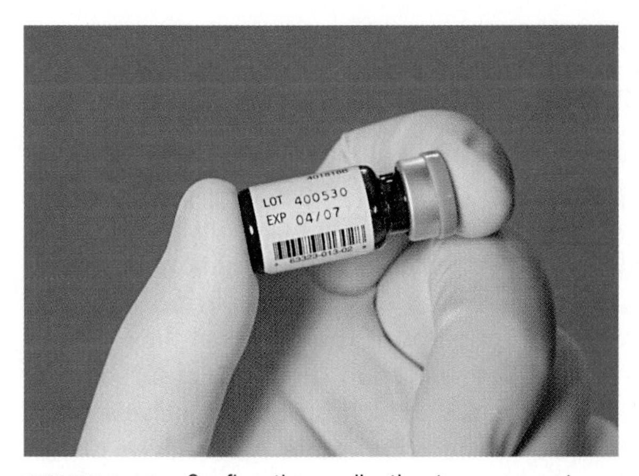

FIGURE 3-16a Confirm the medication type, amount, and expiration date.

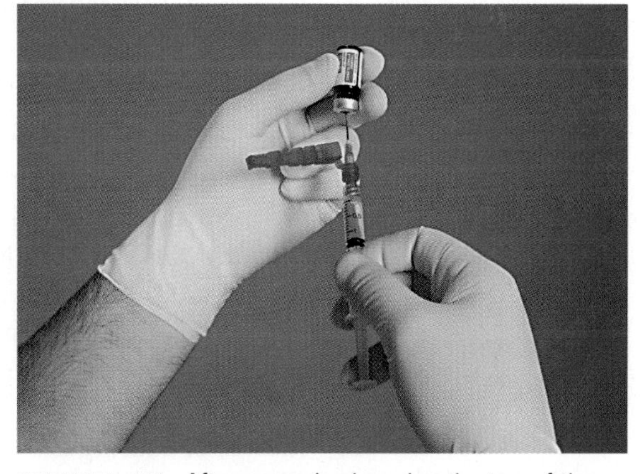

FIGURE 3-16b After properly cleansing the top of the vial, draw the medication into the syringe.

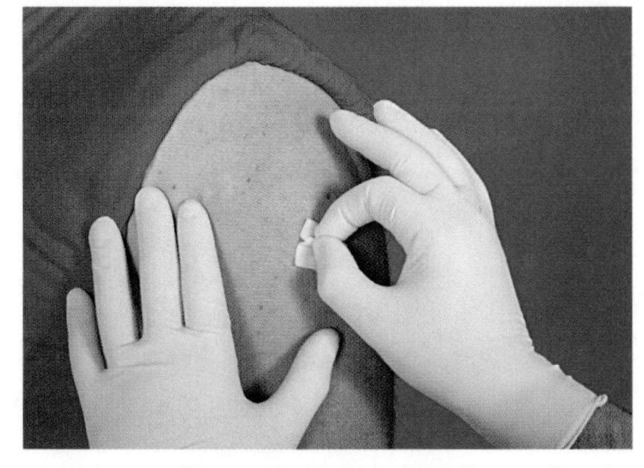

FIGURE 3-16c Cleanse the injection site with an antiseptic.

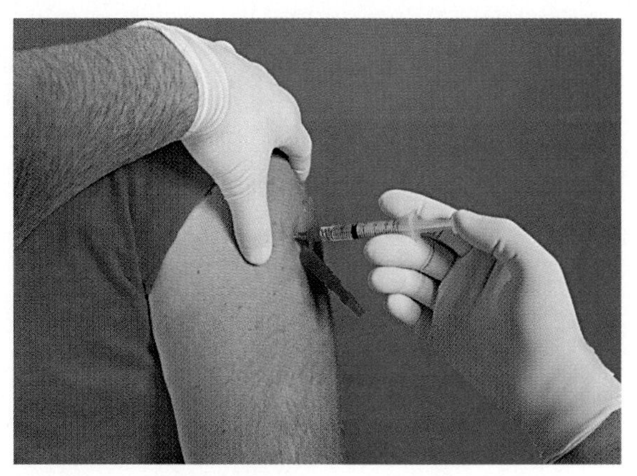

FIGURE 3-16d While holding the skin taut, insert the needle at a 90° angle to the skin. Draw back on the plunger slightly and observe for blood. If none is seen, inject the medication.

Continued on the next page

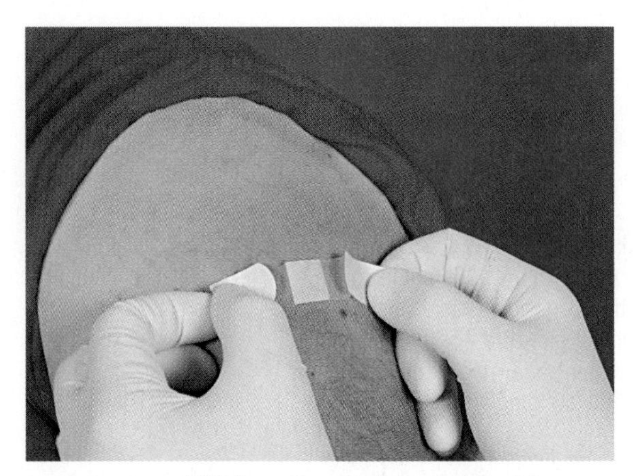

FIGURE 3-16e Withdraw the needle and discard it appropriately in a puncture-resistant biohazard container. Cover the injection site with a sterile dressing.

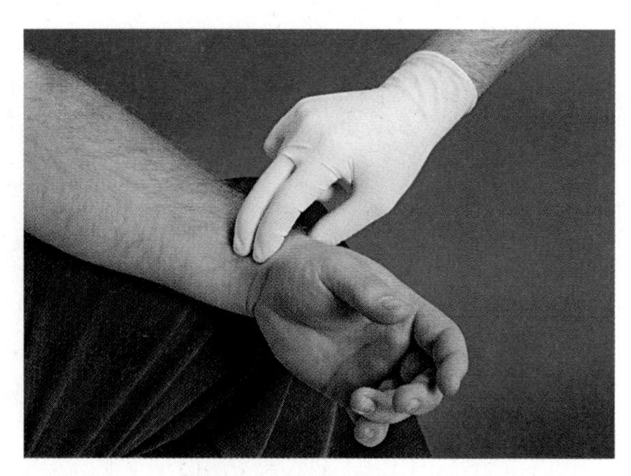

FIGURE 3-16f Reassess the patient.

6. Inject the proper dose into the muscle.
7. Remove the needle and cover the puncture site, if necessary. Dispose of the sharps properly.
8. Monitor the patient, and record the administration time and effects.

Subcutaneous Injection

Subcutaneous (SQ) injections are delivered into the fatty tissue under the outer layers of the skin, using a 5/8-inch, 25-gauge needle and a tuberculin or other syringe with a relatively small volume (Figure 3-17). SQ injections involve small quantities of medications, usually 0.5 to 1 ml of fluid. The medication most commonly administered subcutaneously in the field is 1:1,000 epinephrine.

The SQ route provides slower absorption of medication than the IV route. This may be beneficial in cases where the medication should be absorbed over time. The SQ route also poses fewer risks (e.g., the risk of striking blood vessels and nerves or causing tissue trauma) than other injection routes. Although we discuss the relatively slow speed of this route in relation to the needs of the critical patient, we should also note that, in most cases, SQ injection provides more rapid action than the oral route.

The most common location for SQ injection is the fatty tissue of the upper arm.

There are many locations around the body where SQ injections may be performed. The most common is the fatty tissue of the upper arm. This location provides easy access and requires minimal clothing removal.

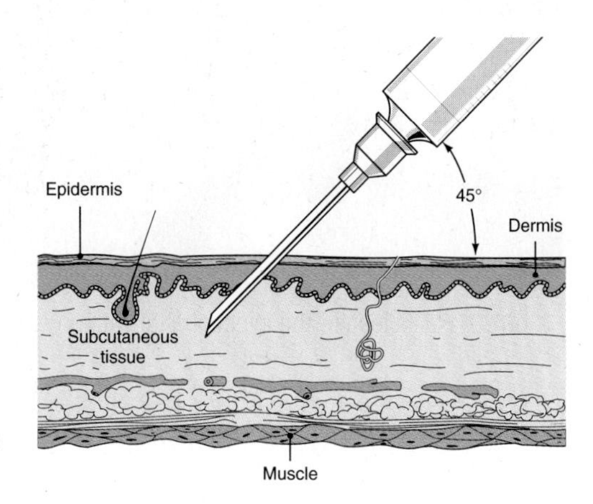

FIGURE 3-17
Subcutaneous injections are delivered at a 45° angle into the fatty tissue beneath the outer layers of the skin. Draw back the plunger slightly to ensure that the needle is not in a blood vessel.

To perform an SQ injection (Figure 3-18a–f),

1. Take body substance isolation precautions.
2. Gather the equipment and medication. Draw the medication into the syringe (or prepare the preloaded device).
3. Prep the site of injection with an alcohol swab.

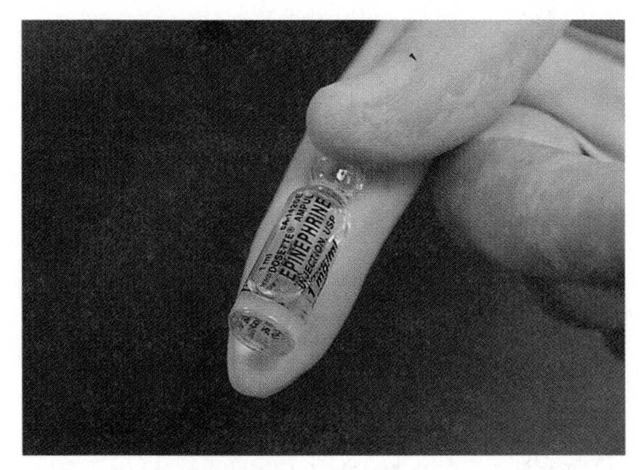

FIGURE 3-18a Check the medication.

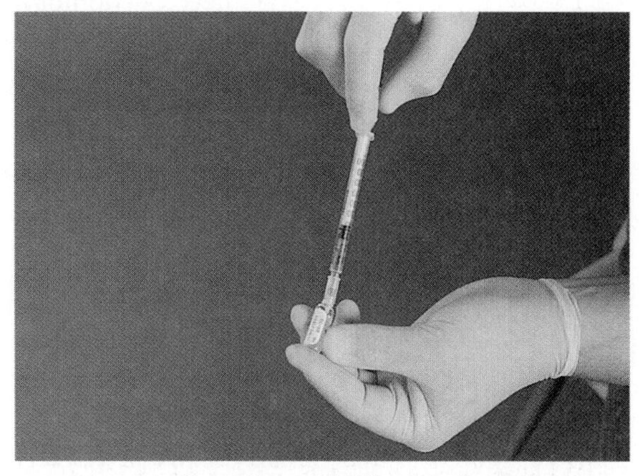

FIGURE 3-18b Draw the medication into the syringe.

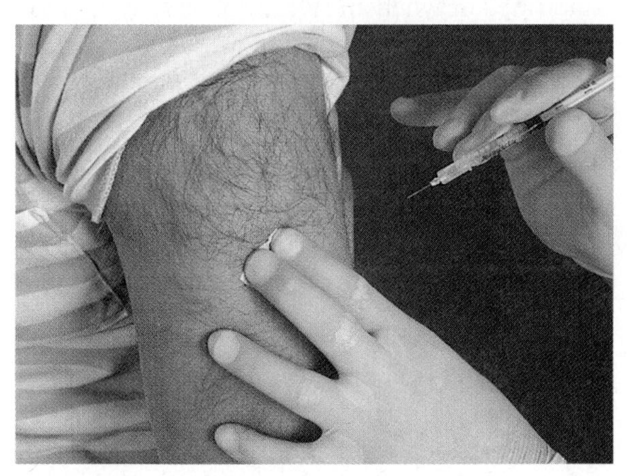

FIGURE 3-18c Prep the injection site.

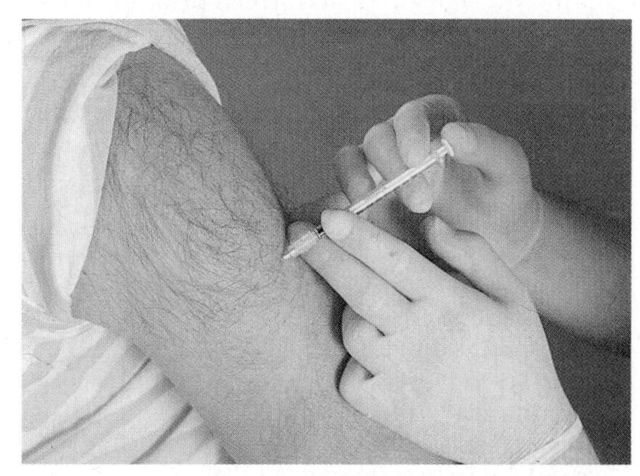

FIGURE 3-18d Insert the needle at a 45° angle. Draw back slightly on the plunger and observe for blood. If none is seen, inject the medication.

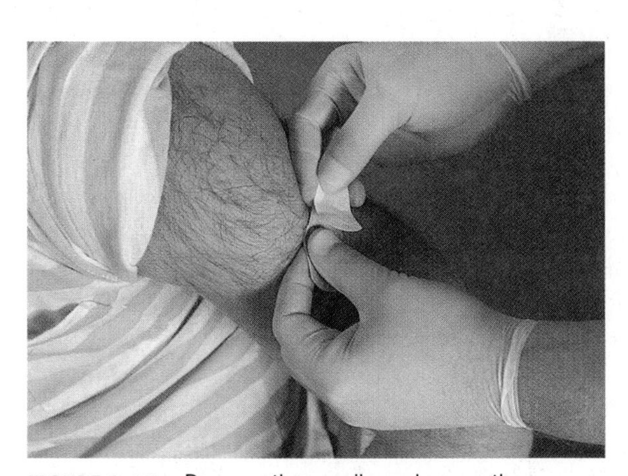

FIGURE 3-18e Remove the needle and cover the puncture site.

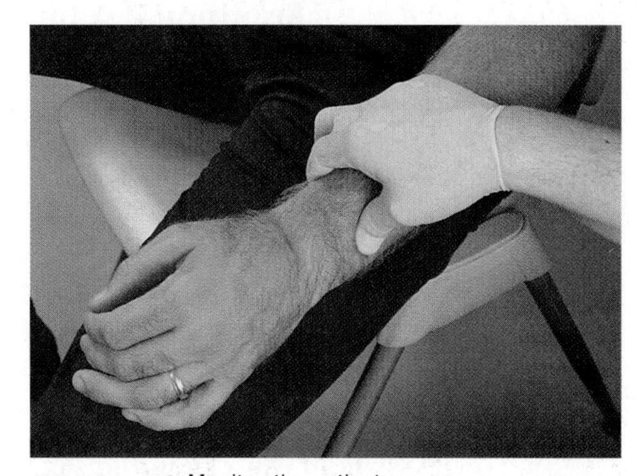

FIGURE 3-18f Monitor the patient.

4. Grasp the fatty tissue of the upper arm (or another appropriate location).
5. Insert the needle into the skin at a 45-degree angle.
6. Release the grasp of the fatty tissue, making sure the needle remains in the SQ tissue.
7. Draw back slightly on the plunger of the syringe to ensure that the needle is not in a blood vessel. If you see blood flow into the syringe, remove the needle—do not inject the medication. Choose another site.
8. Inject the proper dose into the patient.
9. Remove the needle and cover the puncture site, if necessary. Dispose of the sharp properly.
10. Monitor the patient, and record the administration time and effects.

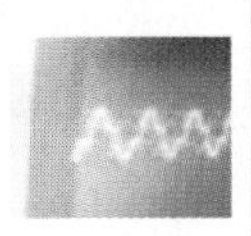

OTHER METHODS OF MEDICATION ADMINISTRATION

Tracheal Administration

Medications may be administered through the tracheal tube. This is usually performed prior to an IV line being established or when an IV cannot be started in the patient who requires intubation. The route of administration and the drugs that are routinely administered suggest that cardiac and respiratory arrest are the most common clinical situations in which this procedure is used.

Clinical Insight

To remember which medications are commonly administered through the tracheal tube, you can "lean" on the mnemonic LEAN, standing for lidocaine, epinephrine, atropine, and naloxone.

The medications that may be administered through the tracheal tube are lidocaine, epinephrine, atropine, and naloxone. The administration of diazepam (Valium) tracheally is controversial; it is not recommended that diazepam be administered via this route.

Generally, medications administered via the tracheal route are given in 2 to 2.5 times their usual strength. The recommended dose of atropine is 1.0 to 2.0 mg. The medication should be diluted in saline to bring the volume up to 10 ml of liquid (if necessary) to ensure adequate delivery of the medication to the lungs. The solution is injected directly into the tube between ventilations. The resumption of ventilations helps deliver the medication. Several authorities recommend three to four successive ventilations to distribute the medication into the lungs.

Sublingual Administration

Medications such as nitroglycerin may be administered sublingually. The vascular oral mucosa provides access for the medication to be absorbed into the circulation. Some risks are worthy of noting here.

Patient compliance is always an issue in the sublingual administration of medications. Lack of understanding, language or hearing barriers, or anxiety can cause the patient to swallow the medication rather than let it dissolve under the tongue. Nitroglycerin will also lose potency in a brief time, especially if exposed to light. Current recommendations are that tablets be replaced every 6 months. The patient does not always do this. If the cardiac discomfort is not relieved by the patient's nitroglycerin and the date of the prescription cannot be verified, a trial with current stock medication from the ambulance or emergency department may be worthwhile. For patients experienced in taking nitroglycerin, a headache

Patient compliance is always an issue in the sublingual administration of medications.

or a bitter taste may also indicate potent medication. Sublingual nitroglycerin sprays have a longer shelf life than tablets. With proper instruction, the compliance problems may also be reduced.

Be sure to monitor the patient carefully after administering nitroglycerin because it may result in a sudden drop in blood pressure. Nitroglycerin is contraindicated in hypotensive patients.

Oral Administration

Oral medications are not frequently given in the field. This is due to the prolonged and unpredictable absorption experienced by patients in shock and the potential inability of the patient to swallow or to protect the airway from aspiration of the medication. Obvious exceptions are medications that are used in oral poisonings: syrup of ipecac and activated charcoal.

Oral medications are the mainstay of medical maintenance at home. The importance of oral (or any) medications in the accurate medical history cannot be overemphasized.

Rectal Administration

Most drugs that are administered rectally are given via this route because other routes are unavailable. Two examples are diazepam, given rectally when an IV cannot be obtained in an actively seizing patient, and promethazine (Phenergan), when the patient cannot tolerate oral medications because of vomiting.

Rectal administration is performed with a 14-gauge IV catheter (needle removed) attached to a syringe containing the medication. Insert the catheter into the rectum and inject the medication. Remove the catheter and hold the buttocks together to retain the medication for absorption. You may also use a lubricated syringe (needle removed) or a pediatric tracheal tube to introduce the medication. In this method, remove the 15/22-mm adapter from the tracheal tube and attach the syringe containing the medication to the proximal end.

SUMMARY

Administration of medications to patients suffering medical problems is a critical part of prehospital care by advanced field care providers. The most common route of administration in the prehospital setting is the IV route. Other routes of administration are used in special circumstances. Parenteral routes (those outside the digestive tract) include IV, IM, SQ, tracheal, IO, inhalation, and transdermal. Enteral (digestive tract) routes include oral, sublingual, and rectal.

Decisions about whether to administer medications in the prehospital setting require clinical judgment that should involve consideration of standing orders, the needs and stability of the patient, and benefit versus risk analysis. The five "rights" must always be ensured: right medication, right dose, right route, right patient, right time.

Administration of medications always places the provider at considerable risk of contact with the patient's body substances, so it is essential always to use appropriate body substance isolation techniques when establishing an IV line, placing a tracheal tube, or performing any of the tasks involved in medication administration.

Many consider peripheral IV cannulation and medication administration to be simple skills. To an extent, they are. But most important, they are part of the decision-making process on which this book is founded. Many times the question is not "*How* do I start an IV?"; rather, it is "*Should* I start an IV?" Other forms of medication administration are the same. IO infusions and IM and SQ injections are relatively simple skills. What to do with them is the key. It is the difference between a technician and a clinician. Technicians can perform these procedures with overwhelming success. Clinicians can not only perform the procedures, but also know the how, when, and why of their use. Use these skills in combination with your clinical decision-making skills for the greatest success as a prehospital clinician.

SCENARIO FOLLOW-UP

You are at the scene for a 59-year-old male who collapsed suddenly after dinner and is in cardiac arrest. Fire department EMTs have already arrived and defibrillated the patient with two sets of three shocks. They continue CPR while your partner prepares to defibrillate again. You prepare to intubate the patient. The patient's cardiac rhythm converts to asystole. You intubate the patient. Your partner sets up a bag of normal saline and attempts an IV in the patient's left arm. The IV attempt is unsuccessful.

The EMTs continue resuscitation as you administer epinephrine down the tracheal tube. Your partner evaluates for other potential IV sites but cannot find any sites in the arms. Standing orders allow for external jugular cannulation for patients in cardiac arrest when other sites cannot be found. With oxygenation and epinephrine, the patient returns to ventricular fibrillation. After an additional shock, you repeat epinephrine and administer lidocaine down the tube.

The external jugular IV attempt is successful, and further medications are administered by this route. You and your partner move the patient to the ambulance as the resuscitation continues. En route to the hospital, the patient regains a pulse but has no respiratory effort. You continue ventilations and careful monitoring of the patient.

The patient continues to maintain a pulse with a blood pressure of 90/50 and is admitted to the coronary care unit (ccu). Respirations have not resumed, and the patient is placed on a ventilator. The patient suffers a second cardiac arrest in the CCU the next day. He dies after a lengthy resuscitation effort.

In this case, IV lines and medication administration were important parts of the patient's care. Your advanced life support team worked together to get all advanced life support tasks—manual defibrillation, intubation, and IV line—completed efficiently. When things do not go as we might like (e.g., when an IV is missed), alternative methods are used for medication administration. Although cardiac arrests are not the most common call, this was a case where IV and medication skills were effectively integrated to give the patient the best possible chance for a positive outcome.

FURTHER READING

1. American Heart Association. *Textbook of Advanced Cardiac Life Support.* 2002.
2. Bledsoe, B., R. Porter, and R. Cherry, "Medication administration," in *Paramedic Care: Principles and Practice—Volume 1.* Upper Saddle River, NJ: Pearson/Prentice Hall, 2000.
3. Bledsoe, B.E., D.E. Clayden, and F.J. Papa. *Prehospital Emergency Pharmacology.* 5th ed. Upper Saddle River, NJ: Pearson/Prentice Hall, 2001.
4. *Medication Administration and I.V. Therapy Manual: Process and Procedures.* 2nd ed. Springhouse, PA: Springhouse Corporation, 1993.
5. Mistovich, J.S., R.W. Benner, and G.S. Margolis. *Advanced Cardiac Life Support.* Upper Saddle River, NJ: Pearson/Prentice Hall, 1998.

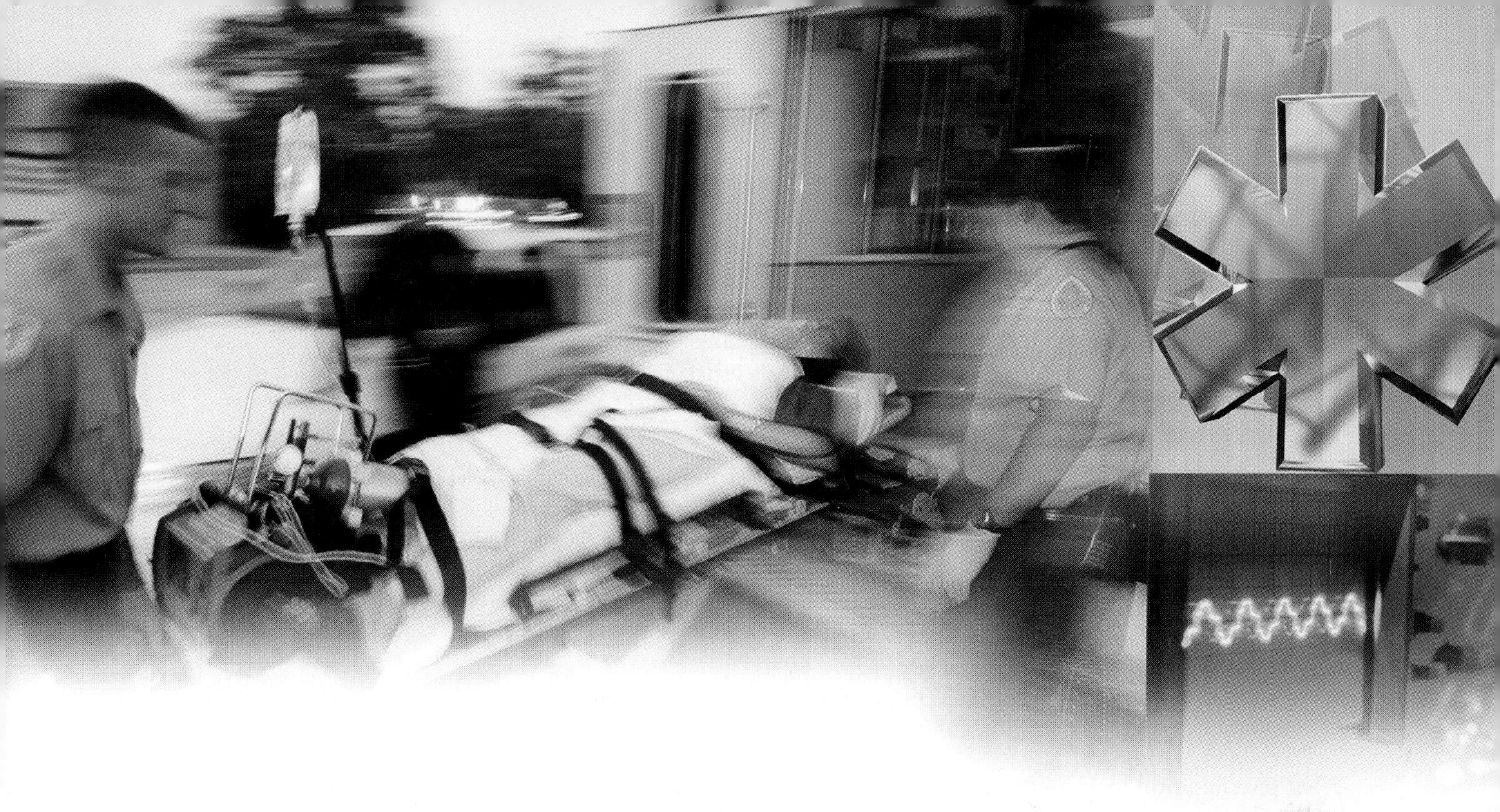

HYPOPERFUSION (SHOCK)

4

Hypoperfusion is the inadequate delivery of oxygen and other nutrients to the body's tissues. It can have many different causes and is the end result of a variety of disease processes. When not recognized and reversed in time, hypoperfusion will result in death. In fact, hypoperfusion (shock) is the major killer of humans. For this reason, the health care provider must understand the circumstances and conditions in which shock is possible, conduct a careful assessment, and recognize the signs and symptoms of shock. Based on these findings, the provider must take appropriate measures to support perfusion and prevent the progression of, or to reverse, shock.

Topics that are covered in this chapter are

- Defining Hypoperfusion and Shock
- Anatomy and Physiology of Tissue Perfusion
- Pathophysiology of Shock
- Differential Diagnosis
- Assessment Priorities
- Management Priorities

SCENARIO

You are called to the scene of a 65-year-old male who suddenly collapsed in his home. On arrival, you find your patient supine on his living room floor. He is awake and appears flushed. As you approach, you note that his breathing seems labored, and he looks uncomfortable. You also note a large dressing on his foot. You introduce yourself and ask the patient what seems to be the problem. He tells you he was watching TV when he felt nauseated and tried to get up but got very dizzy and "passed out." His son was standing beside him, eased him to the floor, and called 911. The patient seems to be alert and oriented but is very anxious.

You ask the patient if he has any pain. He denies pain but tells you "Something's wrong. I feel like I'm jumping out of my skin." You observe that, although he speaks in complete sentences, he is panting after he talks. You assist him in elevating his head and shoulders with a pillow. He tells you that it helps him feel better.

The patient tells you he was just dismissed from the hospital yesterday for a bunion removal and was doing fine until this episode. He is on Vasotec (enalapril) for hypertension and Motrin (ibuprofen) for pain. He takes both regularly, with the last dose of Vasotec taken about 30 minutes ago. He took Motrin last night. He denies any other problem and states he has no allergies that he knows of.

As you observe the patient, you note that he appears flushed all over. You ask if he has been outdoors, and he states that he has not been out for several days and, in fact, rarely goes outside.

What physiological mechanisms are suggested by his chief complaint, history, and initial assessment—and what differential diagnosis do these mechanisms suggest to this point? How would you proceed with further assessment to determine wider or narrower possibilities for your differential diagnosis? How would you begin care of this patient?

DEFINING HYPOPERFUSION AND SHOCK

Perfusion is the delivery of oxygen and other nutrients to the tissues of the body. It is the result of constant and adequate circulation of blood, which also provides for removal of waste products. *Hypoperfusion* is defined as inadequate tissue perfusion.

perfusion the delivery of oxygen and other nutrients to body tissues.

hypoperfusion inadequate tissue perfusion.

Inadequate tissue perfusion can be limited to one organ or tissue, as in the case of a coronary artery blockage that results in inadequate delivery of oxygenated blood to heart tissues, or it can be limited to one extremity, as might result from compartment syndrome or embolus restricting blood flow to an arm or leg. Hypoperfusion can also be systemic; the term *shock* is synonymous with systemic hypoperfusion. Of the various types of hypoperfusion, shock is the one that receives the most attention, is arguably the most frequent, and is the least understood. Throughout the remainder of this chapter, the terms *hypoperfusion* and *shock* are used interchangeably.

shock systemic hypoperfusion; inadequate delivery of oxygen and other nutrients to body tissues.

Shock is a state in which perfusion is inadequate to meet the cellular demands of the body. It can have a variety of causes. It may result from a problem with the lungs, the heart, the blood vessels, the blood, or the nervous system—the systems, organs, and substances that play key roles in perfusion. If allowed to progress uninterrupted, shock will involve every body system and ultimately lead to death. Thus, it is highly important to suspect when states of hypoperfusion may exist and to render treatment correctly and efficiently.

When hypoperfusion exists, the body attempts to compensate. The actions of compensatory mechanisms result in observable signs and symptoms. These signs and symptoms can provide clues to the presence of shock and its degree of severity.

Being able to suspect when states of hypoperfusion exist requires knowledge of the following:

- Mechanisms that cause shock
- Implications of assessment findings
- Diagnostic indicators pertinent for the field

In trauma, the mechanisms that cause shock include mechanisms of injury; in medical emergencies, mechanisms include disease states. In trauma, the mechanism of injury is sudden, definite, and usually obvious (e.g., a car crash, a gunshot wound, even a fall). The majority of clues to a mechanism of injury are found in observing the scene. With a medical problem, however, the mechanism of disease takes time to develop and is usually more subtle than a mechanism of injury. The majority of clues regarding the mechanism of disease are found in the history and require purposeful questioning.

Understanding the implications of assessment findings and diagnostic indicators pertinent for the field requires a thorough knowledge of anatomy, physiology, and pathophysiology.

Treatment of hypoperfusion requires rapid identification in order to implement appropriate therapy early enough to preserve organ function and, ultimately, the life of the patient. The remainder of this chapter is intended to

Hypoperfusion requires rapid identification and early therapy to preserve organ function and, ultimately, the life of the patient.

- Provide a background knowledge of anatomy, physiology, and pathophysiology so you can more readily recognize the indicators of hypoperfusion.
- Emphasize clues to the cause of hypoperfusion that you can find through history-taking and physical assessment.
- Improve your ability to recognize the degree of severity of hypoperfusion.
- Explain interventions you can take to slow the process of hypoperfusion.

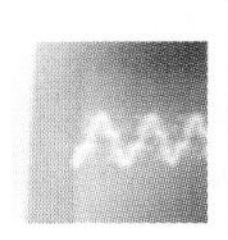

ANATOMY AND PHYSIOLOGY OF TISSUE PERFUSION

The work of perfusion (the exchange of oxygen, nutrients, and waste products between the blood and the cells) occurs at the capillary level. To provide adequate perfusion, the body requires an intact respiratory system (for exchange of oxygen and carbon dioxide), a sufficient amount of oxygen-rich (usually carried by hemoglobin) and nutrient-saturated blood, a functioning heart (to pump the blood), and a system of intact vessels to transport the blood. If any of these systems malfunctions, inadequate perfusion (shock) may occur.

Heart

Adequate tissue perfusion depends on *cardiac output,* which is defined as the amount of blood ejected from the left ventricle each minute. The classic formula for calculating cardiac output (in liters per minute) is *stroke volume* (milliliters of blood pumped by the left ventricle with each beat) times heart rate (beats per minute).

cardiac output the amount of blood ejected from the left ventricle each minute.

stroke volume the amount of blood ejected from the left ventricle with each heartbeat.

$$\text{stroke volume} \times \text{heart rate} = \text{cardiac output}$$

Cardiac output that is adequate to maintain perfusion requires a sufficient amount of blood delivered to the heart as well as a heart that is functioning adequately.

To maintain cardiac output, heart muscle requires sufficient oxygen and glucose to produce enough energy to keep up with the work load. Heart muscle is extraordinarily durable. Its contractions are affected by what is known as the *Frank-Starling mechanism.* In the Frank-Starling mechanism, the more cardiac muscle is stretched, the more strongly it will contract. Because of the Frank-Starling mechanism, the greater the *preload,* or volume of blood delivered to the heart from the venous system, the greater will be the force of contractions if the heart is healthy and adequately nourished. This is the vital mechanism that sustains perfusion when you exert yourself. However, in some patients, cardiac muscle or structure has become damaged (e.g., through a myocardial infarction, cardiomyopathy, or valvular damage) and has lost its ability to fully respond to the stimulus of preload. If cardiac muscle is not healthy or lacks sufficient oxygen or glucose to meet demand, cardiac failure may result.

Frank-Starling mechanism attribute of heart muscle by which the more it is stretched the more strongly it will contract.

preload the volume of blood delivered to the heart.

Vessels

Because the body's vascular system is so extensive (60,000 miles of vessels, including the capillary system) and the total blood volume relatively small (5–6 liters), regulation of blood flow is a constant and critical process. The body regulates blood flow by controlling either the size of the vessels or the amount of flow into the vessels.

The sympathetic and parasympathetic nervous systems are involved in controlling the size of the vessels, both arteries and veins, by constriction and dilation. Arterioles regulate blood flow to the capillary beds (Figure 4-1). At the juncture of the smallest arterioles (metaarterioles) and the capillary beds lies the precapillary sphincters. These sphincters contract and relax to regulate blood flow to the capillary beds. The function of the sphincters is influenced by the cells' demand for oxygen, need for nutrients, and accumulation of metabolic acids. The sphincters relax as needed to allow enough blood to enter the capillary beds to supply oxygen and nutrients and carry away wastes. The sphincters constrict when the need for oxygen and nutrients is reduced. Dilation of vessels in one area may be balanced by constriction in another to maintain the overall size of the vascular container.

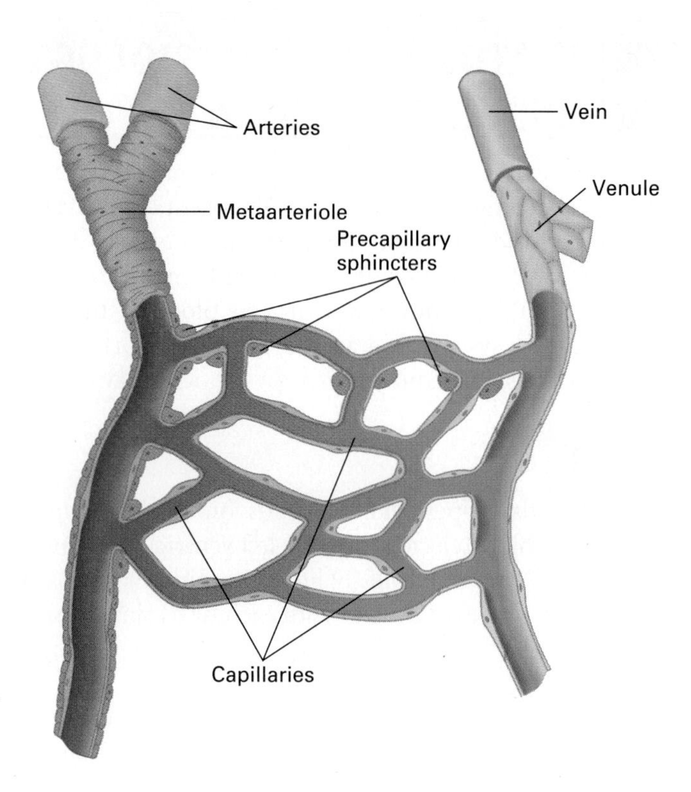

FIGURE 4-1
Capillary bed, showing precapillary sphincters (smooth muscle bands) at the junction of arteriole and capillaries. With sphincters relaxed, blood flows through the capillaries. With sphincters constricted, blood flow through the capillaries is reduced or stopped.

When arteries and veins constrict (vasoconstriction), there is an increase in peripheral vascular resistance (PVR), or *afterload,* which is defined as the resistance against which the heart must pump. Venous constriction also plays an important role in governing preload (the amount of blood reaching the heart), which in turn affects stroke volume and cardiac output. Vasoconstriction, primarily of the veins, can maintain enough pressure in the system to perfuse vital organs (heart, brain, lungs, and kidneys) almost normally, even when as much as 25 percent of the total blood volume has been lost. In shock, shunting blood to the vital organs (those that work to maintain perfusion) becomes the body's priority. Because there are more veins than arteries in the body, veins and venules serve as a blood reservoir when needed. When the mechanism of vasoconstriction fails, this same proportion of veins to arteries may cause a relative hypovolemia.

afterload the resistance against which the heart must pump.

Blood

The blood plays a key role in perfusion, transporting oxygen and glucose to the body's cells and transporting wastes away from the cells. Oxygen is carried to the cells by hemoglobin, the iron-containing pigment of the red blood cells. Waste carbon dioxide is carried to the lungs in the form of carbonic acid dissolved in the plasma of the blood.

Inhaled oxygen diffuses across the walls of the alveoli (the air cells of the lungs) into the adjoining capillaries, to be picked up by the hemoglobin of the blood. At the same time, waste carbon dioxide is diffusing into the lungs to be exhaled. Although inhalation of oxygen is critical to the body's survival, it is important to remember that exhalation of carbon dioxide is equally important. If anything interferes with exhalation of carbon dioxide, the build-up of excess carbon dioxide fosters formation of harmful metabolic acids, causing a condition known as *acidosis.*

acidosis excessive acidity of body fluids.

To keep the organ systems involved with perfusion working smoothly, and also to meet the extreme metabolic demands caused by hypoperfusion, various hormones come into play. These hormones, carried in the bloodstream, enhance the working properties of the organ systems.

PATHOPHYSIOLOGY OF SHOCK

A state of hypoperfusion, or shock, can result from dysfunction of any part of the network of organs, systems, and substances that normally maintain perfusion. For example, a neurological dysfunction that causes dilation of the blood vessels or prevents them from constricting will make the vascular container too large for the existing volume of blood. A severe blood loss will mean that there is not enough blood to fill the vascular container, even with constriction of the vessels. A failure of cardiac function will interfere with the pumping of blood to all organs and tissues.

Because the primary causes of shock differ and body tissues malfunction at different stages of metabolic impairment, signs and symptoms of shock vary and sometimes conflict. Skin color may be flushed, pale, or mottled. Heart rates may be bradycardic, normal, or tachycardic. Lungs may be clear or full of fluid. Core temperature may be hyperthermic, normal, or hypothermic. Sweating may be absent, generalized, or limited to the head and neck.

Because primary causes differ and body tissues malfunction at different stages of impairment, signs and symptoms of shock vary and sometimes conflict.

hypovolemia loss of body fluid that ultimately results in (hypovolemic) shock.

hemorrhagic shock shock resulting from blood loss; a subcategory of hypovolemic shock.

With such a wide variety of seemingly contradictory signs and symptoms, you might conclude that there is no way to know whether a patient is or is not experiencing shock. However, there is a classic shock syndrome—the cluster of signs and symptoms that are associated with *hypovolemia* or, more specifically, *hemorrhagic shock.*

Because hemorrhage is the most common cause of shock, the processes of hemorrhagic shock and the stages the patient suffering from hemorrhagic shock goes through serve as a baseline to which all other types of shock are compared. For field personnel, the processes and stages can be identified by signs and symptoms. Our patients, however, rarely fit into neat little categories. So, you should not only rely on a list of signs and symptoms, but also gain an appreciation for the underlying processes of shock so you can readily recognize it, determine the degree of severity, begin appropriate treatment, and initiate timely transport.

The stages of shock discussed in the following segment are described as they would typically progress in a state of hemorrhagic shock. Other types of shock are discussed in later segments. Although hemorrhagic shock is more commonly encountered in trauma, it does occur from medical causes such as gastrointestinal bleeds or ruptured ectopic pregnancy. Even though other types of shock may more commonly occur from medical causes, remember that hemorrhagic shock illustrates the basic principles of shock to which other types of shock are compared.

The Classic Stages of Shock

Shock is ultimately a cellular event (Table 4-1) that progresses through a series of definable cellular changes. These changes result in observable signs and symptoms that are divided into a series of stages from mild to lethal—from compensated, to progressive (decompensated), to irreversible.

Compensated Shock

A reduction in cardiac output is an integral factor in all types and stages of shock. It may be a cause, an effect, or both. The cycle of hemorrhagic shock begins with blood loss, which causes a decrease in preload, which in turn causes a reduction in cardiac output.

Whatever the triggering event, when shock starts, baroreceptors in the arch of the aorta and in the carotid sinus detect a fall in cardiac output almost immediately, and the body's effort to compensate for shock begins. The pressure receptors in the baroreceptors and carotid sinus stimulate the medullae of the adrenal glands to increase secretion of epinephrine and norepinephrine.

TABLE 4-1 Progression of Cellular Destruction in Shock

I	▪ Normal cell.
II	▪ Hypoxia and cellular ischemia occur; anaerobic metabolism begins; lactic acid production greatly increases, leading to metabolic acidosis; sodium-potassium pump fails.
III	▪ Ion shift occurs; sodium moves into the cell, bringing water with it.
IV	▪ Cellular swelling occurs.
V	▪ Mitochondrial swelling occurs; failure of energy production widespread.
VI	▪ Intracellular disruption releases lysosomes, and breaks in plasma membrane evident.
VII	▪ Cell destruction begins.

Epinephrine and norepinephrine are catecholamines, a type of hormone, which the adrenal glands secrete directly into the bloodstream. Epinephrine and norepinephrine interact with alpha (α_1 and α_2) and beta (β_1 and β_2) receptors located on the membranes of most organs, including the heart, lungs, blood vessels, and sweat glands.

Alpha receptors (both α_1 and α_2 receptors affect the vasculature), stimulated primarily by norepinephrine, cause vasoconstriction, which increases peripheral vascular resistance. As mentioned earlier, the increased peripheral vascular resistance results in increased preload, which increases stroke volume and cardiac output.

Vasoconstriction occurs first in the organs least necessary for immediate survival. Those organs include the intestinal tract and the skin (periphery). The constriction of blood vessels in the skin causes pallor. The degree of vasoconstriction that is needed to maintain cardiac output will govern the degree of pallor you see. Pallor may initially be very subtle in patients with darker skin tones. Usually, pallor is most noticeable in the mucous membranes, the conjunctiva of the eyes and the skin under the eyes, around the mouth and nose, and in the hands, arms, feet, and legs. Vasoconstriction also causes the skin to become cool. Additionally, the loss of blood decreases heat production. Decreased oxygen and glucose contribute to decreased metabolism. Decreased metabolism lowers body temperature.

In addition to causing vasoconstriction, alpha receptor stimulation of sweat glands causes diaphoresis, which is perceived as clammy skin. When it begins, diaphoresis is subtle with early signs of sweating appearing on the upper lip and under the eyes.

Beta receptors, affected primarily by epinephrine, cause bronchodilation (β_2 receptors) and stimulation of cardiac function (β_1 receptors), both of which help compensate for reduced perfusion. Bronchodilation results in more oxygen reaching the alveoli of the lungs and, thus, the body cells, and also boosts removal of waste carbon dioxide. Beta $_1$ effects on cardiac function are summarized in the mnemonic CARDIO:

Beta effects on cardiac function cause an increase of

C = Contractility
A = Automaticity
R = Rate
D = Dilation (of coronary arteries)
I = Irritability
O = Oxygen demand

Together, the vasoconstrictive actions of alpha stimulation and the cardiac effects of beta stimulation increase preload, stroke volume, and heart rate. The result is an increase in cardiac output. In this manner, during the period of *compensated shock,* the body maintains perfusion.

compensated shock the period of shock during which the body is able to compensate for the effects of shock and maintain adequate tissue perfusion.

Keep in mind that the increase in heart rate is relative to the person's own resting heart rate. The increase may not be immediately noticed in those with slower resting heart rates. In patients on certain medications such as beta-blockers, the increase in heart rate may be limited or even prevented.

Combined effects of alpha and beta stimulation in other areas of the body help increase the body's energy supply by converting glycogen to glucose.

In emergency situations and in the field, a rough indicator of cardiac output is blood pressure, and a relatively reliable indicator of perfusion is mental status. Blood pressure is a function of the force of contraction and the resistance against which the contraction must work. If compensatory efforts are successful in sufficiently stimulating cardiac contractility and vasoconstriction, the body will maintain a blood pressure within normal limits. Additionally, the brain will be sufficiently perfused so the mental status will be alert to slightly anxious. A normal blood pressure finding does NOT rule out the presence of shock.

Clinical Insight

Because compensatory efforts will maintain blood pressure within normal limits as shock progresses, keep in mind that a normal blood pressure does *not* rule out the presence of shock.

Progressive (Decompensated) Shock

If shock continues without relief, further compensatory mechanisms are stimulated. The kidneys detect a drop in filtration pressure and release renin, which sets off a chain of compensatory events. Renin is an enzyme that, when released into the blood, stimulates the conversion of angiotensinogen into angiotensin I. This protein travels to the lungs and is converted to angiotensin II, a powerful vasoconstrictor that further constricts arterioles, precapillary sphincters of the capillary beds, and veins; further stimulates the sympathetic nervous system; and also stimulates aldosterone production. Aldosterone acts directly on the kidneys to conserve sodium, which acts to conserve body water. The combination of increased vasoconstriction and conservation of body water further maintains preload, thus maintaining stroke volume and thereby cardiac output.

In the absence of sufficient oxygen, normal aerobic metabolism changes to anaerobic metabolism.

At this point, the cells and tissues supplied by the capillary beds are subject to increasing vasoconstriction and suffer further hypoperfusion. In the absence of sufficient oxygen, normal aerobic metabolism changes to anaerobic metabolism with a corresponding increase in waste products, especially carbon dioxide and metabolic acids. As metabolic acids build up, the respiratory system attempts to compensate by increasing the rate and depth of ventilation. The body can maintain adequate tidal volume at rates up to 30 breaths per minute. However, at rates over 30, the rate overtakes the depth, and rapid, shallow respirations are characteristic of this stage of shock.

The increasing vasoconstriction and corresponding constriction of the precapillary sphincters shunts blood to vital organs but traps the remaining blood, causing pooling in the capillary beds. Pooling may cause mottling of the skin. Pallor progresses to cyanosis as a result of hypoxemia and tissue hypoxia. Cyanosis is usually detected first around the nose, mouth, earlobes, and distal extremities. There may be conditions, such as poor lighting or patients with darker skin tones, that make detection of cyanosis difficult. In such cases, use other clinical findings, such as changes in mental status or appearance of mucous membranes, to evaluate adequacy of perfusion.

progressive shock the period of shock during which the body begins to lose its ability to compensate for shock ("decompensates") and becomes unable to maintain adequate tissue perfusion. Progressive shock is also known as *decompensated shock*.

It is during this stage—*progressive shock* (also known as *decompensated shock*)—that the classic signs of shock are noted: mental status changes (drowsiness, lethargy, or combativeness); cool or cold, clammy skin that is obviously pale or slightly cyanotic; widespread sweating; tachycardia; rapid, shallow respirations; and a falling blood pressure. If the patient is seen at this stage, it is usually very obvious that there is something wrong.

Irreversible Shock

If the process of shock is allowed to continue, cellular damage occurs as the result of the continued buildup of carbon dioxide and metabolic acids. Circulating blood actually becomes toxic to the surrounding cells. Cell membranes start to break down, releasing lysosomal enzymes (highly acidic substances from within the cells). Capillary sphincters become ineffective and dysfunction, releasing highly toxic, pooled blood into the already acidic circulation. Acidic blood causes red blood cells to stack into misshaped chains called rouleaux formation. Unable to bend like normal red blood cells, the rouleaux form microemboli, lodging in the capillary beds of organs and further contributing to organ ischemia. Together, the circulating enzymes, acids, and microemboli contribute to the failure of the organs that are still being perfused, specifically the lungs, brain, heart, and kidneys.

At this stage, most patients are unresponsive (there are, however, exceptions). The pulse disappears, and the susceptible heart may show irritable dysrhythmias (e.g., premature ventricular contractions [PVCs]). The rhythm eventually becomes bradycardic. On the ECG, the P wave disappears, the QRS complex widens, and an idioventricular rhythm progresses into asystole. There is no detectable blood pressure, and respirations become agonal. The skin is frequently gray or mottled, and the hands and feet appear waxen or cyanotic. Production of sweat ceases, but if evaporation has not occurred, the skin will remain clammy. Adult respiratory distress syndrome (ARDS—a disorder resulting from abnormal permeability of the pulmonary capillaries or alveolar epithelium) is especially common. The patient is also likely to suffer hypoxic brain syndrome, kidney failure, and heart failure. Even if the patient is resuscitated at this phase, the mortality rate is still very high. This phase of shock is termed *irreversible shock* because the prognosis is so poor. However, support of the body systems long enough to allow these systems to heal will sometimes result in a positive outcome.

irreversible shock an advanced condition of shock in which cell, tissue, and organ damage cannot be reversed and will, in most circumstances, result in death.

DIFFERENTIAL DIAGNOSIS

As stated earlier, any factor that interferes with cardiac function, vascular integrity, or intravascular volume can cause shock. The initial organ system affected will usually determine the signs and symptoms that occur. Types of shock are known either by the primary organ of dysfunction or by the primary cause of dysfunction. The Weil-Shubin classification of shock is listed here and briefly described in Table 4-2.

Types of Shock

- Hypovolemic shock (includes hemorrhagic shock)
- Obstructive shock (includes cardiac tamponade, tension pneumothorax, and pulmonary emboli)
- Distributive shock (includes neurogenic, anaphylactic, and septic shock)
- Cardiogenic shock

All types of shock, if unrelieved, will progress through compensated, progressive, and irreversible stages, although these stages may manifest differently in different types of shock. The classic manifestations for hemorrhagic shock, as described on earlier pages, are summarized in Table 4-3.

TABLE 4-2 Types of Shock

Hypovolemic Shock	■ Caused by an insufficient amount of blood or body water. The most common cause of hypoperfusion is severe blood loss, or hemorrhage. Hypovolemic shock caused by blood loss is commonly called hemorrhagic shock.
Obstructive Shock	■ Caused by an obstruction, usually mechanical, that prevents return of sufficient blood to the heart (e.g., cardiac tamponade, pulmonary embolism, or tension pneumothorax).
Distributive Shock	■ Caused by an abnormal distribution of blood and insufficient return of blood to the heart resulting from uncontrolled vasodilation, extreme vascular permeability, or a combination of both. There are several types of distributive shock. If the condition results from dysfunction of the nervous system, it is neurogenic shock; if from a severe allergic reaction, it is anaphylactic shock; if from septicemia (the presence of pathogenic bacteria in the blood), it is septic shock.
Cardiogenic Shock	■ Caused by insufficient cardiac pumping power. The most common cause of cardiogenic shock is an acute myocardial infarction, resulting in the injury or death of heart muscle, and the consequent failure of the left ventricle to pump effectively. Other causes include valvular failure and abnormal rates (e.g., too fast or too slow).

TABLE 4-3 Classic Shock Syndrome—Hemorrhagic Shock

Type	Signs and Symptoms					
	Mental Status	**Skin**	**Blood Pressure**	**Pulse**	**Respiration**	**Other**
Compensated Shock **Mechanisms** *Volume depletion* *Body detects fall in cardiac output.* *Sympathetic nervous system stimulates secretion of epinephrine and norepinephrine, which stimulate alpha and beta receptors.* *Alpha stimulation causes vasoconstriction.* *Beta stimulation causes bronchodilation and cardiac stimulation.*	■ Hyperalert progressing to anxious	■ Becoming cool, pale. ■ Sweating begins at upper lip, under eyes, gradually extending to other areas.	■ Normal	■ Normal to rapid	■ Normal to rapid	
Progressive Shock **Mechanisms** *Kidneys secrete substances that simulate further vasoconstriction and conservation of body water.* *Due to increased hypoperfusion, cell wastes and metabolic acids build up.*	■ Drowsiness, lethargy, or combativeness	■ Cool to cold, clammy. ■ Blood pooling causes mottling. ■ Pallor progresses to cyanosis around nose, mouth, earlobes, distal extremities. ■ Delayed capillary return.	■ Begins to fall	■ Becomes rapid	■ Becomes rapid, shallow	■ Decreased urination
Irreversible Shock **Mechanisms** *Compensatory mechanisms unable to maintain perfusion.* *Hypoxia* *Further build-up of metabolic acids and other wastes. Circulation of acids, enzymes, microemboli. Cell damage and death. Organ failure.*	■ Deteriorating to unresponsiveness	■ Gray, mottled, cyanotic, waxen. ■ Sweat production ceases, but skin may remain clammy if evaporation is slow.	■ Decreases, becomes undetectable	■ Slows, then disappears	■ Agonal respirations	■ Irritable heart, prone to dysrhythmias, deteriorates to asystole.

When the cause of shock is something other than blood loss, there will be some differences from the classic syndrome and considerable difference in treatment. Establishing the underlying etiology of shock determines pharmacologic treatment and, in the case of discriminating between anaphylactic and cardiogenic shock, can determine survival.

In the majority of cases, a good history will reveal the likely causes, while the physical exam will confirm what the history has already told you. However, when the history is vague or confusing, the differential diagnosis may be limited to identifying the body system affected rather than a more specific cause for the problem.

Determining which body system needs specific reassessment will point you in the direction of a cause. The patient's respiratory status will be one principal guide to a differential diagnosis, so adequate assessment of the respiratory system is a required skill. Because hearing lung sounds in the back of a moving vehicle is very difficult, the care provider needs to have an idea of precipitating causes prior to leaving the scene, using the early assessment findings, including respiratory effort, as a baseline to which further assessment results will be compared.

The following sections of the text and Table 4-4 summarize the types of shock with an emphasis on how their mechanisms, signs, and symptoms may differ from those of the "classic" shock syndrome that were shown in Table 4-3.

Clinical Insight

It is important to balance the need for assessment at the scene with the need for expeditious transport. Because the lung sounds are a key guide to a differential diagnosis of shock, and hearing lung sounds in a moving ambulance is very difficult, take care to assess a baseline respiratory status before leaving the scene.

Hypovolemic Shock

Hypovolemic shock results from a loss of fluid volume: blood, plasma, or body water. As explained earlier, blood loss is specifically referred to as hemorrhagic shock. This is the classic type of shock described in the previous section. Medical causes of internal bleeding include ruptured cysts, ectopic pregnancies, ruptured aortic aneurysms, gastrointestinal (GI) bleeds, vaginal hemorrhage, and so on.

hypovolemic shock shock resulting from fluid loss: blood, plasma, or body water.

Body-water loss resulting in dehydration is usually due to vomiting and/or diarrhea or excessive sweating or excessive urination as in unrecognized hypoglycemic hyperosmolar nonketotic coma. Third spacing (loss of fluid from the vascular system or cells into the interstitial spaces of the body) is another mechanism of body-water loss that may cause severe edema and that may be due to infection such as peritonitis, protein losses, or other causes. Dehydration is an acute problem often encountered, especially in the very young and the elderly.

Skin vitals in the patient suffering shock from dehydration may vary somewhat from those seen in hemorrhagic shock in that sweating may not be apparent and the skin may have poor turgor. A frequent assessment finding in the dehydrated patient is dry skin with tenting (the skin tending to remain peaked after being pinched and released—Figure 4-2). A common finding seen in hypovolemic shock is thirst. The exception to this is elderly patients, who may have impaired thirst mechanisms.

skin vitals skin color, temperature, and moisture.

You may suspect the presence of hypovolemia after or while you are performing airway control, delivering high-flow, high-concentration oxygen, and assuring adequate tidal volume. If you suspect hypovolemia, start an IV of crystalloid solution for fluid replacement. Appropriate solutions include normal saline (or 0.9 percent sodium chloride) or lactated Ringer's. Administer the solution at a rapid flow rate, usually by bolus, 250 to 500 cc at a time, and then reassess respiratory function, mental status, and vital signs. Research suggests that large amounts of crystalloid dilute clotting factors. A maximum of 3 liters of crystalloid has been suggested to help prevent this effect, although several medical conditions may require larger amounts of fluid. Preventing high systolic pressures has also been proposed in cases of internal bleeding to prevent disruption of clots that may have

TABLE 4-4 Types of Shock—as Contrasted to Classic Shock Syndrome

Type	Signs and Symptoms *Hallmarks of the specific type of shock* *Signs and symptoms that differ from those of the classic shock syndrome*					
	Mental Status	**Skin**	**Blood Pressure**	**Pulse**	**Respiration**	**Other**
Hypovolemic Shock **Mechanism** *Volume depletion*						
From Blood Loss (hemorrhagic shock) *See Table 4-3—Classic Shock Syndrome*						
From Dehydration **Mechanism** *Volume depletion*		■ Sweating absent ■ Poor skin turgor (tenting)				■ Thirst (except in elderly with impaired thirst mechanism)
Obstructive Shock **Mechanisms** *Obstruction that interferes with preload and/or afterload*						
From Pulmonary Embolism **Mechanism** *Pulmonary circulation blocked*	■ Anxiety; sense of impending doom	■ Pallor to cyanosis, especially around nose and mouth				■ Possible chest pain ■ Lung sounds may be clear ■ Possible syncope ■ Possible cardiac dysrhythmias (PVCs, atrial fibrillation) ■ Possible cardiac arrest
From Tension Pneumothorax and Cardiac Tamponade **Mechanisms** *Pressure in thoracic cavity; pressure on aorta, ventricles* *Backup of venous pressure*		■ Cyanosis first around nose and mouth		■ Paradoxical pulse; narrowed pulse pressure	■ Sudden sharp chest pain and shortness of breath in COPD patient with ruptured bleb ■ Clear lung sounds	■ Distended neck and hand veins ■ Discriminating signs: Unequal lung sounds in tension pneumothorax Distant heart sounds in cardiac tamponade—hard to detect in the field

TABLE 4-4 **Types of Shock—as Contrasted to Classic Shock Syndrome** *(continued)*

Type	**Signs and Symptoms** *Hallmarks of the specific type of shock* *Signs and symptoms that differ from those of the classic shock syndrome*					
	Mental Status	**Skin**	**Blood Pressure**	**Pulse**	**Respiration**	**Other**
Distributive Shock Mechanisms *Abnormality in vasodilation or vasopermeability or both—interferes with preload/afterload*						
Neurogenic Shock (from injury to the spinal cord or compromise of nervous system function from drug/poison) **Mechanism** *Vasodilation*		■ In areas of vasodilation: at first becomes warm and dry with normal skin color ■ Later with pooling: mottling of dependent areas, pallor and cyanosis to upper surfaces		■ Highly variable depending on injury or action of the drug/poison: may be abnormally slow or abnormally rapid	■ Severely compromised ■ Becoming slow, shallow, with abnormal patterns ■ Patient may lose stimulus to breathe	■ Hypothermia ■ Pulmonary edema may occur with drug/poison
Anaphylactic Shock (from a severe allergic reaction) **Mechanism** *Vasodilation* *Permeability of vessels* *Fluid shift from vasculature to cells* *Smooth muscle contraction* *Microclotting*		■ Hives ■ Itching ■ Possible petechia ■ Possible flushing or pallor/cyanosis		■ Abrupt fall in cardiac output	■ Rapid, shallow ■ Possible shortness of breath ■ Possible dyspnea with stridor, wheezing, crackles ■ Possible respiratory arrest	■ Swelling of mucous membranes ■ Possible pulmonary edema
Septic Shock **Mechanism** *Overwhelming infection causing build-up of endotoxins*		■ Varies from flushed pink (if fever is present) to pale and cyanotic ■ Possible petechia ■ Possible purple blotches ■ Possible peeling (general or at palms and soles) ■ Red streaks progressing proximally	■ Early: cardiac output increases but toxins may cause loss of peripheral vascular resistance ■ Late: Hypotension; precipitous fall in blood pressure		■ Dyspnea with altered lung sounds	■ Possible high fever (except some elderly and very young patients) ■ Late: frank pulmonary edema

TABLE 4-4 Types of Shock—as Contrasted to Classic Shock Syndrome *(continued)*

Type	Signs and Symptoms *Hallmarks of the specific type of shock* *Signs and symptoms that differ from those of the classic shock syndrome*					
	Mental Status	**Skin**	**Blood Pressure**	**Pulse**	**Respiration**	**Other**
Cardiogenic Shock Mechanisms *Heart (pump) failure; drop in cardiac output*		■ Cyanosis		■ Rate may be bradycardic, tachycardic, or within normal limits	■ Diminishing lung sounds progressing to wheezing and crackles ■ Patient complains of increased difficulty breathing ■ Coughs up white or pink-tinged foamy sputum	■ Pulmonary edema

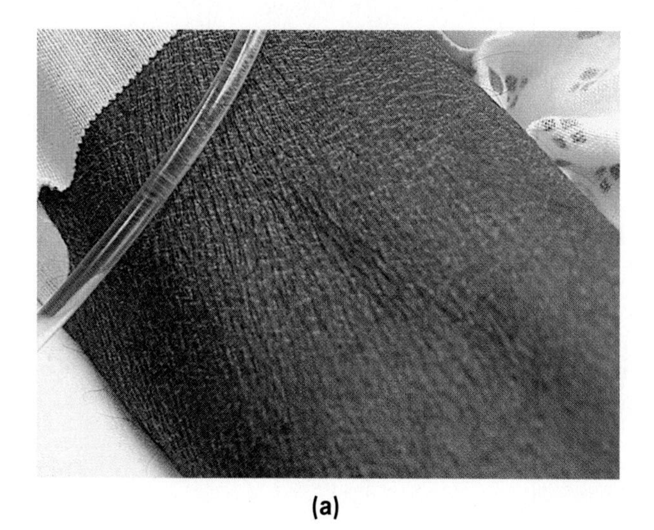

(a)

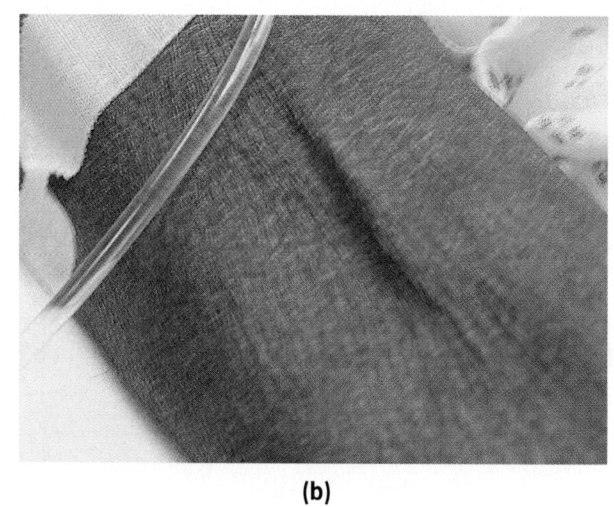

(b)

FIGURE 4-2
Tenting of the skin is a sign associated with dehydration. (a) The arm before the skin is pinched. (b) If the person is dehydrated, the skin remains "tented" after the pinch is released. (© Edward T. Dickinson, M.D.)

formed internally. Sufficient fluid is generally given to support a systolic pressure of 70 to 100 mmHg.

Research supporting these concepts has been done primarily on trauma patients. It is unclear how this will apply to patients with nontraumatic causes of bleeding, the elderly, or those with an underlying history of hypertension. Local medical direction will dictate specific guidelines.

Obstructive Shock

Obstructive shock is a category that includes any mechanical obstruction—such as tension pneumothorax, cardiac tamponade, or pulmonary emboli—that interferes with preload and/or afterload.

obstructive shock shock resulting from a mechanical obstruction of the circulatory system, such as tension pneumothorax, cardiac tamponade, or pulmonary emboli.

Tension Pneumothorax and Cardiac Tamponade

Tension pneumothorax and cardiac tamponade interfere with both preload and afterload. They are frequently associated with trauma but can also occur as a result of medical conditions. *Tension pneumothorax* (Figure 4-3) (air or gas trapped in

tension pneumothorax air or gas trapped in the pleural space with no route of escape.

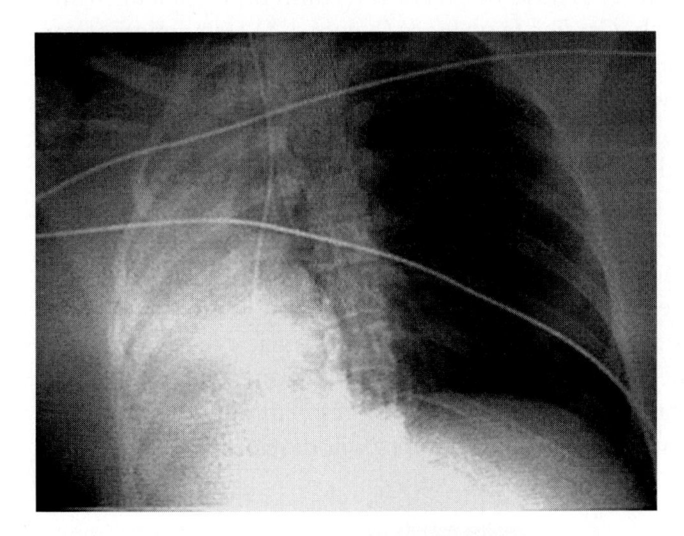

FIGURE 4-3a
With tension pneumothorax, as shown in this X-ray, air enters the chest cavity, collapsing the affected lung, exerting pressure on the opposite lung, and causing deviation of the trachea away from the affected side. (© Howard A. Werman, M.D., FACEP.)

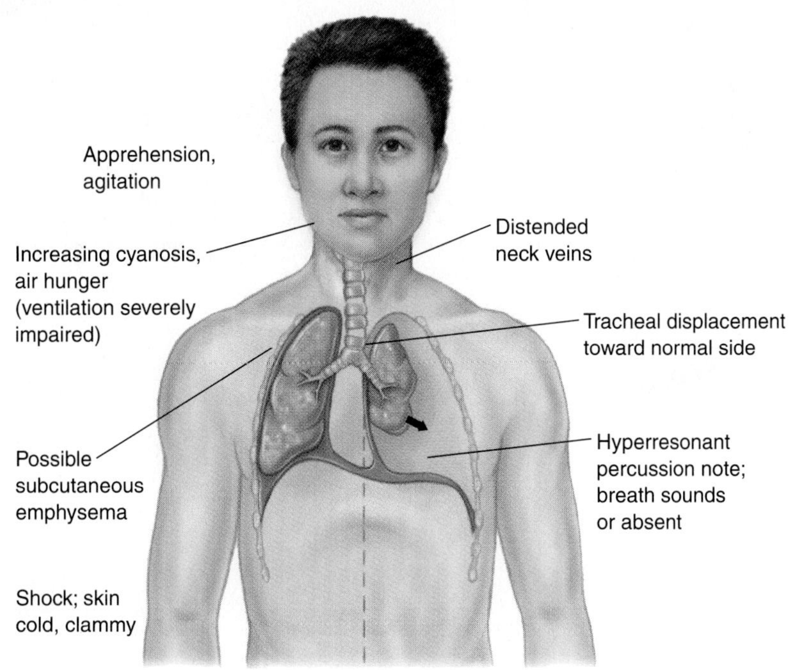

FIGURE 4-3b
The physical findings of tension pneumothorax.

FIGURE 4-4
Cardiac tamponade is an accumulation of fluid in the pericardium.

pleuritic chest pain sharp, stabbing pain, worsened by coughing, sneezing, deep breathing, or movement.

cardiac tamponade accumulation of excess fluid in the pericardium (the sac that encloses the heart).

paradoxical pulse suppression of the pulse at the close of inspiration; also called *pulsus paradoxus*.

the pleural cavity) is seen in patients with COPD when a bleb (a bubble on the surface of the lung) ruptures and there is progressive trapping of pleural air. *Pleuritic chest pain* with sudden, acute shortness of breath is a common complaint with a spontaneously ruptured bleb. *Cardiac tamponade* (Figure 4-4) (restriction of cardiac filling caused by accumulation of fluid in the pericardium) can result from large pericardial effusions, which may occur with pericarditis, ruptured myocardium post MI, ruptured coronary artery post cardiac catherization procedure, leukemia, renal failure, and certain other chronic conditions. However, tamponade is not common outside of trauma.

Tension pneumothorax and cardiac tamponade are both associated with the phenomena of pulsus paradoxus, distended neck and hand veins (Figure 4-5), and a narrowed pulse pressure. A *paradoxical pulse* (suppression of the pulse at the close of inspiration) occurs when the pressure on the ventricles increases, as in cardiac tamponade, or when pressure on the aorta increases due to unilateral pressure increases in the thoracic cavity, as with a tension pneumothorax. A patient with cardiac tamponade or tension pneumothorax will develop a blue-gray skin

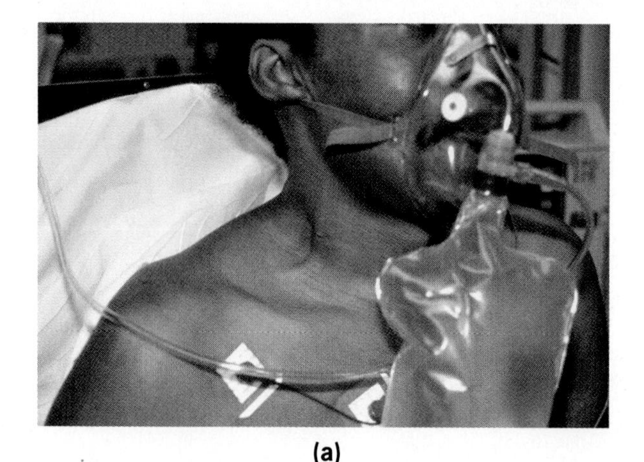

(a)

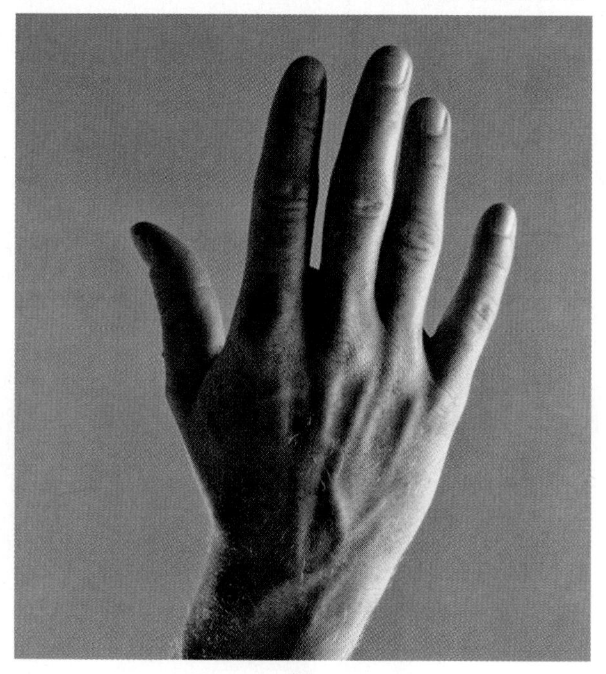

(b)

FIGURE 4-5
(a) Distended neck veins. (© Edward T. Dickinson, M.D.)
(b) Distended hand veins are associated with both tension pneumothorax and cardiac tamponade.

color resulting from hypoxia, usually seen first around the nose and mouth. Both conditions also result in a backup of venous pressure with distended neck and hand veins in the presence of falling, narrowed *pulse pressure* (the difference between the systolic and the diastolic pressure).

pulse pressure the difference between the systolic and diastolic blood pressures.

Cardiac tamponade presents with clear lung sounds. A tension pneumothorax presents with unequal breath sounds. The affected side has a noticeable decrease in both inhalation and exhalation sounds, a discriminating sign that is useful in the field. Cardiac tamponade has distant heart sounds that progress to a complete absence of sounds on the affected side. This is a discriminating sign that may be difficult to assess accurately in the field.

If history and physical assessment suggest a tension pneumothorax, oxygenation is necessary, and positive pressure should not be withheld. However, use of positive pressure will often worsen the problem. The treatment is a needle decompression with a large-bore over-the-needle catheter, 10, 12, or 14 gauge. There are two possible sites. The anterior site is located on the affected side between the second and third ribs, the midclavicular line. The second site is midaxillary on the affected side between the fourth and fifth ribs. Which site is chosen is usually dictated by the situation or by medical direction. In either case, the needle is inserted up and over the lower rib. Going up and over the rib will avoid injury to the intercostal artery, vein, and nerve that are located just under the rib. This should relieve the pressure, and immediate improvements in skin color, heart rate, strength of the pulse, and character of respirations should be noted.

If history and physical assessment suggest cardiac tamponade, the treatment is pericardiocentesis, which is usually performed at the hospital. In the field, a fluid bolus is frequently used to temporarily increase filling pressure of the heart. However, the most appropriate action is to notify the receiving hospital of the signs or symptoms that led you to suspect tamponade as the problem. This will alert them to the condition and allow time to prepare for the patient.

Pulmonary Emboli

The fine capillary network of the lungs serves as a natural filter for microscopic emboli that form in our bodies on a regular basis. (Emboli are usually blood clots, but can also be formed from fat, bone marrow, tumor fragments, amniotic fluid, or air bubbles.) In some cases, emboli that are trapped in the lungs (*pulmonary emboli*) are of significant size or are numerous enough to cause significant alteration in both pulmonary and cardiac function. When this occurs, pulmonary emboli may interfere either with preload to the left ventricle or with sufficient oxygenation of blood.

pulmonary emboli obstructions of pulmonary arteries, usually blood clots.

clot shower occurrence of multiple blood clots.

Chest pain does not always occur with pulmonary emboli; however, if it does, it is often pleuritic in nature. The patient often experiences a sense of impending doom because of hypoxic effects on the brainstem. Tachycardia and tachypnea are frequent findings. The heart rate increases to compensate for decreased preload and to maintain cardiac output, while the respiratory rate increases to compensate for hypoxia. Lung sounds are usually clear but depend on the pattern of the *clot shower* and the time interval. Depending on the type, extent, and distribution of the clot shower, a variety of other signs and symptoms can also occur (e.g., syncope, cardiac arrest, or a fine petechieal rash around the neck, which is more common with fat emboli). Skin changes may range from pallor to cyanosis or a gray tinge, particularly around the nose and mouth, as a result of hypoxia. Additionally, the emboli trigger an inflammatory response, which releases chemicals that can also produce

Emboli rarely occur as a single clot in a single event. More often, they occur as multiple clots and multiple events.

changes in lung sounds (localized wheezing is more common) and coughing, as well as cardiac dysrhythmias. Among the more common dysrhythmias are PVCs and intermittent atrial fibrillation.

If history and physical assessment suggest pulmonary emboli, administering high-flow, high-concentration oxygen, ensuring adequate tidal volume, monitoring cardiac rhythm, and IV access are all field-appropriate measures. If shock is present, cardiac arrest may be imminent. Unfortunately, there is no pharmacologic therapy available for the field treatment of this problem. Treatment is supportive.

Distributive Shock

distributive shock shock resulting from abnormal vasodilation or vasopermeability or both.

Distributive shock is a category of shock that results from an abnormality in vasodilation, vasopermeability, or both. The cause usually determines the presenting signs and symptoms. When vasodilation occurs by itself, the cause is usually neurogenic shock. When vasodilation occurs along with increased permeability, the cause is usually anaphylaxis or sepsis.

Neurogenic Shock

neurogenic shock shock resulting from abnormal vasodilation caused by a loss of sympathetic nervous system response.

Neurogenic shock occurs when there is a severe reduction in peripheral vascular resistance due to widespread vasodilation, which is usually caused by a loss of sympathetic nervous system response. In trauma, this generally results from injury to the spinal cord. Medical causes can include toxins from infection or a poison or a tumor in the brainstem. Neurogenic shock may also result from a massive stimulation of the parasympathetic system, which can occur in a drug overdose or poisoning.

Normally, blood vessels maintain a certain amount of tone, neither totally constricted nor totally dilated. Further, blood vessels in a given tissue will have more or less tone than the vessels in another tissue. When metabolic demand in any tissue increases, the arterioles supplying those capillary beds dilate and the precapillary sphincters relax, supplying more nutrients and oxygen. The venules also expand to accommodate the waste products. When the tissue demand decreases, the arterioles constrict, the precapillary sphincters tighten, and the venules resume normal size.

Ordinarily the vessels of the body do not all dilate at the same time. When some vessels dilate, others constrict. This prevents a loss of pressure within the system while satisfying the metabolic needs of specific body tissues.

When neurogenic shock occurs, a large number of vessels—sometimes, all the vessels of the body—dilate at the same time.

When neurogenic shock occurs, however, a large number of vessels—sometimes, all the vessels of the body—dilate at the same time. In the case of spinal cord interruption, signals to the sympathetic trunk are disrupted, causing specific areas to vasodilate. In the case of a drug overdose or poisoning, the brainstem may be affected. Not only do all blood vessels dilate, but the respiratory and cardiac centers may also be affected.

This type of shock results in signs and symptoms that differ from the classic shock picture. Skin vitals may not fit the usual picture of shock. In the areas of vasodilation, the skin will not immediately become pale, cool, and clammy but rather will remain warm and dry with a normal skin tone. The total blood volume remains the same, but the capacity of the vessels is increased. The result is hypoperfusion of all tissues. Sweating may not occur because of lack of sympathetic stimulation of the sweat glands. Vasodilation may eventually lead to hypothermia because of the inability of blood vessels near the surface of the skin to constrict and conserve body heat. Eventually, blood pools in the dependent parts of the body (the effect of gravity), leaving the upper surfaces pale, sometimes cyanotic, or with a gray cast. Exactly when this change occurs is highly individual and, when a toxin is the cause, may depend on which drug or poison the patient was exposed to and the dose.

In addition, heart rate in neurogenic shock is highly variable. If a drug or poison—for example, heroin or toxic levels of prescribed drugs such as methyldopa or propranolol or exposure to agricultural insecticides such as an organophosphate or carbamate—has interfered with the sympathetic system, the cardiac rate may be slow. If the substance is specific to the vascular system, the rate may become tachycardic in an effort to compensate.

Clinical Insight

When the heart rate slows and preload remains the same or falls, cardiac output falls. If the sympathetic system is blocked or inhibited, blood pressure will fall.

Regardless of the heart rate, most cases of neurogenic shock result in compromised respirations. In most cases of drug-induced neurogenic shock, nervous control of the respiratory system is severely compromised, resulting in an abnormal respiratory rate (usually decreased but may be elevated in some conditions), decreased depth, abnormal breathing patterns, or even a loss of the stimulus to breathe. *Pulmonary edema* may also occur with drug- or poison-induced shock, depending on the physiological actions of the substance that was taken.

pulmonary edema accumulation of fluid in the lungs (further explained under "Lung Sounds").

When the history and physical findings suggest neurogenic shock, effective management of the respiratory system may also have a positive effect on the heart rate by either increasing a slow rate or decreasing a fast rate. If the condition is drug induced and the specific drug is known, an antidote may be available. In the case of narcotics, altered mental status, bilateral constricted pupils, and depressed respiratory drive compose the typical triad of symptoms. However, cerebral hypoxia due to depressed respiratory drive may overwhelm pupil constriction, resulting in bilateral pupil dilation. In either case, when narcotic overdose is suspected, naloxone (Narcan) 2 mg slow IV push is the antidote. In the case of diazepam (Valium), flumazenil is the antidote. Glucagon is used for both beta-blocker (propranolol [Inderal]) and calcium channel blocker (verapamil [Calan]) overdoses, and so on. Access to a poison control center is beneficial, and direct contact with the receiving hospital may help guide your treatment. In the presence of clear lung sounds, fluid boluses are appropriate. Assessing and treating hypoglycemia and monitoring of cardiac rhythms is essential, with management of dysrhythmias according to American Heart Association advanced cardiac life support (AHA ACLS) guidelines.

If pulmonary edema and hypotension continue after the initial fluid bolus, the next drug of choice depends on the substance or toxin. In these cases, contacting a poison control center is wise. In some cases, dopamine may be the drug of choice. Low doses (2 to 5 μg/kg/min) stimulate dopaminergic receptors and preserve the kidneys and mesentery. Doses of 5 to 10 μg/kg/min will stimulate the beta effects of increased contractility and dilation of coronary arteries. If hypotension persists, higher doses of dopamine, 10 to 20 μg/kg/min, will begin to stimulate alpha receptors. Those effects will increase the heart rate and cause vasoconstriction. As doses approach 15 to 20 μg/kg/min, tachycardia and vasoconstriction become more pronounced. Both an increase in heart rate and in vasoconstriction significantly increase oxygen demand.

Anaphylactic Shock

Anaphylactic shock and its cousin anaphylactoid reaction are severe and exaggerated allergic reactions. Mild allergic reactions are usually single system problems (e.g., hives) and are usually more aggravating than life threatening. Occasionally,

anaphylactic shock a severe allergic reaction; an exaggerated response of the immune system.

allergic reactions will extend to multiple body systems. The degree of interference with normal oxygenation and perfusion will determine the severity of the reaction.

Anaphylactic reactions involve multiple body systems and are life threatening. Anaphylactoid reactions are life threatening if they involve the airway or the cardiovascular system. The mechanism of both reactions is closely tied to the body's immune system. Anaphylaxis involves IgE as the trigger for mast cell/basophil degranulation; anaphylactoid reactions do not. In either case, the reaction can occur within seconds or may take up to several hours after exposure to an allergen. The speed of the reaction depends on the degree of sensitivity the patient has previously developed and the route of exposure: injection, ingestion, absorption, or inhalation. Initial signs and symptoms depend on the speed of the reaction and the target organ. Target organs of anaphylaxis usually include the vascular system, lungs, GI tract, and skin. Which organs serve as the target organs is a function of the allergen and the local concentration of mast cells.

When contact with an allergen occurs, mast cells located near mucous membranes and just outside the small blood vessels, as well as basophils in the bloodstream, degranulate and release massive amounts of histamine, tryptase, chymase, leukotrienes, cytokines, and prostaglandins (formerly known as "slow-reacting substance of anaphylaxis" or SRSA), heparin, platelet-activating factors, and other vasoactive chemicals. These substances cause widespread bronchoconstriction, smooth muscle contraction, and extreme vasodilation, and increase permeability of the capillaries (Figure 4-6). A marked loss of fluid from the vasculature into the surrounding tissues occurs, and local smooth muscle cells contract. Histamine is fast acting and triggers the immediate reaction. Leukotrienes, cytokines, and prostaglandins enhance and prolong the reaction. Because of the variety of target organs, a wide variety of abnormal tissue responses can occur, depending on the type of tissue in which the reaction occurs and the speed of the reaction.

In the skin, vasodilation and increased permeability cause generalized flushing and/or urticaria (hives) (Figure 4-7). Severe itching results from the stretching of the skin and associated stretching of nerve fibers caused by the massive fluid shift. Increased permeability causes swelling, especially noticeable in the mucous membranes, including those of the larynx (causing stridor), the trachea, and the bronchial tree. Swelling in the bronchial tree irritates smooth muscle (causing wheezing). Permeability may be extensive enough to cause a fluid shift into the alveoli (causing crackles, or "rales") and sometimes frank pulmonary

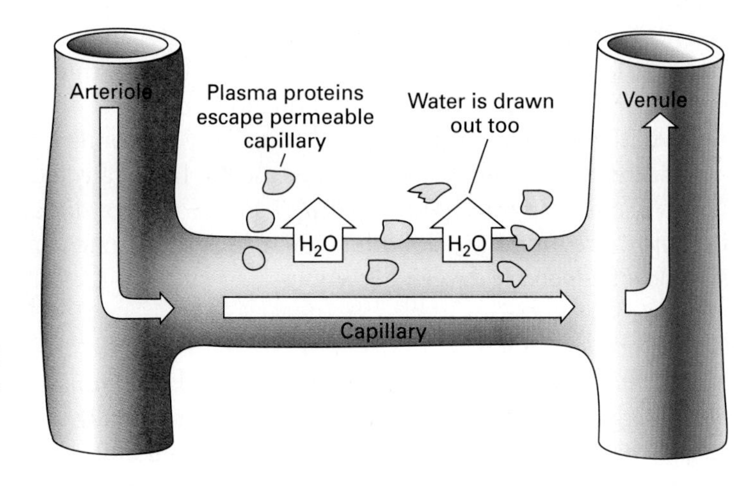

FIGURE 4-6
When capillaries become more permeable, as in anaphylactic reactions, excessive fluid is lost from the vascular system into surrounding tissues, causing edema and, in extreme cases, hypovolemia and shock. (Normally, forces that push fluid out of the capillaries and forces that pull fluid into the capillaries are balanced. When capillary permeability increases, however, plasma proteins escape. These large molecules create a hypertonic solution that draws water to dilute and balance tonicity on both sides of the membrane, inside and outside the capillary. So, when plasma protein molecules escape the permeable capillaries, they also pull fluid out of the capillaries.)

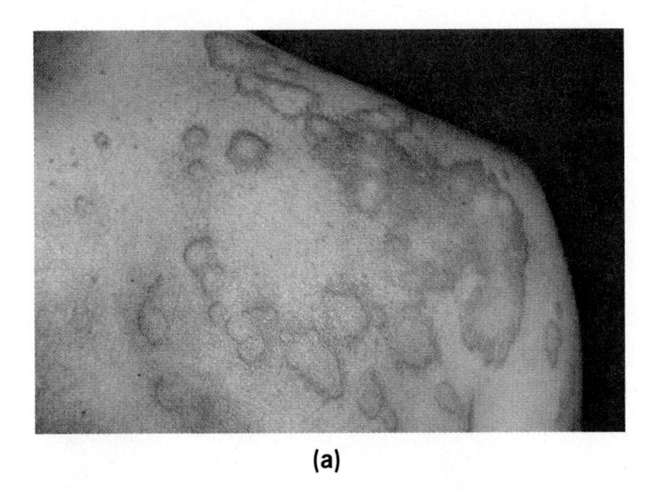

(a)

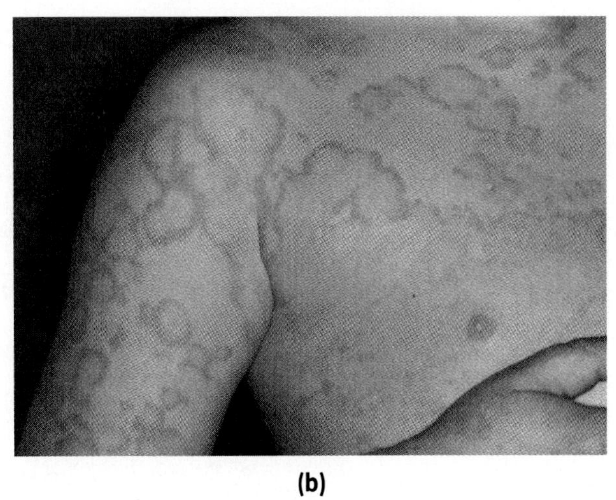

(b)

FIGURE 4-7
(a) Common urticaria (hives). (b) Variation of urticaria. (Both: ISM/Phototake USA)

edema. The permeability and microclotting (from platelet activation) may be so great as to cause petechiae (small hemorrhages under the skin)(Figure 4-8).

The wide variety of reactions may have an equally wide variety of effects on the skin. Skin may be flushed, have urticaria, or both. Petechiae may also be evident. If, however, the skin is not the target organ, the resulting hypoxia may result in pallor and cyanosis.

With anaphylaxis, the wide variety of reactions may have an equally wide variety of effects on the skin.

Smooth muscle contraction, in combination with vasodilation and increased permeability in the GI tract, may result in stomach cramps, vomiting, and protracted diarrhea. In the respiratory tract, the same smooth muscle contraction and permeability may cause bronchospasm (wheezing) and laryngospasm (stridor) or respiratory arrest.

The combination of vasodilation and increased vascular permeability causes an abrupt fall in cardiac output. The heart rate increases to compensate, often reaching 150 to 180 beats per minute. Because effects on body systems usually occur simultaneously, the patient in anaphylactic shock frequently is profoundly hypotensive with varying degrees of dyspnea. On occasion, the target organ may be the vascular system, where resulting hypotension produces extreme pallor rather than the tell-tale flushing or hives. In those cases, it is not uncommon for itching and hives to occur only after sufficient fluid volume restores perfusion.

When the history and physical findings suggest that the problem is anaphylaxis, the respiratory system and cardiovascular system require vigorous support. Pharmacologic therapy depends on the degree to which either or both systems are affected. The initial drug of choice is epinephrine because of its effect on alpha and beta receptors (as a vasoconstrictor and bronchodilator). Its ability to stabilize mast/basophil cell walls and limit the release of histamine and other chemicals is immediate but short acting. Therefore, epinephrine must be followed by additional pharmacologic agents, as is discussed later in this section. Epinephrine can be given subcutaneously, intramuscularly, or intravenously. The SQ and IM adult dose is 0.3 to 0.5 mg of 1:1,000 dilution. The IV dose, 0.1 mg of 1:10,000 dilution, is usually reserved for severe cardiovascular collapse. If a patient who is given epinephrine is also taking a beta-blocker, the response from epinephrine may be incomplete. In these cases, consider administration of glucagon, 0.5 to 1 mg slow IV push.

When history and physical findings suggest anaphylaxis, the respiratory and cardiovascular systems require vigorous support.

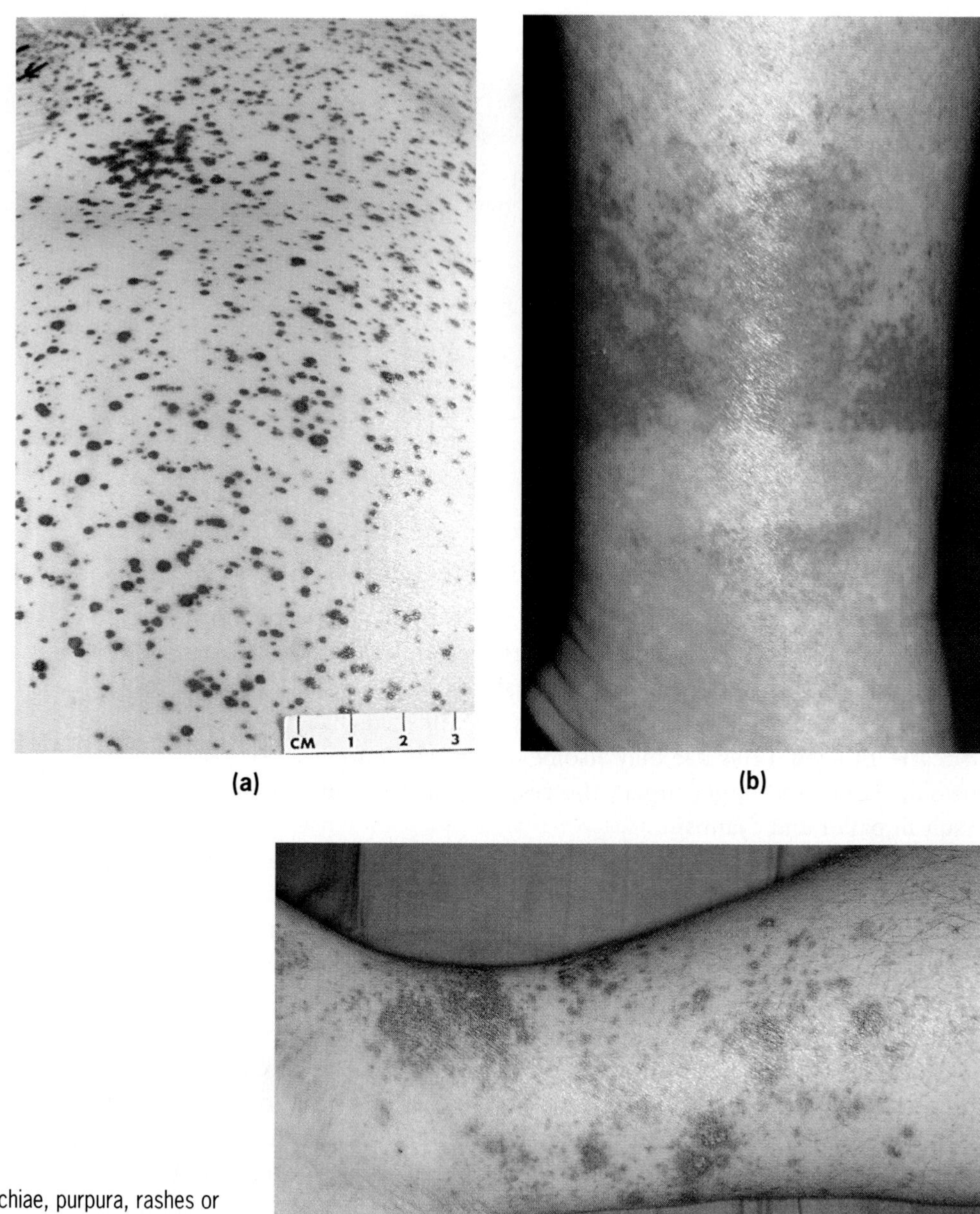

FIGURE 4-8
Skin changes such as petechiae, purpura, rashes or peeling may be associated with sepsis. (a) Petechiae. (© Children's Hospital and Medical Center/CORBIS)
(b) Purpura. (© Dr. P. Marazzi/Photo Researchers, Inc.)
(c) Vascular purpura. (© ISM Phototake USA)

Clinical Insight

Obtaining a good history can be a critical determinant of treatment. For example, in a patient with a cardiac history, administration of epinephrine for a mild allergic reaction could trigger an AMI and, as a result, alternative drugs should be considered.

If the patient's primary sign of allergic reaction is wheezing and the blood pressure is above 70, then a bronchodilator such as albuterol or metaproterenol may be sufficient. However, if severe cardiovascular effects are present, epinephrine is recommended. In such cases, epinephrine should never be withheld.

In milder cases of allergic reaction, however, administration of epinephrine may be questioned due to the age and previous medical history of the patient. Because of several anecdotal cases, it has been suggested that in a patient who is older than age 40 who has a cardiac history (e.g., acute myocardial infarction [AMI] within the last year, angina, congestive heart failure), the alpha and beta effects of epinephrine may exert such an additional strain on the heart that an AMI may result. This is one example of why ascertaining previous history can be a critical determinant of treatment. The exact components that indicate a positive cardiac history are up to local medical direction.

If a patient presents with a mild case of allergic reaction and epinephrine is contraindicated by medical direction, the next drugs of choice include diphenhydramine (Benadryl) or dopamine. Diphenhydramine, which can also be used with epinephrine, is a potent antihistamine that blocks H1 receptors. (H1 receptors, when stimulated by release of histamine during an allergic reaction, cause bronchoconstriction, increased capillary permeability, rhinorrhea, tachycardia, urticaria, and contraction of the gut; H2 receptors, when stimulated by histamine, cause secretion of gastric acids among other things.) Both H1 and H2 receptors are involved with vasodilation. Histamine is also the culprit, with conditions such as headache, flushing, hypotension, and GI effect, such as nausea, vomiting, abdominal cramping, and diarrhea. Stimulation of H1 receptors causes an immediate effect, while stimulation of H2 receptors causes delayed effects. Although H3 and H4 receptors are the least well known, research suggests that they increase motor activity, enhance acid production, and modulate inflammation. It is important to note that diphenhydramine has no effect on the bronchoconstrictive action of leukotriene. This explains why bronchoconstriction may return after initial treatment. Bronchodilators such as metaproterenol or albuterol remain a mainstay of treatment when bronchoconstriction is involved.

Diphenhydramine's onset of action is not as rapid as that of epinephrine, but its effects last longer. Diphenhydramine may be given intravenously or intramuscularly. The dose is 10 to 50 mg slow IV push or 25 to 50 mg IM. Diphenhydramine is also given in addition to epinephrine in the case of anaphylaxis or if a long transport is necessary. With the advent of H2 blockers, such as rantidine (Zantac), famotidine (Pepcid), and cimetidine (Tagamet), many physicians are now advocating initiation of rantidine, famotidine, or cimetidine to control severe reactions. There is a wide range of dosing that may be done; that is, rantidine 50 mg in 50 to 100 ml may be infused over 10 to 15 minutes, famotidine 20 mg in 100 ml over 15 to 30 minutes, while cimetidine 300 mg in 50 to 100 ml may be infused over 15 to 20 minutes.

Along with pharmacologic therapies, fluid boluses are also recommended to replace fluid lost due to third spacing. Fluid losses usually amount to several liters. Normal saline or lactated Ringer's can be used as fluid replacement, with normal saline the more frequent choice. Repeated boluses of 500 to 1,000 ml are usually given.

Along with pharmacologic therapies, fluid boluses are recommended to replace fluid lost due to third spacing.

In cases of persistent hypotension—after epinephrine, fluid boluses, and histamine blockers—dopamine may be chosen. The initial dose is usually within the 5 to 10 μg/kg/min range and increased if there is no or limited response.

Any patient that has suffered an allergic reaction that requires field treatment should be given a steroid such as methylprednisolone (Solu-Medrol) 125 mg slow IV push. This medication should be given as soon as possible after immediate treatment. Methylprednisolone acts to stabilize the cell walls of mast cells and basophils and is long acting. Administration prevents restimulation of the degranulation process of the cell walls.

Septic Shock

Septic shock is the result of an overwhelming infection. Septic shock may not be noticed for some time and may be confused with a wide variety of other conditions. This type of shock begins with an infection that sets in motion an overwhelming systemic response from the immune system, the end results of which are hypotension, hypoperfusion, and end organ dysfunction. The infection can be caused by bacteria, fungus, and some viruses. Gram-negative bacteremia is more likely to cause sepsis (50 percent of infections) compared to gram-positive bacteremia (25 percent of infections). The inflammatory and cellular events are

septic shock shock resulting from an overwhelming infection.

complex and significant. Organisms invade the body through the bloodstream or locally. In either case, the organisms release structural components (commonly referred to as toxins, either endotoxins or exotoxins) that trigger our natural immune system to release its own endogenous mediators (e.g., cytokines from monocytes and prostaglandins from neutrophils, along with histamine, heparin, tumor necrosis factor [TNF], and others).

When released in normal amounts, these substances are beneficial in helping localize and destroy the invading organisms and initiate tissue repair.

systemic inflammatory response syndrome (SIRS) exaggerated, generalized immune system response to infection that extends to healthy tissue with profound effects on the vasculature and organ systems.

However, when this response becomes exaggerated and results in a generalized response extending to healthy tissue, there is a profound effect on the vasculature and organ systems. This generalized response is termed *systemic inflammatory response syndrome (SIRS)*. SIRS is manifested by two or more of the following: (1) temperature > 38°C (102°F) or < 36°C (96.8°F); (2) heart rate > 90/bpm; (3) respiratory rate > 20/min or $PaCO_2$ < 32 mmHg; (4) WBC > 12,000 cells/mm^3 or < 4,000 cells/mm^3 or > 10 percent immature (band) forms. SIRS is often termed the first stage of sepsis, and it can persist for some time before signs of organ dysfunction occur.

When SIRS persists, several things happen. Mediators trigger the clotting cascade in an attempt to wall off the infection, but because the infection is widespread or in the bloodstream, many small clots form. Because the mechanisms to break down blood clots are impaired, tissues, organs, and organ systems become ischemic. In addition, the mediators, which are present in exaggerated amounts, damage the endothelial cells of the vasculature, resulting in leaking of fluid. The total effect on tissues and organ systems is microvascular permeability, vasodilation, organ ischemia/dysfunction, and shock.

Severe sepsis is determined when hypotension, hypoperfusion, and perfusion abnormalities occur. Those are usually recognized when urine production is reduced or ceases, when an acute alteration in mental status occurs, or when lactic acidosis is present. Septic shock is present when hypotension, due to sepsis, is unresponsive to fluid resuscitation in the presence of organ failure or an acute alteration in mental status. In the field, hypotension unresponsive to fluid resuscitation, in the presence of altered mental status, with a history of fever, is highly suggestive of septic shock.

A wide variety of possible signs and symptoms may occur, depending on the location of the infection, the organism of infection, the strength of the immune response, and the presence of preexisting conditions that impair the immune system, such as use of immunosuppressive drug therapies and chronic diseases such as diabetes and cancer.

Attempts have been made to classify septic shock in terms of stages. The first stage is the hypermetabolic stage where the cardiac output is increased but organism toxins causing vasodilation may prevent a higher blood pressure. The patient may appear sick but not critically so. In the last stage, organism toxins have usually built up to the point where they cause such increased permeability of the vascular system that a precipitous fall in blood pressure occurs along with signs of multiple organ system failure.

Septic shock is the most often missed type of shock.

There is a wide variety in progression through the stages and, as a consequence of the subtle effects of various organisms that may be causing the infection, a lack of uniformity in presentation. As a consequence, septic shock is the most frequently missed type of shock in the field. However, some features of septic shock are worth noting.

Many patients present with high fever (> 38°C or 102°F). However, there are exceptions. The elderly and the very young may not have a fever or may even be hypothermic. The skin can be flushed and pink (due to fever) or very pale to cyanotic, especially when the lungs are involved or in later stages of septic shock. Those with darker skin tones may not appear remarkably affected. However, a good history, including recent illness and fever, will help identify this as a likely cause, even when skin appears normal.

Usually, the target organ system is the first to suffer vasodilation with increased permeability. The most susceptible organ systems include the lungs and the intestinal tract. Eventually, marked vasodilation occurs throughout the body. Because the lungs are among the first organs affected, increasing dyspnea with altered lung sounds and hypotension are common early signs of septic shock. These signs may be confused with congestive heart failure, especially in the elderly.

Initially, there is a high cardiac output due to a high metabolic rate (from the infection) and vasodilation elsewhere in the body. However, impaired oxygen and glucose metabolism is widespread, further contributing to tissue ischemia in multiple organ systems (multiple organ system failure), including the brain. As a result, an altered mental status is common.

Development of microemboli in widespread areas of the body, in combination with increased permeability of the vessels, contributes to petechiae (small reddish-purple spots). Specific organisms, such as meningococcus, may result in purpura (large reddish-purple or bluish blotches, which may be considered to be very large petechiae) in a general distribution over the skin. (Review Figure 4-8.) Other organisms may result in rashes or skin peeling in a general pattern over the body or localized in the palms of the hands or the soles of the feet.

The key sign/symptom that should alert the provider to possible sepsis is the presence of altered mental status with a history of fever or illness/infection.

Clinical Insight

The key to possible sepsis is altered mental status with a history of fever or infection.

Septic shock is usually determined based on the history of infection or illness prior to the onset of shock. When the history and physical findings suggest that the problem is septic shock, management of the respiratory system may range from high-flow, high-concentration oxygen by nonrebreather mask to intubation of the unconscious patient. Progressive resuscitation with crystalloid is the first treatment option, followed by dopamine. The dose is the same as for neurogenic shock, with low doses begun and repeated first. An important consideration is monitoring the cardiac rhythm. PVCs are managed by oxygen, with use of lidocaine or amiodarone as a last resort. Ultimately, appropriate antibiotic therapy must be administered.

Cardiogenic Shock

Cardiogenic shock occurs as a result of abnormal heart function. This can be caused by factors such as failure of the heart muscle, valvular insufficiency, or a rhythm disturbance. Of all the causes of cardiogenic shock, failure of heart muscle due to AMI is the most common. However, cardiogenic shock will not occur until at least 40 percent of the left ventricular muscle malfunctions.

cardiogenic shock shock resulting from abnormal function of the heart; failure of the heart muscle, valvular insufficiency, or rhythm disturbance.

Shock from AMI, valvular insufficiency, or a heart rate unable to maintain cardiac output (a rate usually less than 50 or greater than 150 in the adult) will result in similar signs and symptoms.

Clinical Insight

The presence of pulmonary edema is one of the chief indicators of cardiogenic shock as differentiated from hemorrhagic shock.

In cardiogenic shock, one of the biggest differences from hemorrhagic shock is the presence of pulmonary edema. As contractions of the left ventricle become less and less efficient, blood backs up into the pulmonary vasculature. This back pressure disturbs the hydrostatic pressure balance, the capillary fluid pressure exceeding the air pressure in the alveoli. Water from the plasma is forced into the interstitial spaces, irritating the bronchioles and causing bronchoconstriction as a protective mechanism. Eventually, body water enters the alveoli. Early pulmonary edema may present with diminished lung sounds as the fluid enters the interstitial space and exerts pressure on the airways. As the fluid levels increase, wheezes (which are not always heard) and crackles, or rales, may be present. The patient will complain of increased difficulty breathing as this process continues. Eventually, a productive cough of white or pink-tinged foamy sputum will develop. Cyanosis is a typical sign because of two factors that occur together: First, the diffusion of gases across the alveolar membrane is directly inhibited, which reduces the amount of oxygen available to the blood. At the same time, the patient is suffering from hypotension, which decreases circulation and perfusion.

Clinical Insight

Cyanosis is a typical sign of cardiogenic shock because of two factors that occur together: inhibition of oxygen diffusion across the alveolar membrane and hypotension.

When you suspect cardiogenic shock, supplying high-flow, high-concentration oxygen and assuring adequate tidal volume with positive pressure will be a priority. Establish a peripheral IV with normal saline at a TKO rate. Fluid administration is kept to a minimum, while pharmacologic access is maximized.

Cardiogenic shock can be rate related, so it is important to monitor the cardiac rhythm. Correction of a perfusion-altering rate is a priority. Atropine (0.5 mg and repeated to maximum 3 mg) for sinus bradycardia and use of an external pacer for other bradycardias is recommended. Tachycardic rhythms (usually more than 150 beats per minute) that result in cardiogenic shock are managed by sedation and cardioversion in the awake patient. If the blood pressure does not warrant cardioversion, other pharmacologic therapy, such as adenosine and/or diltiazem, is warranted.

Dopamine is the drug of choice for cardiogenic shock not related to rate. Desired doses are between 5 and 10 µg/kg/min. A typical dose is 5 µg/kg/min. The goal is to start low and gradually increase the dose until the systolic pressure is adequate to support perfusion (as indicated by a systolic pressure of 70–100 mmHg and/or improved mental status). Avoiding a rapid heart rate, which increases oxygen demand, is also an important consideration. Doses of 10 to 20 µg/kg/min often trigger tachycardia and a vasopressive effect.

Dobutamine is often considered with dopamine when considering pharmacologic treatments for cardiogenic shock. Dobutamine is a synthetic sympathetic stimulating agent with a few differences. Dobutamine primarily stimulates beta receptors with minimal alpha effect at normal doses (2–20 µg/kg/min). Compared to dopamine, dose for dose, dobutamine exerts a stronger inotropic action (effect on contractile force) with comparatively little chronotropic action (effect on rate). However, at higher doses, dobutamine may induce production of an endogenous norepinephrine, which can have a profound effect on the myocardium. The dose is particularly important, with doses as small as 0.5 µg/kg/min making a significant difference. Precise flow rates are extremely important. Thus, dobutamine is an alternative often limited to use in controlled environments with precise volumetric control.

An additional option is a bolus of fluid, usually 250 to 300 cc of crystalloid. This may help patients with right heart infarction by increasing preload and thus stimulating the Frank-Starling mechanism. Many patients suffering cardiogenic shock have a history of hypertension and have been managed on diuretics. Therefore, they are starting out with a degree of dehydration on top of cardiogenic shock. Sometimes, a fluid bolus will help support perfusion, but it must be judiciously administered with close attention paid to the effects on the respiratory system.

There are times when a fluid bolus can be a field diagnostic test. When lung sounds seem to be clear but the patient is clearly hypotensive, a bolus of fluid with reassessment of lung sounds may help point the direction of treatment (e.g., use of fluids versus pharmacology).

Factors Affecting Shock

The rate at which the signs of shock develop is determined by a number of factors:

- *Type of shock* —Anaphylactic shock may occur within minutes of exposure, while early stages of septic shock might go unrecognized for a day or two.
- *Age* —The younger the patient, the less it takes to induce shock, but the more effective the compensatory mechanisms. In the older patient, especially one older than age 50, it may take longer for compensatory mechanisms to function, and the mechanisms may not be as effective, due to changes of aging.
- *Preexisting diseases* —Compensatory mechanisms may be malfunctioning or not functioning at all.
- *Speed of onset* —In general, the slower the onset of a cause of shock (e.g., a slow GI bleed), the more time the body has to compensate, thus delaying recognition until later stages.
- *Effects of drugs* —Pharmacologic control for preexisting disease states may interfere with the body's compensatory mechanisms (e.g., beta-blockers, ACE inhibitors). Use of alcohol and other recreational drugs can also severely complicate or interfere with the body's normal response to shock. Sometimes, recreational drug use itself will result in neurogenic shock. When the history does not seem to match the physical findings, suspect that there is an additional problem that must be assessed for and treated.

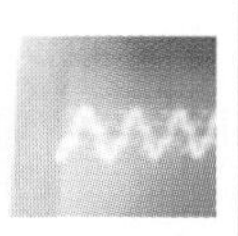

ASSESSMENT PRIORITIES

Initial Assessment

The signs and symptoms of shock may first be observed during your initial assessment of the patient's mental status, the airway, breathing, and circulatory status, and the baseline vital signs assessments. As soon as shock is suspected, assure an open airway and administer high-flow, high-concentration oxygen, assisting ventilations if necessary. Position the patient to best aid perfusion (elevating the head and shoulders if pulmonary edema is suspected), and keep the patient warm.

Focused History and Physical Exam

A thorough and accurate history and physical exam are critical as a basis for determining appropriate further treatment, such as IV fluids and pharmacologic therapy. Use of a particular agent for one type of shock (e.g., epinephrine in anaphylaxis) can be contraindicated for another type (e.g., epinephrine in cardiogenic shock). Decisions will be based on a field impression of which body system is most likely failing or causing the failure.

As you continue the patient assessment through the history and physical findings, be alert to indications of the underlying cause and type of shock the patient may be experiencing. Assessment tools such as obtaining a 12-lead ECG in the case of cardiogenic shock and determining blood glucose levels may be invaluable. This information will help guide you in determining appropriate treatment. Critical body systems must be supported, with the respiratory system the priority.

Keys to History

In the medical patient, history is the key to determining the problem. History should include details regarding the chief complaint. In the case of medical emergencies, the chief complaint may involve symptoms such as chest pain, difficulty breathing, or abdominal pain. Details such as onset, activity at time of onset, associated signs and symptoms, alleviation, severity, radiation, and so on can be valuable clues. Mnemonics such as OPQRST (Onset, Palliation/Provocation, Quality, Radiation, Severity, and Time) are useful in remembering what questions to ask. Finding out the age of the patient and the previous medical history will also be valuable.

In the shock patient, treatment often occurs at the same time as the history-taking and physical assessment, with both the history and physical findings guiding pharmacologic and other treatment.

In the shock patient, treatment often occurs at the same time as the history-taking and physical assessment, with both the history and physical findings guiding pharmacologic and other treatment. The following paragraphs discuss clues to keep in mind that can help point the way.

Hemorrhagic shock in a medical patient usually involves abdominal complaints. Organs that can bleed enough to cause shock are the GI tract, the liver, the spleen, and the ovary or fallopian tube. Vascular problems such as aneurysms can also cause shock. History may reveal a sudden onset of pain, followed by syncope or dizziness. A history of dizziness when going from a lying to sitting or sitting to standing position is highly suspicious for a volume problem (see "Orthostatic Hypotension" later in the chapter).

Pain may indicate potential sources of shock. Radiating pain to the neck or shoulder is due to diaphragmatic irritation, usually from a ruptured or rupturing viscus. Stretching or rupturing of a viscus produces poorly localized visceral pain that is perceived in the abdomen but not well localized. Radiating pain may also be caused by an expanding or ruptured aneurysm of the abdominal aorta. Where the pain is perceived depends on the aneurysm's location, amount of stretching of the vascular wall and, in the rare occasion of dissection, the direction of the separation of aortic wall layers. Aortic aneurysms often occur around the renal area, from which pain may radiate to the flank or back. If the defect is posterior, pain may radiate to the back, or if the defect is anterior, radiation may be from back to front. If the defect extends toward the iliac arteries, pain may radiate down either or both legs.

Clinical Insight

A frequent cause of sepsis in the elderly is a urinary tract infection. The only initial signs may be urinary incontinence and confusion.

A history of illness (e.g., cough, headache, urinary symptoms), suddenly followed by dizziness when arising or shortness of breath, may indicate sepsis. If followed by sudden abdominal pain, an organ, usually the appendix, intestines, or spleen, may have spontaneously ruptured.

A history of diabetes should alert the care provider to special problems. Diabetics are especially prone to septic shock or "silent" (painless) abdominal bleeds. In the diabetic or older patient, a history of illness followed by increasing dyspnea or diaphoresis on exertion may also indicate cardiogenic shock from a silent (painless) AMI. In the diabetic patient with flu-like symptoms, it is frequently difficult to distinguish a silent AMI causing congestive heart failure from septic shock.

History of recreational drug use, or of a sudden change in mental status after a party, may indicate a drug-related etiology. In this hypotensive patient, suspect neurogenic shock. A close assessment of the respiratory and cardiac systems is necessary.

History of contact with an allergen or a sudden onset of dizziness, difficulty breathing, itching (with or without hives), or swelling with low blood pressure in the previously healthy person may indicate anaphylactic shock. Also look for simultaneous nausea/vomiting and diarrhea. Keep in mind that a key difference between food poisoning and a severe allergic reaction is the presence of signs and symptoms of shock, especially with respiratory compromise. Because dehydration is possible in food poisoning, determine the length of time that vomiting and diarrhea have taken place. (In food poisoning, vomiting is often followed by diarrhea, although this is not a hard and fast rule. If shock occurs in the food poisoning patient, it is due to dehydration and usually takes some time to develop in the adult.)

A history of smoking, use of birth control pills, prolonged bed rest, recent surgery, first-trimester pregnancy, and long-bone fracture are all risk factors for pulmonary emboli. When the history also includes a sudden onset of an impending sense of doom and pleuritic chest pain, pulmonary emboli are strongly suggested. These symptoms are often accompanied by tachycardia and tachypnea as the body attempts to compensate for impaired pulmonary function.

A history of COPD (chronic bronchitis or emphysema) in the patient who has a sudden onset of sharp, localized chest pain with difficulty breathing suggests a ruptured bleb, which may lead to a tension pneumothorax. Activity at time of onset may include laughing, coughing, or straining (especially when lifting). A ruptured bleb leading to a tension pneumothorax may also occur when the COPD patient is being ventilated by positive pressure, either by a bag-valve mask or by a mechanical ventilator. An early sign is difficulty bagging or frequent pressure-release-valve warnings.

Patients with a medical cause of cardiac tamponade are not common. Such cases often involve a chronic disease process, such as systemic lupus erythematosus (SLE), or an inflammatory process such as pericarditis. Development of tamponade from a medical cause is a relatively slow process. Recognition usually comes from physical assessment findings.

History and complaints consistent with AMI in the hypotensive patient with pulmonary edema suggest AMI complicated by cardiogenic shock.

Keys to Physical Assessment

A knowledge of the relationships between body systems and of disease states is invaluable in relating physical signs and symptoms to history and pathophysiology, thus helping form an accurate impression of the severity of the situation.

Skin Vitals Skin color, temperature, and moisture are among the first things care providers notice on approach. Skin color is influenced by how close the blood vessels are to the surface and by the presence or absence of pigment.

Vasodilation of peripheral vessels causes a flushed appearance in patients with lighter skin tones. Patients with darker skin tones may appear darker than usual to their family members. There are three primary causes of vasodilation: 1) heat dissipation, 2) sympathetic nervous system inhibition or parasympathetic nervous system stimulation, and 3) interference with normal nervous system function, as in septic shock. Vasodilation with increased permeability, as in anaphylaxis, may cause urticaria, or hives, which appear as large, raised itchy blotches on the skin. The blotches may be concentric or irregular in shape and will blanch when pressed. Extreme permeability may allow red blood cells to leak through the skin, causing petechiae, which appear as a maroon-colored rash that does not blanch, especially in skin folds and the inner aspect of joint spaces. This may also occur in certain forms of septic shock.

Vasoconstriction causes a pale appearance. Constriction occurs as a heat conservation mechanism or as a method to shunt blood volume. In the case of shock, it is a sympathetic response designed to shunt blood to vital organs, caused primarily by the stimulation of alpha receptors. Normally, vasoconstriction will occur only to the degree necessary to increase preload enough to maintain cardiac output.

When the need is relatively small, the degree of constriction may not result in obvious signs.

Areas of the body that are nonessential to survival are the first to be affected by vasoconstriction. This will first be noticeable at the extremities, especially at the feet and hands, and the skin, particularly the skin of the facial area. Pallor occurs more noticeably in the conjunctiva and the area around the eye, the mucous membranes of the mouth, the area around the nose and mouth, and the earlobes. Pallor is more noticeable in these areas because of their relatively high concentration of blood vessels. In the conjunctiva and the mucous membranes of the mouth, the absence of pigment also makes pallor more noticeable. In patients with darker skin tones, vasoconstriction makes the skin appear ashen or gray. In Asian or Indian patients or patients with a tan, the skin takes on a yellow cast.

Skin may also be cyanotic, the characteristic blue color around the nose and mouth and in the nail beds caused by a deficiency of oxygen in the blood. In patients with darker skin, cyanosis appears even darker with a gray cast. In Asian or Indian patients, cyanosis gives a green cast to the skin. Mucous membranes and the conjunctiva are the best places to look for cyanosis. Cyanosis may develop slowly or relatively quickly. Patients with cardiogenic shock, tension pneumothorax, or cardiac tamponade develop cyanosis very quickly.

With some causes of shock, such as pulmonary emboli, a line of demarcation, or color change, may appear.

With some causes, such as pulmonary emboli, a line of demarcation, or color change, may appear. When noted, the patient is in extreme shock and the demarcation is noted usually at the nipple line. An abdominal aneurysm may result in a mottling of the skin over the abdomen as a result of blood pooling in the capillary beds.

Skin temperature and moisture are also directly related to the amount of epinephrine and norepinephrine secreted. With the resulting vasoconstriction and shunting of blood to the core, the skin will lose heat. Vasoconstricted skin decreases metabolism and does not maintain heat. Even though the body's purpose in shunting blood to the core is to maintain an adequate core temperature, the patient may complain of feeling cold. The patient's skin will feel cool or cold to the touch. However, if the ambient temperature is hot (above normal body temperature of 98.6°F), the patient's skin may feel warm to the touch despite the shunting-away of blood from the skin.

Diaphoresis may or may not occur. In hemorrhagic shock, cardiogenic shock, and obstructive shock, such as from cardiac tamponade or tension pneumothorax, sweating is common. With dehydration, pulmonary emboli, or neurogenic shock, sweating is usually not present. In anaphylactic or septic shock, sweating may or may not be present. The presence or absence of diaphoresis does not exclude a hypoperfused state. Rather, the sudden onset of sweating is more indicative of an epinephrine/norepinephrine release and warrants further assessment.

Clinical Insight

The presence of diaphoresis is clinically significant, while the absence of it may not be—because sweating is common with some types of shock but not others. In other words, the absence of sweating does not necessarily mean that shock is not present.

An important point to remember is that in states of widespread vasodilation (as in neurogenic shock or anaphylactic shock), as explained earlier, the body loses heat due to conduction of heat to the environment and is in danger of hypothermia. The general rule of thumb is that the patient in shock must be protected from further heat loss because activation of the body's compensatory heat-generation mechanisms will further consume valuable oxygen and nutrients.

The presence of distended veins (in hands and neck) in the hypotensive patient suggests an obstruction or backup in the venous system. Additionally, a narrowed pulse pressure and an irregular pulse that disappears on inhalation and returns on exhalation are key signs of increased intrathoracic pressure. The patient should be assessed for a tension pneumothorax or cardiac tamponade.

Mental Status The brain is extremely sensitive to hypoxia, either from hypoxemia (insufficient oxygenation of the blood) or from low cardiac output. Because the brain is vital to life, the body maintains perfusion to the brain at all costs. Epinephrine and norepinephrine secreted by the adrenal glands have little effect on the brain or its perfusion. The perfusion of the brain is primarily governed by cardiac output. However, the brain does respond to levels of norepinephrine and dopamine produced locally. These catecholamines act on the reticular activating system in the brainstem, stimulating a state of wakefulness or alertness. This stimulation contributes to the anxiety often seen in the early stages of shock. As the shock state continues, increased levels of catecholamines together with the increasing concentrations of metabolic acids, cerebral hypoxia, and ischemia result in confusion, disorientation, agitation, and, in extreme states, combativeness.

In the later stages of shock, when the levels of norepinephrine and dopamine are exhausted, decreased cerebral perfusion and continued ischemia of brain cells trigger drowsiness and a decreased mental status. Because of the extreme sensitivity of the brain to decreased levels of oxygen and increased levels of carbon dioxide and metabolic acids, a change in mental status is one of the first indicators of an increase or decrease in cardiac output. As the process of shock continues, the mental status continues to change. There are, however, variations. The slower the process of shock, the longer an alert mental status will be maintained. In some patients (e.g., the elderly or brain injured), the patient's baseline alertness may be diminished, thus making these assessments difficult.

Cerebral levels of norepinephrine may be initially inhibited with a fall in cardiac output, thus resulting in a pronounced state of confusion, drowsiness, or even stupor as the presenting level of consciousness.

Vital Signs Vital signs are the pulse, blood pressure, and respirations. Pulse oximetry is also generally included as vital sign measurement, as are skin color or tone, temperature, and moisture, as well as pupil size and reaction. End-tidal CO_2 measurements are typically included in intubated patients.

In healthy hearts, the pulse rate tends to remain within normal limits, even with up to 15 percent volume deficit, as a result of peripheral vasoconstriction and the heart's ability to increase its contractile strength. However, the pulse, along with skin vitals, is one of the first observable indicators of the compensatory mechanisms associated with hypoperfusion. The character of the pulse may reflect the status of perfusion more accurately than the rate. Detection of the pulse may be affected by the degree of peripheral vascular resistance. Increased peripheral resistance tends to weaken the pulse. The pulse may be hard to feel or may feel weak and thready.

Clinical Insight

Pulse character is a more reliable early indicator of impaired perfusion than pulse rate. Compensatory increases in peripheral vascular resistance will tend to support cardiac contractile strength and pulse rate but may make the pulse feel weak and thready.

In some types of shock the heart rate may be slow, as with some causes of neurogenic shock. In obstructive shock (cardiac tamponade or tension pneumothorax), the heart rate may be fast and regular, while the pulse is irregular. The pulse irregularity is due to obstruction of the great vessels resulting in suppression of the pulse at the end of each full inspiration, a phenomenon called a paradoxical pulse, or pulsus paradoxus. Cardiogenic shock can be caused by a heart rate that is too slow, too fast, normal, or irregular. In addition, a sick myocardium is prone to dysrhythmias.

Respirations are stimulated by chemoreceptors in the brainstem that are sensitive to carbon dioxide and blood acid levels. As the shock cycle stimulates anaerobic metabolism and acid production, respirations will increase in depth and rate to increase supplies of oxygen to the hemoglobin and to rid the body of metabolic acids through increased exhalation of carbon dioxide. As the shock cycle continues, the increasing rate will override the depth, and respirations will eventually become rapid and shallow.

Blood pressure is the last vital sign to reflect diminishing cardiac output.

Blood pressure is the last vital sign to reflect diminishing cardiac output. The normal compensatory mechanisms of peripheral vasoconstriction, increased cardiac contractility, and fluid conservation/shifts maintain the systolic pressure until 25 to 30 percent of volume is lost. The slower the development of shock, the longer the systolic pressure will be maintained. However, if the contractility of the heart is affected (as in cardiogenic shock), the onset and progression of shock has a tendency to occur much faster. As mentioned earlier, narrow pulse pressure is a sign of increased intrathoracic pressure, and cardiac tamponade or tension pneumothorax should be suspected.

In the beginning stages of shock, the pulse and respirations are more susceptible to recognizable changes than the blood pressure. Also keep in mind that repeated vital signs measurements, especially in the early stages of shock, are more valuable than a single reading. Patients have a wide range of "normal," especially in heart rates. The average heart rate in normal adults is about 70 beats per minute during sleep and can accelerate to more than 100 during muscular activity or emotional excitement. In well-conditioned athletes at rest, the heart rate is normally about 50 to 60. An increase of 20 beats per minute is unlikely to be recognized as abnormal in the athlete and may not be considered elevated in other persons. Because of this, heart rates are considered to be relative. Therefore, the initial rate serves as a baseline to which later measurements will be compared.

Clinical Insight

Normal vital signs vary from individual to individual. Repeated measurements help identify trends.

If the body's compensatory mechanisms are functioning very well, the initial vital signs may appear normal. Repeated pulse, respiratory, and blood pressure readings will be most valuable when taken in the context of the whole patient. Serial vital signs, considered along with the mechanism of disease if any, history, and other assessment findings will help indicate patient trends. It is the pattern of body responses that must be observed. Recognition of the pattern can provide clues to patient conditions that require aggressive management.

Lung Sounds Lung sounds can provide a valuable clue to possible causes of shock. Disease states that promote a disruption in the hydrostatic pressure balance in the pulmonary vasculature, thus leading to pulmonary edema, usually require specific interventions that may be contraindicated for other disease states. In shock, those treatment choices are critical to outcome. Therefore, being able to determine if pulmonary edema is present is considered mandatory and provides information that will be used to determine treatment.

Determining the presence of pulmonary edema is critical to determining whether fluid administration is appropriate.

Additionally, lung sounds are indicators of cardiac response to increased preload. Cardiac intolerance to increased preload can complicate the problems of the patient who is in shock, especially in the older patient.

Shock states that promote pulmonary edema include cardiogenic shock, septic shock, anaphylactic shock, and drug-induced neurogenic shock. In early stages, fluid leaks out of the capillaries, increasing the distance between the capillary wall and alveolar wall across which oxygen and carbon dioxide must diffuse. As the fluid builds up around the alveolus clusters, the terminal bronchiole is affected, causing spasms, which are detected as wheezes. As the fluid increases and hydrostatic pressure exceeds the balance of air pressure in the alveoli, fluid accumulates in the alveoli, which is detected as crackles, or rales. In general, the lungs will hold approximately 1 liter of fluid before crackles will be heard. Because fluid follows gravity, crackles will be heard first in the most dependent portions of the lung fields and are most easily heard in the back.

There are signs that fluid is building up, however, before crackles are heard. Because water tends to follow gravity, in patient lying supine, body water will settle in the posterior portions of the pulmonary lobes and spread out. This gives the feeling of air hunger. The patient will complain of feeling short of breath and will want to sit up. When sitting, body water is confined to the lower lobes with a limited area to spread, thus increasing the availability of open air spaces, aiding breathing. Maintaining a sitting position, however, must be balanced with maintaining perfusion to the brain. Often, it is best to place the patient supine with head and shoulders elevated. The worse the pulmonary edema, the more upright the patient must sit to breathe. Use of accessory muscles when breathing, or the complaint of difficulty breathing or shortness of breath when flat, is an important clue to the presence of pulmonary edema. Occasionally, a patient will be found in a reclining position with the head and shoulders elevated. If the patient has been sitting in this position and has not moved for a period of time, it is possible that a degree of compensation has been reached to the point that crackles will not be heard until the patient is forced to exert himself (e.g., when transferring to the cot). Because of this phenomenon, lung sounds should be reassessed after movement.

In tension pneumothorax, the lung sounds are a discriminating sign. It is important to listen to both inhalation and exhalation. If lung sounds are assessed early in the process, inspiration of air can be heard bilaterally, but exhalation will not be complete on the affected side. As the process continues and air trapping builds up pressure, both inhalation and exhalation will diminish until, eventually, the affected side will have no air movement. If tension pneumothorax has progressed to this point, there will be no lung sounds on the affected side. This progression may occur very rapidly, especially in the patient who has a lack of ventilatory reserve, such as the patient with COPD.

A sudden onset of air hunger is typical of the patient with a pulmonary embolus. However, air hunger is also a result of hypoxia, and all shock patients will exhibit air hunger at some point. What is important about the air hunger is that it is recognized and oxygen supplied.

Orthostatic Hypotension *Orthostatic hypotension*, also known as postural hypotension, is a drop in blood pressure when the body position changes (e.g., when the patient sits up or stands rapidly). (A comparison of the patient's blood pressure when he is lying down versus after he sits or stands up is known as the "tilt test.") Such changes in body position disturb compensatory mechanisms, which may result in more obvious signs and symptoms. These symptoms include changes in mental status, skin vitals (pallor and sweating), and vital signs (especially tachycardia), as well as patient complaints such as dizziness and nausea.

orthostatic hypotension a drop in blood pressure when the body moves from a lying to a sitting or standing position; also called *postural hypotension.*

Orthostatic hypotension is considered by some to be the chief diagnostic sign for early shock. As such, it can be a useful diagnostic tool for all types of shock. Generally, this is done after a patient has been lying supine and an initial base line pulse and blood pressure have been taken. Then, if vital signs are taken after the patient is raised into a sitting or standing position and the heart rate increases by 20 beats per minute and the systolic drops by 10 mmHg, postural hypotension is considered to exist. In the field, the sudden onset of dizziness, pallor (with or without nausea or a "faint feeling"), and the disappearance of or an increase in the rate of the pulse are enough to strongly suggest a volume deficit.

Occasionally, a patient may rapidly deteriorate when being moved. In the case of internal bleeding, this may result from disturbing an existing clot, causing further internal bleeding. Because of this, patients suspected of being in shock should be handled gently.

MANAGEMENT PRIORITIES

Appropriate treatment of the patient in shock, done quickly and efficiently with rapid transport to the closest appropriate facility, will afford the best possibility for a good outcome. The guiding principles for treatment are

1. Open the airway.
2. Administer high-flow, high-concentration oxygen. This includes a nonrebreather mask with reservoir at 15 lpm or higher if needed to maintain an inflated reservoir bag. In the case of inadequate respiratory effort, assist with a bag-valve mask with reservoir at 15 to 20 lpm at a rate of 10 to 14/min, ensuring a good tidal volume. If end-tidal CO_2 measurement is available, either by nasal cannula or by tracheal tube, both the waveform and the numerical value should be assessed.
3. Establish IV access with normal saline or lactated Ringer's. Administer an initial fluid bolus of 250 to 500 ml. Additional fluid may be warranted based on the type of shock and the response.
4. Apply a cardiac monitor. Attention should be given to whether the rhythm can support perfusion. If the rhythm is the problem, obtain a 12-lead ECG if appropriate, then follow ACLS guidelines.

It is critical to differentiate between cardiogenic and noncardiogenic shock states.

Once the rhythm is one that can support perfusion, a thorough history and physical examination will guide further treatment. The first task is to differentiate between cardiogenic and noncardiogenic shock states. Assessing lung sounds, respiratory effort, and ECG changes are of critical importance.

A history of abdominal pain with clear lung sounds in the presence of a normal or tachycardic supraventricular rate suggests a noncardiogenic problem that may respond to volume support. However, continued monitoring of lung sounds and respiratory effort is necessary to detect cardiac intolerance to increased preload. If lung sounds remain clear, repeated boluses are the treatment of choice. The most important element here is repeated reassessment of lung sounds and respiratory effort.

In the rare case where lung sounds remain clear and respiratory effort is good, but the patient continues to deteriorate, assess for an irregular pulse that seems to diminish or disappear on inhalation (paradoxical pulse) and jugular venous distention. Cardiac tamponade may be the problem, and pericardiocentesis is the treatment of choice. Auscultating for muffled heart sounds is helpful but in the noisy field environment is impractical.

In some cases, pulmonary emboli may also present in this manner. History may help you discriminate between the two, but definitive treatment takes place in the hospital.

If lung sounds are clear but diminished or absent on one side, the problem may be a tension pneumothorax. Distended jugular veins and paradoxical pulse may also be present; however, cardiac tamponade and a tension pneumothorax are differentiated by lung sounds. Treatment of a tension pneumothorax requires a needle decompression on the side with altered lung sounds.

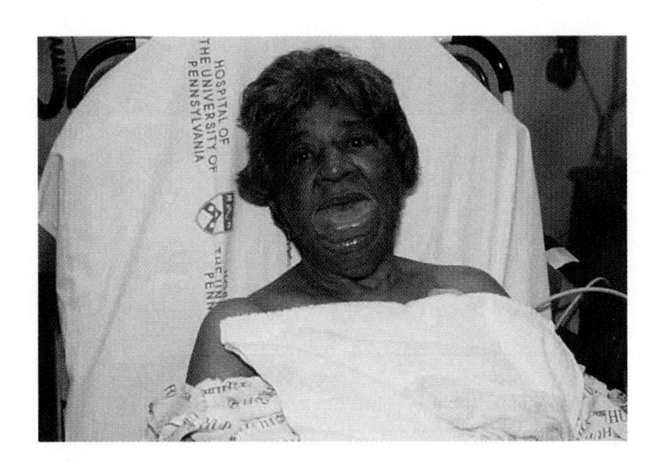

FIGURE 4-9
An allergic response: localized angioedema to the tongue.
(© Edward T. Dickinson, M.D.)

Presence of Pulmonary Edema

If, after a fluid bolus or during your respiratory assessment, wheezes and/or crackles are heard or respiratory effort becomes labored, it will be important to determine if there is cardiac involvement. It is critical to discriminate between shock of cardiac origin and shock due to an allergic reaction. History and attention to skin tones will help.

A history of bee sting, exposure to an allergen, presence of flushed skin, urticaria, or welts in the unresponsive patient will be definitive. Respiratory effects may involve stridor, wheezing, or extreme pulmonary edema. For severe cardiovascular collapse, administer epinephrine, 0.1 mg of 1:10,000 IV push. For less severe reactions (Figure 4-9), administer the adult dose of epinephrine 0.3 to 0.5 mg of 1:1,000 SQ or IM. What qualifies as "severe" is up to local medical direction. For reactions involving massive angioedema or for an additional aid to the effects of epinephrine, consider diphenhydramine, 25 to 50 mg slow IV push and an H2 blocker such as cimetidine or methylprednisolone.

Once the heart rate is corrected (atropine or pacing for bradycardia, adenosine, or cardioversion for supraventricular tachycardia), persistent pulmonary edema suggests cardiac muscle failure. The patient may or may not have a history consistent with AMI because cardiac muscle failure may be due to factors such as overdoses. (If overdose is known, contact the poison control center.) In any case, if cardiac intolerance to preload is present, dopamine at 5 to 10 μg/kg/min is recommended for its cardiac effect. Dopamine at higher doses of 10 to 20 μg/kg/min primarily stimulate alpha receptors for a vasopressor effect.

A similar situation where the history suggests an infection (dysuria, treatment for a urinary tract infection or upper respiratory infection, or presence of an indwelling catheter), the problem may be septic shock. Fluid replacement is a priority with dopamine as the drug of choice. The dose range extends from 5 to 20 μg/kg/min to include both the cardiac and vasopressor effects.

SUMMARY

Shock remains the end result of a variety of disease processes. Many types of shock are preventable. The health care provider must learn to suspect when shock is possible, conduct a thorough assessment, recognize shock when it is present, and choose the most appropriate treatment at the most appropriate time for the best possible outcome (Figure 4-10). This can only be achieved if the care provider not only understands the anatomy, physiology, and pathophysiology of shock, but also recognizes which organ systems are involved, supports the compensatory mechanisms already in place, and addresses immediately treatable causes.

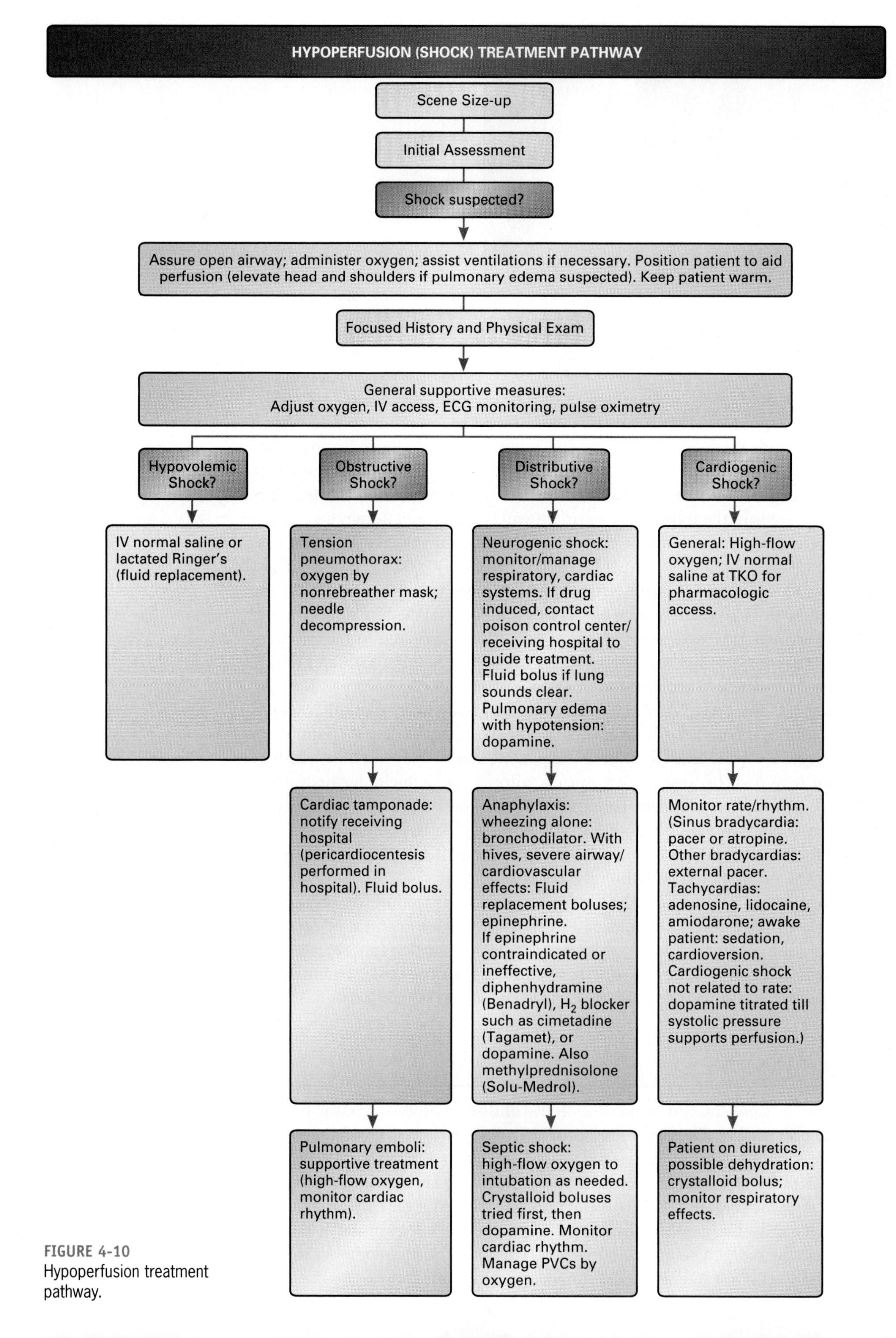

FIGURE 4-10 Hypoperfusion treatment pathway.

SCENARIO FOLLOW-UP

A 65-year-old male, who was recently discharged from the hospital after removal of a bunion, has suddenly had an episode of nausea and syncope. You are called to the scene and, as you approach the supine patient, you note that his breathing seems labored and he looks uncomfortable. He is alert and anxious. He denies pain but says he feels as if he is "jumping out of his skin." He reports that he is on Vasotec (enalapril) for hypertension and Motrin (ibuprofen) for pain. He took Motrin last night and Vasotec about 30 minutes ago. You have noted that the patient appears flushed all over, but he says he has not been outdoors and has no allergies that he is aware of.

As you are gathering the history, your partner has been hooking up oxygen and taking vital signs. Because the patient had a syncopal episode and appears short of breath, you place him on a nonrebreather mask with reservoir and administer oxygen at 15 lpm. Your partner reports that his vital signs are pulse 140 by carotid (radial is rapid and too faint to count), respirations 28, blood pressure 60/palpated.

While your partner applies the monitor, you note that lung sounds are absent in the bases with faint, bilateral wheezes throughout the upper lobes. His ECG is a sinus tachycardia. While your partner readies an albuterol inhalation treatment for your patient's bronchospasm, you attempt to start an IV. An IV of normal saline is started with difficulty, and a bolus of 500 ml fluid is given to replace fluid lost by fluid shift. Lung sounds remain the same, and the patient's blood pressure improves to 76/52.

As you load him for transport, you question the patient further about any new food or medication changes, and he tells you that his Vasotec is a new medication that he just started taking the day before he was dismissed from the hospital.

Because of his widespread vasodilation (evidenced by his flushed skin), anxiety, bronchospasm, and syncope approximately 30 minutes after ingestion of a new medication, you suspect an anaphylactic reaction. While you prepare epinephrine, you ask if he has had any heart problems or chest pain within the last year. The cardiac effects of epinephrine have a high probability of aggravating angina or other preexisting cardiac problems. He denies both, and you give him 0.5 mg of 1:1,000 epinephrine SQ. You chose epinephrine for its antihistamine effect and vasoconstrictive action. You chose the SQ route because his systolic rate is greater than 70.

Within a few minutes the patient tells you he is feeling better, and he looks visibly better. Vital signs 5 minutes after administration of epinephrine are pulse 120, respirations 20, and blood pressure 88/64. His skin is approaching normal color, and he is no longer panting after talking. Because his mental status is intact and he has improved significantly, you decide to administer a second fluid bolus of 500 ml and follow-up treatment with diphenhydramine (Benadryl) 50 mg, slow IV push and methylprednisolone (Solu-Medrol) 125 mg slow IV push. Repeat vital signs are P 118, R 18, and BP 96/72.

On arrival at the hospital, admission vital signs have not changed. Your patient is given a third 500-ml bolus of fluid and 20 mg famotidine (Pepcid) slow IV push. He is admitted for acute anaphylactic reaction and is told not to take Vasotec again. Another medication is prescribed in its place.

FURTHER READING

1. "2005 AHA Guidelines for Cardiopulmonary Resuscitation and Emergency Cardiac vascular Care" *Circulation,* 2005;112(24 supp).
2. Alexander, D. "New concepts in shock management," *Air Medical Journal,* 1996;15(2):85-91.
3. Berkow, R, M.H. Beers, and M. Burs, eds. *The Merck Manual of Diagnosis and Therapy.* 17th ed. Rahway, NJ: Merck & Company, 1999.
4. Bickell, W.H., M.J. Wall, P.E. Pepe, R.R. Martin, V.F. Ginger, M.K. Allen, and K.L. Mattox. "Immediate versus delayed fluid resuscitation for hypotensive patients with penetrating torso injuries," *New England Journal of Medicine,* 1994;331(17):1105-1109.
5. Bledsoe, B., R. Porter, and R. Cherry. "General principles of pathophysiology: hypoperfusion," in *Paramedic Care: Principles and Practice—Volume 1.* Upper Saddle River, NJ: Pearson/Prentice Hall, 2000.
6. Bongard, F.S. "Shock and resuscitation," in F.S. Bongard and D.Y. Sue, eds., *Current Critical Care Diagnosis and Treatment.* Stamford, CT: Appleton & Lange, 1994.
7. Capone, A.C., P. Safar, W. Stezoski, S. Tisherman, and A.B. Peitzman. "Improved outcome with fluid restriction in treatment of uncontrolled hemorrhagic shock," *Journal of the American College of Surgeons,* 1995; 180:49-56.

8. DALTON, A. "Shock," in P.T. Pons and D. Cason, eds., *Paramedic Field Care: A Complaint-Based Approach.* St. Louis: American College of Emergency Physicians, Mosby–Year Book, 1997.
9. FONTANAROSA, P.B. "Abdominal, genitourinary, and back pain," in P.T. Pons and D. Cason, eds., *Paramedic Field Care: A Complaint-Based Approach.* St. Louis: American College of Emergency Physicians, Mosby–Year Book, 1997.
10. GOLDMAN, L. and D. AUSIELLO, eds. *Cecil Textbook of Medicine.* 22nd ed. St. Louis: Saunders, 2004.
11. GUYTON, A.C. and J.E. HALL. *Textbook of Medical Physiology.* 10th ed. Philadelphia: W.B. Saunders, 2001.
12. HAAK, S.W., S.J. RICHARDSON, and S.S. DAVEY. "Alterations of cardiovascular function," in K.L. McCance and S.E. Huether, eds., *Pathophysiology: The Biologic Basis for Disease in Adults and Children.* 4th ed. St. Louis: Mosby, 2002.
13. MARTINI, F.H. and E.F. BARTHOLOMEW. *Essentials of Anatomy and Physiology.* Upper Saddle River, NJ: Pearson/Prentice Hall, 2000.
14. MCPHEE, S.J., V.R. LINGAPPA, and W.F. GANONG, eds. *Pathophysiology of Disease: An Introduction to Clinical Medicine.* 4th ed. Chicago: McGraw-Hill, 2003.
15. RAKEL, R.E. and E.T. BOPE, eds. *Conn's Current Therapy 2005.* St. Louis: Elsevier Saunders, 2005.
16. ROTHENBERG, M.A. *Mechanisms and Treatment of Disease Pathophysiology: A Plain English Approach.* Eau Claire, WI: PESI Healthcare, 2001.
17. SAUNDERS, M.J. *Mosby's Paramedic Textbook.* 2nd ed. St. Louis: Mosby, 2000.
18. THIBIDEAU, G.A. and K.T. PATTON. *Anatomy and Physiology.* 4th ed. St. Louis: Mosby, 1999.

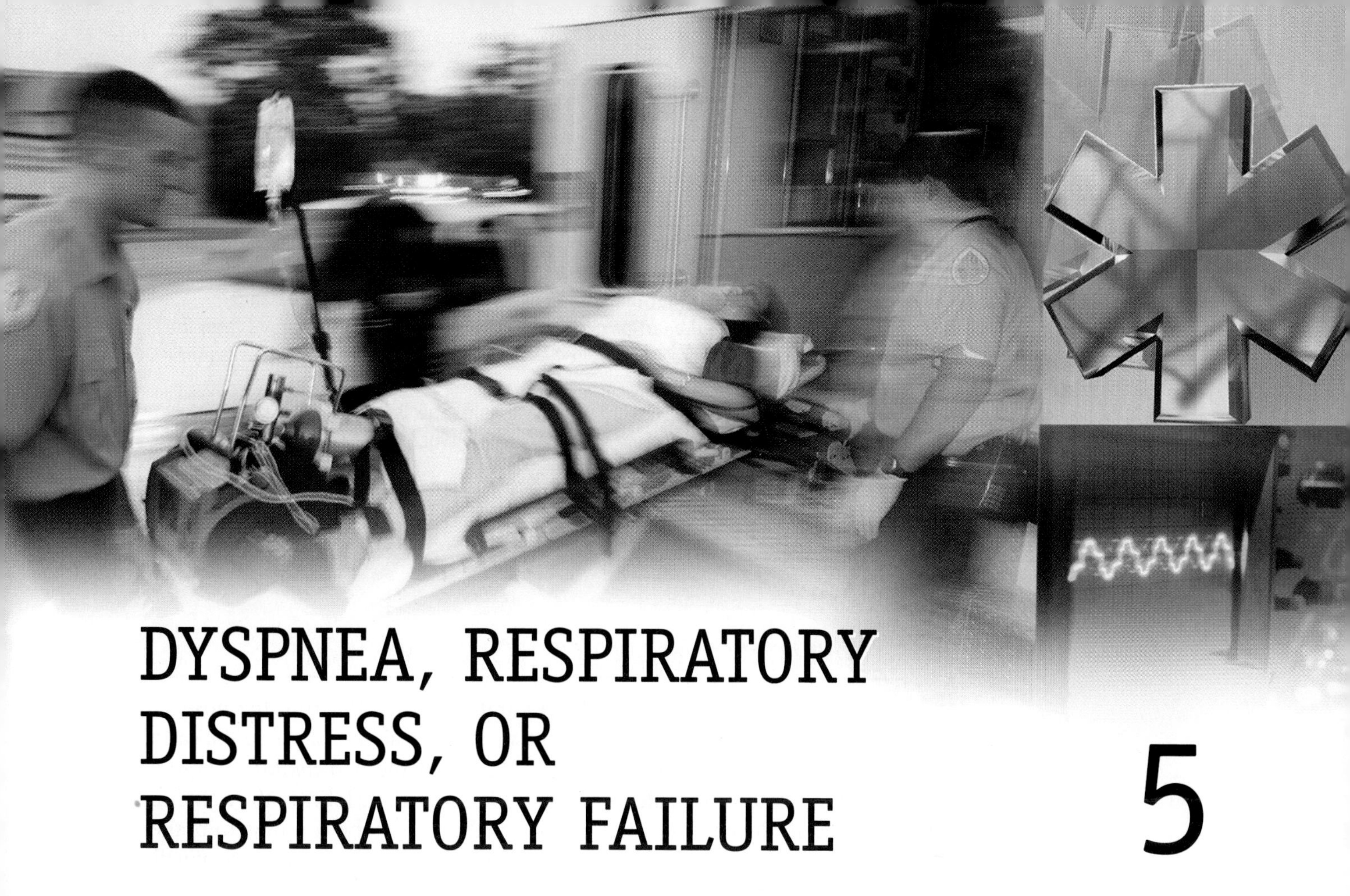

DYSPNEA, RESPIRATORY DISTRESS, OR RESPIRATORY FAILURE

5

A significant number of patients access the emergency care system with respiratory complaints that include shortness of breath, or dyspnea. Patients often describe dyspnea in a variety of ways such as feeling "breathless," "smothering," "can't catch my breath," or "unable to get an adequate breath." The variation in the description of this complaint makes dyspnea difficult to characterize. Although dyspnea can be a complaint primarily attributed to the respiratory system, many other causes outside of the respiratory system are possible. When confronted with a complaint of dyspnea, the health care provider must, as necessary, take immediate measures to support respiration and ventilation. Then, the provider must conduct a thorough assessment aimed at discovering clues to the underlying cause of the patient's respiratory difficulty and provide appropriate treatment.

Topics that are covered in this chapter are

- Anatomy and Physiology
- Determining the Severity of Respiratory Distress or Failure
- Differential Diagnosis and Management Priorities

SCENARIO

You are spending a quiet afternoon in the firehouse when your unit is requested to respond to a patient with "respiratory distress." As you approach the scene, you are met by an elderly gentleman who says that his wife is having trouble breathing. You walk with him toward the house, noting that the area appears free of any immediate dangers.

He tells you that his wife has a history of both lung and heart problems. She was just recently discharged from the hospital after a 2-week course of treatment for "breathing problems." She has a long history of smoking and uses home oxygen at night.

As you approach the patient, you see an uncomfortable-looking elderly female. She is breathing approximately 40 times per minute and appears to be struggling with each breath. There is audible wheezing. She appears confused when you begin to obtain a brief history.

How would you proceed with the immediate care of this patient?

ANATOMY AND PHYSIOLOGY

The *upper airway* consists of the respiratory structures from the nose and mouth to the *carina*; the *lower airway* consists of all structures distal to the carina (Figure 5-1). At the carina, the trachea divides into the two *mainstem bronchi*, which further divide into smaller tubes that give rise to three lobes in the right lung and two lobes in the left lung. The bronchi within each lobe continue to branch until they reach the smallest functional units, the *terminal bronchioles*. Finally, these structures divide into small gas-filled sacs called the *alveoli*. Within the alveoli, inspired gases are separated from the circulatory system by only a thin membrane, allowing exchange of oxygen and carbon dioxide between the body and the atmosphere.

The lungs are sponge-like structures in which the exchange of gases takes place. The outer aspect of the lung is covered by a thin membrane called the *visceral pleura*. The *parietal pleura* is found beneath the ribs and muscles that line the chest cavity. The *pleural cavity* (the space between the visceral and parietal pleura) is normally filled with a small amount of lubricating fluid, but it is also a potential space where blood or other fluids (pleural effusion), air, or infection can accumulate.

The major muscles of breathing (Figure 5-2) are the diaphragm, the intercostal muscles, and the neck muscles, primarily the scalene and sternocleidomastoid muscles. The *diaphragm*, a dome-like muscle separating the thorax and abdomen, performs the majority of the work of respiration. The *intercostal muscles* have motor and sensory innervation from the spinal intercostal nerves. Stretch receptors on these muscles play an integral role in the perception of dyspnea or breathlessness. Remember that the *sternocleidomastoid muscles* of the neck are not normally used during quiet ventilation but become important during strenuous breathing.

dyspnea an abnormal or uncomfortable awareness of breathing.

Dyspnea is defined as an abnormal or uncomfortable awareness of breathing. In general, dyspnea is perceived by the brain when the ventilatory effort does not adequately meet the metabolic demands of the body. Although the exact mechanisms that create a feeling of dyspnea are not completely understood, several factors are known to contribute to the feeling of breathlessness, including receptors in the lungs and respiratory muscles, the blood pH level, and the serum oxygen concentration. It is important to remember, however, that there is not a direct relationship between the level of hypoxia and the sensation of dyspnea; many hypoxic patients will not complain of being short of breath (e.g., COPD patients), while other patients with normal pO_2 levels may complain of dyspnea (e.g., patients with pulmonary emboli).

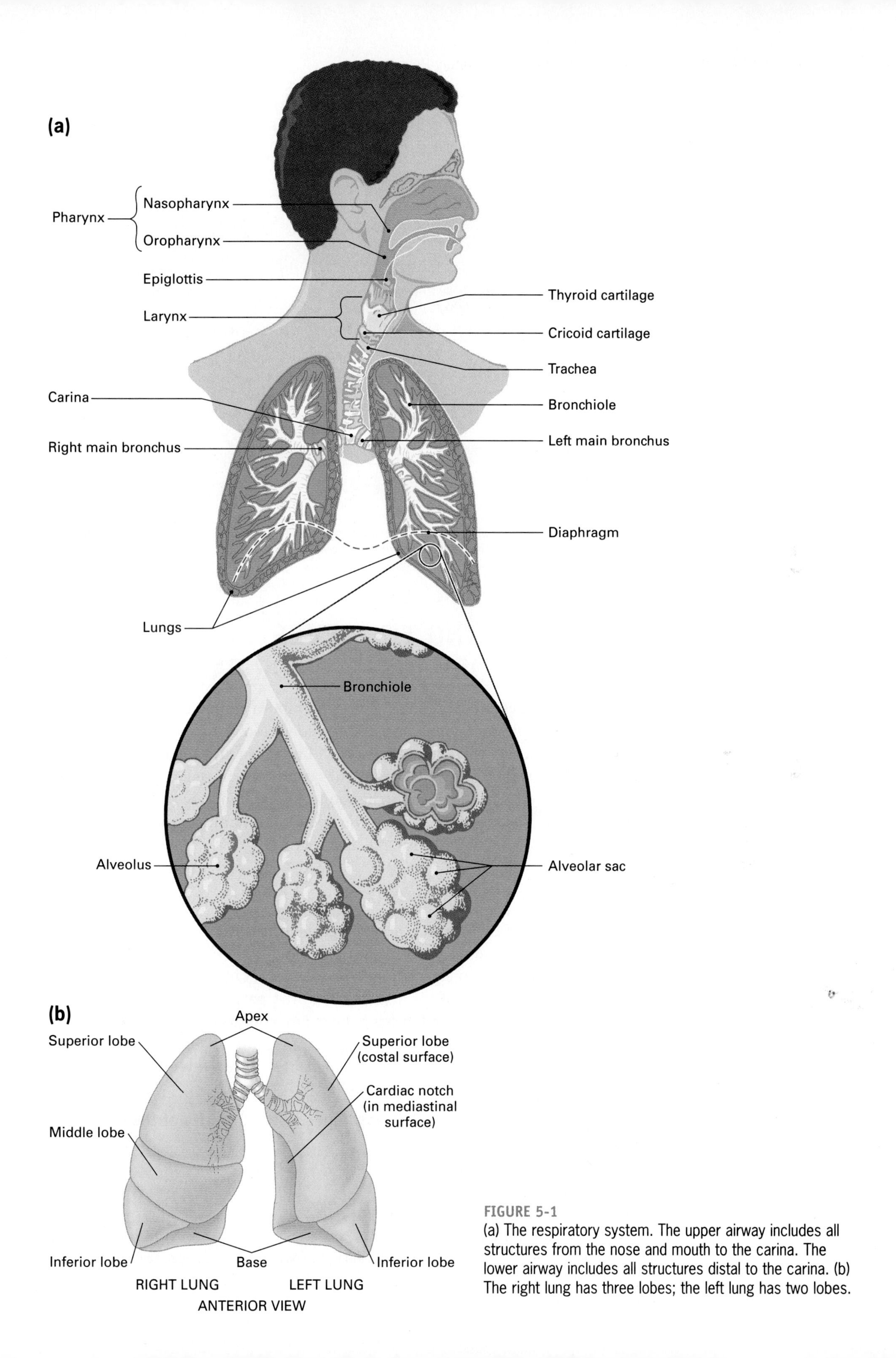

FIGURE 5-1
(a) The respiratory system. The upper airway includes all structures from the nose and mouth to the carina. The lower airway includes all structures distal to the carina. (b) The right lung has three lobes; the left lung has two lobes.

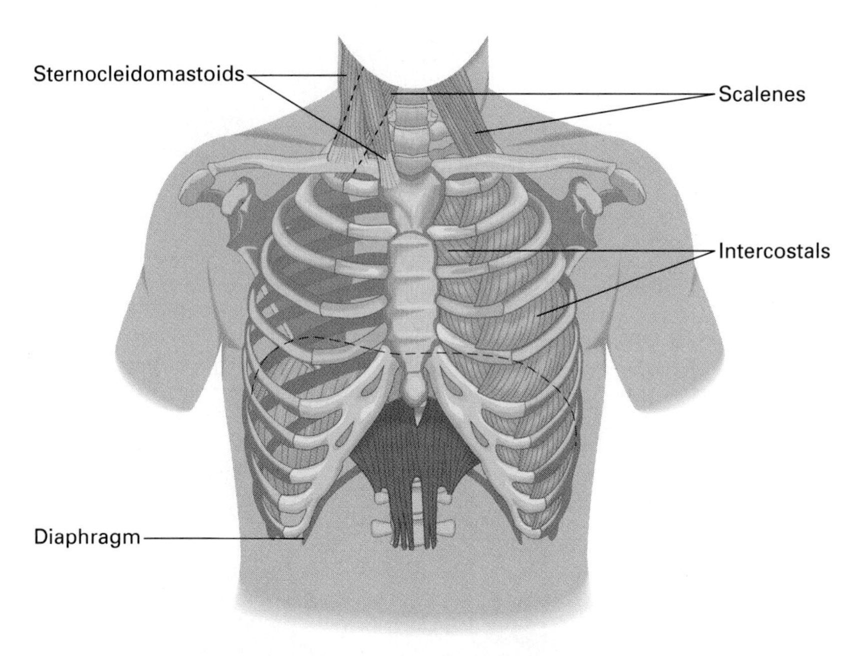

FIGURE 5-2
The muscles of respiration.

Note: Scalenes are posterior to sternocleidomastoids. At anatomical left, sternocleidomastoids are not shown to reveal structure of scalene.

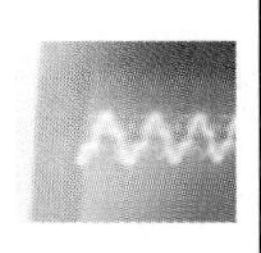

DETERMINING THE SEVERITY OF RESPIRATORY DISTRESS OR FAILURE

The initial assessment of the patient with dyspnea is aimed at determining the severity of the respiratory complaints and the condition of the patient (Table 5-1). The speed with which therapeutic actions will be taken and the thoroughness of your assessment will be based on the patient's condition. In general, the more critical the patient, the sooner you will initiate interventions and the less time you will spend in obtaining a history and performing a physical examination.

In general, the more critical the patient, the sooner interventions will be initiated and the less time will be spent obtaining a history and conducting a physical exam.

Scene Size-Up

As with all other emergency situations, the first step is a scene size-up. As you approach, in addition to assuring the safety of yourself and your fellow emergency care providers, you can obtain some immediate clues about the condition of the patient. Note the patient's position. You would approach a patient who is seated or lying down and appears comfortable in a different manner than the patient who is leaning forward on his arms. View the patient's ventilatory effort as you approach. A normal patient breathes between 8 and 24 times

TABLE 5-1 Respiratory Distress: Clues to the Severity of the Patient's Condition

The following are indications of severe respiratory distress:

- Posture: sitting up, leaning on arms
- Unable to speak complete sentences without pausing to "catch my breath"
- Breathlessness noted at rest
- Imminent respiratory failure or arrest indicated by bradycardia, bradypnea, agonal respirations, apnea

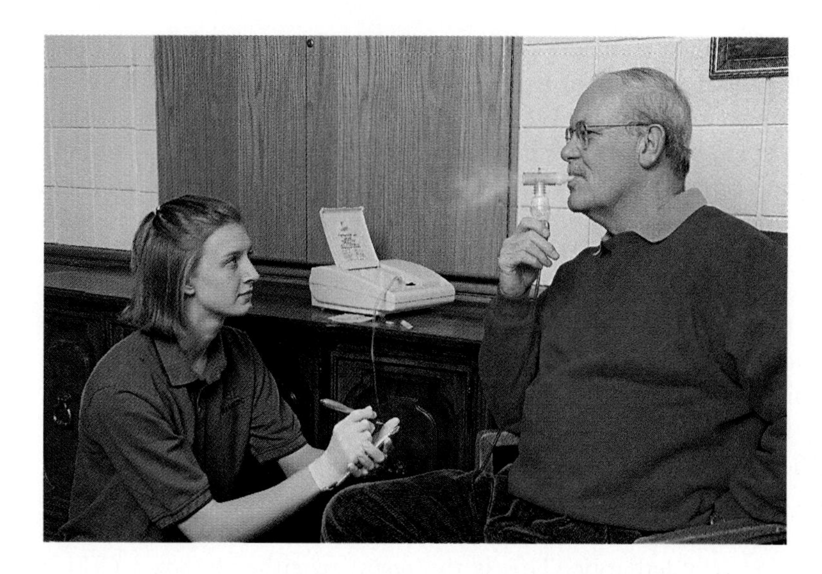

FIGURE 5-3
Home aerosol/nebulizing equipment may be found at the scene of a patient with asthma or COPD.

per minute with a tidal volume of 400 to 800 ml. A patient who is breathing more deeply and rapidly is experiencing respiratory difficulty. Additionally, note the patient's mental status. Patients with significant respiratory distress tend to be agitated, confused, or lethargic. Finally, assess the respiratory effort. The use of sternocleidomastoid and intercostal muscles to assist respiration is a particularly worrisome sign.

You may spot other helpful clues while you are inspecting the scene. Look for home oxygen devices, portable mechanical ventilators, noninvasive ventilation machines (e.g., the continuous positive airway pressure [CPAP] machines), or home nebulizing equipment (Figure 5-3). Additionally, inspect for cigarettes or ashtrays for evidence of cigarette smoking. These may all provide some clues about the patient's underlying medical condition. You should briefly inspect any medications that the patient is taking. Focus particular attention on the use of nitrates, diuretics, digitalis preparations, antidysrhythmic agents, inhalers, steroids, antibiotics, or blood thinners.

Initial Assessment

The scene size-up is followed by a brief initial patient assessment. This would include an assessment of the patient's airway, breathing, circulatory status, and mental awareness. In patients who are dyspneic, the initial assessment should help determine whether there is any obstruction of the airway and/or impending respiratory failure.

The patient's airway is a particular focus of the initial assessment. Airway obstruction from any cause can lead to complaints of breathlessness. Remember that normal respiration is a quiet process. When approaching a patient with respiratory complaints, listen for any upper airway sounds such as grunting, snoring, or stridor that suggest upper airway obstruction.

If there is an obstruction, make an immediate determination as to whether the obstruction is complete or incomplete. Additionally, you must quickly determine if the obstruction has resulted from foreign body aspiration or another cause. In the case of complete obstruction, you will note that the patient will have an ineffective cough, stridor, poor air movement, and decreased mental status or unconsciousness.

Immediately determine if an obstruction is complete or incomplete.

For patients with aspirated foreign material, initiate standard basic life support measures. If the patient is still awake, stand behind the adult victim and perform repeated Heimlich manueuvers in an attempt to remove the foreign body. Perform chest thrusts if the patient is pregnant or obese. If the patient becomes unconscious, perform a jaw-tongue lift and attempt to visualize any foreign body. If one is seen, it should be removed using a finger sweep. Then, after repositioning the airway, attempt rescue breathing, followed by chest compressions. Repeat the entire sequence until the foreign body is removed. A patient who has a tracheostomy should have his airway suctioned, because mucous plugging is a common cause of obstruction in these patients.

Clinical Insight

After the airway, the next priority is impending respiratory failure. Agitation, confusion, and low pulse oximetry readings suggest hypoxia. Confusion and somnolence suggest retention of carbon dioxide in the bloodstream. Ominous signs include a slow respiratory rate (less than 8 breaths per minute), bradycardia, and hypotension. Provide immediate ventilatory support.

Finally, if these attempts are unsuccessful or other causes of obstruction are noted (e.g., infection, laryngospasm, angioedema), then you should attempt to provide a definitive airway. Although tracheal intubation should be attempted, a surgical airway is often required (see Chapter 2, Airway Management, Ventilation, and Oxygen Therapy).

Once you have addressed the airway, turn your attention to the possibility of respiratory failure. Patients with respiratory failure will be found to be agitated, confused, or very lethargic. This is the result of either hypoxia (which leads to agitation) or the accumulation of CO_2 in the bloodstream caused by inadequate elimination of the gas by the respiratory system (which leads to confusion or lethargy). The patient is often seen bobbing the head and will appear sleepy, with drooping eyelids. When respiratory failure is imminent, the patient will develop a slow heart rate (bradycardia), a slow respiratory rate (bradypnea), and poor air movement, which can be noted on auscultation of the lungs. Hypotension is an ominous sign in these patients. Respiratory arrest may occur as a late finding.

Once you have recognized impending respiratory failure, you must provide ventilatory support to the patient (see Chapter 2). Immediate measures may include mouth-to-mask ventilation or bag-valve-mask ventilation. Commonly, tracheal intubation must be performed unless there is an easily reversible cause of the patient's respiratory complaints. The urgency of the situation will prevent the health care provider from performing a more detailed assessment of the patient. In less urgent situations, noninvasive techniques such as CPAP ventilation may be tried, as is discussed later in this chapter.

If airway obstruction and respiratory failure are excluded, general supportive measures should be provided while the history and physical exam are conducted to find the likely cause of the dyspnea. These measures should include supplemental oxygen, IV access, cardiac monitoring, and pulse oximetry.

Focused History and Physical Exam

Having addressed the immediate concerns of airway obstruction and respiratory failure, along with an assessment of circulation, you should next undertake a history and physical examination focused on identifying the immediately treatable causes of dyspnea.

Focused History

In evaluating the patient with dyspnea, conduct a SAMPLE history, using the mnemonic OPQRST (Onset, Palliation/Provocation, Quality, Radiation, Severity, and Time) to help you obtain more complete information about the patient's chief complaint:

1. Onset
   - *Did your shortness of breath develop gradually or suddenly?* A sudden onset would be typical of conditions such as foreign body airway obstruction, anaphylaxis, angioedema, asthma, pneumothorax, or pulmonary embolism. However, conditions such as COPD, pneumonia, congestive heart failure,

or various neuromuscular disorders would be associated with a gradual onset of dyspnea.

2. Palliation/Provocation
   - *What makes your symptoms better? What makes them worse?* Patients with COPD report improvement in symptoms after coughing. Symptoms that improve in the upright position suggest a cardiac cause of dyspnea. Activity will worsen dyspnea in patients with underlying cardiac and respiratory disease.
3. Quality
   - *Can you describe your breathing difficulty? Do have any discomfort along with it? What is the discomfort like?* Patients with asthma may describe tightness in the chest. Patients with pleural effusion, pneumothorax, or pulmonary embolism may report sharp, stabbing, pleuritic pain. Patients with a cardiac problem may describe burning, crushing, or squeezing chest pain.
4. Radiation
   - *If you have pain, does it go anywhere?* Patients with an underlying cardiac problem may describe pain that radiates to the back, jaw, neck, or arms.
5. Severity
   - *How has your breathing problem interfered with your normal activities?* Patients with chronic conditions such as COPD or congestive heart failure should be able to describe how disabling their symptoms are in terms of typical daily activities such as climbing stairs or walking distances. In addition, the patient's speech pattern will lend some clues as to the seriousness of the complaint. If the patient is unable to speak in complete sentences, this is a troubling sign.
   - *Do you notice the breathing difficulty when you are sitting still or resting?* Breathlessness noted at rest usually indicates a more advanced medical condition. For example, patients with stage IV congestive heart failure have symptoms at rest and have the worst prognosis.
6. Time
   - *Over what period of time did your shortness of breath develop?* In general, patients with worsening of COPD, pneumonia, cardiomyopathy, or congestive heart failure will describe a gradual progression of symptoms. In contrast, dyspneic patients with asthma, pulmonary embolism, spontaneous pneumothorax, or foreign body aspiration will report a sudden onset of their complaints.
   - *Have you been treated for similar problems in the past?* The patient's medical history may be an important link to establishing the cause of dyspnea. This is typically true of patients with chronic medical conditions such as asthma, COPD, congestive heart failure, or pneumonia, which may be recurrent in nature. However, remember that other causes of dyspnea may complicate a chronic respiratory disorder. For example, a patient with COPD may suddenly develop a spontaneous pneumothorax. The asthmatic patient may have a relapse of symptoms because of an underlying pneumonia.
7. Additional Considerations
   - *Have you noticed any additional symptoms?* Other associated findings may help distinguish causes of dyspnea. For example, fever, sore throat, and pain on swallowing suggest an infectious cause of airway obstruction in the patient who is short of breath. Chest pain, orthopnea (breathing difficulty when lying flat), and paroxysmal nocturnal dyspnea (PND)

Clinical Insight

Patients classically describe their cardiac pain as squeezing, crushing, or pressure. However, many patients do not have "classic" chest pain. The elderly, women, and diabetics are particularly prone to unusual presenting complaints with acute cardiac syndromes. Dyspnea is commonly the only complaint in these patients.

(sudden awakening at night with breathing difficulty) are more common in patients with congestive heart failure, whereas fever, cough, pleuritic chest pain, and sputum production are seen in patients with pneumonia.

– *What medications are you taking?* Current medications may help the emergency care provider understand the patient's underlying medical conditions. Diuretics, digitalis preparations, and nitrates are commonly used in patients with congestive heart failure. Inhaled agents and steroids are typically seen in asthmatics and patients with COPD. Another important clue is the determination of whether a medication was just started in a patient with an airway obstruction, suggesting an allergic cause. However, the clinician must be careful not to have tunnel vision based on the patient's medications or previous medical conditions.

Focused Physical Examination

The focus of the physical examination is to identify immediately treatable causes of breathlessness. One immediate clue to the severity of the patient's respiratory complaints is to observe the number of words the patient can speak when responding to your questions during the history. You should be concerned about patients who must take time to "catch their breath" after only a few words. The patient's general appearance must also be assessed. Are there any signs of cyanosis? What position does the patient assume? Severely dyspneic patients assume an upright position, leaning forward on their arms (the so-called "tripod" position).

You should be concerned about patients who must take time to "catch their breath" after only a few words.

Also consider the patient's body type. A very thin but barrel-chested and cachectic (emaciated) appearance indicates chronic obstructive respiratory disease (emphysema). A tall, thin individual is more likely to develop a spontaneous pneumothorax.

Begin the focused physical examination with an assessment of vital signs. Patients suffering severe dyspnea tend to demonstrate tachypnea and tachycardia. Bradycardia, bradypnea, or apnea are more ominous signs suggesting respiratory failure. The patient's temperature is important to record because it may indicate an infectious cause of dyspnea such as pneumonia, epiglottitis, or croup. Additionally, patients with pulmonary embolism can have a low-grade fever.

agonal respirations slow, irregular, shallow, gasping breaths seen in respiratory failure or impending respiratory arrest.

Next, consider whether an abnormal respiratory pattern is present (Figure 5-4). *Agonal respirations* are slow, irregular, shallow, and gasping-type breaths that are seen

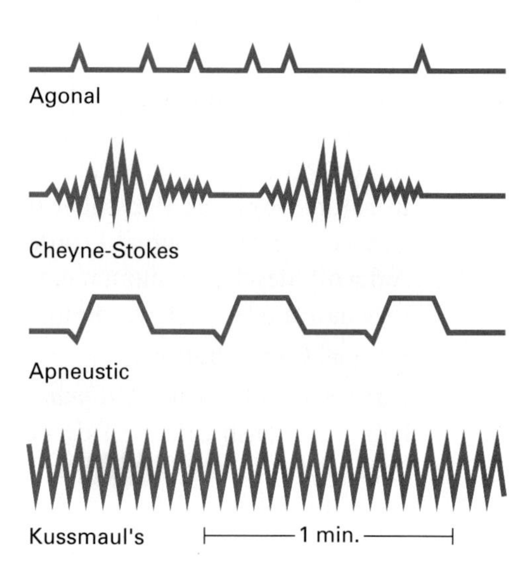

FIGURE 5-4
Abnormal respiratory patterns.

in patients with respiratory failure and impending respiratory arrest. *Cheyne-Stokes respirations* are typical of older patients with metabolic disease or stroke. They are characterized by regular cycles of apnea gradually changing to periods of hyperventilation. No respiratory management is indicated. *Apneustic breathing* is characterized by long, deep breaths separated by periods of apnea. Such breathing is associated with severe central nervous system (CNS) disease and often requires ventilatory support. Finally, *Kussmaul's respirations* are deep, rapid, and regular breaths associated with metabolic acidosis. Patients with this ventilatory pattern may occasionally report dyspnea.

Cheyne-Stokes respirations regular cycles of apnea gradually changing to periods of hyperventilation.

apneustic respirations long, deep breaths separated by periods of apnea.

Kussmaul's respirations deep, rapid, regular respirations.

The body areas you should address during the focused examination include the oropharynx and chest with cardiac examination. Inspect the oropharynx for any obvious foreign bodies or evidence of infection. Two points deserve mention: Use extreme care in attempting to remove suspected foreign bodies that are not visible; blind attempts at removal can worsen the obstruction. Also, you must take care in examining the patient with suspected infection in the supraglottic region. Unnecessary manipulation can lead to laryngospasm and worsening obstruction. Carefully examine the area for redness, swelling, edema, distortion of the normal anatomy, and pus. The patient may be unable to swallow or open the mouth. Examine the neck for tracheal deviation, jugular venous distention, and use of accessory muscles. Remember to suction any patient with a tracheostomy because plugging of the airway from mucus or blood occurs commonly.

Inspect the chest for respiratory effort and symmetric movement. Asymmetry may be seen with pneumothorax, pneumonia, or pulmonary embolism. Palpation of the chest may reveal crepitus or subcutaneous emphysema. Finally, carefully auscultate the chest. The inspiratory and expiratory phases should be free of noise. Stridor, wheezing, crackles (also called rales), or rhonchi are all abnormal sounds that may be heard during respiration. It is important to note whether these sounds are heard in one lung field only or in both lungs. Additionally, expiration should last approximately twice as long as inspiration. Any prolongation of the expiratory phase suggests an obstructive process, such as asthma or COPD.

Finally, examine the heart. Focus particular attention on abnormal heart sounds such as gallop rhythms or murmurs. A crunching sound heard with each beat is called Hamman's sign and indicates air in the mediastinum. Distant or muffled heart sounds may indicate a pericardial effusion. Also assess the regularity of the heart. Any irregularities may suggest impaired cardiac function and resultant congestive heart failure. (It should be noted that cardiac assessment takes skill on the part of the examiner and may be difficult because of significant background noise in the prehospital environment.)

A more complete history and physical examination may be indicated if the previously mentioned findings do not reveal an obvious source of dyspnea. As a general rule, supportive measures constitute the treatment for other causes of dyspnea in the prehospital phase of care.

DIFFERENTIAL DIAGNOSIS AND MANAGEMENT PRIORITIES

The main causes of dyspnea can be divided among upper airway obstruction, respiratory disease, cardiac disease, neuromuscular disease, and other causes, including anemia, hyperthyroid disease, and metabolic acidosis (Table 5-2). Psychogenic hyperventilation is diagnosed after excluding all other causes of breathlessness and should not be considered a primary diagnosis in the prehospital environment.

Underlying causes of dyspnea may include obstruction, respiratory, cardiac, or neuromuscular diseases, and others.

TABLE 5-2 **Causes of Dyspnea**

Upper Airway Obstruction	Foreign body
	Infections
	    Croup
	    Epiglottitis
	    Ludwig's angina
	    Retropharyngeal abscess

Respiratory Causes	Aspiration
	Asthma
	COPD
	    Chronic bronchitis
	    Emphysema
	Pneumonia
	Noncardiogenic pulmonary edema
	Pleural effusion
	Pleuritis; pleurodynia
	Pneumothorax
	Pulmonary embolism
	Toxic inhalation

Cardiovascular Causes	Acute pulmonary edema/congestive heart failure Acute myocardial infarction Cardiomyopathy Pericardial tamponade Cardiac dysrhythmias
Neuromuscular Diseases	Muscular dystrophy Amyotrophic lateral sclerosis (Lou Gehrig's disease) Guillain-Barré syndrome Myasthenia gravis
Other Causes	Anemia Hyperthyroid disease Metabolic acidosis Psychogenic hyperventilation

Airway Obstruction

Early airway obstruction usually presents with an initial complaint of dyspnea. Stridor or wheezing may accompany this complaint. A history of foreign body sensation in the throat or chest noted after eating strongly suggests a case for a food foreign body, which is the most common cause of airway obstruction. The onset of symptoms may be acute if a foreign body or allergic reaction is the cause of obstruction. Any complaint of dyspnea or respiratory distress in a patient who has a tracheostomy should prompt suspicion of an airway that is obstructed from mucous plugging.

However, the onset may be more insidious if infection is the cause. Infections involving the tissues below the tongue (Ludwig's angina), the epiglottis (epiglottitis), below the glottis (croup), or behind the pharynx (retropharyngeal abscess) may also lead to airway obstruction. Fever, pain on swallowing, and difficulty opening the mouth all suggest an infectious cause.

Patients on blood-thinning medications such as warfarin (Coumadin) may also develop airway obstruction from the spontaneous development of hematomas within the soft tissues of the neck.

Finally, swelling of the tissues as the result of anaphylaxis or angioedema may result in an obstructed airway. The sudden onset of symptoms after ingesting food or medication or after an insect bite raises the suspicion of *anaphylaxis* as the cause. Associated findings include a rash that itches, wheezing in the lung fields, hypotension, nausea, abdominal cramps, or an inability to urinate. *Angioedema* may result from hereditary factors that are aggravated by stress, trauma, or surgery. The result is sudden onset of swelling about the face (including the airway), hands, and abdominal organs. Certain drugs, particularly angiotensin-converting enzyme (ACE) inhibitors, may also cause angioedema.

Laryngospasm is the sudden closure of the glottic opening, which may be triggered by infection, irritants, or manipulation. This may also result in a clinical picture of airway obstruction.

Treatment of these conditions depends on the patient's symptoms at the time of presentation. For patients who are complaining of mild dyspnea, establish supportive measures such as supplemental oxygen and intravenous access while you are seeking a cause. Closely watch the patient for a sudden deterioration in the status of the airway. Epinephrine given subcutaneously (0.3 to 0.5 mg) or intravenously (0.1 to 0.5 mg), diphenhydramine (Benadryl) (25 to 50 mg), and methylprednisolone (Solu-Medrol) (125 mg) may all be used in the prehospital management of anaphylaxis and angioedema. If the patient is unable to control the airway or there is concern about progression to complete obstruction, definitive airway management is indicated, including possible need for a surgical airway (see Chapter 2).

anaphylaxis severe allergic reaction.

angioedema swelling or hives affecting the skin, mucous membranes, or viscera. There are various causes, possibly hereditary, including sensitivity to certain foods, drugs, or other substances or environmental conditions.

laryngospasm sudden closure of the glottic opening.

Respiratory Diseases

Various respiratory diseases and conditions can lead to a patient complaint of breathlessness.

Asthma

Asthma is a common cause of dyspnea that can usually be reversed by appropriate therapy. The underlying problem in asthmatics is increased responsiveness of bronchial smooth muscle (bronchoconstriction) to a variety of stimulants and an inflammatory response within the tracheobronchial tree. These inciting stimuli can include allergens, weather changes, exercise, respiratory infections, foods, and medications.

asthma disease characterized by increased responsiveness of the tracheobronchial tree to a variety of stimulants, resulting in paroxysmal constriction of the bronchial airways.

The classic symptoms of asthma include dyspnea, cough, and wheezing. Patients may occasionally complain of shortness of breath with exertion and chest tightness, which may lead to confusion with cardiac causes of dyspnea. Patients will initially present with wheezing heard on auscultation. Eventually, prolongation of the expiratory phase of respiration is noted. In severe cases, the patient will be noted to use accessory muscles of respiration (sternal and intercostal retraction) and to have *less* wheezing due to diminished air flow.

Prehospital therapy for dyspnea due to asthma includes supportive measures such as oxygen supplementation, intravenous access, and monitoring of pulse oximetry. Beta-adrenergic agents such as albuterol (2.5 to 5.0 mg), levalbuterol (0.63 to 1.25 mg), or metaproteranol (0.2 to 0.3 ml) are effective in prehospital treatment of asthma. Subcutaneous epinephrine (0.3 mg) or terbutaline (0.25 mg) is used in selected settings. Other agents used include steroids given parenterally (methylprednisolone 125 mg) or orally (prednisone 60 mg) and anticholinergic agents given by inhalation (ipratropium bromide [Atrovent] 0.5 mg).

chronic obstructive pulmonary disease (COPD) a blanket term for diseases that impede the functioning of the lungs. These include **chronic bronchitis** (increased mucous production in the bronchial tree) and **emphysema** (abnormal increase in size of alveoli and destruction of alveolar walls).

Chronic Obstructive Pulmonary Disease

Chronic obstructive pulmonary disease (COPD) is another leading cause of dyspnea. Cigarette smoking is implicated as a cause of COPD in most patients. Other patients develop COPD because of occupational exposures, pollutants, recurring infections, and genetic predisposition (e.g., alpha-1 antitripsin deficiency).

COPD is further classified into chronic bronchitis and emphysema. Patients with *chronic bronchitis* tend to present with symptoms of chronic productive cough. Because these patients tend to be somewhat obese and have chronically low blood oxygen concentrations, they have a characteristic appearance that causes them to be known as "blue bloaters." In addition to wheezing, crackles or rales and rhonchi are typically heard on examination of the lungs. When they become ill, these patients tend to present with increasing somnolence resulting from increasing blood levels of carbon dioxide.

Emphysema patients are typically thinner with large, barrel chests. Symptoms are caused by progressive destruction of the lower airway structures. These patients tend to hyperventilate to maintain normal blood oxygen concentrations, leading to their description as "pink puffers." With disease flares, these patients tend to breathe through pursed lips in order to maintain positive pressure that will keep the alveoli open. Breath sounds seem very distant in these patients.

Most COPD patients have elements of both chronic bronchitis and emphysema. Acute presentations are characterized by cough, wheezing, sputum production, and hypoxia. A change in the patient's baseline cough is often reported. Worsening of the underlying disease is typically caused by infections, poor compliance with prescribed medications, weather changes, environmental exposures, and certain medications, such as narcotics, sedatives, and so on.

Prehospital treatment of COPD symptoms includes high-flow, high-concentration oxygen therapy (along with careful monitoring of pulse oximetry and mental status), beta-adrenergic agents (albuterol 2.5 to 5.0 mg, levalbuterol [Xopenex] 0.63 to 1.25 mg, metaproteranol 0.2 to 0.3 ml, epinephrine 0.3 mg), and anticholinergic agents (ipratropium bromide [Atrovent] 0.5 mg). Parenteral steroids (methylprednisolone [Solu-Medrol] 125 mg) are often administered in the hospital setting.

Recently, the use of noninvasive positive-pressure ventilation techniques such as bilevel positive airway pressure (BiPAP) and continuous positive airway pressure (CPAP) have been used to avoid intubation in patients with acute COPD exacerbations. However, there has been little prehospital experience with these techniques. BiPAP and CPAP (Figure 5-5) are considered to be forms of noninvasive ventilation. Positive-pressure ventilation is provided via a tight-fitting mask. The major difference between CPAP and BiPAP is that the positive pressure in CPAP remains constant throughout inspiration and expiration, whereas with BiPAP the inspiratory pressure is at least 3 cm H_2O higher than the expiratory pressure.

Noninvasive ventilation provides at least two benefits to the patient. During inspiration, the positive pressure decreases the work the patient must exert to initiate a breath. During expiration, the positive pressure serves to keep the alveoli open and, therefore, more available for gas exchange. To benefit from noninvasive ventilation, the patient must be awake and able to tolerate the device. The patient must not require constant suctioning. CPAP is more widely available in the out-of-hospital setting and has shown benefit in patients with congestive heart failure in the prehospital environment where it has been well studied. Other potential uses are in exacerbations of COPD, pneumonia, asthma, and early respiratory failure. Complications include facial trauma from the mask, aspiration, and barotraumas, such as pneumothorax.

Clinical Insight

It is often very difficult to distinguish between bacterial pneumonia and pulmonary embolism. Clinically, bacterial pneumonia tends to be found in older patients, although many young patients develop acute cases. Symptoms such as pleuritic chest pain and dypsnea are common to both diseases. Fever, tachycardia, tachypnea, and crackles may be found with both. Fortunately, the prehospital management of both conditions is primarily supportive.

pneumonia inflammation of the lungs caused by bacteria, viruses, or chemical irritants.

Pneumonia

Pneumonia is an infection of the lower respiratory tract that can frequently lead to complaints of dyspnea. As emphasized previously, dyspnea may be out of proportion to the level of hypoxia as measured by pulse oximetry in these patients.

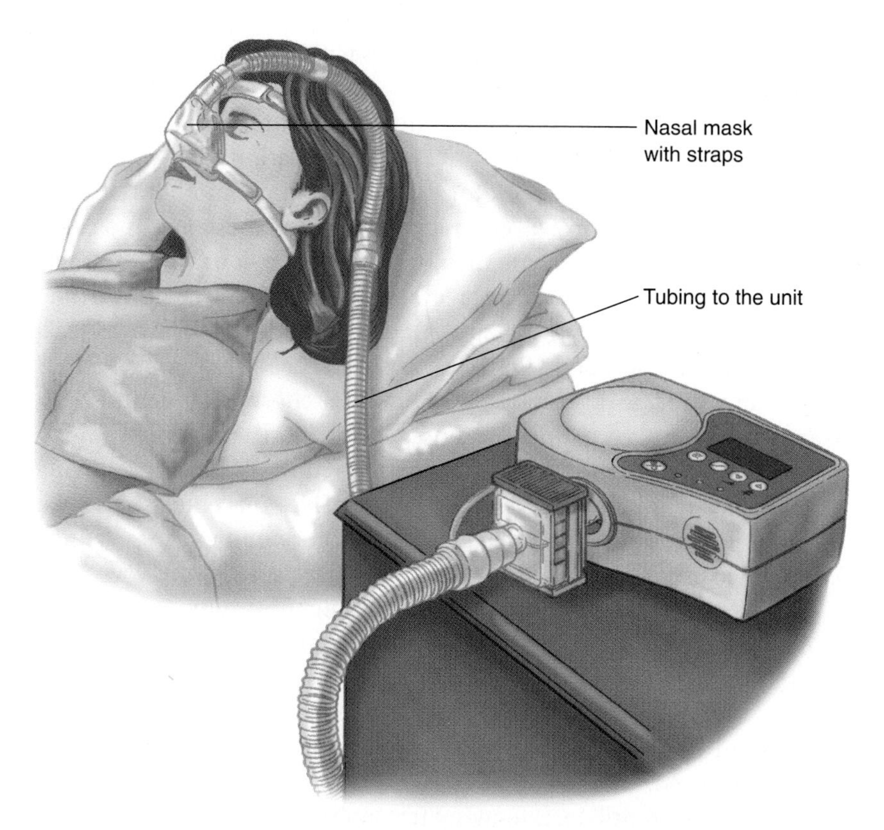

FIGURE 5-5
Noninvasive positive-pressure ventilation devices such as BiPAP and CPAP may be useful in avoiding intubation in patients with acute COPD exacerbations.

Pneumonia is classically divided between bacterial causes and nonbacterial causes (e.g., mycoplasma, chlamydia, viral, tuberculosis). Patients with decreased mental function and CNS disease develop aspiration of anaerobic bacteria and develop pneumonias caused by these organisms. Patients with pneumonia will describe shaking chills, fevers, and pleuritic chest pain, in addition to shortness of breath. Other symptoms such as malaise, body aches, and headache are more common with nonbacterial illness. Physical findings include an elevated temperature, tachycardia, and tachypnea. The lung examination will reveal crackles or rales, rhonchi, and decreased breath sounds in the affected lung areas. Localized wheezing may also be noted.

Prehospital management of pneumonia includes supportive care such as oxygen supplementation, intravenous access, and pulse oximetry monitoring. Intravenous or oral antibiotics are typically administered after a likely organism is identified following X-rays and emergency department evaluation.

pleural effusion accumulation of blood or other fluids, air, or infection (pus) in the pleural space.

Pleural Effusions

Pleural effusions develop when there is an abnormal collection of fluid in the pleural cavity. Dyspnea is caused by compression of the lung tissue by a large collection of fluid. The other major symptom from the pleural effusion is pleuritic chest pain. Other symptoms reflect the underlying disease that caused the pleural effusion. These diseases include congestive heart failure, infection, pulmonary embolism, inflammatory diseases, pancreatitis, cancer, and kidney and liver disease.

Physical examination findings are characterized by a decrease in breath sounds on the affected side, as well as dullness on percussion of the chest on the side of the effusion. Prehospital management is supportive.

pneumothorax abnormal collection of air in the pleural space; **tension pneumothorax** is a pneumothorax in which air enters but cannot escape the pleural space, creating increased pressure, collapse of the affected lung, and compression of mediastinal structures.

Pneumothorax

A *pneumothorax* is an abnormal collection of air in the pleural space. Although this can occur as the result of traumatic injury to the chest, it can also occur spontaneously in young individuals, particularly males with a tall, thin body type. In addition, certain diseases such as asthma, pneumonia, and COPD predispose the patient to the development of a pneumothorax due to thinning of the lung tissue. Finally, any patient who is receiving positive-pressure ventilation (bag-valve-mask ventilation, CPAP, or intubation) is at risk for developing a pneumothorax.

Patients with a pneumothorax will complain of pleuritic chest pain and dyspnea. The onset of pain is usually sudden, often occurring after coughing or straining. In addition, there will be diminished breath sounds, particularly in the lung apices. A bass drum-like quality may be appreciated when the chest is percussed (hyperresonance), but this is more commonly associated with tension pneumothorax. These findings may be difficult to detect in the prehospital environment.

Prehospital treatment of a pneumothorax is primarily supportive, with oxygen supplementation. Definitive therapy for pneumothoraces occupying more than 10 percent of the involved hemithorax involves placement of a tube thoracostomy (chest tube). Carefully observe for the development of a *tension pneumothorax,* which develops when air enters the chest via a one-way valve mechanism. With tension pneumothorax, air in the pleural cavity builds up to such an extent that it collapses the affected lung and compresses mediastinal structures, including the superior and inferior vena cava, causing a significant reduction in venous return to the heart. This results in marked hypotension. Later in the course of this condition, the trachea becomes shifted and the uninvolved lung is compressed. Marked respiratory distress occurs, and the patient becomes more difficult to ventilate. Lifesaving treatment involves decompression of the tension pneumothorax by inserting a large-bore catheter in the second intercostal space along the midclavicular line. This is a temporizing measure until the patient can have a chest tube inserted in the receiving emergency department.

Pulmonary Embolism

pulmonary embolism obstruction of a pulmonary artery or arterial branch, usually by a blood clot carried from a lower extremity.

Pulmonary embolism is caused by an arterial blockage to the pulmonary circulation. Classical teaching has been that the clot arises from pelvic or deep femoral veins. However, any venous clot (including a calf-vein clot) can be the source of an embolus. The disease is more common in patients with recent immobility of the lower extremities (recent surgery, casting, or long-distance travel), those taking estrogen-containing medications (oral birth control pills), or patients with hereditary coagulation disorders. In addition to blood clots, embolisms can be formed from fat, bone marrow, tumor fragments, amniotic fluid, or air bubbles carried in the bloodstream. Pulmonary embolism is the third leading cause of death in the United States and second behind coronary artery disease as a cause of sudden death.

Patients with pulmonary embolism will typically present with symptoms that include dyspnea, pleuritic chest pain, and cough. Tachycardia and tachypnea are commonly seen. Occasionally, syncope, hemoptysis (coughing up blood), and even chest wall tenderness are reported. It should be remembered that symptoms of the disease are both nonspecific and quite variable, and autopsy studies demonstrate that the diagnosis is often missed on initial presentation. Physical findings in the chest are rare and not specific for pulmonary embolism. A loud second heart sound is occasionally reported and findings of deep venous thrombosis (leg swelling, tenderness, and a palpable hardness along the course of the vein) may be noted. Massive pulmonary embolism can produce hypotension from poor venous return to the left ventricle. Prehospital treatment for pulmonary embolism is supportive. In the hospital, anticoagulation, fibrinolytic agents, and surgical removal of the clot are the treatments for this condition.

Other Respiratory Conditions

Several other respiratory conditions can lead to complaints of shortness of breath. *Pleuritis* and *pleurodynia* are inflammatory conditions of the chest wall. Patients may be dyspneic as a result of pain caused by deep inspiration. An occasional friction rub (which sounds like pieces of dried leather being rubbed together) is noted with respiration. *Toxic inhalation* of certain chemicals can lead to dyspnea from irritation of the bronchial passages, thermal injury, bronchospasm, and accumulation of fluid in the alveoli. *Primary pulmonary hypertension* is a rare disorder in which the pressure in the pulmonary artery is elevated. There is no known cause. The disease is most commonly found in young women of child-bearing age, although there is a second peak in the fifth and sixth decade of life. Dyspnea is seen in as the presenting symptom in more than half of the patients with this disorder. The disease is typically fatal. Prehospital therapy is primarily supportive. Patients with the condition may be maintained on a constant infusion of the drug epoprostenal (Flolan), which is a pulmonary vasodilator. This requires infusion through an external pump attached to an indwelling central venous port.

pleuritis/pleurodynia inflammatory condition of the chest wall. Pleuritis is an inflammation of the pleura; pleurodynia is an inflammation of the chest muscle fasciae.

toxic inhalation breathing in of chemical irritants or poisonous substances.

primary pulmonary hypertension elevated pressure in the pulmonary artery with no known cause.

Finally, noncardiac causes of pulmonary edema (e.g., ARDS) can also cause dyspnea because of the accumulation of fluid in the alveolar space as the result of changes in pulmonary fluid balance. *Adult respiratory distress syndrome (ARDS)* is the presence of pulmonary edema in a patient without evidence of volume overload or left ventricular failure. A variety of causes, including sepsis, trauma, aspiration, inhaled gases, drugs, high altitude, hypothermia, obstetric complications, and CNS disease, can lead to noncardiac pulmonary edema. In these disease states, prehospital treatment is supportive with supplemental oxygen, cardiac and pulse oximetry monitoring, and intravenous access. Intubation may be required with 100 percent inspired oxygen and positive end-expiratory pressures added to assure adequate oxygenation. Noninvasive ventilation has been used in mild cases of ARDS.

adult respiratory distress syndrome (ARDS) the presence of pulmonary edema without evidence of volume overload or left ventricular failure.

Cardiac Diseases

Several cardiac disease states may also present with a chief complaint of dyspnea.

Ischemic Heart Disease

Although patients with ischemic heart disease (*angina pectoris* or *acute myocardial infarction*) classically present with a complaint of chest pain, some patients may present with breathlessness as their initial symptom. This is particularly true of patients with underlying diabetes, women, or elderly patients. Associated symptoms, including nausea, sweating, fatigue, dizziness, and weakness, are often present.

angina pectoris chest pain caused by a deficiency in oxygen supply to heart muscle.

acute myocardial infarction (AMI) death of heart muscle resulting from blockage of blood supply and consequent lack of oxygenation.

Seek a careful history concerning current or past episodes of chest pain or discomfort. You may be able to identify a history of other risk factors, including obesity, high blood levels of cholesterol, family history of coronary artery disease, hypertension, smoking, male gender or female in postmenopausal state, or high-strung personality.

Typically, there will be few abnormal physical findings in patients with ischemic heart disease. Crackles, or rales, may be heard in the lung bases if there is any element of left-sided heart failure. Findings such as a soft first-heart-sound, split second-heart-sound, or gallop rhythms are difficult to appreciate in the prehospital setting. In addition to the usual supportive measures (oxygen supplementation, intravenous access), initiate careful cardiac monitoring if you suspect ischemic heart disease.

Abnormal cardiac rhythms should be treated aggressively. Give careful attention to the patient's hemodynamic status. Cardiogenic shock is treated with careful fluid challenges and inotropic agents such as dopamine (5 to 20 μg/kg/min) or dobutamine (10 to 20 μg/kg/min). Prehospital measures for chest pain include supplemental oxygen, as well as nitrates given sublingually (0.4 mg) or by intravenous infusion (10 to 100 μg/min) and aspirin (81 to 325 mg). Morphine sulfate (2 to 5 mg intravenously) is given to relieve pain, reduce preload, and prevent anxiety. Screen patients with suspected myocardial infarction for fibrinolytic administration and establish early contact with the receiving institution.

Congestive Heart Failure

congestive heart failure (CHF) condition caused by impaired pumping ability of the heart, resulting in failure to meet the metabolic demands of the body.

Congestive heart failure (CHF) can also produce a complaint of dyspnea. CHF occurs when the ventricular output is insufficient to meet the metabolic demands of the body. A variety of conditions can lead to CHF, including ischemic heart disease, valvular heart disease, cardiomyopathy, cardiac dysrhythmias, hyperthyroidism, and anemia. Any environmental stress in a patient with these conditions can lead to acute pulmonary edema (acute left heart failure).

Cardiomyopathy is characterized by primary dysfunction of the cardiac muscle. Three types of cardiomyopathy are described: dilated, restrictive, and hypertrophic. Dilated cardiomyopathy, by far the most common, may result from a variety of insults to the myocardium, including coronary artery disease, alcohol, pregnancy, drugs (particularly cocaine), toxins, thyroid disease, and infection. Patients with dilated cardiomyopathy have poor systolic function. Cardiomyopathy is associated with two major complications: CHF and dysrhythmia.

Dyspnea is the result of a variety of factors in CHF, including increased work of ventilation and underlying hypoxia. Symptoms include dyspnea at rest or respiratory difficulty that is worse when lying flat (orthopnea) or at night (PND). The classic finding in patients with acute heart failure is crackles, or rales, in the lung fields, although occasionally wheezing may be more pronounced (cardiac asthma). Patients may also be noted to have ankle edema and an enlarged liver. There may be JVD, which may be made more pronounced by pressing on the liver (hepatojugular reflux [HJR]). A gallop rhythm may be heard on cardiac examination.

Clinical Insight

Many older patients have a medical history of both COPD and CHF. Distinguishing these two conditions in an older dyspneic patient can be quite challenging. Wheezing can be seen in both conditions. In addition, with severe COPD, breath sounds can be distant and thus difficult to interpret. Because of both right heart failure and pulmonary hypertension, hepatomegaly and peripheral edema are common in both conditions. Often, prehospital providers are left treating BOTH conditions by administering supplemental oxygen, betaagonists by inhalation, nitrates to reduce BP and preload, and diuretic agents.

Prehospital therapy for acute heart failure includes immediate administration of supplemental oxygen and establishment of intravenous access as well as heart monitoring and pulse oximetry. Furosemide (Lasix) (40 to 80 mg intravenously) is given because of its diuretic and preload-reducing properties. Nitroglycerin is used via the sublingual (0.4 mg), local (0.4 mg), or intravenous route (10 to 100 μg/min) to reduce both preload and afterload. Morphine sulfate (2 to 5 mg intravenously) is used cautiously to reduce preload and relieve anxiety. Caution is also advised in the use of this drug if the patient is hypotensive or there is danger of respiratory depression. If these therapies are ineffective, inotropic agents such as dopamine (5 to 20 μg/kg/min), dobutamine (10 to 20 μg/kg/min), and epinephrine (0.1 to 5.0 μg/kg/min) are used to increase the effectiveness of cardiac contraction. Morphine sulfate (2 to 5 mg intravenously) is used cautiously to reduce preload and relieve anxiety, although this practice is controversial in CHF.

Many prehospital systems have used CPAP effectively in patients with CHF. Two other agents deserve mention, although neither is commonly used in the out-of-hospital setting. ACE inhibitors are used to counteract some of the pathophysiological changes that occur in the failing heart. Enalapril is the only available intravenous ACE inhibitor. Additionally, niseritide is a recombinant form of human natriuretic peptide that is also used in patients with CHF. The drug's action is primarily in reducing preload and afterload. There is conflicting evidence about the benefits of niseritide in the setting of CHF.

A diagnostic dilemma develops in the patient who has wheezing in the face of acute heart failure. This is particularly difficult in that many elderly patients have elements of both COPD and CHF. Definitive diagnosis is only established after diagnostic studies such as chest radiography are obtained in the hospital setting. It is reasonable to give the patient in CHF who presents with wheezing an inhaled beta agonist (albuterol 2.5 mg, metaprolol 0.2 to 0.3 ml) to treat his bronchospasm until more definitive diagnostic studies, such as brain natriuretic peptide (BNP) levels, are performed. Finally, any contributing cardiac dysrhythmias that lead to impaired cardiac output should be treated according to appropriate ACLS guidelines.

Cardiac Tamponade

A related clinical entity that causes breathlessness is *cardiac tamponade.* This is a life-threatening complication of acute pericarditis in which the pericardial sac becomes filled with fluid, restricting cardiac filling. Major causes of pericarditis include infection (both viral and bacterial), renal failure, cancer, drugs, and connective tissue disease such as lupus. The major symptoms of cardiac tamponade are dyspnea, orthopnea, and PND. The jugular veins may be distended, the liver may be enlarged, and the patient may be hypotensive. A drop in the systolic blood pressure of more than 10 mmHg may be found with inspiration (pulsus paradoxus). This, however, is not a unique finding in pericardial tamponade and is not always present. A pericardial friction rub may be heard and the heart sounds may appear distant, but these findings are very difficult to appreciate in the prehospital setting. Prehospital management is primarily supportive. A pericardiocentesis or surgical "window" may ultimately be performed to relieve the problem.

cardiac tamponade abnormal accumulation of fluid in the pericardium.

Neuromuscular Disorders

Several neuromuscular disorders can create a sensation of dyspnea. The mechanism for breathlessness in these disease states is the inability of the weakened respiratory musculature to produce the ventilatory effort to meet the patient's metabolic demands. This is particularly true if the patient is affected by an upper respiratory infection, pneumonia, other infections, stress, or increased demand due to physical exertion.

Several neuromuscular disease states that present with dyspnea include congenital *muscular dystrophies,* degenerative disorders such as *amyotrophic lateral sclerosis* (*ALS,* or *Lou Gehrig's disease*), *myasthenia gravis,* or immunologic conditions such as *Guillain-Barré syndrome.*

Patients with ALS present with a chronic, steadily progressive wasting of the muscles. The proximal extremity muscles, muscles of swallowing and speech, and respiratory muscles are primarily affected. Mental function and sensory nerves are, however, preserved.

Patients with Guillain-Barré, in contrast, present with a weakness that extends from the distal portion of the body (hands and feet) to the more proximal regions, including the chest muscles. There may be sensory loss and absent or diminished reflexes. Typically, Guillain-Barré syndrome is preceded by a viral infection.

Diseases such as myasthenia gravis affect the juncture where nervous impulses interact with the muscles (motor endplate). These patients have weakness of the proximal musculature and facial muscles that is worsened by repeated use and improved by rest. Visual changes are common. Patients can develop a myasthenic crisis in which there is a pronounced muscular weakness that includes the respiratory muscles.

Prehospital treatment of these neuromuscular conditions is supportive, with careful attention to supporting ventilation and providing supplemental oxygen.

muscular dystrophy wasting disease of the muscles.

amyotrophic lateral sclerosis (ALS) a muscular dystrophy caused by degeneration of motor neurons of the spinal cord. Also called **Lou Gehrig's disease.**

myasthenia gravis disease characterized by muscular weakness and fatigue worsened by repeated use and improved by rest.

Guillain-Barré syndrome a disease of unknown etiology, characterized by pain and weakness beginning in the distal extremities and progressing to involve entire limbs and possibly the trunk.

Patients with CNS depression as the result of drugs, stroke, or head injury may be either hypoxic or hypercarbic but, because of altered mentation, rarely report dyspnea despite these conditions.

Other Causes of Dyspnea

anemia condition that exists when the hemoglobin content of the blood is inadequate to supply the body's oxygen demands.

hyperthyroidism condition resulting from excessive thyroid gland secretion leading to increased metabolic activity.

metabolic acidosis excessive acidity of body fluids that may result from metabolic changes.

Finally, several other conditions can cause dyspnea. *Anemia* can result from a variety of medical conditions (blood loss, iron or vitamin deficiency, malignancy, chronic illness). Patients may be tachycardic, and where significant blood loss has occurred, hypotension is noted. The classic physical finding in the anemic patient is pale skin and mucous membranes. Dyspnea is caused by increased respiratory effort as a response to the reduced availability of hemoglobin (decreased in anemic patients) to carry oxygen to the tissues. Additionally, severe anemia can lead to congestive heart failure, which may further lead to dyspnea.

Hyperthyroid patients may also be dyspneic as the result of the body's increased respiratory drive. The increased respiratory rate results from the increased metabolic demands caused by excessive circulating thyroid hormone. These patients are typically thin with oily skin and hair loss. Nervousness, tremors, and diarrhea are reported. A swollen thyroid gland may be appreciated, and brisk reflexes may be noted.

Clinical Insight

In a patient who demonstrates deep labored breathing but who demonstrates clear lung fields on auscultation, you should immediately think about metabolic causes of dyspnea. A new-onset diabetic with DKA can be diagnosed using this clinical clue.

Patients with *metabolic acidosis* may also be short of breath. This condition can result from various causes, including infection, kidney failure, drugs including aspirin, alcohol, carbon monoxide and cyanide intoxication, and diabetes. Patients will typically present with deep, rapid respirations (Kussmaul's respirations) and have clear breath sounds. Dyspnea is caused by an uncomfortable awareness of the effort of breathing as a response to the accumulated body acids.

Psychogenic hyperventilation is an abnormal ventilatory pattern brought about by psychological causes. Dyspnea may be an accompanying complaint. The diagnosis is established after medical causes of respiratory distress have been eliminated. Because this cannot be done with certainty in the prehospital environment, patients suspected of having this condition should receive general supportive measures, including supplementary oxygen during transport. It is inappropriate to treat these patients by having them rebreathe their exhaled carbon dioxide (i.e., do not have them breathe into a paper bag).

psychogenic hyperventilation increased ventilation caused by mental status such as anxiety. The diagnosis is established only after other possible causes of the hyperventilatory activity have been ruled out.

SUMMARY

All patients with complaints of respiratory distress should be approached in the same systematic manner in order to avoid missing a significant underlying cause of their complaint. The initial focus begins with the scene size-up, which is directed at obtaining a cursory idea of the severity of illness and collecting as many helpful clues as possible to establish the basis for the patient's complaints. A focused initial assessment is conducted, addressing the patient's airway and identifying any signs of impending respiratory failure. Impending respiratory failure is suggested by such findings as mental status changes (lethargy, confusion, agitation), loss of muscle tone, and a diminished respiratory effort. At this point, attention is addressed to establishing a definitive airway and providing ventilatory support.

If airway obstruction and respiratory failure are excluded, general supportive measures should be instituted while a focused history and physical exam are conducted to establish the likely cause of the patient's dyspnea (Table 5-3). These supportive measures should include oxygen supplementation, intravenous access, and cardiac and pulse oximetry monitoring.

TABLE 5-3 Causes of Dyspnea: Typical Findings

Causes of Dyspnea	Typical Findings		
Airway Obstruction	**Scene Size-up**	**History**	**Physical Exam**
Foreign body	Evidence of a meal or snack	Sudden onset while eating; foreign body sensation in throat	Possible visible foreign body
Infection		Gradual onset; pain on swallowing	Fever, difficulty opening mouth
Anaphylaxis	Evidence of a meal, medication, or outdoor environment (insect bite)	Sudden onset after ingesting food or medication or after insect bite	Itchy rash, wheezing, hypotension, nausea, abdominal cramps, inability to urinate
Angioedema		Sudden onset; taking ACE inhibitor medication	Sudden swelling about the face, hands, abdominal organs
Other causes		Blood-thinning medication (e.g., Coumadin), causing hematomas in neck	Evidence of infection, irritants, manipulation leading to laryngospasm
Respiratory Causes	**Scene Size-up**	**History**	**Physical Exam**
Asthma	Asthma medications (inhalants)	Sudden onset; dyspnea with exertion; chest tightness; history of treatment for asthma	Cough, wheezing, eventual prolongation of expirations (more than three times inspirations)
COPD (chronic bronchitis; emphysema)	Home oxygen equipment; inhalants	Gradual onset; dyspnea interferes with normal activities (stair climbing, walking distances); improvement after coughing; history of treatment for COPD	Appearance: Thin with barrel chest. Chronic bronchitis: obese, low blood oxygen ("blue bloaters") Emphysema: normal blood oxygen, tendency to hyperventilate ("pink puffers") Both: wheezing, sputum, productive cough
Pneumonia		Gradual onset; shaking chills, pleuritic chest pain	Fever, tachycardia, tachypnea, crackles, rhonchi, decreased breath sounds in affected lung areas
Pleural effusion		Gradual onset; pleuritic chest pain. Other symptoms associated with underlying cause (e.g., CHF, infection, pulmonary embolism, inflammatory disease, pancreatitis, liver disease)	Decreased breath sounds and dullness of percussion on affected side
Pneumothorax		Sudden onset; pleuritic chest pain	Diminished breath sounds especially in apices of lungs; bass drum-like quality on percussion tension pneumothorax: shifted trachea, hypotension, increasing difficulty in ventilating patient
Pulmonary embolism		Sudden onset; pleuritic chest pain; history of recent surgery or immobility of lower limbs, estrogen-containing medication (birth control pills), hereditary coagulation disorders	Cough; occasional syncope, coughing up blood, chest wall tenderness

TABLE 5-3 Causes of Dyspnea: Typical Findings *(continued)*

Respiratory Causes	Scene Size-up	History	Physical Exam
Pleuritis; pleurodynia		Gradual onset	Occasional friction rub
Cardiac Causes	**Scene Size-up**	**History**	**Physical Exam**
General		Past episodes of chest pain; history of diagnosed cardiac disease or dysfunction; history of obesity, high blood cholesterol; family history of cardiac disease; male or postmenopausal female; high-strung personality	Crackles at lung bases with left-sided heart failure; soft-first-sound; split-second-sound; gallop rhythm; other abnormal rhythm

Underlying causes of respiratory distress include airway obstruction, respiratory diseases, cardiac disease, neuromuscular disease, and other causes such as anemia, metabolic acidosis, hyperthyroid disease, and psychogenic hyperventilation. Specific diseases that should be identified in the prehospital setting include reactive airway disease (e.g., asthma, COPD) in which beta agonist inhaled agents can be administered by emergency care personnel. Airway obstruction as the result of anaphylaxis should be treated with epinephrine and inhaled beta agonists, as well as aggressive fluid resuscitation. Acute pulmonary edema associated with CHF should be treated with diuretic agents, nitrates, and morphine sulfate to reduce both afterload and preload and make the heart function more effectively. Finally, dyspnea from ischemic heart disease should be treated with nitrates and morphine sulfate. All other conditions require supportive care and aggressive attention to the airway and ventilatory status. (Figure 5-6)

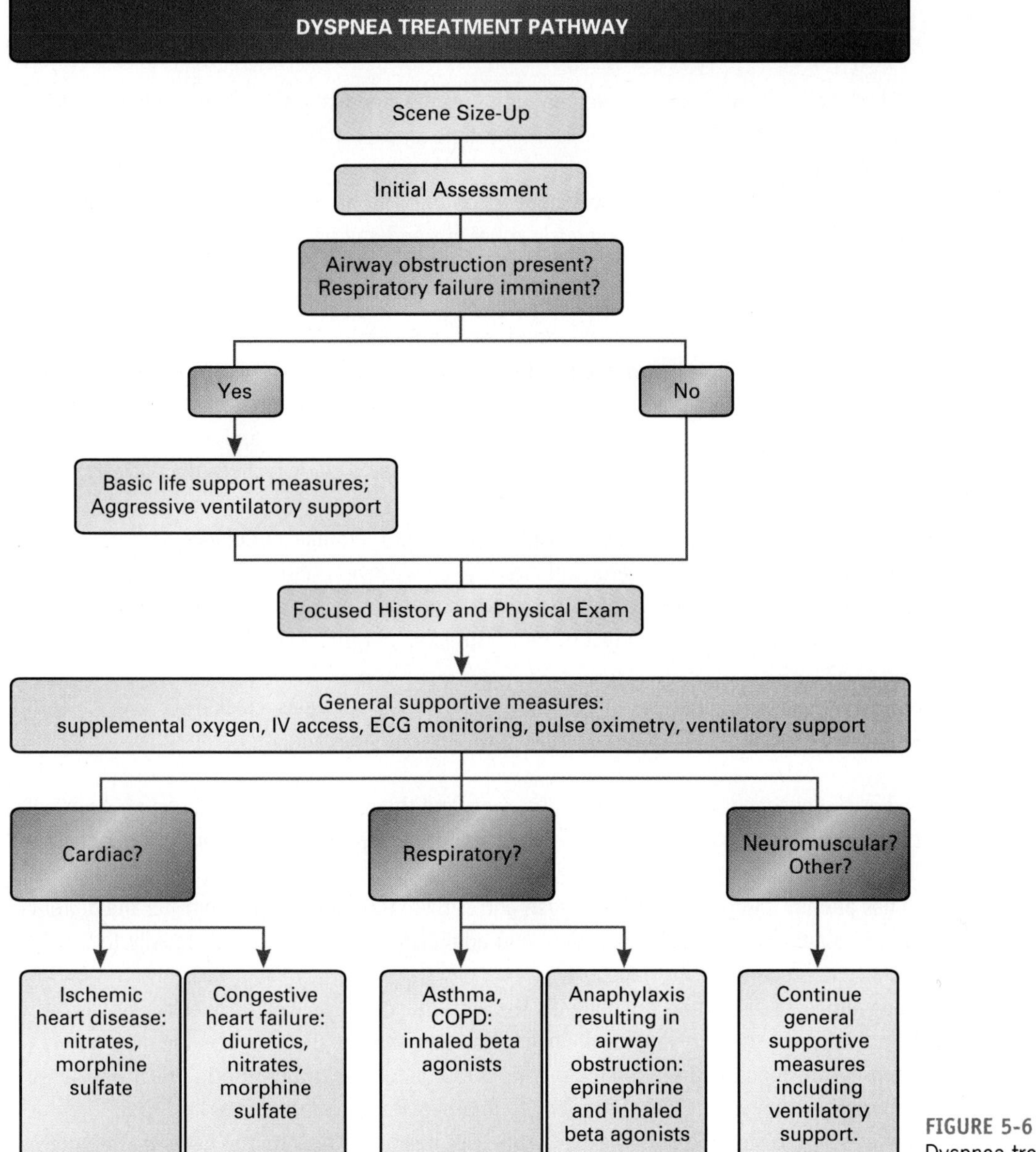

FIGURE 5-6
Dyspnea treatment pathway.

SCENARIO FOLLOW-UP

Your unit has been dispatched to the home of an elderly woman with "respiratory distress." You learn from her husband that she has a history of lung and heart problems. She is a long-time smoker and uses home oxygen at night. She looks very uncomfortable when you arrive.

As you approach, you determine that the patient's airway appears patent. Her breathing is rapid (40 breaths per minute) and labored. Wheezing is audible. You note some cyanosis at her lips and nail beds. She seems confused when you attempt to gather a history from her.

Because the patient's dyspnea, cyanosis, and altered mental status all indicate possible hypoxia, you instruct your coworker to apply 100 percent oxygen by nonrebreather mask. You keep the patient in a position of comfort; as with many dyspnea patients, this patient indicates that she can breathe better sitting up. Other airway supplies remain close at hand. You instruct your partner to obtain vital signs while you confirm wheezing throughout both inspiration and expiration. You administer albuterol 2.5 mg by aerosol, because of its bronchodilating action, and also begin an intravenous line with normal access. You apply a cardiac monitor, which demonstrates a sinus tachycardia with a rate of 120.

You now begin to direct questions to the patient's husband. At the same time, you take a brief look at the patient's medications, which are close at hand. They include albuterol and ipratropium (Atrovent) inhalers, an antibiotic, digoxin, and a diuretic agent (Lasix). The patient's husband relates that she has had to sleep in a chair the last few nights and that "her legs are getting all swole up." During her most recent hospitalization, she was told that she had "water in her lungs."

You perform a brief, focused physical examination, which reveals distended neck veins, crackles or rales in both lungs heard approximately halfway up each lung, and a gallop heart rhythm. As you examine her legs, you note pitting edema in both ankles.

The information provided by the husband, the patient's medications, and the physical exam findings of abnormal lung sounds, a gallop heart rhythm, and pitting edema to the patient's ankles indicate that the patient is probably suffering from CHF, COPD, or both.

By this time, the patient has already improved with the oxygen and aerosol treatment. You administer the diuretic furosemide 80 mg intravenously to help relieve fluid congestion, and administer nitroglycerin sublingually to reduce cardiac preload and afterload as you prepare her for transport.

Your treatments have been aimed at supporting the patient's tissue oxygenation, as well as opening airway passages, relieving fluid congestion, relieving the workload of the heart, and generally helping her breathe more easily.

During transport, you continue to monitor the patient's mental status and respiratory effort, which appear to improve steadily. You are prepared to administer CPAP if she fails to improve. Her respiratory rate falls to 32 breaths per minute, and she no longer appears to struggle during each breath. Her heart rate falls to 104 beats per minute.

On arrival at the hospital, you give your report to the receiving staff, who are very familiar with the patient and thank you for your efforts.

FURTHER READING

1. Conklin, B. "B-type natriuretic peptide: a new measurement to distinguish cardiac from pulmonary causes of acute dyspnea." *J Emerg Nursing,* 2005;31(1): 73–75.
2. Laack, T.A. and D.G. Goyal. "Pulmonary embolism: an unexplained killer," *Emerg Med Clin NA,* 2004; 22(4):961–983.
3. Michelson, E. and S. Hollrah "Evaluation of the patient with shortness of breath: an evidence based approach," *Emerg Med Clin NA,* 1999;17(1):221–237.
4. Manning, H.L., and R.M. Schwartzstein. "Pathophysiology of dyspnea," *NJEM,* 1995; 333(23):1547–1553.
5. Thomas, P. "'I can't breathe': assessment and emergency management of acute dyspnoea," *Austral Fam Physician,* 2005;34(7):523–529.
6. Werman, H.A. "Dyspnea," in P.T. Pons and D. Cason, eds., *Paramedic Field Care: A Complaint-Based Approach.* St. Louis: American College of Emergency Physicians, Mosby–Year Book, 1997.

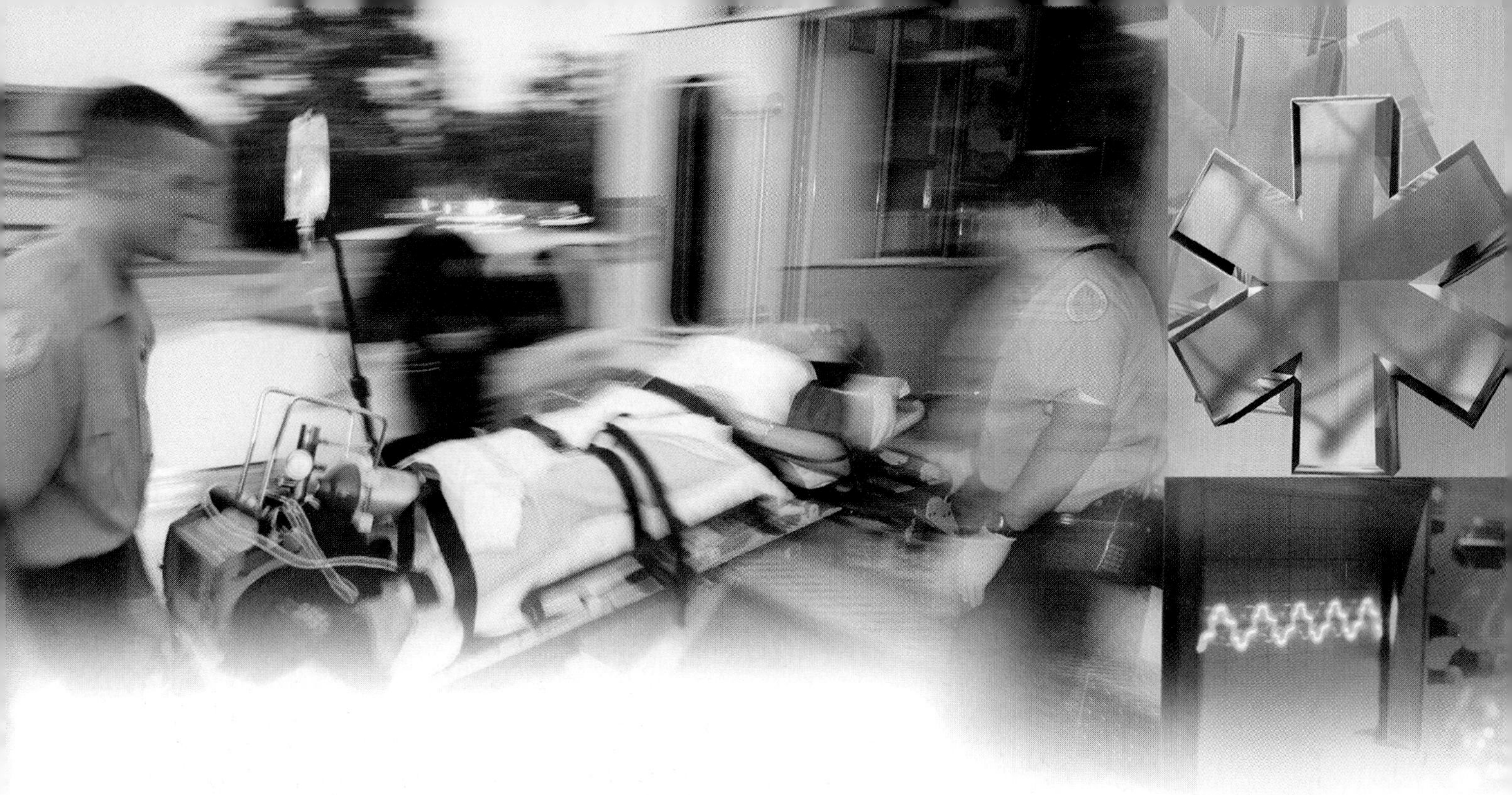

CHEST DISCOMFORT OR PAIN

6

Chest discomfort is one of the most common reasons that patients seek emergency medical care. More than 1.5 million people are admitted to coronary care units each year, and this number represents only a fraction of the patients who seek medical attention for evaluation of chest discomfort, which can be caused by a wide variety of underlying conditions. Patterns of associated findings may help the provider narrow the possibilities to one or more probable causes. However, the key tasks are first to support vital functions and then to focus on identifying a possible myocardial infarction, prompt recognition of which is critical to a successful outcome for the patient.

Topics that are covered in this chapter are

- Anatomy and Physiology
- Initial Approach to Chest Discomfort or Pain
- Differential Diagnosis and Management Priorities

Note: Chest discomfort is a term that includes pain as well as sensations the patient may describe in other ways, including burning, aching, or squeezing. The words *discomfort* and *pain* are both used in this chapter, with *discomfort* being the broader term that includes pain.

SCENARIO

You are dispatched to evaluate a call for a complaint of chest discomfort. On arriving at the dispatched location, you find the 45-year-old patient sitting on a bench outside a crowded office. He is a heavyset African American male whose tie has been loosened by bystanders and who appears slightly sweaty. The patient is able to answer your questions, although he does admit to experiencing some shortness of breath.

You ask him to describe what he is feeling. He tells you that he is experiencing an aching in the middle of his chest that is also noticeable in his back. The sensation (he does not describe it as "pain") began about an hour ago. It is unlike any other discomfort that he has experienced and has become progressively more severe.

How would you proceed in your assessment of this patient? What other questions would you ask? What treatments would you begin?

INTRODUCTION

There are a variety of medical conditions that can present with a complaint of chest discomfort. Although some conditions, such as costochondritis (inflammation of the ribs and cartilage supporting the rib cage) are quite benign, other conditions, including acute myocardial infarction and aortic dissection, are truly life threatening. Determining the cause of chest discomfort in the field can be quite difficult. Remember that up to 5 percent of all patients who turn out to have acute myocardial infarction are initially discharged from the hospital emergency department, even after electrocardiograms, chest radiographs, and laboratory evaluation have been performed. Therefore, you should approach all patients who complain of chest discomfort as if they have a serious medical condition.

somatic pain pain that originates from nerve fibers located in the skin or parietal pleura, typically perceived as sharp and well located.

ANATOMY AND PHYSIOLOGY

Any disease process that affects structures lying within the thoracic cavity (Figure 6-1) can produce chest discomfort. These structures include the heart, pericardium, lungs, pleural cavity, esophagus, aorta, diaphragm, ribs, thoracic spine, chest wall and associated muscles, fascia, and skin. Also, any structure that lies in proximity to the thorax or that is neurologically related to the structures within the thorax can produce chest discomfort. For example, the same nerves that provide sensation to the stomach also provide sensation to the lower portions of the heart. This explains how a gastric ulcer can produce substernal discomfort. Similarly, a herniated cervical disc can present with chest discomfort felt in the upper thorax.

pleura membrane that covers the lungs and walls of the thorax and diaphragm. The visceral and parietal pleura are separated by a serous secretion that reduces friction during respiratory movements of the lungs. Certain injuries or diseases may cause the visceral and parietal pleura to be separated by fluid or air that enters the space between them.

parietal pleura portion of the pleura that covers the inner walls of the thorax.

Stimulation of peripheral pain nerve fibers in the chest results in the perception of pain or discomfort by the brain. Nerve fibers may be stimulated by ischemia, infection, inflammation, or mechanical obstruction of the thoracic organs. For example, the discomfort of myocardial disease is typically caused by local ischemia created by a critical narrowing of the coronary arteries.

Chest pain can be characterized as either somatic pain or visceral pain. *Somatic pain* originates from well-localized nerve fibers located in the skin or *parietal pleura.* Such impulses enter the nerve root at a single spinal cord segment and are precisely mapped in the brain. As a result, the pain is typically well localized and is usually described as sharp in nature. An example of somatic chest pain is the sharp, localized pain noted after a rib injury.

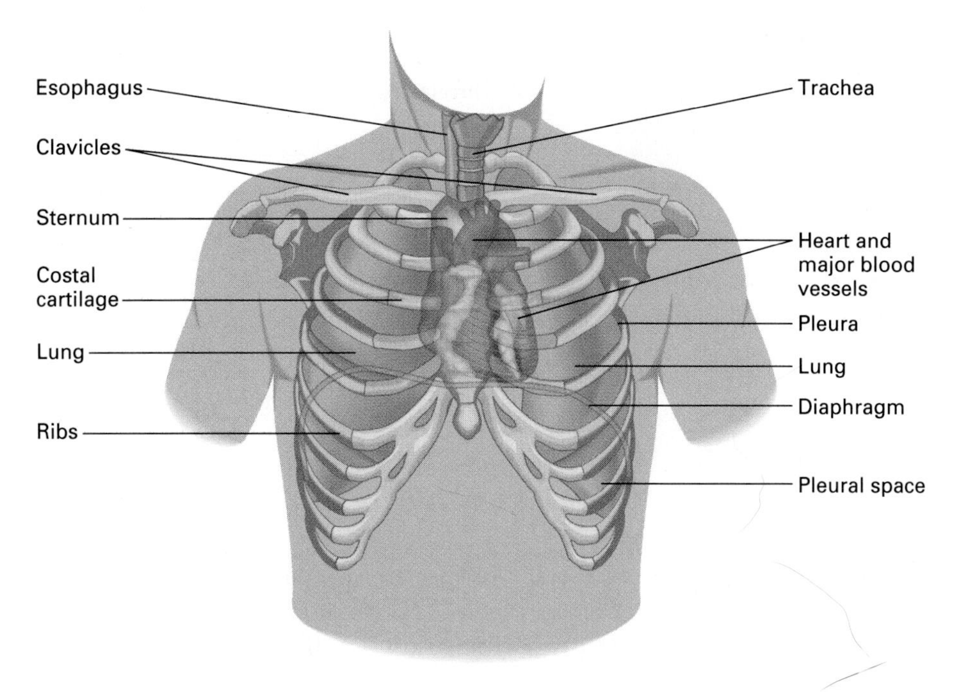

FIGURE 6-1
Structures of the thorax.

Visceral pain can originate from any of the organs in the chest. Pain fibers are located within these organs or along the *visceral pleura.* Impulses from these organs are carried to the brain by what are termed "slow" nerve fibers that cause a general perception of pain but only a vague perception of its location. An inflammatory or infectious response within these organs results in stimulation of several sensory nerves that enter multiple segments of the spinal cord, producing discomfort that is poorly localized and indistinct in character. Often, several organs share similar sensory pathways. This explains why it may be difficult to determine the exact location or organ from which the sensation is arising. Typically, visceral discomfort or pain is described as pressure, heaviness, burning, or aching.

The sensation of visceral discomfort or pain may be misinterpreted by the brain as originating from a specific somatic nerve, resulting in what is called "referred pain." An example of this phenomenon is the perception of shoulder pain that results from irritation of the diaphragm. Similarly, gallbladder pain is often appreciated between the scapulae. The visceral branches that supply the thoracic organs enter the spinal cord in the lower cervical and upper thoracic regions; that is why pain that originates in a thoracic structure is often felt in the neck, jaw, or upper torso.

visceral pain pain that originates from pain fibers in organs or the visceral pleura. The pain is perceived as poorly localized and indistinct in character, often described as pressure, heaviness, burning, or aching.

visceral pleura portion of the pleura that covers the lungs.

Clinical Insight

For patients with suspected AMI, priorities are a focused history and prompt treatment. Measure any intervention that extends prehospital time against the benefit of prompt care (including fibrinolytic therapy or percutaneous coronary intervention) in the hospital setting. Remember that "time is muscle."

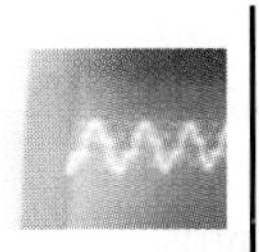

INITIAL APPROACH TO CHEST DISCOMFORT OR PAIN

Immediate Priorities

The initial priority in management of patients with chest discomfort is to determine whether the patient has a life-threatening condition. Specifically, you should focus your attention on the possible presence of an acute myocardial infarction. This is due to the fact that acute myocardial infarction is the most common life-threatening cause of chest discomfort and because the recent focus on early

TABLE 6-1 Causes of Chest Pain

Potentially Life Threatening	Non-Life Threatening
Acute myocardial infarction	Pericarditis
Unstable angina	Costochondritis
Aortic dissection	Pleuritis
Pulmonary embolism	Pneumonia
Esophageal rupture	Simple pneumothorax
Cardiac tamponade	Esophageal spasm
Tension pneumothorax	Esophageal reflux
	Acute cholecystitis
	Mitral valve prolapse

fibrinolytic (clot-busting) drug therapy or mechanical (percutaneous coronary) intervention has made prompt recognition of this condition a priority. However, there are other life-threatening causes of chest discomfort that merit equal attention (Table 6-1).

Another important point to make about the evaluation of chest discomfort is that, although there are "classic" descriptions of discomfort that characterize distinct underlying diseases that cause chest discomfort (e.g., the tearing pain of a dissecting aneurysm), there is significant overlap in the discomfort patterns associated with these conditions. For example, patients with costochondritis classically describe a sharp pain that is reproducible on palpation of the chest. However, a significant number of patients with acute myocardial infarction and pulmonary embolism also present with reproducible chest wall pain.

With these considerations in mind, the patient with chest discomfort should be initially approached to answer the following questions:

1. ***Is there any immediate indication of compromised airway, breathing, or circulation?***
2. ***Does the patient have a potentially life-threatening medical condition (see Table 6-1)?***
3. ***Is there a cardiac cause for the patient's discomfort?***

You should consider all patients with chest pain to have a serious underlying medical condition.

You should consider all patients with chest discomfort to have a serious underlying medical condition.

In the patient with chest discomfort, as with all other medical conditions, an open airway must be ensured. Next, you should assess the patient's ventilations and address any ventilatory compromise (see Chapter 5, Dyspnea, Respiratory Distress, or Respiratory Failure). Then you should assess the patient's circulation. Determine the quality and rate of the radial pulse. Assess the skin vital signs. Finally, determine the patient's mental status. Immediately treat any disturbance of heart rhythm or suspected hypoperfusion (see Chapter 4, Hypoperfusion).

Focused History and Physical Exam

Once you have addressed the ABCs, conduct a more thorough focused history and physical examination to make a preliminary determination of the underlying cause of the patient's complaint.

Focused History

In the vast majority of cases, a thorough SAMPLE history is helpful in developing an early diagnostic impression. Your history should focus on a careful characterization of the patient's chest discomfort. (Remember, however, that the patient's description is not always reliable in localizing the involved organ.) You should also determine the presence of any risk factors that make certain underlying medical conditions more likely.

To determine the character of a patient's discomfort, several important questions must be addressed. The mnemonic OPQRST can be used to assure that all points are carefully assessed. Use the word *pain* if the patient himself complains of pain. Use the word *discomfort* if the patient denies pain or describes other sensations such as aching, burning, or squeezing.

1. Onset
   - *Was the onset abrupt or gradual?* The onset of discomfort of an acute myocardial infarction, pulmonary embolism, and aortic dissection is typically abrupt. In contrast, the onset of discomfort with pericarditis or pneumonia is more gradual. Ask the patient about any factors that were noted immediately before the onset of discomfort. For example, sharp pain noted after heavy lifting or coughing suggests pneumothorax. Ask the patient about any recent history of chest trauma. Also, ask the patient about any drugs (particularly cocaine) used before the discomfort developed.
2. Palliation/Provocation
   - *What relieves the discomfort? What makes the discomfort worse?* Patients with chest discomfort from unstable angina typically continue to obtain relief with nitroglycerin, whereas those with acute myocardial infarction have incomplete or no relief with nitroglycerin. The discomfort or pain of pneumonia, pneumothorax, pulmonary embolism, and pericarditis has a pleuritic (also called respirophasic) component; that is, it tends to get worse with deep inspiration.

     Two additional points should be made. Relief of discomfort with nitroglycerin does not necessarily confirm a cardiac cause of chest discomfort. Patients with esophageal spasm may experience substernal discomfort similar to cardiac discomfort, and it may be relieved with the administration of nitroglycerin. The discomfort of esophageal disease may be indistinguishable from cardiac discomfort and even occurs with a similar age distribution. Thus, one should be very cautious of making a diagnosis of esophageal spasm in the field. Conversely, relief of discomfort with antacids is not exclusively associated with gastrointestinal conditions. Some patients with acute myocardial infarction and unstable angina have described improvement of discomfort after receiving antacids.
3. Quality
   - *Where is the discomfort located? What is the discomfort like? Is the discomfort sharp, tearing, burning, squeezing, aching, or pressure?* Remember that patients who fear they may be having a myocardial infarction tend to be in denial. Some—especially those who are experiencing a more generalized discomfort—will deny that they are having "pain" at all. The pain of aortic dissection is classically described as a tearing pain; however, atypical presentations are also reported.

Clinical Insight

Nitroglycerin has many beneficial effects that make it effective for treatment of a number of disorders that cause chest pain. In acute coronary syndromes, nitroglycerin improves collateral blood flow to ischemic portions of the heart, reduces both preload and afterload, and is a vasodilating drug. This improves oxygen delivery to the heart while reducing oxygen requirements. Nitroglycerin is a smooth muscle relaxant, which explains why patients with esophageal spasm improve following administration. Even patients with a dissecting thoracic aneurysm will improve with nitroglycerin due to its effects on blood pressure, which will reduce intraaortic pressures and thus reduce pain and help prevent further dissection.

4. Radiation
   - *Where does the pain go?* The pain of acute myocardial infarction classically radiates down the arms or into the neck or jaw. Aortic dissection pain typically radiates straight through to the back. The pain of acute cholecystitis (gallbladder infection) may be felt between the scapulae.
5. Severity
   - *On a scale of 1 to 10, how severe is the discomfort?* The patient should be asked to grade the level of discomfort based on a scale of 1 to 10. The patient is told that 10 is the "worst pain he has ever felt" and 1 is minimal discomfort. This allows for continuous evaluation of the patient's discomfort during the entire course of treatment and helps determine the effectiveness of each intervention.
6. Time
   - *How long have you had the discomfort?* With chest discomfort, the questions about onset, listed previously, are likely to be more useful than questions about how long the discomfort has been present. The patient often will not be able to remember exactly when the discomfort began. However, establishing the exact onset of discomfort in a patient with acute myocardial infarction will be an important factor in determining eligibility for fibrinolytic therapy or cardiac catheterization.
7. Associated Symptoms
   - *What other symptoms or problems have you noticed?* Specifically, the patient should be questioned about symptoms such as shortness of breath, nausea, vomiting, sweating, hemoptysis (coughing up blood), syncope, feelings of doom, and rashes.
8. Preexisting Medical Conditions
   - *Do you have any medical conditions that you know about? Have you ever had discomfort like this before?* Finally, question the patient about any preexisting medical conditions that would favor one underlying cause of chest discomfort over others. If you suspect possible acute myocardial infarction or unstable angina, question the patient about underlying risk factors that make coronary artery disease more likely. These include a history of previous angina or myocardial infarction, hypertension, diabetes mellitus, smoking, or elevated cholesterol. A history of coronary artery disease in a close family member (parent or sibling) is another risk factor.

     Patients with a history of prolonged immobilization after surgery or travel, history of deep venous thrombosis (blood clot in the deep veins of the thigh or pelvis) or pulmonary emboli, recent pregnancy, smoking, underlying cancer, clotting disorder, or use of estrogen preparations have an increased risk of pulmonary emboli. Patients with cancer, renal failure, or other inflammatory conditions are at risk of developing pericarditis. A patient with cancer is also at risk of developing a large pericardial effusion (collection of fluid around the heart), leading to cardiac tamponade. You should determine whether the patient has underlying hypertension or *Marfan syndrome;* both conditions are risk factors for aortic dissection.

Marfan syndrome a hereditary disorder of connective tissues producing laxity of joints, aortic dissection, and problems with the optic lens.

Focused Physical Examination

The physical examination offers few specific findings in identifying the cause of the patient's chest complaints. Perhaps the most important finding on examination is the general appearance of the patient. Emergency care personnel should be immediately

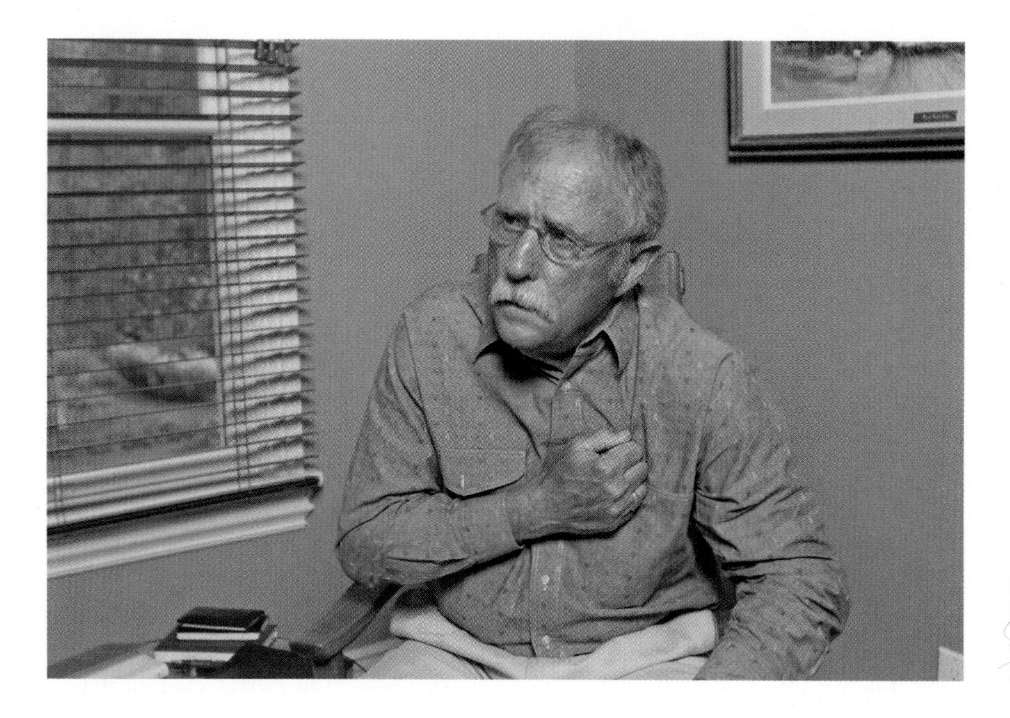

FIGURE 6-2
Levine's sign—fist clenched over sternum—suggests cardiac disease.

concerned about any patient who appears anxious, dyspneic, diaphoretic, and uncomfortable. A patient who is clenching a fist over the sternum (called Levine's sign, Figure 6-2) suggests cardiac disease.

The patient's vital signs should be assessed to determine clues to the possible cause of the complaint. The temperature may be elevated if there is an infectious cause of chest discomfort such as pneumonia or pericarditis. However, patients with pulmonary embolism and acute myocardial infarction can also present with a slight temperature elevation. Hypertension and tachycardia, usually seen in patients who have any significant cause of chest discomfort, are the result of a catecholamine (adrenaline) response to the underlying disease. Tachypnea is also commonly seen. Hypotension should cause immediate concern; it may be seen with pulmonary embolism, aortic dissection, cardiac tamponade, acute myocardial infarction, or esophageal rupture. A narrow pulse pressure and pulsus paradoxus are found in cases of pericardial tamponade. Blood pressure readings should be recorded in both arms if there is a suspicion of aortic dissection. Occasionally, a significant difference (more than 20 mmHg) may be detected in patients with active dissection.

You should perform a careful lung examination. Crackles, or rales, indicate fluid in the alveoli and may be present with pneumonia. Crackles may also be audible in some cases of pulmonary embolism and acute myocardial infarction. Patients with simple pneumothorax or tension pneumothorax present with diminished breath sounds on the involved side. This may be difficult to detect during the field examination, particularly in subtle cases. A pleural *friction rub,* heard during each breath, may be appreciated in cases of pulmonary embolism.

friction rub sound heard when dry surfaces rub together (e.g., when pleural or pericardial tissues are inflamed).

In addition to auscultating the chest, also palpate the chest wall for tenderness. Localized pain may be seen in musculoskeletal causes such as costochondritis or chest wall injury but may also be noted in cases of acute myocardial infarction and pulmonary embolism or pleuritis.

A careful cardiac examination can be useful to determine an underlying cause of chest discomfort, but again, this may be difficult to perform in the field. One of the classic findings in cardiac tamponade is muffled heart sounds (Figure 6-3). Extra systoles, gallop rhythms, or murmurs can be noted in cases of acute myocardial

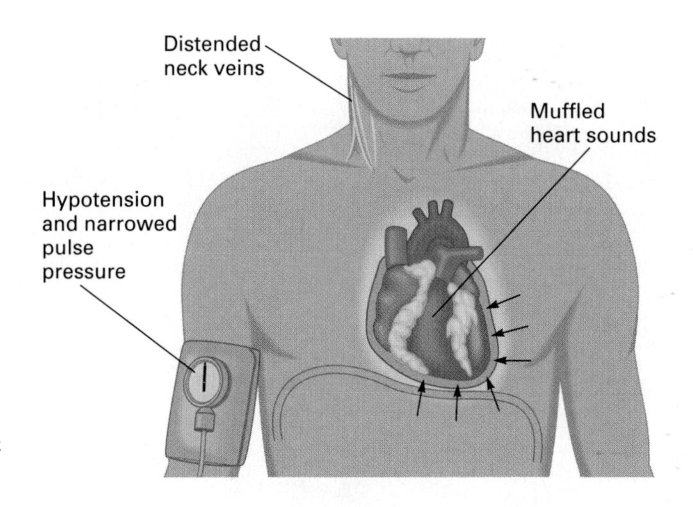

FIGURE 6-3
Signs of cardiac tamponade.

infarction. A murmur may also be heard in cases of aortic dissection if the aortic valve is involved. A difference in pulses in the upper extremities is also associated with this condition. A midsystolic click is classically seen in mitral valve prolapse. A friction rub that varies with the heartbeat is seen with acute pericarditis and occasionally in esophageal rupture.

A careful examination of the abdomen should be included in the assessment of any patient with chest discomfort to rule out an intraabdominal cause of chest discomfort (see Chapter 8, Acute Abdominal Pain).

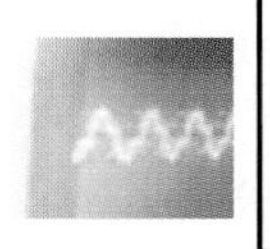

DIFFERENTIAL DIAGNOSIS AND MANAGEMENT PRIORITIES

There has been considerable emphasis on avoiding needless delays in the care of patients with chest discomfort, especially those with acute myocardial infarction. This is because, in these cases, the early use of fibrinolytic (clot-busting) drug therapy or mechanical (percutaneous coronary angioplasty) intervention can significantly improve the patient's chances for survival. Other conditions, particularly aortic dissection, pulmonary embolism, and esophageal rupture, also require early diagnosis and intervention.

Pay particular attention to the possibility of acute myocardial infarction, and treat these patients in a timely manner.

For any patient with nontraumatic chest discomfort, establish intravenous access, administer supplemental oxygen, and provide continuous cardiac monitoring and pulse oximetry, if available. It is important to establish intravenous access because the patient may require drug therapy or a fluid bolus. Hypotension can be present with several of the potentially life-threatening causes of chest discomfort, including pulmonary embolism, aortic dissection (in approximately one in five cases), esophageal rupture, cardiac tamponade, and acute myocardial infarction (particularly with right ventricular infarction). Out-of-hospital management of patients with these conditions includes administration of fluid boluses and possible pressor support.

You should give supplemental oxygen to any patient who complains of chest discomfort. Several of the conditions that cause chest complaints may present with some degree of hypoxia. These include pulmonary embolism, pneumonia, pneumothorax, pleural effusion (fluid in the cavity that surrounds the lung), and acute myocardial infarction. Monitor the patient with continuous pulse oximetry, if this is available; otherwise, observe the patient for clinical evidence of hypoxia such as confusion, agitation, or cyanosis. Give oxygen by nasal cannula or nonrebreather mask to maintain an adequate clinical response. In other conditions, evidence of shock (see Chapter 4) may be present. In these cases, administer 100 percent oxygen via nonrebreather mask to maximize oxygen delivery to the tissues.

Finally, as in all other serious conditions, you should monitor the patient's rhythm continuously. Many underlying causes of chest discomfort can result in heart rhythm disturbances (e.g., acute myocardial infarction, aortic dissection, pulmonary embolism), particularly if there is associated hypoxia.

Acute Myocardial Infarction

Once the measures described previously have been initiated, you must direct your attention to whether the patient's chest complaint is of cardiac origin. This is important for two reasons: 1) therapy can be initiated in the field for cardiac chest discomfort, and 2) rapid identification of acute myocardial infarction may have a significant impact on the patient's survival.

Always suspect an *acute myocardial infarction* (AMI) when you are treating any appropriately aged patient (males older than 30 years, females older than 40 years) who complains of chest discomfort. Any prior history of coronary artery disease should immediately heighten your suspicion, as should the presence of other risk factors for heart disease, including diabetes, hypertension, smoking, obesity, elevated cholesterol, or family history of coronary artery disease. Acute myocardial infarction is the most significant presentation along the spectrum of diseases more broadly called acute coronary syndromes. This broad syndrome includes unstable angina, non-ST segment elevation (non-Q wave) myocardial infarction, and ST segment elevation myocardial infarction (STEMI) (see Appendix B on ECG interpretation).

acute myocardial infarction death of a portion of heart muscle caused by insufficient oxygen supply, usually resulting from blockage of one or more coronary arteries.

Patients with acute myocardial infarction (Figure 6-4) will classically describe midsternal or epigastric discomfort, burning, crushing, pressure, or squeezing. Remember, however, that only half of the patients describe their chest discomfort in these terms. One in four patients who are later proven to have suffered an acute myocardial infarction will report sharp or stabbing pain. The pain may radiate into the arms or left side of the neck or jaw.

Symptoms associated with acute myocardial infarction include sweating, shortness of breath, nausea, or dizziness. In older patients or diabetics, these associated

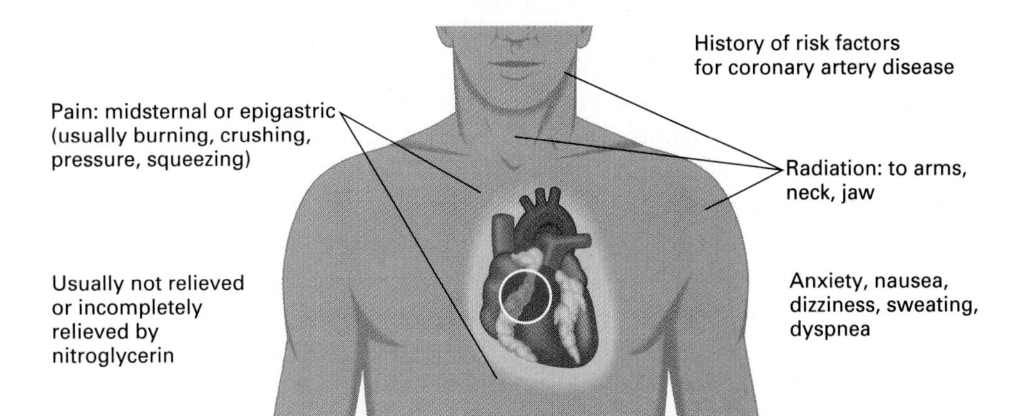

FIGURE 6-4
Signs and symptoms of acute myocardial infarction.

symptoms may be the predominant complaint ("silent heart attack"—a myocardial infarction without classic chest pain). Additionally, women will often present with dyspnea or nausea as their presenting complaint. When chest discomfort does occur in women, it is not typically described as a pressure sensation. As a result, the diagnosis of acute myocardial infarction is more commonly delayed or missed in females when compared to male patients.

A careful history is essential to establish the diagnosis of acute myocardial infarction. Physical findings are very nonspecific. Additionally, in the majority of cases, the initial electrocardiogram may not demonstrate the classic ST segment changes associated with this disorder.

In addition to the general supportive measures outlined previously, out-of-hospital treatment of patients with acute myocardial infarction includes administration of nitroglycerin 0.4 mg sublingually or by spray every 5 minutes for a total of three doses, or less if there is relief of discomfort. Some out-of-hospital systems will initiate an intravenous infusion of nitroglycerin 10 to 100 μg/min if there is no improvement with the previously described methods of nitroglycerin administration. Care should be exercised in the use of nitroglycerin for patients with right ventricular infarction. Such patients may present with hypotension and will require fluid administration to improve ventricular filling prior to the use of nitroglycerin. Additionally, males should be questioned about the use of medications for erectile dysfunction—e.g., sildenafil (Viagra)—because the administration of nitroglycerin in conjunction with these medications can produce profound hypotension.

Clinical Insight

A right ventricular infarction is typically seen in association with acute inferior myocardial infarction. You should consider an RV infarction in any patient with an acute inferior MI who presents with unexplained hypotension. The diagnosis is established by obtaining an ECG with the precordial leads placed across the right side of the chest. Classic ST segment elevations in the right precordial leads are diagnostic. The treatment of hypotension in the face of an RV infarction is to administer fluids. This leads to improved right-sided filling pressure and, thus, better cardiac output. Nitroglycerin can cause a significant drop in blood pressure in these patients.

Aspirin may also be administered; the patient chews and swallows four baby ASA tablets (81 mg). This agent is used to inhibit platelet aggregation, which is an important component of arterial occlusion seen in acute coronary syndromes. Newer agents called GP IIb/IIIa inhibitors are more specific agents that are used to prevent platelet aggregation. The role of beta-blocking agents has also been emphasized in these patients. Administration of both GP IIb/IIIa inhibitors and beta-blockers are delayed until a definitive diagnosis is established.

Morphine sulfate may also be administered in 2 mg intravenous increments every 5 to 10 minutes. Morphine has several advantages when used for patients with suspected myocardial infarction, including reducing pain and anxiety and decreasing preload, which improves myocardial performance. The acronym MONA has been used to remind providers of the important elements of care for acute coronary syndromes: morphine, oxygen, nitroglycerin, and aspirin. Beta-blocking agents such as metaprolol or atenolol administered within the first 12 to 24 hours have been shown to reduce the mortality of acute myocardial infarction.

Where possible, transmission or interpretation of a 12-lead ECG in a patient with suspected myocardial infarction should be considered (see Appendix B on ECG interpretation). This may allow early identification of patients with true myocardial infarction who may benefit from prompt administration of fibrinolytic agents or coronary angioplasty. These two modalities cause chemical (fibrinolytic agents) or mechanical (angioplasty) disruption of the clot that is commonly present in the setting of acute myocardial infarction. In some areas with advanced care providers and transport times in excess of 30 to 60 minutes, fibrinolytic agents have been recommended for use in the out-of-hospital setting. Although older agents such as streptokinase and alteplase [tPA] are still commonly used, two newer agents that can be administered by bolus (retevase, tenectaplase [TNKase]) have made administration of fibrinolytic agents far more reliable. These systems also perform screening histories to determine if contraindications to fibrinolytic therapy exist (Table 6-2).

TABLE 6-2 Contraindications and Cautions for Fibrinolysis Use in ST Elevation Myocardial Infarction*

Absolute Contraindications

- Any prior ICH
- Known structural cerebral vascular lesion (e.g., AVM)
- Known malignant intracranial neoplasm (primary or metastatic)
- Ischemic stroke within 3 months, EXCEPT acute ischemic stroke within 3 hours
- Suspected aortic dissection
- Active bleeding or bleeding diathesis (excluding menses)
- Significant closed head or facial trauma within 3 months

Relative Contraindications

- History of chronic severe, poorly controlled hypertension
- Severe uncontrolled hypertension on presentation (SBP greater than 180 mmHg or DBP greater than 110 mmHg)†
- History of prior ischemic stroke greater than 3 months, dementia, or known intracranial pathology not covered in contraindications
- Traumatic or prolonged (greater than 10 minutes) CPR or major surgery (less than 3 weeks)
- Recent (within 2 to 4 weeks) internal bleeding
- Noncompressible vascular punctures
- For streptokinase/anistreplase: prior exposure (more than 5 days ago) or prior allergic reaction to these agents
- Pregnancy
- Active peptic ulcer
- Current use of anticoagulants: the higher the INR, the higher the risk of bleeding

AVM, arteriovenous malformation; CPR, cardiopulmonary resuscitation; DBP, diastolic blood pressure; ICH, intracranial hemorrhage; SBP, sysolic blood pressure.

*Viewed as advisory for clinical decision making and may not be all inclusive or definitive.

†Could be an absolute contraindication in low-risk patients with ST elevation myocardial infarction.

Source: *Circulation,* 2004;110:588-636.

Unstable Angina

Patients with *angina* typically present with discomfort that is similar in character to the discomfort of other acute coronary syndromes. The discomfort generally lasts between 5 and 15 minutes and is promptly relieved by rest or sublingual nitroglycerin. There are many variances from this classic description, and distinguishing unstable angina from acute myocardial infarction in the field is very difficult.

The patient's anginal pattern is unstable when the symptoms occur with greater frequency, are noted with less exertion, occur at rest, or are new in onset. This is a particularly troubling history that suggests a 10 to 20 percent risk for progression to acute myocardial infarction. The initial management of these patients generally parallels the care described for patients with suspected myocardial infarction. These patients are generally hospitalized and are placed on intravenous nitroglycerin and heparin with evaluation of coronary blood flow.

angina pectoris literally, "pain in the chest," caused by insufficiency of blood and oxygen to meet the increased workload of the heart; **stable angina** is promptly relieved by rest, oxygen, or nitroglycerin; **unstable angina** is a more frequent and severe occurrence of anginal pain that may occur at rest and may be the precursor of acute myocardial infarction.

Aortic Dissection

Aortic dissection is a rare but life-threatening cause of chest pain. It is found in 1 in 1,000 hospital admissions. Patients with this condition have a mortality of 1 to 2 percent per hour in the first 24 to 48 hours of hospitalization and an overall mortality of 90 percent. The disease is most commonly seen in hypertensive males between the ages of 40 and 70 years. The condition may be seen in younger patients who have rare connective tissue diseases such as Marfan syndrome or

aortic dissection a disruption in the integrity of the wall of the aorta that may result in rupture of the vessel.

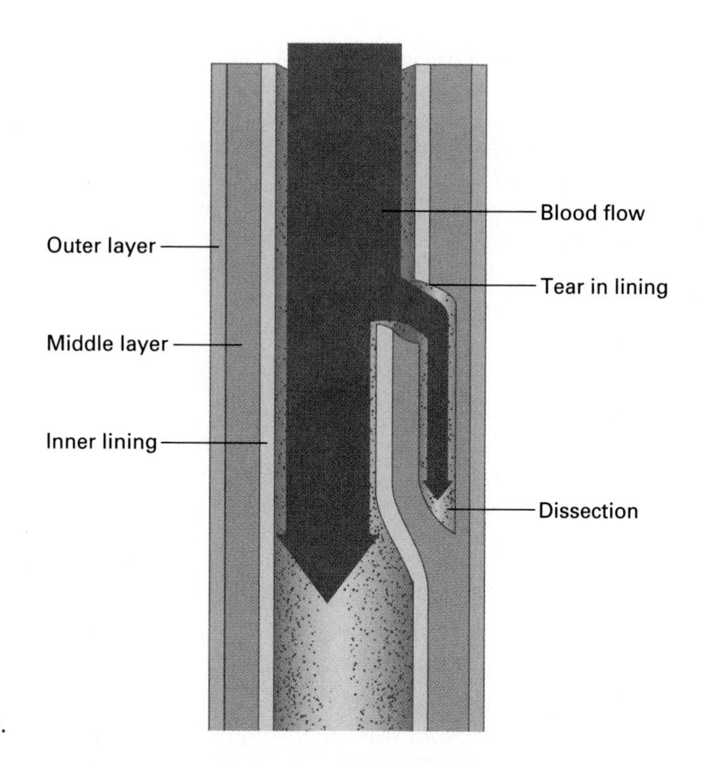

FIGURE 6-5
Aortic dissection.

Ehlers-Danlos syndrome a hereditary disorder of connective tissues producing easily bruised skin, hyperextensible joints, and visceral malformations, among other effects.

Ehlers-Danlos syndrome. The cause of aortic dissection is an underlying tear in the inner lining of the aorta (intimal tear). The pressure of blood flow through the aorta causes a separation of the intimal lining from the muscular layers of the aorta, creating a false pathway in which blood attempts to flow (Figure 6-5).

The pain of aortic dissection is classically described as "tearing" in character with radiation to the back, flank, or arm. Other descriptions of the pain include "cutting" or "ripping." The pain is most intense at onset. Some patients can feel progression of pain down the back as the false channel extends down the aorta.

The symptoms associated with aortic dissection depend on the location of the intimal tear and are directly related to compromise of the major arterial branches of the aorta. If the aortic arch is involved, compromise of the carotid and subclavian arteries may produce stroke-like symptoms or a pulseless upper extremity. If the dissection progresses proximally, the patient can develop occlusion of a coronary artery, hemopericardium (blood in the pericardial sac), cardiac tamponade, or aortic valve insufficiency. Physical findings are associated with compromise of the major branches of the aorta and include neurologic abnormalities (carotid artery) or loss of upper extremity pulses (subclavian). Aortic valve compromise produces a diastolic heart murmur and signs of left-sided heart failure. More proximal dissection may result in cardiac tamponade associated with hypotension, distended neck veins, and muffled heart sounds (Beck's triad, review Figure 6-3). Rarely, the dissection can produce damage to the kidneys and spinal column.

Aortic dissection represents a true medical emergency. Out-of-hospital management of an aortic dissection involves general supportive care. It may be difficult to distinguish this condition from an acute myocardial infarction because both the description of pain and ECG findings are similar for both conditions. In addition, aortic dissection can directly lead to an acute myocardial infarction if the coronary arteries are compromised by the dissection. Fortunately, treatments for acute myocardial infarction, such as nitroglycerin and morphine sulfate, will control blood pressure and anxiety and thus be helpful to the patient with aortic dissection. The goal of therapy for aortic dissection is to maintain a systolic blood pressure

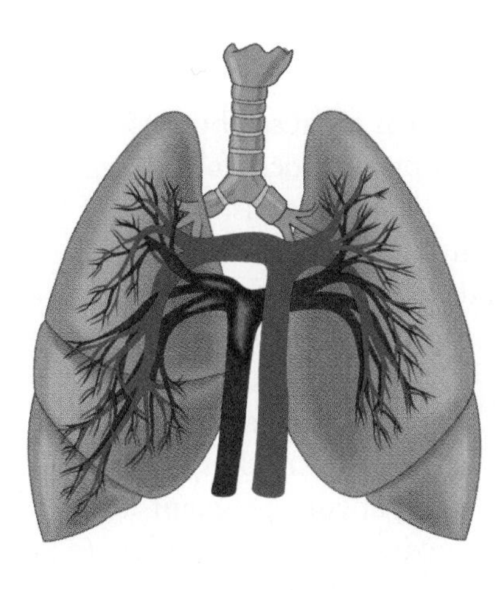

FIGURE 6-6
Pulmonary embolism. A fat deposit is invading and obstructing pulmonary arteries.

between 100 and 120 mmHg while maintaining cerebral, cardiac, and renal perfusion. In-patient management depends on the location of the dissection. If the aortic arch is involved, surgical repair with placement of a graft is used. For dissections involving the descending aorta alone, medical management of hypertension in an intensive care setting is used.

Pulmonary Embolism

Pulmonary embolism (Figure 6-6) is a potentially life-threatening condition that can produce chest pain. The most life-threatening forms of this condition occur when more than half of the pulmonary vasculature is affected by clot. You should suspect the diagnosis after a careful history; however, the diagnosis is confirmed only by using special radiological testing. A dislodged clot that originates from a pelvic or lower extremity vein is the cause of pulmonary embolism in the vast majority of cases; however, a thrombus in any vascular structure can produce a pulmonary embolism. Although embolisms are usually blood clots, an embolism can also be formed from fat, bone marrow, a tumor fragment, amniotic fluid, or an air bubble carried in the bloodstream.

pulmonary embolism obstruction of the pulmonary artery or arterial branches by matter carried in the bloodstream, normally a blood clot that has become dislodged from a vein in the lower extremities and traveled to the pulmonary vasculature.

Several risk factors increase the likelihood of pulmonary embolism, including a history of immobility, pregnancy, recent trauma or surgery, underlying cancer, oral estrogen preparations such as birth control pills, congenital clotting disorders, and smoking. You should remember, however, that one in five patients who present with a pulmonary embolism has no risk factors.

Patients with pulmonary embolism often describe sharp, pleuritic chest pain, which may be associated with dyspnea (see Chapter 5), tachypnea, and tachycardia. The pain of pulmonary embolism is believed to be the result of distention of the pulmonary arteries. Hypoxia is often present. A normal pulse oximetry reading, however, does not exclude a diagnosis of pulmonary embolism. Rarely, patients present with hypotension (see Chapter 4). Physical findings are not prominent and may include crackles or rales, a pleural rub, and a warm, reddened, tender lower extremity. The most suggestive physical finding is a warm, tender venous cord in a lower extremity (deep venous thrombosis); however, a venous cord is often absent.

Out-of-hospital management consists of supportive care, including the measures previously described. Hospital management consists of heparin administration to prevent further clot development, placement of mechanical barriers against the clot, and administration of fibrinolytic agents, or surgical removal of the clot in the most severe cases.

Esophageal Disruption

esophageal disruption rupture of the esophagus, usually caused by a sudden, forceful rise in intraabdominal pressure as from forceful vomiting or coughing.

Esophageal disruption is a life-threatening condition that is caused by perforation of the esophagus. This condition is typically caused by a sudden, forceful rise in intraabdominal or intrathoracic pressure leading to complete disruption of the esophageal lining. Gastrointestinal contents leak into the mediastinum, producing chest pain and overwhelming infection. Fluid tends to accumulate as the result of the acids present in the mediastinum, and this results in fluid loss in the intravascular space.

The pain associated with this condition is a sharp, steady pain that is felt in the anterior chest, back, or epigastric region. Radiation to the neck is common. A history of forceful vomiting (particularly in alcoholic patients, pregnant females, and bulimic patients), coughing, or any recent medical instrumentation (e.g., nasogastric tubes, endoscopy) increases the risk of esophageal rupture. Pain on swallowing or occasional hemoptysis (bloody sputum) are associated with this condition. Physical findings include fever, tachycardia, tachypnea, and hypotension. A pleural friction rub may be heard with auscultation of the chest. This is distinguished from a pericardial friction rub by the fact that it is heard during the phases of respiration.

Out-of-hospital care consists of aggressive fluid resuscitation and electrocardiographic monitoring. Hospital management consists of aggressive fluid resuscitation, intravenous antibiotics, surgical drainage, and careful monitoring in an intensive care unit. This disease carries a high mortality.

Cardiac Tamponade

cardiac tamponade accumulation of excess fluid in the pericardium that may result from injury or from pericarditis or other medical conditions.

Cardiac tamponade is a life-threatening medical condition caused by the accumulation of fluid within the pericardial sac. The accumulated fluid ultimately compromises the heart's ability to fill with blood and thus prevents an adequate cardiac output. When the fluid accumulates as the result of an infectious or inflammatory condition such as pericarditis, chest pain may be an associated symptom. Other entities such as malignant or uremic pericardial effusions are not typically associated with chest pain. Generally, the causes of cardiac tamponade are similar to those conditions that cause pericarditis, and the pain is similar to that associated with acute pericarditis.

In addition to chest pain, cardiac tamponade is recognized by the triad of distended neck veins, hypotension, and muffled heart sounds (Beck's triad, review Figure 6-3). Associated signs and symptoms include dyspnea, tachycardia, and tachypnea. A narrow pulse pressure and pulsus paradoxus are also associated with this condition.

Out-of-hospital management consists of the general supportive measures listed previously. Fluid boluses are often required to maintain cardiac filling pressure. Emergent management includes performing a pericardiocentesis, which involves advancing a large-bore catheter into the pericardial sac and removing some of the surrounding fluid. Prehospital use of this procedure should be guided by your local protocols and approved by the medical direction physician.

To perform an emergent pericardiocentesis, attach a long 16- or 18-gauge catheter to a syringe. Cleanse the area around the patient's left xyphoid process with an antiseptic solution and, where possible, anesthetize the area. Introduce the catheter into the left subxyphoid region and direct it toward the inferior portion of the left scapula. Maintain negative pressure on the syringe until either fluid is withdrawn or you see signs of cardiac irritation (ST segment changes are seen on the monitor or ventricular ectopy is noted). You should withdraw enough fluid to produce clinical improvement. In some cases, the catheter is advanced over the needle and left in place with a three-way stopcock allowing for further withdrawal of fluid as needed.

In patients with medical causes of cardiac tamponade, the fluid may vary from thin, straw-colored fluid to thick, cloudy fluid. Signs of cardiac irritation suggest that the catheter is directly striking the outer layer of the heart.

Pericardiocentesis serves two purposes: 1) Removal of even a small amount (30 to 50 ml) of fluid will result in a dramatic improvement in cardiac output, and 2) the fluid can be analyzed to determine the underlying cause of the condition. Definitive management may involve placing a small "window" into the pericardium to drain the fluid or complete surgical removal of the pericardial sac.

simple pneumothorax abnormal collection of air in potential space between the parietal pleura and the visceral pleura; **tension pneumothorax** is a pneumothorax in which air enters but cannot escape the pleural space, creating increased pressure, collapse of the affected lung, and compression of mediastinal structures.

Simple Pneumothorax/Tension Pneumothorax

A *simple pneumothorax* occurs when air enters the potential space between the parietal pleura and the visceral pleura that contains the serous fluid that lubricates the lungs. A *tension pneumothorax* occurs when a simple pneumothorax develops a one-way valve mechanism. In this setting, air is allowed to enter the chest during inspiration but not able to leave during expiration. A pneumothorax usually develops in a patient who has a congenital or acquired weakening of the lung tissue. These conditions are also seen in patients with chronic obstructive lung disease, lung cancer, or lung infections.

The pain of a simple pneumothorax develops suddenly and is usually sharp and pleuritic in nature. Patients will breathe fast and shallowly because deep inspiration is more painful. The development of a tension pneumothorax is heralded by the findings of neck vein distention, severe respiratory distress, tracheal deviation (a late sign), markedly diminished breath sounds and, in extreme cases, hypotension (Figure 6-7).

A tension pneumothorax is not commonly seen in a spontaneously breathing patient. It is far more common when a patient is given positive-pressure ventilations by bag-valve-mask device, noninvasive techniques such as CPAP or BiPAP,

Clinical Insight

The earliest and most sensitive finding in a patient with a developing tension pneumothorax who is receiving positive-pressure ventilation is increasing difficulty in bagging the patient or persistent high-pressure alarms on a mechanical ventilator. Tracheal deviation and asymmetry of breath sounds may be difficult to determine early on in the course of a developing tension pneumothorax. Hypotension and cyanosis are late findings. You should first assure that the tracheal tube or airway has not become occluded when ventilation is difficult. Needle decompression should then be performed if allowed by local protocol.

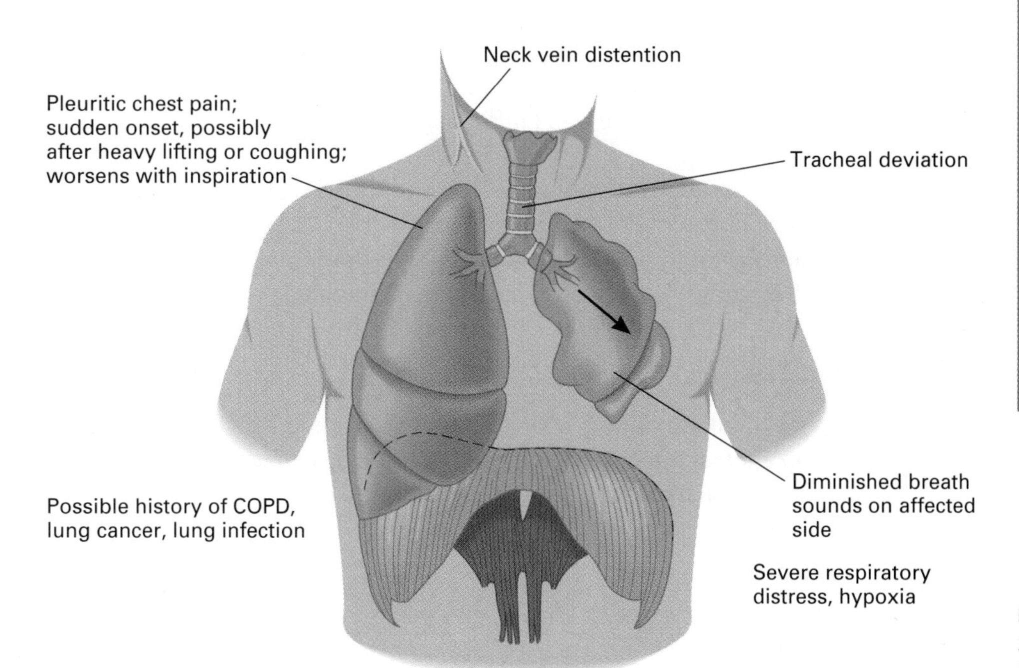

FIGURE 6-7
Signs and symptoms of tension pneumothorax.

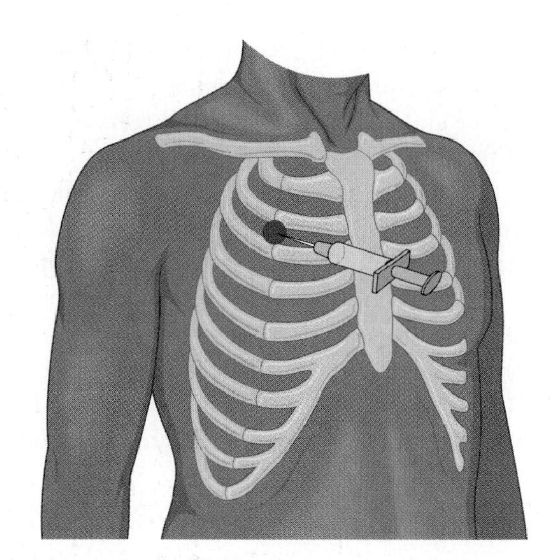

FIGURE 6-8
Needle decompression of a pneumothorax. Place a large-bore needle above the third rib in the midclavicular line.

or through a tracheal tube, particularly when the patient has any of the predisposing conditions listed previously. Once this condition is identified, you should immediately decompress the involved lung using a large-bore (14- or 16-gauge) needle placed above the third rib in the midclavicular line (Figure 6-8). Prehospital use of this procedure should be guided by your local protocols and approved by the medical direction physician.

Pericarditis

pericarditis inflammation of the pericardium, the sac that surrounds the heart.

Pericarditis is an inflammatory condition that produces a steady, burning retrosternal pain that may radiate to the back, neck, scapula, or jaw. The pain can be worsened by deep respiration and may occasionally be noted with each phase of the cardiac cycle. It is worse in a lying position and is improved by sitting up or leaning forward.

The pain is typically of longer duration than myocardial pain. The pain associated with pericarditis is produced by irritation of the pericardial sac; extension to the parietal pleura results in the pleuritic nature of the pain. An intermittent rub that varies with the cardiac cycle may be heard, but this may be difficult to appreciate in the out-of-hospital environment. The ECG monitor may demonstrate ST segment elevation or depression similar to findings seen with acute myocardial infarction (Figure 6-9).

The out-of-hospital treatment of this condition is supportive; definitive treatment includes nonsteroidal antiinflammatory drugs such as ibuprofen. This diagnosis is established only after acute coronary syndromes that also present with chest pain and ST changes on the ECG have been eliminated.

Costochondritis

costochondritis inflammation of the ribs and/or cartilagenous structures of the ribs.

Costochondritis is an inflammation of the ribs and cartilage supporting the rib cage that may develop after an upper respiratory infection. The pain associated with this condition is typically sharp in character and is made worse by movement of the

FIGURE 6-9
ECG findings with pericarditis and AMI may be similar: (a) ST segment elevation or (b) ST segment depression.

(a)
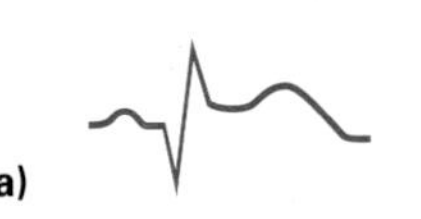

(b)
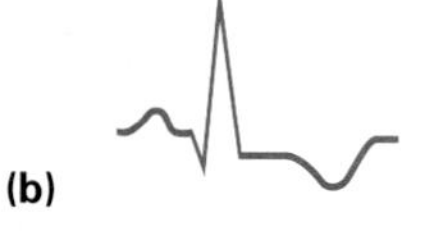

chest wall. Activities such as deep breathing or lifting the arms will also make the pain more intense. Physical examination will reveal pain on direct palpation of the chest wall. You must remember that a small percent of patients with pulmonary embolism and acute myocardial infarction may also have chest wall tenderness. Therefore, the diagnosis of costochondritis is made after excluding other significant causes of chest pain. Definitive treatment includes the use of heat or cool compresses and nonsteroidal antiinflammatory drugs.

Pleurodynia

Pleurodynia is an inflammatory condition of the parietal pleura. Patients with this condition complain of sharp, pleuritic pain. There are few associated symptoms. Physical examination rarely reveals any positive findings, although a pleural rub may be heard. As with costochondritis, treatment includes heat or cool compresses and nonsteroidal antiinflammatory drugs.

pleurodynia inflammation of the parietal pleura.

Gastrointestinal Diseases

Gastrointestinal disorders such as peptic ulcer disease, acute cholecystitis, esophagitis, esophageal spasm, and gastroesophageal reflux can also produce chest discomfort. This is because of the sensory nerve fibers shared between abdominal structures and organs in the thorax. The discomfort associated with gastrointestinal disease is often described as a retrosternal burning that is similar in character to the discomfort associated with acute myocardial infarction. Pain may radiate into the throat, and there is often an associated acid taste described as "heartburn." The discomfort may be worse at night, particularly when lying down or leaning far forward. On physical examination, you may find discomfort on palpating the epigastric region or the upper quadrants of the abdomen. This is a very nonspecific finding and may be found with other more significant problems.

Gastrointestinal disorders can also produce chest pain. This is because of the sensory nerve fibers shared between abdominal structures and organs in the thorax.

Esophageal spasm is a particular dilemma because the discomfort is indistinguishable in nature and character from cardiac discomfort and will improve with the administration of nitroglycerin. It should also be remembered that some patients with acute myocardial infarction may report improvement of symptoms after administration of antacids. This suggests that the use of nitroglycerin and antacids is not reliable in distinguishing among the various causes of chest discomfort.

Because of the significant overlap between the symptoms of acute myocardial infarction and some cases of gastrointestinal disease, you should initiate general supportive measures. Consider the possibility that a life-threatening condition may be the cause of the patient's complaints and treat accordingly.

For more about gastrointestinal disorders, see Chapter 8, Acute Abdominal Pain, and Chapter 9, Gastrointestinal Bleeding.

Mitral Valve Prolapse

Mitral valve prolapse can occasionally produce episodes of chest pain. In this condition, the elastic mitral valve expands into the left atrium during systole. Chest pain is believed to be due to stretching of the muscular and tendonous attachments (chordae tendinae and papillary muscles) on the valves. These patients may also complain of dizziness, dyspnea, palpitations, and syncope. Physical findings that

mitral valve prolapse expansion of the mitral valve into the left atrium during systole.

suggest the diagnosis include a systolic murmur or a midsystolic "click." Cardiac dysrhythmias may also be found in this condition. The vast majority of patients with mitral valve prolapse are asymptomatic.

Out-of-hospital treatment includes the supportive measures described previously until more significant causes of chest pain can be eliminated.

SUMMARY

Chest discomfort is a common presenting complaint for a variety of medical illnesses. In addition to disease processes affecting structures that lie within the thorax, any disease process that affects structures in close proximity or with a neurologic relationship to the thorax can result in a complaint of chest discomfort. Although there are characteristic patterns associated with certain diseases, there is enough variation to suggest that the quality of chest discomfort is not specific enough to identify the medical cause of chest discomfort with any certainty. Physical findings are rarely helpful in distinguishing the different causes of chest discomfort (Table 6-3). Keep in mind that acute myocardial infarction may present with a patient complaint of chest discomfort rather than pain (the patient may deny chest pain) or may simply present with symptoms such as sweating, dyspnea, dizziness, or nausea—particularly in women, in diabetics, or in elderly patients.

In approaching a patient complaining of chest discomfort (Figure 6-10), you should first address the patient's airway, breathing, and circulatory status. Once this has been addressed, you should establish general supportive measures, including intravenous access, oxygen supplementation, and electrocardiographic monitoring. You should then focus on the possibility of an acute myocardial infarction. This is important to identify because out-of-hospital treatment can be of benefit to the patient and because prompt identification can improve the patient's ultimate outcome. Specific out-of-hospital treatments may include oxygen, nitrates, aspirin, and morphine sulfate. Transmission or early interpretation of a 12-lead ECG can be helpful in readying hospital personnel to begin early fibrinolytic therapy.

TABLE 6-3 Causes of Chest Pain: Typical Findings

Causes of Chest Pain	History	Physical Exam
Acute myocardial infarction	Sudden onset; pain typically midsternal or epigastric with radiation to arms, neck, or jaw; typically described as discomfort, burning, crushing, pressure, or squeezing, sometimes sharp or stabbing (or pain may be denied); usually *not* relieved by nitroglycerin; anxiety, nausea, dizziness; history of or risk factors for coronary artery disease (including diabetes, hypertension, smoking, obesity, elevated cholesterol, or family history)	Sweating; dyspnea; possible hypotension, hypoxia, slight fever, crackles, localized chest wall tenderness, extra systoles, gallop rhythms, or new murmurs; initial ECG may not show ST segment changes typical of AMI
Unstable angina	Pain similar to AMI; generally 5–15 min duration; usually relieved by rest or nitroglycerin; presence of risk factors for coronary artery disease; pattern is "unstable" when symptoms occur more frequently, with less exertion or at rest, or are new in onset (10%–20% risk of AMI with unstable angina symptoms)	Difficult to distinguish from AMI in the out-of-hospital setting

TABLE 6-3 Causes of Chest Pain: Typical Findings *(continued)*

Causes of Chest Pain	History	Physical Exam
Aortic dissection	Sudden onset; pain typically described as "tearing," "cutting," or "ripping," most intense at onset; sometimes felt progressing downward; typically radiates straight to the back, flank, or arm; underlying hypertension	Possible hypotension, diastolic heart murmur; difference in upper extremity pulses, heart rhythm disturbance. Difficult to distinguish from AMI in the out-of-hospital setting
Pulmonary embolism	Sudden onset; pleuritic pain; usually worsens with deep inspiration; history of immobility, deep venous thrombosis, recent pregnancy, smoking, underlying cancer, use of estrogen preparations (but often occurs without risk factors)	Friction rub; often with cough, dyspnea, tachypnea, tachycardia, hypoxia, possible fever, crackles, chest wall tenderness, coughing up blood, syncope, heart rhythm disturbance. Rarely with hypotension. Suggestive findings: warm, reddened, tender venous cord in lower extremity
Esophageal disruption	Sudden onset; sharp, steady pain in anterior chest, back, or epigastric area, commonly radiates to neck; possible pain on swallowing; history of forceful vomiting or coughing or recent nasogastric tube, endoscopy, or other medical instrumentation	Possible fever, tachycardia, tachypnea, hypotension, friction rub, bloody sputum
Cardiac tamponade	Chest pain may or may not be present; possible pain if inflammatory cause such as pericarditis; other causes may not produce pain	Beck's triad: distended neck veins, hypotension, muffled heart sounds. Associated findings: dyspnea, tachycardia, tachypnea, narrow pulse pressure, and pulsus paradoxus
Simple pneumothorax/tension pneumothorax	Sudden onset, possibly after heavy lifting or coughing; pleuritic pain, usually worsens with deep inspiration, cancer, or lung infections	Diminished breath sounds on one side; tension pneumothorax characterized by severe respiratory distress, neck vein distension, tracheal deviation, hypoxia, and hypotension in extreme cases
Pericarditis	Gradual onset; steady, burning, retrosternal pain, may radiate to back, neck, scapula, or jaw; usually worsens with deep inspiration; sometimes noted with each phase of cardiac cycle; worse when lying down, improved by sitting up or leaning forward; typically longer duration than myocardial pain; history of cancer, renal failure, or other inflammatory conditions	Friction rub that varies with the heartbeat; possible temperature elevation; ECG may demonstrate ST segment changes similar to AMI
Costochondritis	Gradual onset; sharp pain, typically worsened by chest wall movement as with deep breathing or lifting the arms	Localized chest wall tenderness; possible fever
Pleurodynia	Gradual onset; pleuritic pain; few associated symptoms	Possible pleural rub
Pneumonia	Gradual onset; pleuritic pain, usually worsens with deep inspiration; chills	Fever, tachycardia, tachypnea, crackles, rhonchi, decreased breath sounds in affected lung areas; hypoxia
Gastrointestinal diseases	Pain and other symptoms often similar to AMI	May be difficult to distinguish from life-threatening cardiac condition in out-of-hospital setting
Mitral valve prolapse	Episodes of chest pain; possible dizziness, palpitations, syncope	Midsystolic click; possible heart rhythm disturbance; possible dyspnea

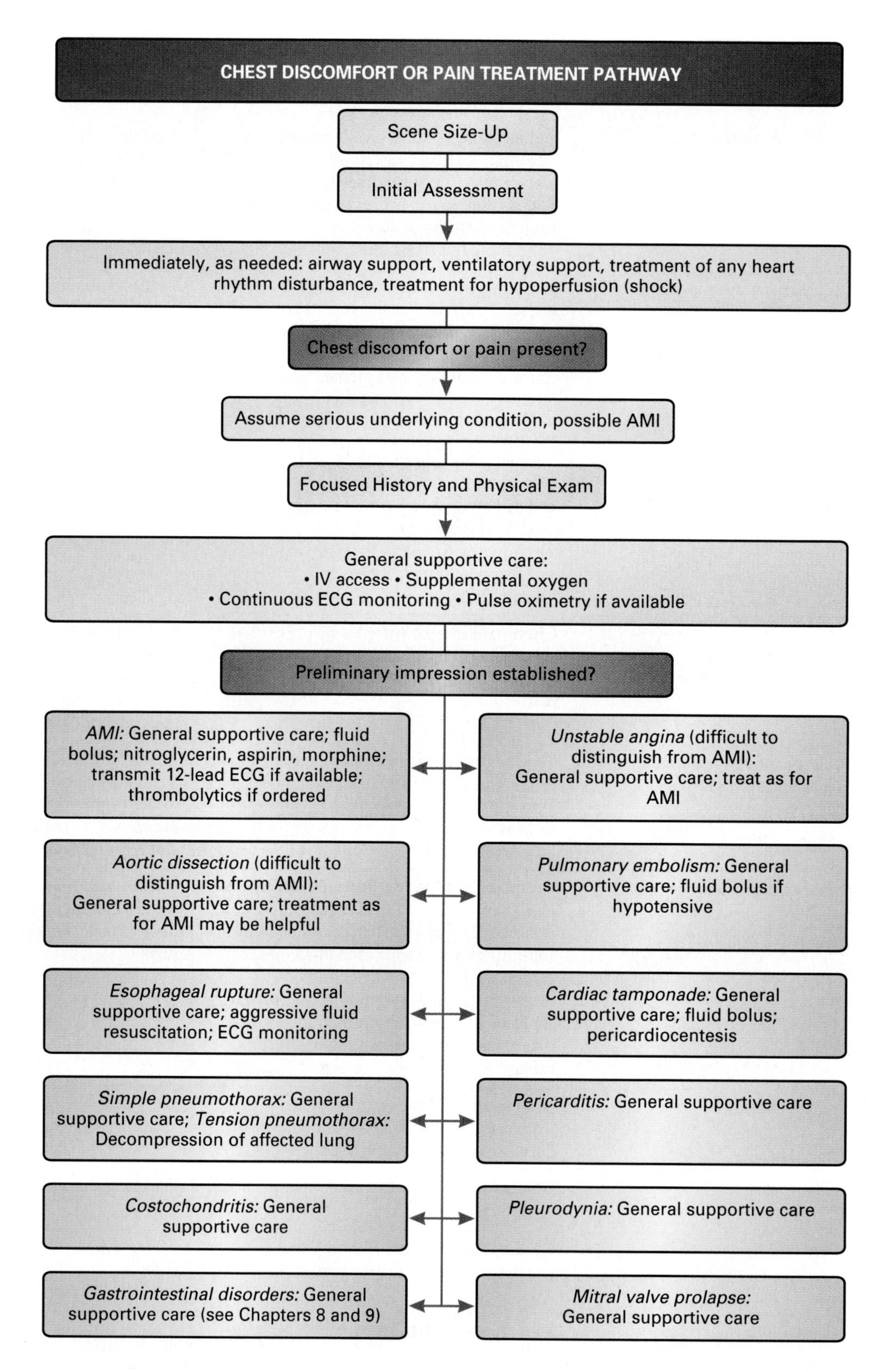

FIGURE 6-10
Chest discomfort or pain treatment pathway.

SCENARIO FOLLOW-UP

In responding to a call for a complaint of chest discomfort, you find a 45-year-old heavyset African American male sitting on a bench outside an office. His tie has been loosened by bystanders, and he appears slightly sweaty. He admits to some shortness of breath but is able to answer your questions.

The patient describes an "aching" in the middle of his chest that is also noticeable in his back. (He does not use the word "pain.") The sensation began about an hour ago and has gotten progressively more severe. It is unlike any other discomfort that he has ever experienced.

Because the patient is able to provide a brief history, you are able to note that he is maintaining a patent airway. You also note that he has an easy respiratory pattern without an increase in the depth or rate of breathing. His radial pulse is bounding at a rate of approximately 60 beats per minute.

On further questioning, you learn that the patient works in a high-pressure job and smokes approximately 10 cigarettes daily, mostly while at work. His past medical history is notable only for hypertension, for which he is taking Procardia 60 mg XL once daily, and a remote history of an ulcer. He has been on this medication for approximately 15 years. He is particularly worried about the aching in his chest because his father died of a "heart attack" in his early fifties.

A brief physical examination reveals few abnormal findings. The patient's lung sounds are clear. He has a regular cardiac rhythm with a bounding apical impulse. His distal radial pulses are symmetric, and he has no pedal edema. Your partner records his vital signs as heart rate 60, respirations 18, and blood pressure 170/100 in both arms.

As you would for any patient with a complaint of chest discomfort, you instruct your partner to place the patient on supplemental oxygen by nasal cannula at 4 lpm and a cardiac monitor while you establish an intravenous line with 0.9 normal saline. You ask the patient to rate his chest discomfort on a scale of 1 to 10; he reports his discomfort at a level of "7."

You tell the patient that because of his age, history of high blood pressure, and family history, you are concerned about an acute myocardial infarction. You explain your concerns and inquire about the use of Viagra or related medications. Because AMI is suspected, your partner places a sublingual nitroglycerin 0.4 mg tablet under the patient's tongue and also gives him four baby aspirins to chew and swallow. You warn the patient that he may experience a slight headache, a common side effect of nitroglycerin, but that he must tell you about any changes in his chest complaint. You and your partner also obtain a 12-lead electrocardiogram, which is transmitted telemetrically to the receiving hospital.

You move the patient into the vehicle for transport to the local emergency department. You begin to review your prehospital chest discomfort checklist. En route, your medical control advises you to give two additional sublingual nitroglycerin 0.4-mg tablets and monitor the patient's blood pressure, cardiac rhythm, and pulse oximetry. The patient's vital signs remain unchanged during transport, although his discomfort declines to a level of "3" by the time you arrive.

The emergency department staff confirms that the patient has evidence of an acute inferior myocardial infarction on your transmitted electrocardiogram. Because the patient has had some recent surgery and also reports a history suggestive of ulcer disease, a decision is made to take the patient directly to the cardiac catheterization lab. The patient undergoes successful angioplasty and stenting of a completely occluded right coronary artery and has an uneventful recovery.

Several months later, you see the patient jogging by the fire station. He reports that he is exercising daily, has lost 40 lb, and quit smoking.

FURTHER READING

1. Antman, E.M., D.T. Anbe, P.W. Armstrong, E.R. Bates et al. ACC/AHA guidelines for the management of patients with ST-elevation myocardial infarction—executive summary. A report of the American College of Cardiology/American Heart Association Task Force on Practice Guidelines (Writing Committee to revise the 1999 guidelines for the management of patients with acute myocardial infarction). *J Am Coll Cardiol,* 2004;44(3): 671–719.
2. Bhatt, D.L., M.T. Roe, E.D. Peterson, Y. Li, et al. Utilization of early invasive management strategies for high-risk patients with non-ST-segment elevation acute coronary syndromes: results from the CRUSADE Quality Improvement Initiative. *JAMA,* 2004; 292(17): 2096–2104.
3. Green, G.B., and P.M. Hill. "Approach to chest pain," in J.E. Tintinalli, J.S. Stapczynski, and G.D. Kelen, eds., *Emergency Medicine: A Comprehensive Study*

Guide. 6th ed. New York: McGraw-Hill, 2004, pp. 333–343.

4. GOLDHAUBER, S.Z., and C.G. ELLIOT. "Acute pulmonary embolism: part I: epidemiology, pathophysiology, and diagnosis," *Circulation,* 2003;108(22): 2726–2729.
5. GORGAS, D.L. "Prehospital diagnosis and treatment of acute coronary syndromes and the management of prehospital chest pain," in J.W. Hoekstra, ed., *Handbook of Cardiovascular Emergencies.* Boston: Little, Brown and Company, 2001, pp. 151–158.
6. HOLLANDER, J.E. "Acute coronary syndromes," in J.E. Tintinalli, J.S. Stapczynski, and G.D. Kelen, eds., *Emergency Medicine: A Comprehensive Study Guide.* 6th ed. New York: McGraw-Hill, 2004, pp. 343–352.
7. BROWN, J.E., and G.C. HAMILTON. "Chest pain," in P. Rosen and R.M. Barkin, eds, *Emergency Medicine: Concepts and Clinical Practice.* 5th ed. St. Louis: Mosby, 2002, pp. 162–171.
8. WAYNE, M.A., and R. CARRERO. "Chest pain," in G.R. Schwartz, B.K. Hanke, and T.A. Mayer, eds., *Principles and Practice of Emergency Medicine.* 4th ed. Philadelphia: Lippincott Williams & Wilkins, 1998.
9. ZALENSKI, R., and R. ROBERTS. "Chest pain," in A.L. Harwood-Nuss, C.H. Linden, R.C Luten, S.M. Sheppard, and A.B. Wolfson, eds., *The Clinical Practice of Emergency Medicine.* 3rd ed. Philadelphia: Lippincott Williams & Wilkins, 2005, pp. 58–62.

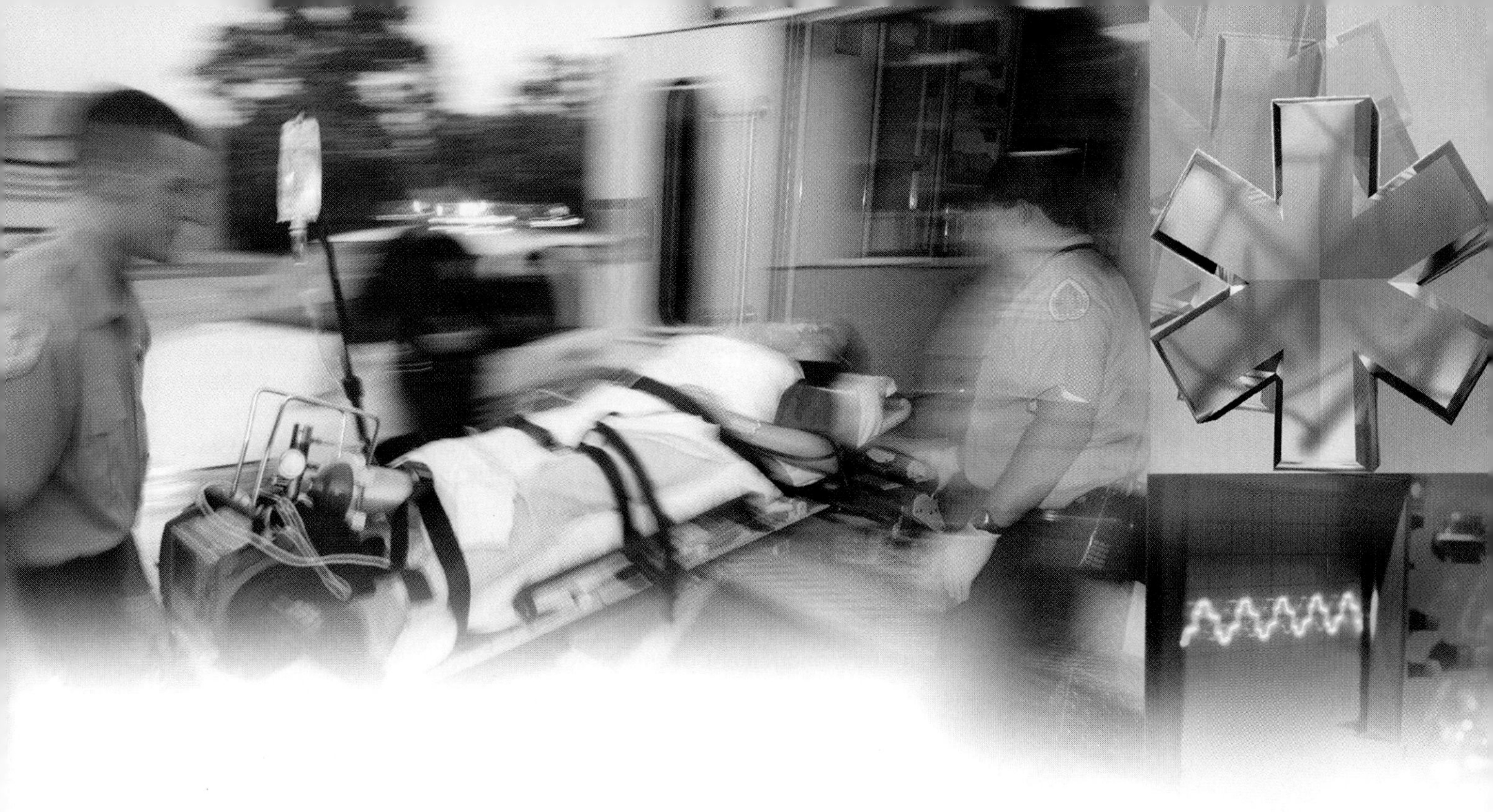

7 ALTERED MENTAL STATUS

Altered mental status is any behavior or response that diverges from the normal, indicating impaired mental function. Presentations vary enormously—from a patient who is just a little confused to one who is totally unresponsive. Altered mental status can result from any number of causes and is a "red flag" sign of physiological instability. The challenge to the care provider is not only to support basic functions, especially airway patency, but also to be able to quickly identify and manage the probable cause.

Topics that are covered in this chapter are

- Terminology and Altered Mental Status
- The Pathophysiology of Altered Mental Status
- General Assessment and Management of Altered Mental Status
- Differential Diagnosis: Intracranial Causes of Altered Mental Status
- Differential Diagnosis: Extracranial Causes of Altered Mental Status

SCENARIO

Early in your shift, you are called to a neighborhood residence for a male patient exhibiting altered mental status. On arrival, you are greeted by anxious family members who inform you that the patient is in an upstairs bedroom. While evaluating the scene for hazards, you make your way to the bedroom and find the patient supine on a bed, making loud gurgling noises. As you pass a nightstand, you note cigarette-filled ashtrays and medicine containers labeled Lovastatin and Vasotec.

The patient is a 68-year-old male who is unresponsive and who displays flexion to painful stimuli. Your rapid assessment of the airway reveals vomitus pooling in the oral cavity. As your partner aggressively suctions the oropharynx, you note Cheyne-Stokes respirations with inadequate ventilation and oxygenation. An initial pulse oximetry reading reveals an arterial saturation of 78 percent. You instruct your partner to place an oropharyngeal airway and begin high-flow, high-concentration oxygen therapy with tracheal intubation to follow. You continue with the initial assessment and note a slow radial pulse accompanied by cool, slightly diaphoretic skin with a capillary refill of 2 seconds.

How would you continue the assessment and management of this patient?

INTRODUCTION

altered mental status a deficiency in level of consciousness, cognitive ability, or general orientation; any behavior or response that diverges from the normal and is indicative of impaired mental function.

Altered mental status is frequently encountered in the prehospital setting. By definition, altered mental status is a deficiency in level of consciousness, cognitive ability, or general orientation. Accordingly, the number of specific behaviors comprising altered mental status is virtually limitless.

Altered mental status is not a disease in itself. Rather, altered mental status is a sign of an underlying abnormality in need of correction. The diseases and injuries that can cause an altered mental status are as numerous and varied as the presentations of altered mental status. Many of these underlying abnormalities are life threatening and in need of immediate intervention. Therefore, it is paramount that the prehospital care provider combine thorough assessment skills with a strong knowledge of the effects of various diseases on mental status.

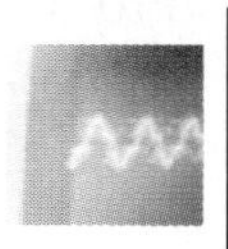

TERMINOLOGY AND ALTERED MENTAL STATUS

Altered mental status can be signaled by any of a multitude of behaviors and responses that diverge from the normal. Because manifestations of impaired mental function are so varied, describing a patient's behavior precisely is paramount in conveying the exact nature and severity of the altered mental condition.

In addition, it is critical to note any change—whether improvement or deterioration—because initial and differential diagnoses are often influenced by the specific progression of the patient's outward mental presentation. Again, precise terminology is required to depict the progression accurately and to assist in the confirmation or exclusion of certain diagnoses.

An exact description of altered mental status is clinically important and must be conveyed without any room for misinterpretation.

So, an exact description of altered mental status is clinically important and must be conveyed without any room for misinterpretation. The following are terms commonly employed in the medical description of altered mental status:

- *Amnesic State.* Amnesia is the loss of memory, the inability to recall past events. A patient with amnesia generally presents with a normal to decreased level of consciousness. Specifically, amnesia is described as retrograde (prior to an event), anterograde (after an event), or general (not pertaining to an event at all).

- ***Coma.*** A coma is an absolute state of unresponsiveness. The patient cannot be aroused by external stimulus. In some usages, as in the Glasgow Coma Scale (GCS), there are varying levels of coma as indicated by degree of responsiveness to stimuli. A GCS score of 8 or less in a patient with no eye opening to verbal stimuli is an accepted definition of coma.
- ***Confusion.*** An individual who exhibits a relative level of consciousness but is disturbed in the perception or remembrance of person, place, time, or events is said to be suffering confusion.
- ***Decreased Level of Consciousness.*** This term applies to any state in which the patient presents as anything other than alert with full orientation and normal cognition.
- ***Delirium.*** Delirium is a state of confusion characterized by disorientation from time and place that is often accompanied by auditory or visual hallucinations and/or incoherent or irrelevant speech. The patient may exhibit a normal to decreased level of consciousness.
- ***Dementia.*** Dementia is associated with a progressive deterioration of memory and cognitive impairment.
- ***Lethargy.*** This term pertains to a normal to decreased level of consciousness associated with the inability to react or respond to stimuli with normal perception or speed. Lethargy also describes a condition of drowsiness or indifference.
- ***Somnolence.*** Somnolence in general usage means sleepiness. In clinical use, the term refers to a prolonged state of drowsiness, possibly resembling a trance, which may last for days.
- ***Stupor.*** Stupor is an unresponsive state from which the patient can be transiently aroused by means of external stimuli. When the stimulus ceases, the patient lapses back into unresponsiveness.
- ***Unconsciousness.*** A state of being unaware, without consciousness; unresponsiveness.

Appropriate terminology assures that your description will be universally understood. In addition, it is an effective tool for the rapid and accurate communication of medically relevant information. The importance of using precise terminology to describe an altered mental status cannot be overemphasized.

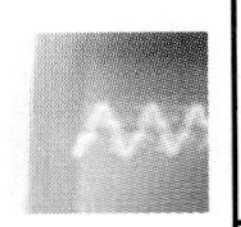

THE PATHOPHYSIOLOGY OF ALTERED MENTAL STATUS

Consciousness, or the ability to perceive ourselves and the environment in which we exist, is a direct function of the cerebrum and the reticular activating system (RAS).

consciousness a state of awareness of oneself and one's environment.

The Cerebrum

The *cerebrum* comprises approximately 40 percent of total brain mass. It is divided into right and left hemispheres and is covered by a convoluted gray matter called the *cerebral cortex*. The cerebrum is responsible for memory, thought, speech, voluntary movement, and sensory perception. Different portions of the cerebrum are responsible for different functions (Figure 7-1). Damage to, or dysfunction of, the cerebrum results in alterations of these functions. Both cerebral

cerebrum the largest portion of the brain, consisting of right and left hemispheres, responsible for memory, thought, speech, voluntary movement, and sensory perception.

cerebral cortex the covering of the cerebrum.

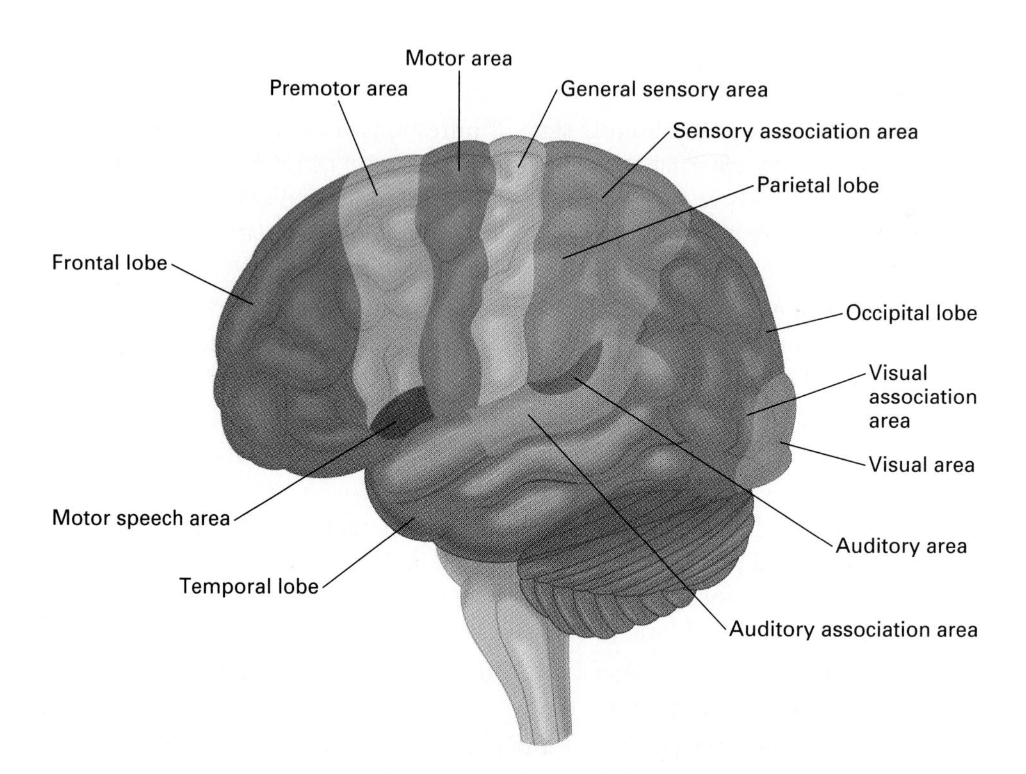

FIGURE 7-1
The cerebrum (left hemisphere).

hemispheres must malfunction to result in significant altered mental status or unconsciousness.

The Reticular Activating System

reticular activating system (RAS) nerve fibers extending from the brainstem to the cerebral cortex that are responsible for initiating and maintaining states of arousal and awareness.

Unlike the cerebrum, the *reticular activating system RAS* (Figure 7-2) is not a distinct, readily identifiable structure. Rather, the RAS is comprised of ascending sensory nerve fibers originating within the brainstem and proceeding on to the thalamus. From the thalamus, these fibers are directed to specific regions of the cerebral cortex for final interpretation. The continual direction of sensory information

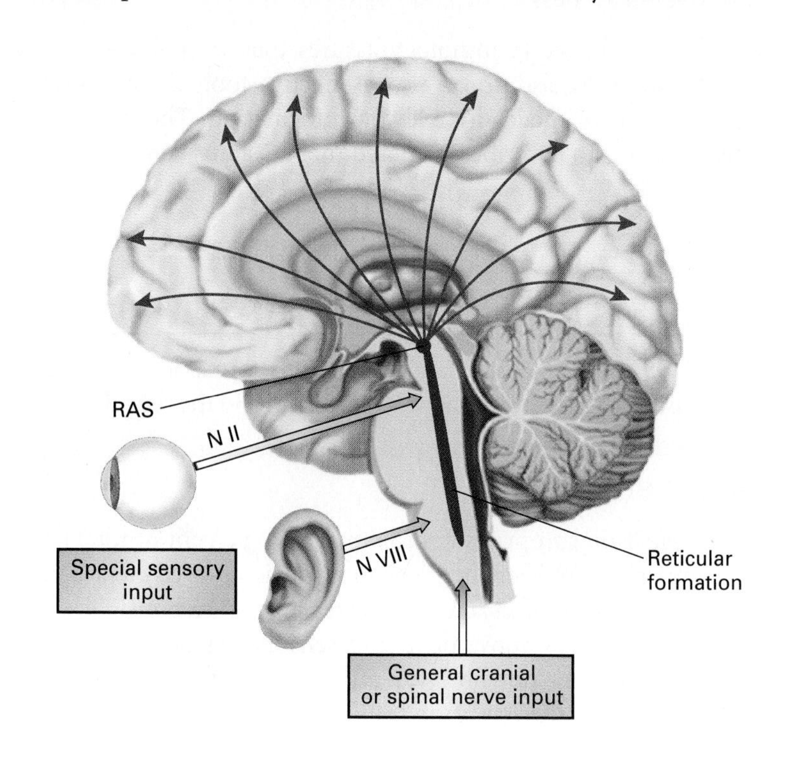

FIGURE 7-2
The reticular activating system.

to the cerebral cortex by the RAS maintains the cerebrum in a state of constant awareness, or consciousness.

The majority of altered mental and comatose states are explained in reference to dysfunction of the RAS and/or cerebrum. Generally, a conscious individual with normal cognition and full orientation has an intact RAS and two intact cerebral hemispheres. Altered mentation and coma become evident when a patient loses function in the RAS and/or both cerebral hemispheres.

Because the RAS receives and relays ascending sensory information, any breakdown within the RAS blocks the transmission of these vital stimuli. As a result, information does not reach the cerebral cortex and the state of arousal is diminished or lost. Even if the cerebrum is intact, the end result is coma.

Similarly, dysfunction of both cerebral hemispheres will lead to a serious alteration in mental status and, quite possibly, coma, as an intact RAS relays sensory information to a nonintact cerebrum. If there is dysfunction in just one cerebral hemisphere, however, depending on the severity, the patient will retain consciousness but exhibit behavioral alterations and/or the loss of specific neurologic abilities. An example would be a stroke patient who has suffered damage to one cerebral hemisphere and is confused and has impaired motor ability on the opposite side.

As long as an individual has an intact RAS and at least one functional cerebral hemisphere, a level of consciousness will be maintained.

As long as an individual has an intact RAS and at least one functional cerebral hemisphere, consciousness will be maintained.

Structural and Metabolic Alterations

Numerous conditions can result in the dysfunction of the RAS and/or cerebrum. These conditions can be categorized as either structural or metabolic:

- *Structural Alteration.* Structural alterations that result in dysfunction of the RAS or the cerebrum are lesions (areas of physical damage) that occur directly to the central nervous system (CNS). Trauma, brain tumors, strokes, and encephalitis are examples of conditions that cause structural alterations.
- *Metabolic Alteration.* Metabolic conditions originate outside of the CNS. As such, metabolic alterations affect the brain indirectly. Generally, metabolic alterations produce a chemical environment that is incompatible with normal brain function. Depending on the degree of severity, changes in mental status resulting from metabolic conditions can present anywhere along the spectrum from confusion to coma. Hypoxia, hypoglycemia, and electrolyte imbalances are examples of metabolic alteration.

A good understanding of the relationship between structural or metabolic damage to the brain and altered mental status can enable the health care provider to rapidly identify causes of altered mental status and treat them appropriately. Often, accurate identification with appropriate intervention will stabilize or correct the underlying abnormalities and save a life.

Clinical Insight

In assessing the patient with an altered mental status, consider that the underlying cause may be structural (e.g., damage from trauma, tumor, stroke, or encephalitis), metabolic (e.g., from toxic ingestion, hypoglycemia, or electrolyte imbalance), or environmental (heatstroke or hypothermia).

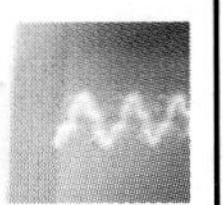

GENERAL ASSESSMENT AND MANAGEMENT OF ALTERED MENTAL STATUS

Because there are so many possible etiologies of altered mental status, it is extremely important to use a systematic method of patient assessment, as described in Chapter 1, Assessment of the Medical Patient. The following section provides a general framework, presenting points that are common to assessment and management of a patient with altered mental status, regardless of cause. The remainder of the chapter deals with differential diagnosis of various causes of altered mental status and specifics about their assessment and management.

Note: Throughout this chapter, assessment steps are presented in the sequence that is appropriate if the patient, because of an altered mental status, is unable to provide a SAMPLE history. As discussed in Chapter 1, when the patient is unable to provide a history, the physical exam should be conducted before the history is gathered from family members or others. If the patient is alert and oriented enough to provide a history, the history should be obtained before the physical exam is conducted—and before a deteriorating mental status prevents gathering information from the patient. With partners working together, or with an experienced provider who can effectively multitask, the history and the physical exam are often conducted simultaneously.

When the patient is alert, obtain the history before conducting the physical exam—and before a deteriorating mental status prevents gathering information from the patient.

Scene Size-Up

Be aware that any condition that alters mental status can produce alterations in patient perception resulting in unintentional aggression and violent behavior toward those attempting to assist. If the patient becomes hostile or aggressive so that you feel personally endangered, leave the scene and call for appropriate assistance.

Once scene safety is assured, actively seek clues in the immediate environment that may shed light on the cause of the patient's altered mental status. Awareness of items such as glucometers, medications, oxygen, prosthetic limbs, drug paraphernalia, or adverse living conditions can prove helpful as you try to formulate or confirm an initial diagnosis.

Initial Assessment

The initial assessment is aimed at identifying and managing immediate life threats and setting patient priorities. Altered mental status is likely to accompany any life-threatening condition such as shock or respiratory or cardiac failure. A patient with acute altered mental status is always a high priority for rapid transport, with the exception of the hypoglycemic patient who responds appropriately to the administration of 50 percent dextrose or the narcotic overdose patient who responds positively to Narcan and is no longer physiologically unstable.

General Impression

When approaching the patient, gear your attention toward establishing an initial impression of the patient's status, any immediate life threats, and any overt signs of illness. For example, obvious flaccidity or flexion (decorticate posturing) may be the first clue to brain injury as can occur in a stroke, subdural bleed, or infectious process such as meningitis or encephalitis. The presence of an acetone odor or Kussmaul's respirations might indicate diabetic ketoacidosis.

Patient position can also provide valuable clues to the immediate status and possible underlying problem. Cardiac patients tend to remain very still, while patients with hyperthyroidism, hypoxia, or in a postictal state following a seizure may exhibit erratic, uncoordinated movement. Patients in respiratory distress tend to assume a tripod position in an effort to maximize tidal and minute volume.

The patient's facial expression is of particular importance. A look of anguish or anxiety is possibly indicative of severe distress. The face may also provide clues such as circumoral (around the lips and nose) cyanosis, indicating severe hypoxia that may be associated with a significant respiratory or cardiovascular compromise, or facial drooping, suggestive of some sort of CNS difficulty. A dystonic reaction to medication (twisting, twitching, or the like) is also easily observed when you first approach the patient and see his face.

As you approach, you may also be able to make an initial evaluation of the patient's airway and breathing status, especially if sonorous or stridorous sounds are audible.

The amount of information you can gather before making physical contact with the patient can be considerable and invaluable in assisting your formulation of the problem underlying the patient's altered behavior. However, this information can be subtle. You have to make an effort to look for it.

Clinical Insight

Watch the patient's face. A look of anxiety, cyanosis around the mouth, twitching facial muscles—all can provide clues to the presence or cause of altered mental status.

Chief Complaint

The chief complaint is the major clue to the underlying cause of altered mental status. For example, the patient with altered mental status complaining of chest pain may be suffering from a serious cardiac dysrhythmia, congestive heart failure, or left ventricular dysfunction with a decreased cardiac output. Along similar lines, a complaint of fever with neck stiffness may indicate meningitis, while the complaint of anorexia (loss of appetite) may point toward electrolyte or glucose disturbances. Difficulty in speaking may be the initial clue to a cerebral problem such as stroke, tumor, or abscess.

Unfortunately, not all patients with altered mental status are able to accurately convey a chief complaint, or any complaint at all. Even if a chief complaint is produced, you may have to declare the patient unreliable and look to other sources, such as family, friends, or other witnesses.

If the appropriate sources of information are not available, you must then document a nonspecific complaint such as inappropriate behavior, decreased level of consciousness, or simply confusion. In such cases, you will have to rely on clues you gather during the remainder of the patient assessment, including historical medical information, the physical exam, and evaluatory interventions, coupled with your general knowledge, to formulate an opinion as to the underlying abnormality.

Clinical Insight

Keep in mind that altered mental status is not a disorder in itself; it is a sign of an underlying disorder. The chief complaint, if offered, is usually the most important clue to the underlying cause of an altered mental status. For example, chest pain would point to a cardiac cause, fever to infection, or aphasia to stroke.

Baseline Mental Status

On reaching the patient's side, you should quickly establish an initial *level of consciousness.* The AVPU method, as described in Chapter 1, represents a fast, widely accepted method of accomplishing this task:

A Alert (patient's eyes are spontaneously open)

V Responds to verbal stimuli

P Responds to painful stimuli

U Unresponsive

level of consciousness state of awareness; may be estimated by the AVPU method or by measures such as the Glasgow Coma Scale.

AVPU

A – Patient is alert (eyes are spontaneously open)
V – Patient responds to verbal stimuli
P – Patient responds to painful stimuli
U – Patient is unresponsive

The ABCs

Airway Depending on the precipitating condition and level of consciousness, a patient with altered mental status has the potential for airway compromise. For a patient who is talking without difficulty, this is not a complicated evaluation. A patent airway can be assumed.

However, any situation involving significant structural or metabolic damage to the brain can seriously impede the patient's ability to swallow, clear secretions, or protect his airway. Examples of cerebral damage include stroke, intracranial infection, and cerebral tumors, among many others. Also, accumulating secretions pose the danger of total airway obstruction and/or pulmonary aspiration. Additionally, the stuporous or comatose patient can lose muscular support of the mandible. With no muscular support, the tongue falls to the posterior pharynx, creating an airway occlusion.

The patient with altered mental status has the potential for airway compromise.

Visualize the airway to appreciate any additional problems, such as tongue deviation, that may accompany cerebral damage or *herniation.* Also, relative hydration can be evaluated in the oral mucosa and tongue. Additionally, you may note particular odors, such as acetone, common to certain diabetic complications, or the musty smell frequently associated with liver disease.

herniation extrusion of the brain through the foramen magnum, the tentorium, the falx cerebri, or the cranial wall.

Immediately correct any shortcoming in airway patency. Initiate any appropriate interventions, such as suctioning or placing an oropharyngeal or nasopharyngeal airway. The nasopharyngeal airway is relatively well tolerated by a patient with an intact but depressed gag reflex and is easy to place. Insert one of these adjuncts, even if you plan to initiate tracheal intubation, so the patient can be preoxygenated with positive-pressure ventilation before the tracheal tube is introduced.

Kussmaul's respirations a pathological pattern of rapid, deep respirations; often associated with acidosis.

Biot's (ataxic) respirations pathological respirations with no coordinated pattern; often associated with stroke.

Breathing The respiratory rate, depth, adequacy, and pattern may also help reveal the underlying abnormality. Pathological respiratory patterns are important clues (Table 7-1). For example, *Kussmaul's respirations* (deep, rapid respirations) are a sign of a metabolic acidosis that the body is attempting to compensate for by elimination of carbon dioxide. Acidosis may have any of a variety of etiologies, such as diabetic ketoacidosis, metabolic acidosis, or acidosis related to toxic ingestion. *Biot's (ataxic)* respirations (highly irregular in rate and depth) or *central*

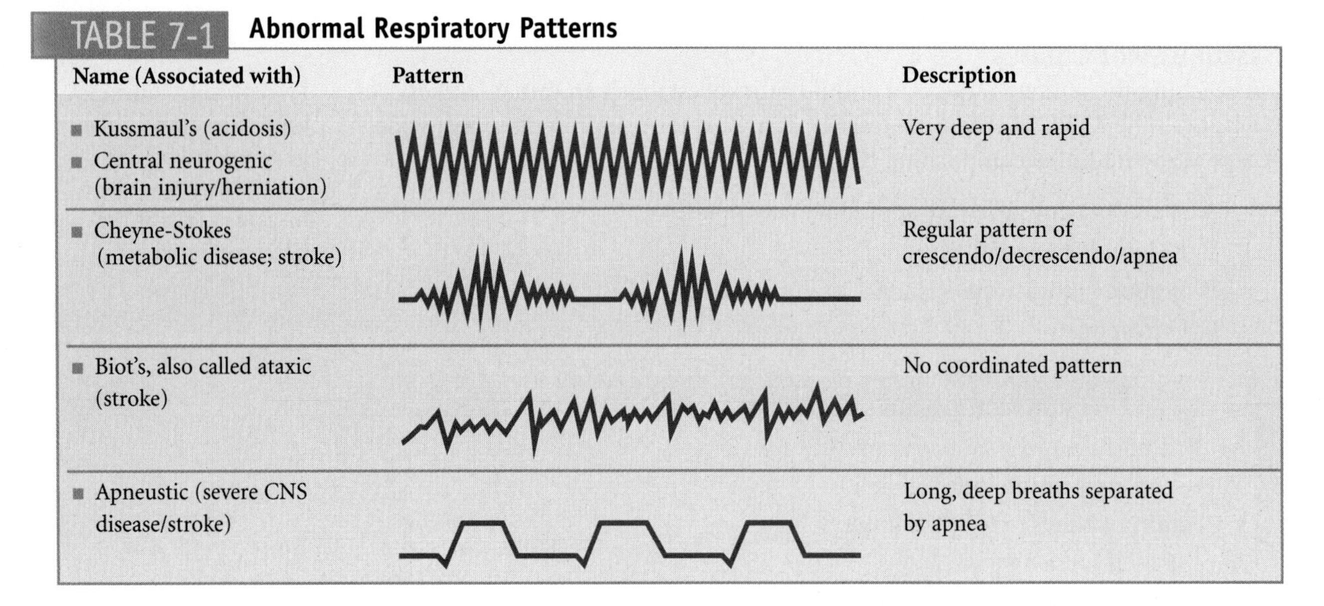

TABLE 7-1 Abnormal Respiratory Patterns

Name (Associated with)	Pattern	Description
■ Kussmaul's (acidosis) ■ Central neurogenic (brain injury/herniation)		Very deep and rapid
■ Cheyne-Stokes (metabolic disease; stroke)		Regular pattern of crescendo/decrescendo/apnea
■ Biot's, also called ataxic (stroke)		No coordinated pattern
■ Apneustic (severe CNS disease/stroke)		Long, deep breaths separated by apnea

neurogenic hyperventilation (very deep and rapid, similar to Kussmaul's respirations) may suggest brain injury or cerebral herniation secondary to causes such as stroke, hepatic failure, electrolyte imbalances, or intracranial infections.

central neurogenic hyperventilations a pathological pattern of rapid, deep respirations; often associated with brain injury or herniation.

Hypoventilation or bradypnea may indicate CNS depression or respiratory failure, with profound hypoxia and CO_2 retention being the cause of the altered mentation. Certain drugs, such as narcotics or barbiturates, can also cause hypoventilation with associated hypoxia from CNS depression.

On evaluation of respiratory and ventilatory status, any and all deficiencies should rapidly be supported or corrected to maintain oxygen saturation levels of 95 to 100 percent. Methods of delivery may include devices such as the nasal cannula, nonrebreather face mask, or positive-pressure ventilation and tracheal intubation when indicated.

If possible, a pulse oximeter should be attached prior to oxygen therapy to establish a baseline quantification of the patient's oxygenation status on room air. However, in cases of suspected hypoxia, the use of pulse oximetry must not delay the application and delivery of high-flow, high-concentration oxygen. Also, remember that certain conditions leading to altered mental status, such as carbon monoxide poisoning, may result in an inaccurate pulse oximetry reading.

In cases of hypoventilation or noted hypoxia, the use of pulse oximetry must not delay the application and delivery of much-needed oxygen.

Circulation Assessment of circulation and perfusion may also shed light on the specific cause of altered mental status.

Palpating the radial or carotid pulse for general pulse rate can be revealing. Initial stages of hypovolemia or accelerated metabolic states associated with infection, hyperthyroidism, hyperthermia, or postictal seizure status may present with tachycardia. Excessive tachycardia, as seen with supraventricular dysrhythmias, can compromise cerebral perfusion secondary to decreases in cardiac output arising from decreased ventricular filling time. Causes of bradycardia include cerebral herniation, certain medications and drugs, and cardiac dysrhythmias such as heart blocks and other electrical disturbances. Bradycardia may cause decreased cerebral perfusion if cardiac output is severely compromised by the slow rate.

Pulse strength, or intensity, may provide clues to relative volume or fluid load and hydration status but is highly variable and difficult to assess reliably.

Pulse regularity is easily noted through basic palpation and may be the first clue to dysrhythmias that decrease cardiac output and, consequently, cerebral perfusion. There are many causes of cardiac dysrhythmias, including electrolyte imbalances, pH disturbances, hypoxia, and toxic ingestion. It is prudent to apply the cardiac monitor for exact evaluation of myocardial electrical status with appropriate management following.

While assessing pulses, you may find it convenient to assess simultaneously for the relative status of peripheral perfusion by way of skin color, temperature, moisture, and capillary refill.

Skin that is warm to hot may indicate the fever of infection such as sepsis, meningitis, or pneumonia. Pale, cool, diaphoretic skin may indicate decreased cardiac output in association with cardiac abnormalities, as discussed previously, or shock. Environmental or internal temperature extremes may be the cause of hot or cold skin. Respectively, such extremes may indicate external changes in temperature or internal changes in homeostatic function, such as sometimes seen with thyroid or liver dysfunction.

Skin color should also be observed. For example, the presence of jaundice may suggest liver or kidney failure, while mottling may provide another clue to decreased peripheral circulation. Cyanosis would suggest a respiratory deficit responsible for the altered mental status.

Patient Priority

At the conclusion of the initial assessment, you must determine whether the patient is a high priority for expeditious transport or whether more time may be spent with the patient on the scene. Patients with acute altered mental status should almost always be considered a high priority for transport.

Focused History and Physical Exam

Physical Exam

Most of the information about the possible cause of altered mental status will come from the initial assessment and the history. The physical exam is useful when you are looking to further confirm a suspected cause or to obtain additional information when the underlying abnormality remains elusive. As noted earlier, the history should precede the physical exam if the patient is alert enough to provide reliable information. If not, the physical exam takes priority, with the history gathered from family or others afterward (or, perhaps, simultaneously if partners are working together).

Examples of physical exam findings pertinent to altered mental status would include the palpation of a goiter (enlarged thyroid gland) in cases of suspected thyroid-induced altered mental status or the finding of incontinence as it applies to the stroke or postictal seizure patient. Other examples include jugular vein distention (JVD) and peripheral edema in the patient with right-sided heart failure, or a barrel chest indicating COPD. Slow-healing wounds or provisional amputations may lead you to consider diabetic complications. It is necessary to link the patient presentation and suspected condition with the appropriate body systems for evaluation during the physical exam.

Further Mental Status Assessment Throughout the entire patient assessment and management, you must make a conscious effort to continually monitor the patient's mental function. In addition to the level of consciousness (see the earlier discussion of AVPU), you should also strive to describe the patient's cognitive ability and orientation. A patient has normal cognition when he is able to interpret and respond to questions in a logical and smooth process—as opposed to providing inappropriate, scattered responses. The patient has normal orientation when he can identify time, place, events, and self. Note any changes in these parameters.

Another tool for describing a patient's mental status is the Glasgow Coma Scale (Figure 7-3). The GCS quantifies eye opening, verbal response, and motor response as indicators of mental function. A major advantage in using the GCS is that it is universally understood among field and hospital personnel. Additionally, the GCS can effectively illustrate patient improvement or decline.

Neurologic Exam Any patient with altered mental status and a satisfactory level of consciousness should be given a neurologic examination to further evaluate the activity of the brain and cranial nerves. The neurologic exam can easily be incorporated into the physical exam, with findings assisting in identification of the underlying abnormality or the severity of a known abnormality.

Much of the neurologic examination will already have been accomplished with reference to the level of consciousness, cognitive ability, and general orientation,

Glasgow Coma Scale

Eye Opening	Spontaneous	4	
	To Voice	3	
	To Pain	2	
	None	1	
Verbal Response	Oriented	5	
	Confused	4	
	Inappropriate Words	3	
	Incomprehensible Words	2	
	None	1	
Motor Response	Obeys Commands	6	
	Localizes Pain	5	
	Withdraws (Pain)	4	
	Flexion (Pain)	3	
	Extension (Pain)	2	
	None	1	
Glasgow Coma Score Total			

FIGURE 7-3
The Glasgow Coma Scale.

as described previously. However, during the physical exam, further testing should occur as listed in Table 7-2.

An additional test for neurologic deficit that can easily be conducted in the field is the pronator drift test. The patient is asked to hold his hands out in front of him, palms up, as if begging, and to close his eyes. The hand on the side with a neurologic deficit will turn over, palm down, and drift downward.

Also review the neurologic exam suggestions in Chapter 1.

Vital Signs

As part of the physical exam, a baseline set of vital signs must be obtained. Variations in pulse and respiration can be important indicators of the possible cause of altered mental status, as pointed out in the previous discussion of the

TABLE 7-2 Neurologic Exam

Tests of Cranial Nerve Function	
Check for . . .	**To assess function of . . .**
Visual disturbances	Optic nerve/II cranial nerve
Pupillary size, equality, and response	Oculomotor nerve/III cranial nerve
Facial droop	Facial nerve/VII cranial nerve
Swallowing difficulty	Glossopharyngeal nerve/IX cranial nerve
Tongue deviation	Hypoglossal nerve/XII cranial nerve
Additional Neurologic Function Tests	
Check for . . .	
Motor function (grip)	
Sensory ability in the extremities	
Strength in the extremities	
Gait ataxia	
Incontinence	

initial assessment. Blood pressure can also be revealing. For example, increases in blood pressure may sometimes be associated with a stroke or a hyperthyroid- or toxic-related altered mental status. Decreases in blood pressure may assist in the confirmation of hypovolemia, hypothyroidism, sepsis, or cardiac failure. A rectal temperature must be taken in any patient with significant altered mental status or coma to identify possibly life-threatening hyper- or hypothermia.

History

If obtainable, a history will be invaluable in helping determine the underlying cause of altered mental status, while effectively ruling out other possible causes. However, as stated earlier, information from the patient with an altered mental status may be unavailable or unreliable. Keep in mind that information given by a confused patient, or secondhand through others not intimately familiar with the patient, may not be very accurate and should be evaluated on a case-by-case basis.

If the patient is unable to provide a medical history, you must look toward other sources, such as family, friends, bystanders, or, when available, on-scene clues such as glucometers, medications, home oxygen, walkers, hospital beds, metered-dose inhalers, and drug paraphernalia, or environmental parameters such as temperature or living style. Additionally, information about the patient's medical history may be obtained during the physical exam (e.g., provisional amputations as found with diabetes or extensive scar tissue on the extremities from chronic parenteral drug abuse).

The SAMPLE method provides an excellent framework for compiling a medical history:

Signs and Symptoms. A description of signs and symptoms surrounding the altered mental status may be useful in determining the base cause. For example, altered mental status accompanied by the feeling of weakness to one side of the body would be indicative of a CNS ailment such as a stroke or brain tumor, while altered mental status with deep, rapid respirations may indicate an acidotic condition.

Allergies. It is extremely important to know about any allergy to medication so you can avoid administering a medication to which the patient is allergic. Additionally, if the patient has taken a medication that is closely related to the agent to which the patient is allergic, this may be the cause of the altered mental status. Once obtained, this information must be conveyed to hospital personnel.

Medications. Medications the patient has been taking provide important insight into the patient's past medical history and possibly into the cause of the altered mental status. Keep in mind that medications in which levels of therapeutic worth fall within a narrow range can be toxic at levels outside this range. Interactions between drugs may be observed, and natural side effects of some medications, such as electrolyte imbalances, may be at play. Illicit drugs can also be placed in this category.

Past Medical History. The past medical history can provide dramatic insight into the patient's medical makeup, and you may be able to identify exacerbation of a preexisting problem as the cause of the present emergency and the altered mental status. This may be noted with COPD, diabetes mellitus, and cardiac conditions. Also, existing medical conditions may predispose the patient to other medical difficulties as, for example, hypertension predisposes a patient to stroke or kidney failure.

Last Oral Intake. The patient's last intake of food and/or fluid may be important in assessing certain types of altered mental status. For example, a frequent victim of altered mental status is the insulin-dependent diabetic who has not

Clinical Insight

In a patient with altered mental status, it is critical to find out and, if possible, bring to the hospital all drugs the patient may be taking, whether prescribed medications, over-the-counter medications, nutritional supplements, or recreational/illicit drugs. First, the specific drugs a patient is taking may point to an underlying condition that has caused the altered mental status, such as an allergic reaction, cardiovascular crisis, or diabetic emergency. Second, the drug itself, if inappropriately taken, may have created a toxic environment that is causing a cerebral disturbance.

eaten after administering exogenous insulin. It is important to gauge the blood glucose reading in relation to the last oral intake. You would expect a blood glucose reading of 100 to 120 mg/dl in a patient who recently ate a large amount of carbohydrates and not the 60 to 80 mg/dl blood glucose reading that is typical in the 8- to 12-hour fasting patient. Also, information about general dietary habits and nutrition can be important. Because many electrolytes and vitamins are obtained through dietary and fluid intake, such information can provide clues to an electrolyte disturbance as the cause of altered mental status. Additionally, you may be able to gauge the possibility of emesis by determining the last oral intake. This information is especially important to the surgical staff if emergency surgery is warranted.

Events Prior to Illness. The behavior or complaints of the patient surrounding the onset of abnormal behavior can be valuable in identifying the cause of the altered mental status. The complaint of a headache immediately preceding the onset of unresponsiveness may suggest a hemorrhagic stroke, while a persistent fever associated with a headache and stiff neck may suggest meningitis. Information such as acute or gradual onset and patient activity at the time of onset can further assist in determining the cause.

Adjunctive Equipment and Interventions

The pulse oximeter, cardiac monitor, and glucometer are important adjuncts to assessment that can also help in identifying causes of altered mental status. Interventions such as intravenous access, drawing of blood specimens, fluid therapy, and tracheal intubation should be considered, based on patient presentation.

Evaluation of blood glucose level is especially important for patients with altered mental status.

Evaluation of blood glucose level is especially important for patients with altered mental status. In the field, blood glucose evaluation is readily accomplished with a glucometer. Readings below 60 mg/dl with signs and symptoms, or less than 50 mg/dl with or without symptoms, may indicate hypoglycemia, while any reading greater than 200 mg/dl may be considered hyperglycemia.

Keep in mind that blood glucose levels can fluctuate secondary to conditions such as diabetes mellitus or any situation that increases metabolic activity, as found with fever, seizure activity, liver disease, and hyperthyroidism. These conditions can rapidly consume glucose reserves and produce a state of relative hypoglycemia. Therefore, it is paramount to evaluate the blood glucose level of anyone with altered mental status, even one who is not a confirmed diabetic.

Clinical Insight

To arrive at a field diagnosis of a patient with an altered mental status, you need strong assessment skills and an internal database of disease processes. Keep in mind, however, that the etiology of altered mental status may be difficult to diagnose in the field. So, focus your primary efforts on support of vital functions, gathering information for the hospital staff, and providing expeditious transport.

Ongoing Assessment

After the initial assessment and the focused history and physical exam, ongoing assessment is performed to determine any changes in the patient's condition—improvement or deterioration—and to assess the effectiveness of care provided so far. It is a continuous monitoring of the patient that is conducted until the patient is transferred to the care of the hospital staff. To perform ongoing assessment, you will repeat the initial assessment (including evaluation of mental status), reassess vital signs, repeat the physical exam, and check interventions.

Despite the properly performed assessment, the etiology of altered mental status may not be readily apparent in the field setting. For this reason, you should bend all efforts toward 1) supporting vital functions (e.g., airway, oxygenation, ventilation, control of bleeding, hydration), and 2) conveying any and all information obtained to hospital personnel.

As discussed earlier, to identify and effectively manage the root cause of altered mental status, you will need two things: strong assessment skills (summarized in the previous section) and an internal database of disease processes to which you can relate your assessment findings. The differential diagnosis information in the remainder of this chapter is intended to help you form such a database.

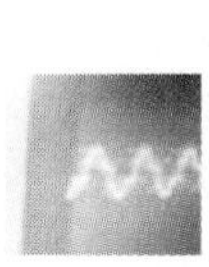

DIFFERENTIAL DIAGNOSIS: INTRACRANIAL CAUSES OF ALTERED MENTAL STATUS

The etiologies of altered mental status are numerous and varied. Eventually, any condition that afflicts the human body will alter the patient's mental status in one way or another. Altered mental status can be subdivided into those etiologies that occur within the brain and its supporting structures and those that occur outside of the brain. Respectively, these classifications are described as intracranial and extracranial. (Review "Structural and Metabolic Alterations.")

Intracranial causes of altered mental status are generally structural in nature, directly affecting the brain and its supporting structures. Several of the more common intracranial causes of altered mental status are head trauma, strokes, infection, and tumors.

Traumatic Head Injuries

Although this chapter is centered on the medical origins of altered mental status, the incidence of head and brain trauma deserve brief mention. The health care provider must recognize that even minor injury to the head can precipitate altered mental status. Furthermore, the appearance of altered mental status stemming from a traumatic injury can lag days to weeks to even months after the actual event, causing frequent misidentification as a medical event. Types of traumatic head injuries include

- *Cerebral concussion*
- *Cerebral contusion*
- *Epidural hematoma*
- *Subdural hematoma*
- *Intracerebral hemorrhage*

cerebral concussion force from a blow to the head that is transmitted to the brain.

cerebral contusion bruising of the brain.

epidural hematoma a swelling or mass of blood formed above the dura mater.

subdural hematoma a swelling or mass of blood formed beneath the dura mater.

intracerebral hemorrhage bleeding within the brain tissue.

It is difficult to distinguish among these conditions in the out-of-hospital setting.

Of particular interest is the subdural hematoma. A subdural hematoma is produced when the veins below the arachnoid meninges are torn (Figure 7-4). Hemorrhage occurs at a slow but steady rate. Occasionally, the rate of hemorrhage is so slow that the injury does not become symptomatic for weeks to months. As the cerebral spinal fluid inhibits normal blood clotting, the expanding hematoma gradually compresses the brain tissue until herniation occurs, resulting in neurologic and mental status changes. Elderly and alcoholics are more prone to delayed presentations of subdural hematoma.

Because of a lengthy delay in the appearance of symptoms, the patient or family may not be aware of the traumatic cause. During assessment, you must aggressively inquire as to any history of head injury and not discount it as minor based on the passage of considerable time.

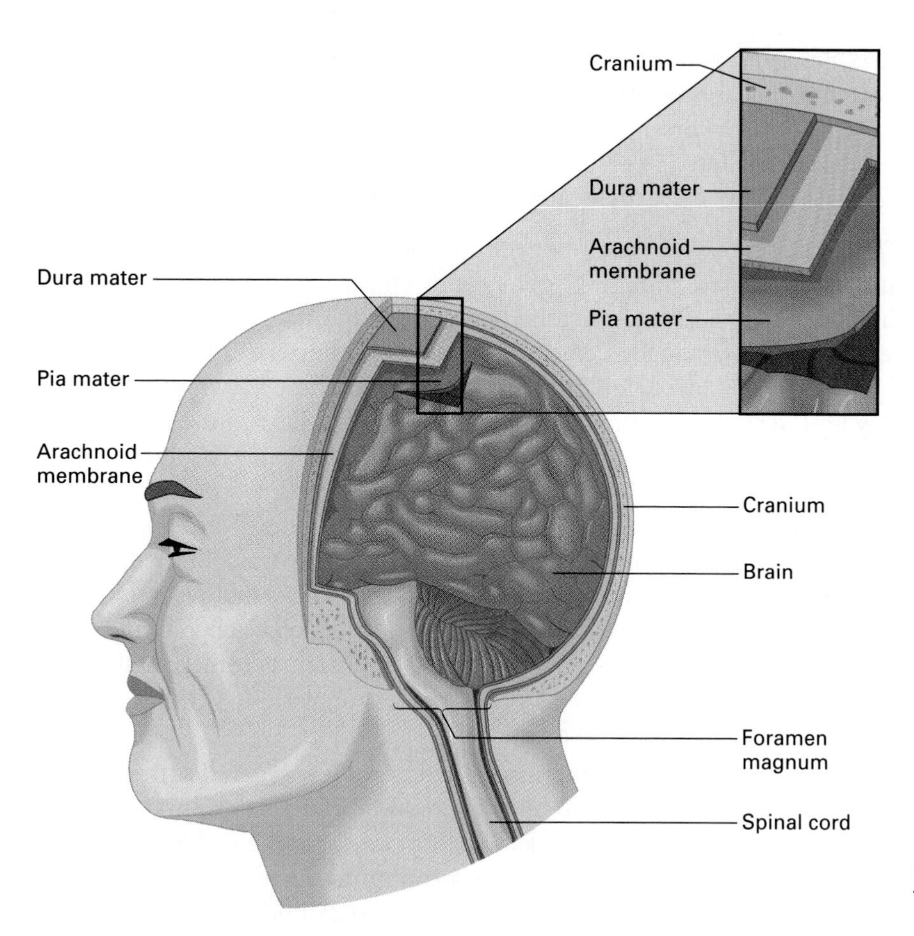

FIGURE 7-4
The meninges of the brain.

Assessment and care of the acute traumatic head injury is essentially identical to that for stroke, with the addition of appropriate spine immobilization. (If the history does not indicate recent trauma or if the trauma history is remote—weeks or longer—then spine immobilization is usually not necessary.)

Stroke

A stroke—often called a "brain attack"—is a structurally based cause of mental and/or neurologic deficits. It can affect any part of the brain, including the cerebrum and/or the RAS. Commonly, there is a disruption of blood supply to an area of the brain. The resulting loss of oxygen and other nutrients causes cellular damage, which becomes evident through changes in mental and/or neurologic status. If blood flow is not restored, cellular death, or infarction, results. Once infarcted, the brain tissue has no chance for salvage. (The reasons a stroke is sometimes called a "brain attack" are the parallels to a heart attack in the cause—oxygen starvation, often resulting from atherosclerotic disease—and the progression from *ischemia* to *infarction.*)

ischemia deficiency of blood supply to the tissues.

infarction death of tissues as a result of cessation of blood supply.

Recall that the majority of sensory and motor nerves to and from the cortex cross over at the lower portion of the brainstem, or medulla. Consequently, the left and right hemispheres control opposite, or contralateral, sides of the body. So, for example, a stroke affecting the right cerebral hemisphere will generally cause deficits on the left side of the body.

Strokes are classified as either ischemic or hemorrhagic.

Ischemic Stroke

An ischemic stroke occurs secondary to the occlusion, or blockage, of a cerebral artery. Blood flow through the artery is severely decreased, depriving all distal cells of oxygen, nutrients, and waste removal. As a result, ischemic brain cells quickly infarct with no hope for restoration. In the occlusive stroke, mental and neurologic disturbances tend to worsen progressively but eventually stabilize within 24 to 72 hours. Approximately 75 percent of strokes are considered ischemic.

Ischemic strokes are further categorized according to cause:

thrombus a blood clot that develops in and obstructs a blood vessel.

- *Thrombotic Stroke.* A thrombotic stroke occurs secondary to the development of a localized *thrombus*, or blood clot, within a cerebral artery. The condition develops as deposits of atherosclerotic plaque narrow the lumen of the cerebral artery, gradually decreasing the supply of arterial blood. Once it is significantly narrowed, inflammation of the diseased area within the vessel may lead to rupture of the plaque. The body views this rupture as an injury and initiates a clotting process at the injury site. Platelets adhere to the roughened surface, creating a thrombus that occludes the artery.

  When you interview the patient or family members, you may uncover a history of gradual progression of mental and/or neurologic changes. You may also obtain a history of transient neurologic deficits that resolved, called transient ischemic attacks (TIAs). This is because cellular ischemia and damage can occur long before the thrombotic occlusion becomes total. Many thrombotic strokes occur during periods of rest or at night, without any history of precipitating physical exertion.

embolus a solid, liquid, or gaseous mass carried to a blood vessel from a remote site.

- *Embolic Stroke.* Similar to the thrombotic stroke, an embolic stroke arises from the occlusion of a cerebral artery. However, occlusion in an embolic stroke results as an *embolus* breaks free from a remote site and lodges within a cerebral artery. The carotid artery is a common source of emboli. (This is why it is important to check for bruits prior to carotid massage—to avoid causing a stroke.) The end result is identical: Arterial occlusion occurs, depriving all cells downstream of oxygenated blood.

  In contrast to a thrombotic stroke, the onset of an embolic stroke is typically abrupt, without warning signs. The patient experiences immediate impairment when the embolus lodges in a cerebral vessel. Physical exertion sometimes triggers the onset because exertion increases circulatory blood flow, creating a greater potential for dislodging a thrombus or fragment of plaque. However, most embolic strokes occur without a history of exertion. As with occlusive stroke, the altered mental status and neurologic deficits in an embolic stroke can progress over the next 24 to 72 hours before stabilizing.

Depending on the location of the blocked artery, occlusive strokes can present in a variety of ways. When it exists, altered mental status can present anywhere from confusion to stupor or coma. Neurologically, an occlusive stroke typically affects motor, sensory, and speech functions, and these changes may be readily observable. Also, altered mental status may exist independently of neurologic changes and vice versa. Most strokes present with focal neurologic changes (e.g., motor, sensory, speech) as opposed to mental status changes. The patient may understand what is happening but be unable to express himself or to respond clearly.

Transient Ischemic Attack

A transient ischemic attack (TIA) is a thrombotic or embolic occlusion that, as its name suggests, is transient, or temporary. In these cases, the body is able to "lyse," or dissolve, the offending occlusion, restoring blood flow to the brain. The altered mental status and/or neurologic deficits secondary to the occlusion correct themselves when the occlusion dissolves. The brain incurs no residual damage, and all mental and neurologic changes return to normal. However, the TIA serves as a warning of underlying problems. One-third of those who experience a TIA suffer a debilitating stroke soon thereafter.

Atherosclerotic disease is a primary cause of ischemic stroke and TIA. Factors that contribute to atherosclerotic disease include hypercholesteremia, diabetes mellitus, genetics, obesity, and physical inactivity. In addition, agents such as oral contraceptives and cigarette smoking alter blood clotting, which predisposes the individual to thrombus and embolus formation. It is important to understand that TIA and stroke are the same disease; however, TIA is a mild, temporary manifestation, while stroke is severe and possibly permanent. The TIA signs and symptoms typically resolve within 1 hour after the onset.

Hemorrhagic Strokes

A hemorrhagic stroke occurs secondary to the rupture of a cerebral vessel. A hemorrhagic stroke is classified as an intracerebral hemorrhage, where the bleeding occurs within the brain tissue itself, or as a subarachnoid hemorrhage, where the bleeding occurs below the arachnoid layer. The dangers associated with a hemorrhagic stroke are twofold. Without arterial blood, brain cells become ischemic and eventually infarct. Additionally, blood from ruptured vessels accumulates and forms an intracranial hematoma. The hematoma rapidly expands, compressing and herniating the brain tissue. Without expedient intervention, death may result.

Hypertension is the primary cause of hemorrhagic strokes. Over time, hypertension weakens portions of the cerebral artery wall, leaving it prone to sudden rupture. Sections of an artery wall can form aneurysms, or balloon-like outpockets. Aneurysms are very unstable and are prone to rupture independently, let alone in conjunction with increased blood pressure. Also, some persons are born with aneurysms, and these can rupture spontaneously at any time in life.

Hypertension is the primary cause of hemorrhagic strokes.

The onset and evolution of a hemorrhagic stroke is rapid. Although hemorrhagic strokes can occur at any time, they happen more frequently during episodes of increased blood pressure such as may result from exertion or stress. Because the hemorrhagic stroke is so abrupt and severe, the decline in mental status is sudden, exhibited by confusion that rapidly progresses to stupor and coma. The patient may complain of a severe headache just before the hemorrhagic stroke occurs. In a subarachnoid hemorrhage, the patient typically complains of "the worst headache" he or she has ever experienced. This is a key assessment finding associated with a hemorrhagic stroke.

Assessment of Possible Stroke or TIA

The following section describes specifics about assessment of a patient suffering a stroke (Table 7-3). These are intended to fit within the generic framework for assessment of a patient with altered mental status that was presented previously in the chapter. The points raised here may either apply to the way you conduct your assessment when you already suspect a stroke or may bring out factors that would point to stroke as a cause of the patient's altered mental status.

Scene Size-Up When conducting a scene size-up, actively search for clues that relate to existing medical problems. Because strokes are often closely related to diabetes or coronary artery disease, look for insulin containers or other medications, glucometers, or home oxygen as soon as you enter the scene. Additionally, observe the patient for signs of advanced brain injury, such as flexion (decorticate

TABLE 7-3 Stroke and Altered Mental Status: Typical Findings

Scene Size-up	Initial Assessment	Physical Exam/Vitals	History
Flexion/extension; facial droop; signs of diabetic or hypertensive history (e.g., insulin, antihypertensives)	Airway compromise (e.g., inability to swallow) Pathologic respiratory patterns (Cheyne-Stokes, central neurogenic, Biot's, apneustic) Cardiac dysrhythmias, pulses difficult to locate	Visual disturbances, pupillary dysfunction; facial droop, swallowing difficulty, tongue deviation, weakness or sensory deficit in extremities, gait ataxia, incontinence Vital signs can vary dramatically; however, blood pressure is typically normal to elevated	Signs/symptoms: headache, hemiplegia, hemiparesis, dysphasia or aphasia, cardiac symptoms, nausea/vomiting, syncope, declining or improving mental or neurologic status Antihypertensive, diabetic, or cardiac medications History of previous TIA or stroke, head trauma, hypertension, coronary artery disease, aneurysm or AV malformation, diabetes, smoking Gradual onset (typical of thrombotic stroke) or sudden onset (typical of embolic or hemorrhagic stroke)

posturing) or extension (decerebrate posturing) (Figure 7-5). Listen for possible airway obstructions as you approach because the stroke patient may lose the ability to swallow or effectively clear secretions.

Clinical Insight

To distinguish confusion from aphasia in a suspected stroke patient, have the patient follow simple commands.

Initial Assessment The chief complaint related to a stroke can vary. The initial stages of an ischemic stroke may present with neurologic change. Aphasia (difficulty speaking) is common and may be mistaken for confusion; however, the aphasic patient can often understand the provider and follow simple commands, which allows differentiation of aphasia from confusion. An intracerebral hemorrhage can account for the sudden onset of severe headache, inappropriate behavior, or loss of consciousness. Neurologic deficits may exist independent of any mental status changes and vice versa. If the patient presents unresponsive, the chief complaint will be derived from other sources, such as family, friends, or witnesses, when available.

(a)
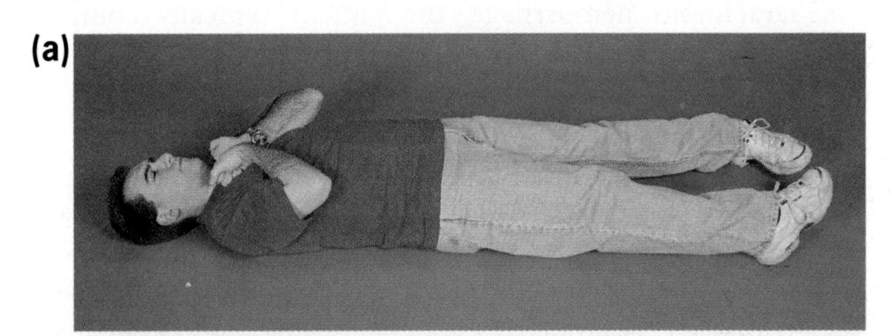

(b)
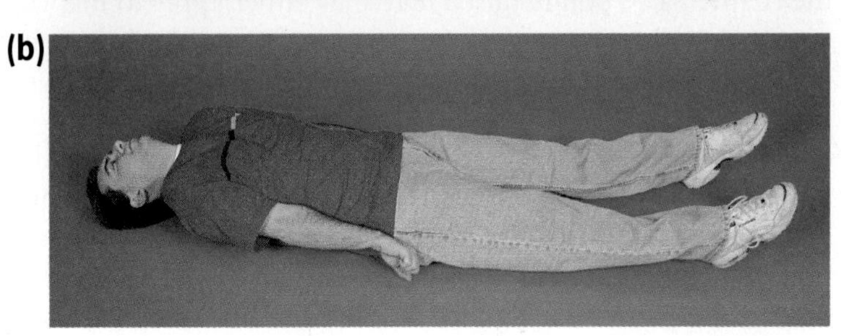

FIGURE 7-5
(a) Flexion (decorticate posturing) and (b) extension (decerebrate posturing).

If the onset of altered mental status occurs hours after the onset of the signs and symptoms of stroke, suspect an increasing intracranial pressure (ICP) associated with an intracerebral or subarachnoid hemorrhage. If the patient presents in a stuporous state or with coma early after stroke onset, suspect a large cerebral infarct or a stroke that has affected the brainstem. Stuporous states and coma are not commonly seen in ischemic strokes. If coma is present in a stroke patient, suspect that either the RAS within the brainstem or both cerebral hemispheres have been affected. If the patient becomes comatose at the onset of the stroke, the patient has most likely suffered a severe hemorrhagic stroke or the basilar artery has been occluded. Suspect possible brain herniation in any patient presenting with an altered mental status after the onset of stroke signs and symptoms.

Airway control in the stroke patient is critical in that brain damage can substantially reduce one's ability to swallow. Accumulating secretions or vomitus present the dangerous prospect of total airway obstruction or pulmonary aspiration. Additionally, the stuporous or comatose patient can lose submandibular tonicity. With no muscular support, the tongue falls to the posterior pharynx, creating an occlusion.

Pay careful attention to respiratory status. Adequacy and patterns of ventilation deserve careful attention. Increased intracranial pressure (ICP) and associated cerebral herniation can produce many outward changes, including the emergence of pathological respiratory patterns. Pathological respiratory patterns associated with stroke include the following (review Table 7-1):

- *Cheyne-Stokes respirations*
- *Central neurogenic hyperventilation*
- *Biot's (ataxic) respirations*
- *Apneustic respirations*

Cheyne-Stokes respirations a pathological pattern of respiration characterized by a regular cycle of crescendo, decrescendo, apnea; often associated with a brain injury, such as stroke.

central neurogenic respirations a pathological pattern of rapid, deep respirations; often associated with brain injury or herniation.

Biot's (ataxic) respirations pathological respirations with no coordinated pattern; often associated with stroke.

apneustic respirations a pathological pattern of long, deep respirations followed by apnea; often associated with severe central nervous system disease or stroke.

Significantly, mortality associated with a stroke is primarily respiratory related.

A stroke or TIA is capable of provoking cardiac complications from direct brain injury, increased ICP, or hypoxia, so full evaluation of the circulatory status is warranted. Radial and/or carotid pulse evaluation may reveal dysrhythmias or other deficits that decrease the heart's ability to adequately perfuse the brain. If cardiovascular collapse has occurred secondary to cerebral herniation, pulses may be quite difficult to locate.

Physical Exam A physical and neurologic exam should be conducted on anyone with a suspected stroke or TIA. Refer to the "Physical Exam" section and Table 7-2, Neurologic Exam, earlier in this chapter, and refer to the description of the Cincinnati Prehospital Stroke Scale (CPSS) and the Los Angeles Prehospital Stroke Screen (LAPSS) in Chapter 1, Assessment of the Medical Patient. In your physical exam, it is important to assess for a facial droop or facial asymmetry (Figure 7-6), weak grip strength, arm drift (Figure 7-7), and speech abnormalities. Have the patient say "You can't teach an old dog new tricks" to test the speech pattern. Assess neurologic function and record the Glasgow Coma Score. Also assess motor and sensory function.

Vital Signs The vital signs associated with a stroke can vary dramatically. Depending on the location of the lesion and the presence of ICP, a variety of respiratory patterns and adequacy can present. Pulse rates are easily increased by the sympathetic nervous system or decreased to bradycardic rates.

Regardless of the type of stroke, blood pressure associated with a stroke is typically normal to elevated. The presence of hypotension should signal you to search for a condition other than a stroke. Medications such as antihypertensives,

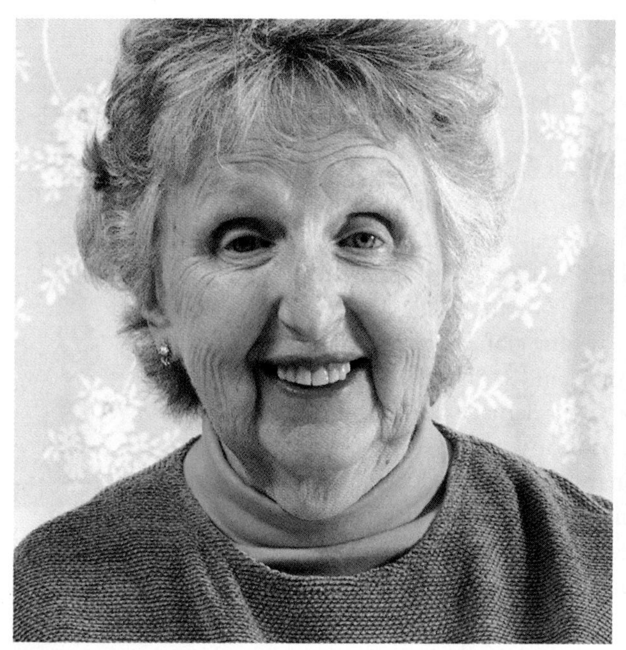

(a)

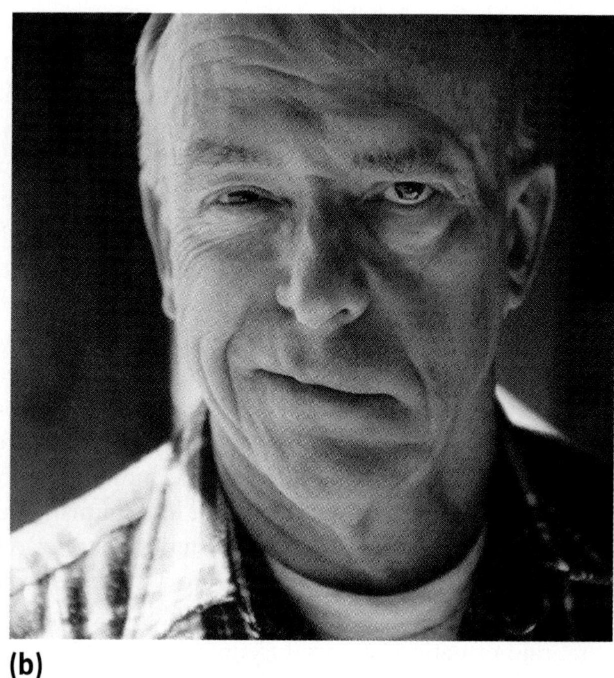

(b)

FIGURE 7-6
(a) The face of a nonstroke patient has normal symmetry. (b) The face of a stroke patient often has an abnormal, drooped appearance on one side. *(Both: © Michal Heron)*

beta-blockers, or diuretics work to decrease the blood pressure. Therefore, pay attention to whether such medications have been used and their potential effects.

Focused History When readily obtainable, a focused medical history, especially a description of events surrounding the onset of altered mental status, can be helpful in confirming the presence of a stroke and differentiating the specific type. The following information, compiled in a SAMPLE format, proves useful when applied to the stroke patient.

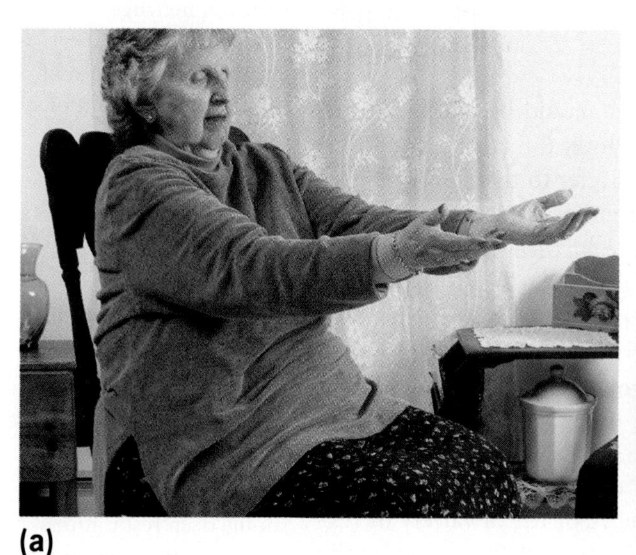

(a)

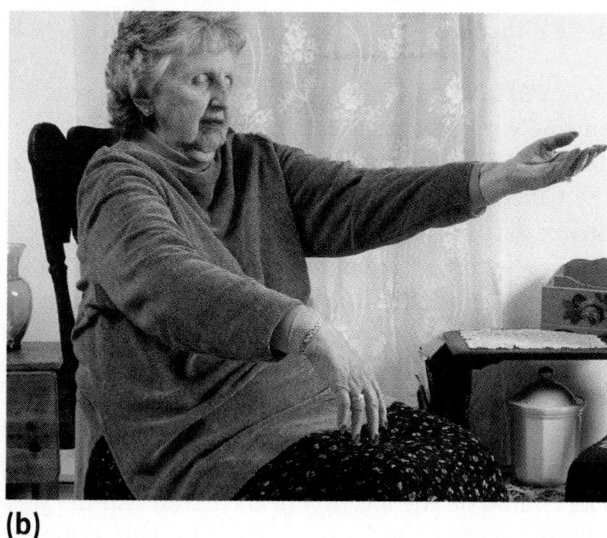

(b)

FIGURE 7-7
(a) A patient who has not suffered a stroke can generally hold arms in an extended position with eyes closed. (b) A stroke patient will often display "arm drift"; that is, one arm will remain extended when held outward with eyes closed, but the other arm will drift or drop downward. *(Both: © Michal Heron)*

In the stroke patient, it is imperative to determine the time of onset of the signs and symptoms due to the narrow window in which fibrinolytic drugs can be administered. The time of onset of the first signs and symptoms is referred to as "time zero." If a patient is found or wakes with signs or symptoms of stroke, time zero becomes the last time in which the patient presented as being normal or without signs and symptoms of stroke. Because this information is crucial to treatment, be sure to relay it to the receiving hospital, include it in your oral report, and document it on your prehospital care report. You may also want to transport a family member, the caregiver, or any other person who last witnessed a normal state of the patient to definitely establish time zero.

Signs and Symptoms. The presence or absence of the signs and symptoms in the following list can help confirm the presence and severity of a stroke:

- Headache
- Declining or improving mental or neurologic status
- *Hemiplegia*
- *Hemiparesis*
- *Dysphasia* or *aphasia*
- Motor or expressive aphasia (Broca's aphasia)—patient understands and knows what to say but cannot form the words
- Receptive aphasia—patient cannot understand what is being said or asked and does not respond or does not respond appropriately
- Cardiac involvement (chest pain, shortness of breath, or dizziness)
- Nausea or vomiting
- *Syncopal episodes*
- Unilateral pupil dilation (Figure 7-8)—indicates brain herniation
- Fixed and dilated pupil—if found in an alert patient with severe headache it may indicate a hemorrhagic stroke

hemiplegia paralysis to one side of the body.

hemiparesis weakness to one side of the body.

dysphasia impairment of speech.

aphasia absence of the ability to communicate through speech.

syncopal episode an episode of fainting.

Allergies. Note any medical allergies the patient may have.

Medications. Identifying medications gives insight into the patient's past medical history. In particular, be cognizant of medications that relate to diabetes or the cardiovascular system. Such medications include

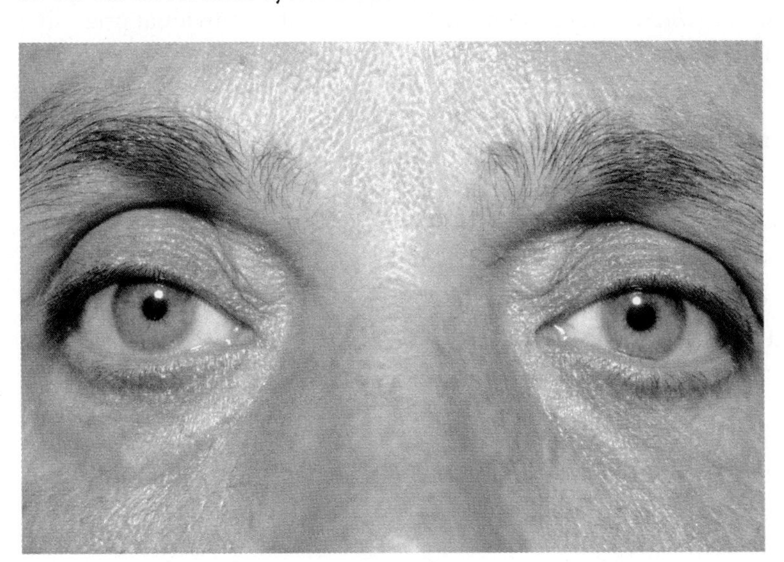

FIGURE 7-8
Unilateral pupil dilation indicates brain herniation. *(© Medscan/Corbis)*

- Anticoagulants or antiplatelets (aspirin, Coumadin)
- Antihypertensives
- Anticholesteremics
- Cardiac medications
- Insulin or oral antihyperglycemics
- Oral contraceptives

Medications that indicate a propensity for thrombus formation (anticoagulants, antiplatelets, anticholesteremics) or preexisting hypertension (antihypertensives) are particularly noteworthy. Also, cardiac drugs may reveal the presence of atrial fibrillation or other dysrhythmias that increase the chance for clot and subsequent embolus creation. The same applies to oral contraceptives.

Past Medical History. Many medical conditions increase one's chances of incurring a stroke. Therefore, all underlying medical problems, especially cardiovascular or diabetic conditions, should be obtained. Inquire about the following factors:

- Previous stroke or TIA
- Hypertension
- Atherosclerosis, coronary artery disease
- Hypercholesteremia
- Cardiac dysrhythmia (especially atrial fibrillation)
- Aneurysms or AV malformations
- Diabetes mellitus
- Cigarette smoking
- Carotid surgery

A past medical history that includes any of these factors is important in reinforcing the suspicion of a stroke or TIA. This information must be relayed to the hospital staff.

Last Oral Intake. The patient's last ingestion of food is significant so that the possibility of vomiting and aspiration can be gauged, if it has not already occurred. Additionally, if surgical intervention is required, the hospital staff must have this information.

Events Prior to Illness. The events or behavior of the individual preceding the onset of the stroke or TIA can help identify the type of stroke that has occurred:

- Gradual or acute onset
- Time of onset
- Improving or declining mental or neurologic status
- Complaints preceding the incident (headache, confusion, dizziness, falls)
- Occurrence during rest or with exertion
- Associated seizure activity

Management of the Stroke or TIA Patient

Treatment of an ischemic or hemorrhagic stroke centers on the support of lost function. Securing a patent airway and ensuring adequate ventilation and oxygenation are the initial priorities. Expedited transport to an appropriate medical facility—one with computed tomography (CT) scanning, fibrinolytic medication administration capabilities, and access to interventional neuroradiology—is critical. In some cases, the effects of an ischemic stroke can be greatly mitigated or reversed if treated quickly. As with a heart attack ("time is myocardium"), time is a critical element in treatment of many strokes ("time is brain cells").

Note that aggressive hyperventilation of the head-injured patient, or the patient with increase ICP, is not recommended. Overzealous hyperventilation will result in a significant decrease in the $PaCO_2$, which will result in excessive cerebral vasoconstriction and decreased cerebral perfusion pressure with a resultant decrease in cerebral blood flow.

The current recommendation for hyperventilation in the severely head-injured patient with evidence of herniation or increased ICP is 20 ventilations/minute. The following would be signs that would warrant hyperventilation at 20/ventilations per minute: 1) unilateral or bilateral dilated pupil; 2) asymmetric pupil reactivity; and 3) nonpurposeful posturing (flexion, also called decorticate posturing, or extension, also called decerebrate posturing). If none of these signs is present, the patient should be ventilated at 10 to 12 ventilations/minute. The keys to treatment are to maintain a patent airway and adequate alveolar ventilation; administer supplemental oxygen; reverse and prevent hypoxia, hypercarbia, hyperthermia, and acidosis; prevent or reverse hypotension by maintaining a systolic blood pressure of 90 mmHg or greater; and prevent or immediately control seizures.

Use an isotonic crystalloid when establishing intravenous access. Unless massive hemodynamic collapse exists, IV fluid administration should be maintained at a TKO rate to limit unnecessary increases in ICP. Avoid dextrose-containing solutions because cerebral edema and worsened neurologic outcomes have been reported as sugar metabolization forces hypoosmolar fluid shifts from the vessels into the brain tissue. Therefore, do not indiscriminately give D_{50} or any other glucose to patients with altered mental status; it is too big a risk if the patient is having a stroke. Research has shown a worsened neurologic outcome following the administration of glucose in patients with intracranial pathology. Always assess the blood glucose with a glucometer before administering dextrose to be sure the patient receiving the dextrose is experiencing a hypoglycemic diabetic emergency, not a stroke or TIA.

As recent advances in the early treatment of stroke have been realized, expeditious transport, preferably to a stroke center or the nearest medical facility capable of managing stroke patients, is paramount. Notify the receiving facility as promptly as possible to permit the staff adequate time to prepare for your patient. Continually monitor changes in mental, neurologic, respiratory, and circulatory status, stabilizing them as needed. Follow your local protocol in performing stroke assessments (LAPSS, CPSS) and required reporting criteria.

As recent advances in the early treatment of stroke have been realized, expeditious transport to the hospital is paramount.

Proper treatment of stroke-induced hypertension is an important consideration. Previously, for a hypertensive patient who has suffered a hemorrhagic stroke, guidelines recommend reduction of the blood pressure to prehemorrhagic levels. However, research indicates that the brain may need the hypertension in the face of a stroke in order to maintain cerebral perfusion. Indiscriminate blood pressure reduction may be perilous. Adhere to local protocols and consult medical direction.

Ongoing Assessment

Until transfer to the hospital staff, continuously monitor the patient by repeating the initial assessment, reassessing vital signs, and checking interventions. Note and manage any changes in the patient's condition, such as seizures, rising ICP, hypoventilation, or airway obstruction.

Cranial Infection

When a pathogen circumvents the body's natural defenses and establishes residence, infection occurs. Infection of the brain or its supporting structures represents a structural alteration with consequent mental or behavioral disturbances. Although many infectious processes have the potential to afflict the brain, meningitis, encephalitis, and cerebral abscess occur with greater frequency.

Meningitis

Meningitis is the infection and inflammation of the meningeal membranes that surround and protect the brain (review Figure 7-4). Meningitis can be caused by a bacterium, virus, fungus, or any pathogen that gains access to the meningeal membranes. Upon infection, a wide array of alterations in mental and behavioral status can be observed.

Because the cranial vault is closed, inflammation of the meningeal layers increases ICP. Associated compression of brain tissue destroys neurons, while compression of cerebral vessels deprives other regions of the brain of adequate blood flow. Along similar lines, increased ICP can obstruct the flow of cerebral spinal fluid, thus decreasing the nutritional bath required by the brain. Depending on severity, the infection may spread to the brain itself and cause a cerebral abscess or encephalitis.

As the infectious process encompasses the entire meninges, the patient may exhibit alterations in mental status that range from drowsiness to stupor to coma and seizure activity. In addition to fever, nausea, and extensive vomiting, the patient may also acknowledge a persistent headache. Because the meninges surround the brain and spinal cord, nuchal rigidity, or neck stiffness, may be noted. Intolerance to light, sound, or ocular movement is a common finding in the patient with meningitis.

Signs of meningeal inflammation may include flexion of the head that causes neck pain and a reflexive flexion of the hips and knees (*Brudzinski's sign*). Flexion of the extremities with pain and resistance on subsequent straightening (*Kernig's sign*) also suggests meningeal inflammation. However, meningitis *can* be present in the absence of these findings. If the inflammation compresses a particular region of the brain, neurologic signs such as hemiparesis or flaccidity may be observed.

Brudzinski's sign flexion of the head that causes neck pain and a reflexive flexion of the hips and knees.

Kernig's sign flexion of the extremities with pain and resistance on subsequent straightening.

Encephalitis

Encephalitis is an infection of the brain tissue itself. Although it can be caused by various bacterial pathogens, the most frequent origin of encephalitis is viral. Encephalitis generally results from an infectious process that occurs elsewhere in the body but gains access to the brain by way of the peripheral nerves or blood vessels. Herpes is an example of a viral pathogen that can cause encephalitis; a less common example is rabies.

Once infection gains a foothold within the brain, inflammation and tissue destruction cause alterations in cerebral function. Over time, continued neuronal degeneration and vascular congestion produce complaints that include fever, headache, personality changes, and confusion. Progression of encephalitis involves agitation, seizures, and stupor. As the entire cerebrum or RAS becomes involved, coma will result.

Depending on the extent of infection, specific neurologic deficits may be noted. *Ataxia*, pupil irregularities, visual disturbances, and facial or ocular palsies may be observable. Encephalitis may also present with nuchal rigidity. You will note that these signs are similar to those for meningitis. Accordingly, encephalitis is very difficult to distinguish from meningitis in the field.

ataxia defective muscular coordination.

Cerebral Abscess

A cerebral abscess is a localized accumulation of purulent material, or pus, within the brain. A cerebral abscess develops when the residue from a bacterial invasion liquefies and accumulates leukocytes, tissue debris, and proteins from the body's immune response. To contain the byproducts, a fibrous capsule forms around the pus. As purulent material within the capsule accumulates, expansion results in the destruction of brain tissue and compression of blood vessels.

The patient with a cerebral abscess may exhibit overt changes in mental status associated with a chronic headache that worsens as ICP increases. Also, focal neurologic deficits can occur specific to the affected region of the brain. If the abscess ruptures, meningitis or encephalitis is a distinct possibility.

Frequently, a cerebral abscess begins as an infection of the nasal cavity, middle ear, or mastoid cells that communicate directly into the brain. Open skull fractures or intracranial operations can also precipitate a brain abscess.

Assessment of Possible Cranial Infection

The following section describes specifics about assessment of a patient suffering an intracranial infection (Table 7-4)—within the generic framework for assessment that was presented earlier in the chapter. The points raised here may apply to the way you conduct your assessment when you already suspect an intracranial infection, or may bring out factors that would point to intracranial infection as a cause of the patient's altered mental status.

The assessment of infection occurring within the cranial vault is quite similar to that for a patient suffering a stroke. Like a stroke, infection of the brain and/or supporting structures can alter mental status and cause neurologic dysfunction. Subsequently, once an infection is suspected, the assessment should work toward describing where it has established itself within the brain and the severity to which it has progressed.

Scene Size-Up During the scene size-up, search for clues that relate to existing medical problems. In particular, the presence of antibiotics or other medications that suggest a recent infection may point to a cranial infection as a cause of altered mental status. Once an infectious cause is suspected, personal protective equipment, including mask, should be worn.

TABLE 7-4 Cranial Infection and Altered Mental Status: Typical Findings

Scene Size-up	Initial Assessment	Physical Exam/Vitals	History
Antibiotics	Airway compromise (vomiting is common) Pathological respiratory patterns may result from increased intracranial pressure Tachycardia from hypermetabolic state; hot, dry, flushed skin	Similar to stroke: Visual disturbances, pupillary dysfunction; facial droop, swallowing difficulty, tongue deviation, weakness or sensory deficit in extremities, gait ataxia, incontinence Nuchal (neck) rigidity; Brudzinski's and Kernig's signs Early vital signs elevated; late vital signs decreased with possible Cheyne-Stokes or central neurogenic respirations	Signs/symptoms: fever, headache, hemiplegia, hemiparesis, visual deficits, hearing loss, nausea/vomiting, syncope; declining or improving mental or neurologic status Antibiotic medications History of recent sinus, ear, or oral cavity infection; history of prior intracranial infection; possible associated seizure activity

Initial Assessment With meningitis or encephalitis, depending on the severity of infection, a chief complaint of persistent headache associated with fever, neck stiffness, or visual disturbances may accompany the outward display of altered mental status. Because a cerebral abscess tends to remain isolated within a particular region of the brain, the chief complaint may mimic a stroke in terms of localized impairments in neurologic function. In severe cases of intracranial infection, lethargy, stupor, or coma may be the chief complaint.

Quickly evaluate airway patency. Vomiting is common in intracranial infections and prompts a concern for aspiration. Again, as neurologic control can be impaired, you must be alert for the loss of swallowing ability with its associated complications.

Assess and classify the respiratory status as either adequate or inadequate. As with a stroke, maintain special watch for pathological respiratory patterns that signify increased ICP with associated herniation of the cerebral contents.

Assessment of circulatory status can provide valuable information about possible intracranial infection. Typically, infections produce tachycardic pulse rates because the body has enacted a hypermetabolic state. Hypermetabolism is a compensatory response that serves to increase the overall core temperature, thus creating a less hospitable environment for invading pathogens. Consequently, the skin will appear hot, dry, and flushed.

If the infection has maintained residence for a period of time, dehydration may also be present. Tenting of the skin when pinched, thirst, prolonged capillary refill time, and decreased pulse rate and blood pressure are indications of possible dehydration.

Physical Exam Because of the structural alterations, the assessment of meningitis, encephalitis, and cerebral abscess is very similar to that for a stroke or TIA. A physical exam with neurologic assessment is paramount. Refer to the "Physical Exam" section and Table 7-2, Neurologic Exam.

Vital Signs Depending on the stage of infection and structural involvement, vital signs associated with a cranial infection will vary. Early in the infectious process, elevated vital signs may be noted as a hypermetabolic state increases cardiac rate and output. Accordingly, blood pressure may be normal to slightly elevated, as will the respiratory rate.

As the infection progresses, the body that is unable to compensate for fluid loss or septicemia may show a decrease in cardiac output and blood pressure. If ICP has forced herniation, an increase in blood pressure may be accompanied by a decrease in heart rate as the brainstem incurs damage. At this point, pathological respiratory patterns such as Cheyne-Stokes or central neurogenic hyperventilation may also become evident.

Focused History A thorough history is important in pinpointing a possible intracranial infection. Placed within a SAMPLE format, pertinent information should include, but is not limited to, the following.

Signs and Symptoms. Signs and symptoms surrounding the cranial infection are extremely important in determining the severity or progression of the cranial infection:

- Headache
- Fever
- Declining or improving mental or neurologic status

- Hemiplegia
- Hemiparesis
- Visual deficits
- Hearing loss
- Nausea or vomiting
- Syncopal episodes

Allergies. Obtain and document any medical allergies the patient may have.

Medications. All medications that the patient is taking should be documented and relayed to emergency department personnel. Pay particular attention to medications such as antibiotics that may signify a recent infection.

Past Medical History. Obtain information about any underlying medical problems. Pay particular attention to a recent history of sinus, ear, or oral cavity infections because these can communicate into the meninges and precipitate cerebral abscess or meningitis. Assess for the presence of an indwelling cerebrospinal fluid shunt.

Additionally, keep in mind that once an intracranial infection has occurred, recurrence is not uncommon. So, it is important to find out whether the patient has had any prior occurrence of this type of infection.

Clinical Insight

Intracranial infections may recur, so it is important to obtain a history of any prior occurrence.

Last Oral Intake. The patient's last ingestion of food and/or fluid is important in gauging the possibility of vomiting and aspiration. Also, you can evaluate a recent history of adequate or inadequate dietary and fluid intake.

Events Prior to Illness. The events or behavior surrounding the onset of meningitis, encephalitis, or cerebral abscess are important. Again, ascertain any history of recent illness that may have communicated into the cranial vault:

- Gradual or acute onset
- Time of initial onset
- Associated fever and/or general malaise
- Improvement or decline in mental status since onset
- Persistent headache throughout
- Associated seizure activity

Management of the Cranial Infection Patient

Treatment of meningitis, encephalitis, and cerebral abscess involves emotional support and resuscitation of decreased or lost vital function. As with other medical emergencies, establishing and maintaining a patent airway, adequate ventilation, and oxygenation are priorities of care.

As discussed previously, the patient with increased ICP should be ventilated at a rate of 10 to 12 ventilations/minute unless there are signs of herniation, in which case you would ventilate at 20 per minute. Apply the cardiac monitor and treat any dysrhythmias. Establish intravenous access with an isotonic crystalloid such as 0.9 percent normal saline solution. As with stroke patients, avoid dextrose-containing solutions because cerebral edema and worsened neurologic outcomes have been reported with use of such solutions.

Occasionally, fever and hypermetabolic activity associated with an intracranial infection can cause dehydration. Significant dehydration should be treated with fluid boluses of an isotonic solution at 20 ml/kg. Take care during fluid resuscitation to guard against fluid overload that may lead to an increase in ICP. In the absence of dehydration, run the fluid at a TKO rate. While obtaining IV access, draw blood for laboratory analysis, and evaluate existing glucose levels in relation to the body's hypermetabolic state and possible decreased dietary intake.

Expedited transport is important. Cranial infections, especially meningitis, are time sensitive. Minutes can count. Early antibiotic treatment improves outcome. During transport, the responsive or intubated patient should be positioned in a semi-Fowler's position so gravity can help control ICP. For the unresponsive patient who cannot be intubated, placement in the recovery (lateral recumbent) position is essential to help evacuate vomitus from the airway.

Personal protective equipment should be worn as soon as an infectious agent is suspected. In case of unprotected contact with meningitis, the health care provider needs to exercise a high degree of surveillance and prophylaxis to avoid becoming infected or to obtain prompt treatment if infection is suspected.

Ongoing Assessment

Continually observe the patient for changes in mental, respiratory, and hemodynamic status, and intervene as appropriate.

Seizure Activity

A seizure is an elaborate and uncontrolled electrical discharge of the cerebral neurons. Because the disorganized electrical activity can affect any and all parts of the brain, altered mental status is frequently observed. Depending on the location and/or degree of cerebral involvement, the outward presentation of a seizure ranges from brief lapses in attention to bizarre psychogenic behavior to severe convulsions. It is important to note the etiology of the seizure as being a primary seizure that is associated with epilepsy or another known seizure disorder or as being a secondary seizure that results from a condition influencing neuron function, such as severe hypoxia or hypoglycemia.

See Chapter 10, Seizures and Seizure Disorders, for a complete discussion of the pathophysiology of seizures and their assessment and management.

Intracranial Tumor

Whether malignant or benign, brain tumors alter mental processes and pose a critical situation. A brain tumor is a growing mass within the enclosed cranial cavity that can be located within or on any cerebral structure. The tumor expands at the expense of the brain matter, increasing ICP. The compression of the tissue and cerebral vessels leads to damage and herniation as brain tissue is eventually forced from the skull.

The mental status of an individual with a brain tumor depends on the tumor's size, location, and rate of growth. Common complaints include confusion, amnesia, lethargy, and/or sudden changes in personality. As ICP rises, signs and symptoms such as headache, vomiting, or seizure activity develop. If herniation ensues, decreased levels of consciousness will progress to stupor and/or coma. Additionally, depending on size, location, and place of residence, brain tumors can produce focal neurologic deficits.

Assessment of Possible Intracranial Tumor

The following section details specifics about assessment of a patient suffering an intracranial tumor (Table 7-5)—within the generic framework for assessment

TABLE 7-5 Intracranial Tumor and Altered Mental Status: Typical Findings

Scene Size-up	Initial Assessment	Physical Exam/Vital	History
Patient presentation/ behavior (may range from docile to violent or comatose; possible flexion or extension posturing)	Chief complaint may reveal patient awareness of brain tumor Airway compromise (secretions, vomitus, tongue) Pathological respiratory patterns may result from cerebral herniation Bradycardia or other dysrhythmias	Similar to stroke: Pathological respiratory patterns Vital signs vary with size, location, progression of tumor; pulses may be bradycardic; occasionally normal or tachycardic; blood pressure hypotensive, hypertensive, or normal	Signs/symptoms: headache, hemiplegia, hemiparesis nausea/vomiting, syncope, dizziness, changes in vision, hearing, or sense of smell; declining or improving mental or neurologic status History of brain tumor; possible associated seizure activity; changes in coordination, memory, sensory perceptions

presented earlier in the chapter. The points raised here may apply to assessment when you already suspect an intracranial tumor, or may bring out factors that would point to intracranial tumor as a cause of the patient's altered mental status.

Because any intracranial tumor can cause cognitive and/or neurologic dysfunction, the assessment described here closely parallels that for a stroke. Prehospital assessment of the intracranial tumor revolves around discovering the presence, relative location, and effects that the tumor has on neurologic status or vital function.

Scene Size-Up Brain tumors can alter mental and behavioral status in various ways. Make special note of the patient's status on entrance into the scene because behavior can range from docile to violent to comatose.

Initial Assessment Similar to stroke and cranial infection, intracranial tumors are capable of inducing cerebral damage through compression and herniation. As you approach the patient and form your general impression, evaluate the overall mental and physical status of the patient. Flexion or extension (decorticate or decerebrate posturing) is evidence of advanced CNS compromise, as are other signs of obvious neurologic deficit.

Patients with brain tumors may already be aware of their presence, and the chief complaint may reflect this awareness. A patient who lacks knowledge of the tumor may complain of altered mental status, chronic headache, vision disturbances, or a gradual onset of neurologic deficits. If family or friends are the ones who called for EMS, the chief complaint may be stated as changes in personality, confusion, or erratic behavior.

For the patient whose tumor is responsible for lethargy, stupor, or coma, evaluation of the airway is paramount. As with any patient exhibiting a decrease in consciousness, secretions, vomitus, or the tongue can cause obstruction. A compromised airway should be immediately corrected. It should be remembered, however, that some tumors will present with seizure. The patient's mental status and ability to protect his airway may improve as the postictal state resolves.

Evaluate respiratory status in reference to adequacy or pathological patterns such as Cheyne-Stokes, apneustic, or central neurogenic hyperventilation. As previously stated, such patterns suggest a tumor that has forced cerebral herniation or is located within the brainstem itself. Establish and maintain a patent airway and adequate ventilation and oxygenation. Do not allow the patient to become hypotensive because this will result in a decrease in cerebral perfusion pressure and cerebral blood flow.

A tumor that has forced herniation or affected the brainstem can also adversely impact the heart and circulatory system. Herniation and destruction of the medullary cardiac center can result in various dysrhythmias, including bradycardia. In addition, hypoxia from inadequate ventilation can also manifest as cardiac difficulties. A cardiac monitor must be placed to determine the electrical status of the myocardium.

Physical Exam Similar to the examination of the stroke patient, the physical exam for the suspected intracranial tumor patient is geared toward the brain and its ability to support neurologic function. The exam should include the neurologic examination outlined in Table 7-2. Information gathered from the neurologic exam can be used to evaluate the presence, location, and general effects of the tumor.

Vital Signs Vital signs associated with an intracranial tumor will vary depending on the size, location, and degree of progression of the tumor. As discussed previously, respiratory patterns associated with cerebral compression and herniation can vary dramatically. Additionally, pulse rates may present as bradycardic secondary to destruction of the brainstem or compression of the vagus nerve. Normal or tachycardic heart rates may also present.

With increased ICP, hypertension may be evident as the body attempts to force perfusion of the hypoperfused brain. Medullary vasomotor center destruction may result in hypertension or hypotension. In the absence of increased ICP or medullary destruction, the blood pressure may present as normal. Recall that anxiety may elevate all vital signs as a result of stimulation of the sympathetic nervous system.

Focused History A pertinent medical history may provide valuable clues that reinforce suspicion of an intracranial tumor. Information as compiled within the SAMPLE format should include, but is not limited to, the following.

Signs and Symptoms. Inquire as to neurologic deficits accompanying the altered mental status. Obtain information about the following signs and symptoms:

- Headache, especially in the morning
- Declining mental or neurologic status
- Hemiplegia
- Hemiparesis
- Seizures
- Nausea or vomiting
- Syncopal episodes
- Dizziness
- Changes in vision, hearing, sense of smell, or sensation (e.g., paresthesia)

Allergies. Note and relay any medical allergies that the patient may have.

Medications. Medications such as anticancer drugs, steroids such as dexamethasone (Decadron), chemotherapy, or radiation therapy are important to note as clues to previous or active cancerous growth.

Past Medical History. Document any underlying problems, particularly an active history of brain or spinal cancer. Pay particular attention to a history of cancer, such as primary lung or breast cancer, that may have metastasized, or spread, to the brain.

Last Oral Intake. The patient's last ingestion of food is important in gauging the possibility of vomiting and aspiration. Also, this information is helpful in evaluating general nutrition.

Events Prior to Illness. Ascertain the events or behavior preceding the onset of altered mental status. Many times, this information can help confirm an intracranial tumor or suggest an alternative cause of the altered mental status:

- Gradual versus acute onset
- Time of onset
- Improving or declining mental status
- Complaints preceding the incident (headache, confusion, dizziness, falls)
- Associated seizure activity
- Changes in coordination, memory, smell, hearing, or vision

Management of the Intracranial Tumor Patient

Management of a patient with an intracranial tumor focuses primarily on the support of decreased respiratory and cardiovascular function.

Establish and maintain an a patent airway and adequate ventilation, oxygenation, and circulation. Do not allow the patient to become hypotensive. When indicated, increased ICP is best managed as previously discussed under "Management of the Stroke or TIA Patient."

Patients with intracranial tumors are prone to seizure activity, which should be managed as described in Chapter 10. These seizures are of a secondary nature and require management with a benzodiazepine to immediately stop the seizure activity.

Transport the patient with an intracranial tumor in a semi-Fowler's position to help decrease ICP. If the patient is not intubated, transport the patient in the recovery position to assist in draining vomitus and avoiding aspiration.

Ongoing Assessment

Continued observation of mental status, airway, breathing, and circulatory parameters is necessary throughout transport, with changes managed as appropriate.

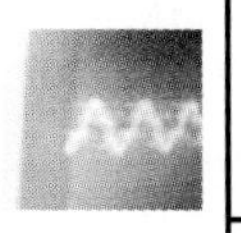

DIFFERENTIAL DIAGNOSIS: EXTRACRANIAL CAUSES OF ALTERED MENTAL STATUS

Extracranial etiologies of altered mental status are those that originate outside the brain and tend to be metabolic in nature. Several of the more common extracranial causes of altered mental status are discussed next.

Pulmonary Causes

Although physically removed from the CNS, the pulmonary system plays a direct role in brain function. The pulmonary system provides for the intake of oxygen and the excretion of carbon dioxide, a byproduct of normal cellular metabolism. Brain activity is highly metabolic and inextricably dependent on the delivery of oxygen for use in the production of the cellular fuel ATP (adenosine triphosphate). Neurons of the CNS are unable to store reserve ATP. Consequently, the brain is highly sensitive to any decrease in oxygen availability.

As with any body cells, the unavailability of oxygen to brain cells produces a state of hypoxia. In response, the cells resort to anaerobic metabolism instead of normal aerobic metabolism. In the short term, anaerobic metabolism is effective in producing minimal levels of ATP for the cellular energy requirements. However, anaerobic metabolism is significantly less efficient than aerobic metabolism and beyond the short term proves destructive, if not fatal, to the brain's cells and activities.

Mild cerebral hypoxia results in restlessness, confusion, or changes in personality ranging from euphoria to irritability. Moderate to severe hypoxia exhibits itself through the impairment of judgment and/or motor ability and may even result in delirium, coma, and death. Essentially, any condition that changes the function of the pulmonary system can induce hypoxic alterations in mental status. Hypoxia typically produces agitation in patients.

Alterations in pulmonary status can also affect the CNS in other ways. During normal cellular metabolism, carbon dioxide and water are produced as waste. Failure of the pulmonary system to excrete carbon dioxide as quickly as it is produced results in the retention of carbon dioxide and the creation of an acidotic environment.

hypercapnia abnormal retention of carbon dioxide.

The abnormal retention of carbon dioxide within the human body is called *hypercapnia*. Generally, carbon dioxide levels are measured through an evaluation of arterial blood and fall within the range of 35 to 45 torr. Any measurement of arterial carbon dioxide greater than 45 torr indicates hypercapnia.

Brain cells are very sensitive to hypercapnia, and significant increases in CO_2 lead to changes in mental status. An acidotic environment alters normal cellular activity and promotes the depression of cerebral function. In addition, carbon dioxide is a potent vasodilator, which serves to improve cerebral blood flow but may also increase ICP. Typically, hypercapnia is evidenced by headache, blurred vision, confusion, somnolence, and fatigue or weakness. In the absence of intervention, cerebral damage and death can result.

Conditions with the potential for the creation of hypoxic and hypercapnic environments include

- Pulmonary hypertension
- COPD
- Cystic and pulmonary fibrosis
- Pulmonary edema (from both cardiogenic and noncardiogenic causes)
- Pneumonia and bronchitis
- Asthma
- Toxic inhalation
- Cancerous tumors
- Tuberculosis
- Muscular dystrophy

Review Chapter 5, Dyspnea, for a discussion of the assessment and management of respiratory complaints.

Cardiac Causes

The heart's sole purpose is to pump blood throughout the circulatory system. While the left ventricle ejects oxygenated blood into the arterial system for delivery to all cells and tissues, waste-ridden blood is delivered by the right ventricle to the lungs for the removal of carbon dioxide and reoxygenation. Without adequate myocardial pumping, circulation is compromised. Cells dysfunction as the absence of oxygen leads to anaerobic metabolism and the accumulation of acidic waste.

As stated previously, the brain is a highly metabolic organ that depends on the bloodborne delivery of oxygen and removal of waste. Even if adequate levels of oxygen are present in the lungs, compromised circulation results in hypoperfusion of the body and the brain. Anaerobic metabolism ensues. Again, anaerobic metabolism is a short-term, stop-gap measure that quickly becomes destructive if the underlying cause is not corrected.

Hypoperfusion secondary to the heart's inability to provide an adequate cardiac output results in cerebral hypoxia. Outward signs of this deficiency are readily observable through changes in mental status. Cardiac conditions related to altered mental status include

Hypoperfusion secondary to the heart's inability to provide an adequate cardiac output results in cerebral hypoxia.

- Cardiac arrest
- Cardiac dysrhythmias
- Ischemia/myocardial infarction
- Cardiomyopathy
- Aortic stenosis
- Orthostatic hypotension
- Carotid sinus syncope (technically, a bradydysrhythmia)
- Left ventricular failure/cardiogenic shock
- Pulmonary embolism (not cardiac, but flow related)

Review Chapter 6, Chest Discomfort or Pain, for a discussion of the assessment and management of cardiac complaints.

Diabetes Mellitus

Glucose, the end product of carbohydrate digestion, represents the primary energy source required by the human body. In the presence of oxygen, all cells use glucose in the production of the cellular fuel ATP. Normal cellular function, including that of the cerebral neurons, depends on a continual supply of glucose. In its absence, ATP levels drop, with a subsequent decline in cellular activity.

Glucose molecules cross cell membranes by way of facilitated diffusion. Insulin, a hormone secreted by the beta cells of the pancreas, is one of the key controlling hormones that regulates this passage of glucose across the cellular membrane. Insulin attaches to a receptor site on the cell membrane and opens a protein channel that, in turn, allows the glucose to be carried across the cell membrane by a protein carrier.

Unlike other body cells, the cerebral neurons rely almost exclusively on glucose and do not fare well with alternative energy sources such as fats and lipids. Also, brain cells do not require the presence of insulin for glucose to cross the blood–brain barrier because ample amounts of glucose independently diffuse across the cellular membrane. Unlike other cells, brain cells have no internal stores of glucose (glycogen). As a highly metabolic tissue, the brain does not readily tolerate shortages of glucose. Inadequate amounts of cerebral glucose result in alteration of mental status that ranges from mild confusion to coma. Ultimately, without cerebral glucose, the neurons will not be able to produce adequate amounts of ATP. If ATP levels are inadequate, the sodium/potassium pump will fail to regulate the amount of intracellular sodium. The intracellular sodium levels will rise and will attract water within the cell membrane. The cell will swell and eventually rupture and die.

Type I Diabetes Mellitus

Type I diabetes mellitus (DM) is a condition in which there is complete absence of insulin secretion by the pancreatic beta cells. The type I DM patient typically contracts the diabetic condition before the age of 30 and requires administration of exogenous insulin. The type I DM patient is more prone to two types of diabetic emergencies, hypoglycemia and diabetic ketoacidosis, than are type II DM patients.

Hypoglycemia Hypoglycemia is the net result of insulin administration without the consumption of complimentary glucose. Causes include the lack of dietary intake following insulin intake or the rapid utilization of ingested glucose as occurs during exertion or fever.

The result of such events is hypoglycemia, or low blood glucose levels. The overbalance of insulin moves too much glucose into the body cells, causing a deficit of glucose in the bloodstream. As the brain relies almost exclusively on bloodborne glucose as an energy source, any decrease in blood glucose level impairs its ability to continue normal function. An alteration in mental status is quickly witnessed and progresses from irritability to confusion to stupor and coma.

In addition to an altered mental status, the health care provider will note signs and symptoms that relate to a sympathetic nervous system response referred to as a hyperadrenergic response. Epinephrine is considered a glucoregulatory hormone, that is, one that attempts to increase the blood glucose level. Epinephrine will decrease or cease the secretion of insulin by the beta cells in the pancreas. Also, epinephrine will increase glycogenolysis, the conversion of stored glycogen in the liver into glucose, and gluconeogenesis, the conversion of noncarbohydrate substances into glucose. The typical signs and symptoms associated with epinephrine, such as tachycardia, palpitations, normal to slightly elevated blood pressure, and pale, cool, diaphoretic skin, are all side effects of the release of epinephrine from the adrenal medulla in an attempt to increase the blood glucose level. The patient may also experience hunger, generalized weakness, a sensation of warmth, and dizziness as a result of the hyperadrenergic resonse.

Hypoglycemia was historically referred to as "insulin shock." This was because of the hypoglycemic patient's presentation of pale, cool, clammy skin and tachycardia, the same signs that are seen in the patient with hypovolemic shock. The reason the two patients present alike is the release of epinephrine in both conditions. In hypovolemic shock, the epinephrine is attempting to shunt blood to the core of the body, preserve volume, and increase blood pressure, whereas in hypoglycemia the epinephrine is released in an attempt to raise the circulating blood glucose level. However, as noted, the two patients present with like signs.

A second set of signs and symptoms exhibited in hypoglycmemia is referred to as neuroglucopenic. These result from the loss of an adequate amount of glucose in the brain cells, which leads to neural dysfunction. These signs and symptoms include altered mental status, bizarre behavior, stupor, confusion, disorientation, focal neurologic deficits, seizure, and coma. The onset of the signs and symptoms is usually very quick, occuring within minutes to hours. An evaluation of the blood glucose level frequently reveals a reading less than 40 mg/dl.

Diabetic Ketoacidosis The undiagnosed diabetic or the insulin-dependent diabetic who fails to take exogenous insulin as prescribed is prone to the development of diabetic ketoacidosis (DKA). In the absence of insulin necessary to move glucose into the body cells, glucose accumulates in the bloodstream, resulting in hyperglycemia. The elevated blood glucose level results in a higher osmotic pressure and draws water from the interstitial and intracellular compartments. This action essentially dehydrates the cells and changes their ability to function in a routine manner.

As the hyperglycemic blood reaches a glucose level greater than 180 mg/dl, the kidneys are unable to reabsorb the excess glucose. Osmotic diuresis ensues as glucose spills over into the urine. Because the urine contains excessive glucose, the kidneys also excrete water, resulting in voluminous urinary output, or polyuria. The net result is profound dehydration. The brain gets plenty of glucose in DKA because insulin is not required to move glucose across the blood–brain barrier. However, over a period of usually 2 to 3 days, the patient begins to display alterations in mental status. This is not directly related to glucose disturbances in the brain, because the brain has large amounts of glucose, but is a direct result of the dehydration of brain cells from intravascular osmotic changes and excessive urination, as well as from metabolic acidosis associated with the metabolism of fats.

The starving cells look toward other sources of energy for the production of ATP, and the body begins to metabolize proteins and fats, which results in the accumulation of ketones. Ketones are a group of very strong organic acids that rapidly drop the blood pH to an acidotic state referred to as ketoacidosis or ketosis.

Sensing an acidotic state, the medullary respiratory center increases the rate and depth of ventilation. Known as Kussmaul's respirations, the deep and rapid respirations are an attempt to return the blood pH to normal by exhaling large amounts of carbon dioxide and thus reducing the carbonic acid level. A small amount of acetone, a byproduct of ketosis, is excreted through the lungs and accounts for the presence of a "fruity" odor on the DKA patient's breath.

At the same time, the kidneys excrete the negatively charged ketone bodies. Unfortunately, because the ketones are strong organic acids, they need to be buffered with positively charged sodium or potassium. This excretion creates further complications through an electrolyte imbalance.

Eventually, Kussmaul's respirations are unable to compensate, and the ketoacidosis progresses to metabolic acidosis. In combination, profound dehydration, electrolyte imbalances, and acidosis severely depress the CNS. If uncorrected, death will occur. This process is slow and may take days to weeks.

As a result of the pathophysiology underlying DKA, you may observe an alteration in mental status that ranges from confusion to lethargy to coma. Signs and symptoms stemming from dehydration are readily evident in terms of tachycardia, decreased blood pressure, dry mucous membranes, and poor skin turgor. In addition, the presence of Kussmaul's respirations coupled with a sweet acetone odor is critical in the identification of DKA.

As a result of the pathophysiology underlying DKA, you may observe an alteration in mental status that ranges from confusion to lethargy to coma.

Many people mistakenly think that the term *diabetic* implies a glucose disturbance; however, *diabetic* really refers to an increase in urine output and does not address a glucose issue. *Mellitus* means "sweetness." Thus, the patient who suffers from DM is experiencing a condition with both an increase in urine output (diabetic) and an increase in glucose in the blood (mellitus). It is the high blood glucose level that increases the urine output.

Diabetes insipidus is another example where understanding the termininology helps in understanding the condition. With diabetes insipidus, it is a reduction in the secretion of antidiuretic hormone from the posterior pituitary gland that leads to excessive urination. There is no disturbance in the glucose level. Again, *diabetes* means an increase in urine output, while *insipidus* means "tasteless." In the older days, diabetes was checked by tasting the urine for sweetness. In diabetes insipidus, because there is no glucose in the urine and a large amount of urine is being produced, the urine would be tasteless rather than sweet.

The term *diabetic ketoacidosis* also tells you the condition's underlying pathophysiological problems. As noted, *diabetic* means the patient is urinating a large amount of fluid. Because it is related to a hyperglycemic condition, the increase in urine output is from osmotic diuresis. The increased urination causes a severe fluid loss, so you would expect to see signs and symptoms of dehydration. *Ketoacidosis* refers to the production of ketone bodies with a resultant metabolic acidosis, which produces typical signs of metabolic acidosis.

Type II Diabetes Mellitus

Type II DM occurs in the individual who produces inadequate levels of insulin or who produces adequate or high levels of insulin but exhibits resistance to insulin utilization within the body. Generally, the onset of type II DM occurs later in life and requires control through dietary modification, exercise, and the administration of oral antihyperglycemics. The type II DM patient is more prone to the complication of hyperglycemic hyperosmolar nonketotic syndrome (HHNS) and hypoglycemia. HHNS has also been known as hyperglycemic hyperosmolar nonketotic coma (HHNC). DKA rarely occurs in the type II DM patient.

Hyperglycemic Hyperosmolar Nonketotic Syndrome Although the body of the type II DM patient is capable of producing insulin, the amount produced is insufficient or is not sufficiently effective in relation to cellular demand. Following the ingestion of food, the circulating glucose rapidly exceeds the ability of available insulin to promote cellular absorption and storage. As a result, partial cellular nourishment occurs with a simultaneous increase in blood glucose.

Similar to DKA, hyperosmotic blood causes a fluid shift from the extravascular to the intravascular space. Again, cellular dehydration results. The dehydration is especially prominent in the brain, where fluid deficits precipitate cerebral dysfunction. As the blood glucose continues to rise, the kidneys begin the excretion of the excessive glucose accompanied by body water (polyuria). The result is profound dehydration, therein worsening cerebral dysfunction.

Because enough insulin exists to promote some glucose transmission across the cellular membrane, the excessive and overwhelming metabolization of fat with the production of ketone bodies does not take place. In the absence of ketosis, significant metabolic acidosis does not occur. Therefore, dehydration and electrolyte imbalances are the basic causes of mental and behavioral changes. As a result, treatment of the HHNS patient centers around the administration of insulin and aggressive fluid therapy.

When observing the HHNS patient, you will observe a confused to stuporous or comatose patient exhibiting the signs and symptoms of dehydration. These signs and symptoms include tachycardia, dehydrated mucous membranes, normal blood pressure or hypotension, and the absence of acetone on the breath. Additionally, the blood glucose level is often greater than 800 mg/dl.

Again, a look at the condition's name—hyperglycemic hyperosmolar nonketotic syndrome—provides a clue to the pathophysiology. *Hyperglycemic* indicates that the condition is a result of an excessively high blood glucose level. The excessive amount of circulating glucose in the blood is producing a *hyperosmolar* state in the blood. Because the blood is hyperosmolar, it will draw in fluid and begin to dehydrate the interstitial and intracellular spaces. Because the blood is hyperosmolar and the blood glucose is excessively elevated, the kidneys will begin to excrete glucose, leading to dehydration. Look for signs and symptoms of dehydration. *Nonketotic* indicates that an overwhelming number of ketones are not being produced. Without excessive ketones, there is no metabolic acidosis, and the signs and symptoms of metabolic acidosis will not be present. The patient will not have the Kussmaul's respirations, fruity odor on the breath, or flushed skin seen in the DKA patient. As noted previously, HHNS was once refered to as HHNC, with the "C" indicating coma. Because not all patients present with coma, the name was changed to HHNS with the "S" implying it is a syndrome comprised of numerous signs and symptoms. With dehydration as the primary pathophysiological problem, rehydration is the primary treatment.

Assessment of Possible Diabetic-Induced Altered Mental Status

The following section details specifics about assessment of a patient suffering a diabetic emergency (Table 7-6)—within the generic framework for assessment presented earlier in the chapter. The points raised here may apply to assessment when you already suspect that the patient is diabetic, or may bring out factors that would point to a diabetic cause of the patient's altered mental status.

As discussed previously, diabetic complications are varied. Differentiation of diabetic complications relies on a working knowledge of the individual pathophysiologies and strong assessment skills.

Scene Size-Up As you size up the scene, note the presence of items such as hypodermic syringes, insulin, glucometers, or lower extremity prosthetic devices, which are tip-offs as to the presence of diabetes.

Initial Assessment As you approach the diabetic patient, formulate a general impression as to current mental status. If the patient is seemingly unresponsive, listen for adventitious noises relating to airway occlusion. In addition, there may be a pervasive smell of ketones that would signify the possibility of DKA.

The conscious diabetic who is unaware that he is diabetic or that his condition is related to his diabetes may offer a chief complaint of confusion, restlessness, or weakness. Even if the patient knows he is diabetic, confusion may prevent him from relaying this information. Some diabetics will be familiar with the signs of fluctuation in blood sugar and relay the chief complaint accordingly.

If the patient is unresponsive, you must question family, friends, or bystanders when available. If there is no one to offer a chief complaint, you will have to obtain it through a thorough assessment and strong index of suspicion.

Evaluate and assure airway patency. The unresponsive diabetic patient can vomit or lose muscular control of the tongue. The respiratory status can provide invaluable information as to the type of diabetic complication that may be present. In addition to evaluating adequacy, look for the deep and rapid pattern of Kussmaul's respirations. Kussmaul's respirations are typically seen in the acidotic condition of DKA as the body attempts pH stabilization by excreting mass quantities of carbon dioxide.

Pay attention to the strength and regularity of radial or carotid pulses. Weak, rapid pulses are commonly associated with DKA and HHNS, while rapid, full pulses typically accompany hypoglycemia. Peripheral perfusion parameters are

Clinical Insight

For a patient with previously diagnosed diabetes, the presence of insulin or other diabetic medications, injection sites, a glucometer, or a medical alert bracelet will alert you to the patient's condition. However, if these clues are not present, do not rule out diabetes as a possible underlying cause of altered mental status until you have measured the blood glucose level. Many diabetics have not been diagnosed, and the current emergency may be their first indication of the condition.

TABLE 7-6 Diabetic-Induced Altered Mental Status: Typical Findings

	Scene Size-up	Initial Assessment	Physical Exam/Vitals	History
Hypoglycemia	Presence of syringes, insulin, glucometers, lower extremity prosthetic devices	Chief complaint may reveal patient or family awareness of diabetic condition; may complain of confusion, restlessness, weakness Acute onset Airway compromise (vomitus, tongue) **Full, rapid pulses** **Diaphoresis**	**Pupils normal to dilated*** Abdomen and extremities: insulin administration sites; medical alert jewelry Slow-healing wounds, distal neuropathy, poor peripheral perfusion; scarring of fingers; provisional amputations **Vital signs: full, rapid pulses; normal-to-shallow respirations; normal blood pressure**	Signs/symptoms: weakness, lethargy, confusion; hunger, thirst, polyuria; chest pain, shortness of breath, dizziness (with cardiac involvement); nausea, vomiting, diarrhea; malaise; abdominal pain (with electrolyte shifts) History of diabetes, cardiac, renal, or vascular disease, obesity, endocrine problems; exertion, infection
Diabetic Ketoacidosis (DKA/hyperglycemia)	Presence of syringes, insulin, glucometers, lower extremity prosthetic devices	Chief complaint may reveal patient or family awareness of diabetic condition; may complain of confusion, restlessness, weakness Gradual onset **"Fruity" smell of ketones on patient's breath** Airway compromise **Kussmaul's respirations** **Weak, rapid pulses** **Poor skin turgor, pallor, delayed capillary refill related to dehydration**	**Sunken orbits related to dehydration** **Ketone odor** Injection sites; medical alert jewelry Slow-healing wounds, distal neuropathy, poor peripheral perfusion; scarring of fingers; provisional amputations **Poor skin turgor (dehydration)** **Vital signs: weak, rapid pulses; Kussmaul's respirations; low blood pressure in later stages**	Signs/symptoms: weakness, lethargy, confusion; hunger, thirst, polyuria; chest pain, shortness of breath, dizziness (with cardiac involvement); nausea, vomiting, diarrhea; malaise; abdominal pain (with electrolyte shifts) History of diabetes, cardiac disease, renal disease, vascular disease, obesity, endocrine problems; family history of diabetes

*Items in bold type are those that can help distinguish hypoglycemia from hyperglycemia (DKA).

Note: Hyperglycemic hyperosmolar nonketotic syndrome (HHNS) presents like DKA/hyperglycemia, except that ketone odors and Kussmaul's respirations will be absent and respirations will be normal to shallow.

also revealing in that significant dehydration associated with DKA and HHNS will produce poor skin turgor, pallor, and a delayed capillary refill. The presence of diaphoresis suggests hypoglycemia.

Physical Exam The physical exam of the diabetic patient may also help confirm one complication over another. Because glucose fluctuations may mimic the early signs of a stroke, a neurologic assessment as described previously may prove helpful in ruling out a stroke. Concerning the diabetic with altered mental status, important aspects of the physical exam are

- ***Head***
  - Pupils (normal to dilated in hypoglycemia)
  - Orbits (sunken eyes in significant dehydration)
  - Oral cavity (hydration quality)
  - Acetone odor (DKA)
- ***Chest.*** Auscultation of breath sounds may reveal possible aspiration
- ***Abdomen.*** Look for insulin administration sites, which may appear to be very small bruises

- *Extremities*
  - Insulin administration sites
  - Medical alert bracelet or necklace
  - Slow-healing ulcerations or wounds
  - Distal neuropathy (sensory loss in the extremities)
  - Poor peripheral perfusion
  - Provisional amputations
  - Scarring of fingers from repeated punctures for blood glucose
  - Poor skin turgor (decreased relative hydration)

Vital Signs In the diabetic, vital signs can help differentiate the type of complication at play. As stated previously, weak, rapid pulses are commonly associated with DKA and HHNS, while rapid, full pulses typically accompany hypoglycemia. Kussmaul's respirations suggest DKA, while a normal to shallow respiratory status is more indicative of HHNS or hypoglycemia.

Blood pressure can vary, depending on the current hemodynamic status. Hypotension occurs in the later stages of DKA and HHNS, secondary to acidosis and dehydration, respectively. Hypoglycemic patients tend to maintain a normal blood pressure throughout.

Focused History The history is important in confirming the suspicion of diabetic complication and differentiating the type of complication. Using the SAMPLE format, helpful information should include, but is not limited to, the following:

Signs and Symptoms. Information obtained should include

- Weakness or lethargy
- Confusion
- Hunger, thirst, or voluminous urination
- Chest pain, shortness of breath, or dizziness (cardiac involvement)
- Nausea, vomiting, diarrhea
- General malaise
- Abdominal pain (electrolyte shifts)

Allergies. Note and document any allergies that the patient may have.

Medications. Look for the presence of insulin or any oral antihyperglycemics. Determine whether the patient has been compliant in taking the medications as prescribed. Because certain medications are capable of producing fluctuations in glucose levels, obtain and document any and all medications that the patient is taking.

Past Medical History. Diabetes tends to precipitate many problems throughout the body. If the diabetes itself is not at play, associated diabetic complications may be responsible for the altered mental status or may compound it. Information obtained should include

- Diabetes (type I or II)
- Cardiac disease
- Renal disease

- Vascular disease
- Obesity (usually associated with type II DM)
- Genetic history of diabetes (usually associated with type II DM but not type I DM)
- Any endocrine problem

polyuria voluminous output of urine.

polyphagia excessive eating.

polydipsia excessive thirst.

Be aware that *polyuria* (excessive urination), *polyphagia* (excessive eating), and *polydipsia* (excessive thirst) are all signs of undiagnosed diabetes.

Last Oral Intake. Determining the last oral intake, especially with the insulin-dependent diabetic, is paramount. Administration of exogenous insulin without supplemental food will rapidly precipitate a state of hypoglycemia. Ask about the frequency and amounts of food that the patient has been eating, keeping in mind that polyphagia is a sign of undiagnosed diabetes.

Events Prior to Illness. Events precipitating the onset of altered mental status can prove helpful in differentiating the cause:

- Gradual onset (DKA, 2 to 3 days; HHNS, up to 12 days)
- Acute onset with hypoglycemia (usually within minutes to hours)
- Weight loss
- Polyuria, polyphagia, polydipsia (undiagnosed diabetes, DKA, HHNS)
- Exertion—rapid utilization of available glucose (hypoglycemia)
- Vomiting—loss of food substance (hypoglycemia)
- Infection—increased utilization of glucose (hypoglycemia)

Management of the Patient with Diabetic Complications

Field treatment will vary, depending on the type of diabetic complication present. Although hypoglycemia is readily correctable in the prehospital environment, correction of DKA and HHNS require insulin and electrolyte alignment (hypokalemia is a common complication of DKA), both of which are reserved for the hospital setting. For such patients, out-of-hospital intervention is geared toward rehydration and support of decreased respiratory and cardiac function.

Regardless of the type of diabetic complication, airway patency and ventilation with adequate oxygenation must be assured. Protection against aspiration is paramount in the patient who is vomiting. Tracheal intubation of the comatose DKA or HHNS patient is useful in such protection and can assist in stabilization of ketone-induced acidosis as endogenous carbon dioxide is excreted. For the hypoglycemic patient who is not vomiting and is supporting a patent airway, tracheal intubation may be deferred because the underlying condition is relatively easily reversed.

Carefully establish intravenous access with an isotonic crystalloid. Generally, an 18-gauge angiocatheter anchored in a sturdy vein is suggested because aggressive fluid therapy is often required.

For the fluid-deficient DKA or HHNS patient, 20 ml/kg boluses should be aggressively administered with hemodynamic reevaluation following each. Recall that diabetics tend to have multiple medical problems, including heart failure and renal complication. Consequently, careful administration of fluid is necessary so as to avoid fluid overload and pulmonary and cerebral edema. Pulmonary auscultation must follow each administration.

Obtaining blood specimens early is particularly important in the diabetic patient because any administration of prehospital dextrose or other medications will significantly change the chemical makeup. Evaluation with a glucometer will quickly reveal an estimated blood glucose level. Any blood glucose reading of less than 60 mg/dl associated with altered mental status or 50 mg/dl without symptoms warrants immediate consideration of hypoglycemia.

Obtaining blood specimens early is particularly important in the diabetic patient because any administration of prehospital dextrose or other medications will significantly change the chemical makeup of subsequent blood samples.

Because diabetics tend to incur a disproportionate incidence of cardiac problems, apply a cardiac monitor for electrical evaluation. If correction of dehydration, hypoglycemia, hyperglycemia, or acidosis fails to abolish a cardiac dysrhythmia, undertake corrective measures. Supplemental dextrose provides the best means for reversing hypoglycemia. For the hypoglycemic who merely displays confusion and has the ability to swallow and obey your commands, oral ingestion of food, drink, or instant glucose is in order. For any lethargic, stuporous, or comatose hypoglycemic patient or for one who is unable to swallow and to understand or obey your commands, who would possibly aspirate oral glucose, intravenous administration of 50 percent dextrose (25 g) is indicated. Remember that administration of dextrose must *not* be undertaken "blind"—that is, without a obtaining a glucometer reading confirming hypoglycemia.

If a peripheral IV line cannot be established, 1 mg of glucagon can be administered intramuscularly. Glucagon liberates stored glycogen from the liver, thus increasing the overall blood glucose level. Unfortunately, hepatic glycogen has often already been depleted by natural mechanisms, rendering the glucagon ineffective. Additionally, if stored glycogen is available, the onset of action for glucagon is delayed because peak effects occur 10 to 20 minutes after administration.

In the past, it was recommended that a hypoglycemic who appears malnourished or who is an alcoholic should have thiamine administered in close proximity to the dextrose. However, thiamine administration in the field has become quite controversial because there is no reliable scientific evidence supporting its use. Follow local protocols and consult medical direction in this regard.

With hypoglycemia, administration of glucose should bring about a rapid and observable improvement. Following administration, reevaluate the blood glucose level for confirmation. Some EMS services have a treat-and-release policy for acute hypoglycemia/altered mental status that is reversed by administration of D_{50}. Again, follow local protocols and consult medical direction.

Ongoing Assessment

During transport of any patient with diabetic complications, constantly reevaluate the airway, breathing, and circulatory parameters. Closely monitor vital signs.

Hepatic Encephalopathy

Changes in liver function secondary to chronic or acute hepatic, or liver, disease can affect mental presentation. The liver is an essential organ with many tasks that include the conversion of ammonia into urea. Ammonia is produced as amino acids are broken down for utilization. In the liver, the toxic ammonia is converted into less toxic urea for excretion by the kidneys.

Failure of the liver to convert ammonia causes increases in circulating ammonia levels that are quite toxic to the brain. Increased ammonia levels were once believed to be the cause of altered mental status related to hepatic encephalopathy. However, research has shown that ammonia is not the chief toxin that causes altered mental status in hepatic encephalopathy. In fact, there is a poor correlation between ammonia levels and the degree of altered mental status. Other, as yet unclear, causes are at play in altered mental status associated with hepatic encephalopathy.

In addition to altered mentation, the patient with hepatic *encephalopathy* will exhibit other signs of liver failure that include *jaundice, ocular icterus, spider angiomas,* and *edema* or *ascites* secondary to portal hypertension. The patient may also show global wasting as the digestive assistance of the liver has been lost. Of particular clinical significance is the presence of *fector hepaticus,* a musty odor on the patient's breath.

encephalopathy any disease or dysfunction of the brain.

jaundice yellowing of the skin or other tissues.

ocular icterus yellowing of the sclerae.

spider angiomas branched growths of dilated capillaries on the skin.

edema fluid accumulation in the tissues; swelling.

ascites fluid accumulation in the abdomen.

fector hepaticus a musty odor on the breath associated with rising ammonia levels in the blood resulting from a disorder of the liver.

Hepatic encephalopathy occurs in those with chronic liver disease and liver failure. Accordingly, hepatic encephalopathy must be considered for any patient with changes in mental status accompanied by a history of alcoholism, cirrhosis, or hepatitis. Note that hepatic encephalopathy takes days to weeks to develop.

Assessment and treatment of hepatic encephalopathy is discussed with the assessment and treatment of uremic encephalopathy.

Uremic Encephalopathy

Uremic encephalopathy is a condition that results from renal, or kidney, failure. Uremia, which literally means "urine in the blood," affects all organ systems of the body, including the CNS. As such, uremia causes alterations in mental and behavioral status.

The kidneys are responsible for the collection and excretion of metabolic wastes. Renal failure causes the accumulation of these wastes, many of which prove toxic in sufficient amounts. In renal failure, nitrogenous metabolic byproducts quickly accrue in a condition known as azotemia. In addition, the body suffers electrolyte imbalances, fluid shifts, and accumulation of many other unfriendly substances. Acidosis ensues and blood pH plummets.

Secondary to acidosis, electrolyte imbalances, and accumulation of toxins, the uremic patient will exhibit changes in mentation that range from lethargy and confusion to seizures and coma. Other signs and symptoms of uremia include nausea, vomiting, cramping, neuromuscular disorders, malaise, and Kussmaul's respirations. Without intervention, death will result. Note that uremic encephalopathy takes days to weeks to develop.

Assessment of Possible Hepatic or Uremic Encephalopathy

The following section describes specifics about assessment of a patient suffering hepatic or uremic encephalopathy (Table 7-7)—within the generic framework for assessment that was presented earlier in the chapter. The points raised here may apply to the way you conduct your assessment when you already suspect hepatic or uremic encephalopathy, or may bring out factors that would point to hepatic or uremic encephalopathy as a cause of the patient's altered mental status.

In that hepatic and uremic complications are not overtly revealing, a thorough, methodic assessment is helpful in the identification of either of these types of encephalopathy.

Scene Size-Up When entering the scene, actively look for clues that will assist in identification of the underlying problem. Evidence of alcoholism suggests liver complications associated with hepatic encephalopathy. Also, diabetics and patients with poorly controlled hypertension run increased risks of kidney disease that may underlie uremic complications. Therefore, the presence of syringes, insulin, home blood pressure cuffs, or a glucometer should start you thinking along such lines.

TABLE 7-7 Hepatic or Uremic Encephalopathy and Altered Mental Status: Typical Findings

Scene Size-up	Initial Assessment	Physical Exam/Vitals	History
Evidence of alcoholism (possible liver/hepatic problem) Evidence of diabetic history (e.g., insulin, syringes, glucometer) Obvious emaciation or jaundice	Chief complaint: general malaise or weakness, possible confusion or behavior alterations (complaints tend to be vague or elusive) Musty odor on breath (fector hepaticus associated with liver failure) Pathological respiratory patterns (e.g., Cheyne-Stokes, central neurogenic, Kussmaul's) Pulses normal or slightly elevated early; slower pulses later from kidney shutdown or intracranial pressure Skin warm, flushed, diaphoresis may or may not be present	Pupillary changes (with herniation), scleral or general jaundice, musty odor on breath, facial palsy or droop, pathological respiratory pattern, presence of dialysis shunt, emaciation, right upper quadrant abdominal distention or tenderness (liver damage), peripheral edema, possible signs of diabetes; possible motor, sensory, or perfusion deficits (with herniation) Vital signs can vary: normal to elevated blood pressure early, decreasing blood pressure late; possible bradycardia	Signs/symptoms: headache, nausea/vomiting, decreased urinary output, weight loss (liver), abdominal pain (liver), back and flank pain (kidneys); declining or improving mental or neurologic status Medications associated with liver or kidney problems History related to liver or kidney problems (e.g., alcoholism, cirrhosis, hepatitis, kidney failure), changes in urinary output, acute weight loss, diabetic complications

As you approach the patient, formulate a general impression as to current mental and physical status. Pay particular attention to pathological respiratory noises that indicate acidosis or airway obstruction in the stuporous or unresponsive patient. Obvious emaciation or jaundice may be the first clues to a possible history of liver disease.

Initial Assessment The chief complaint as to hepatic or uremic encephalopathy may be quite elusive and demand a high index of suspicion for identification. Complaints may center around general malaise and weakness, or be revealed through confusion or isolated alterations in mental and behavioral status with no other information forthcoming.

Hepatic and uremic encephalopathy will manifest in a variety of manners that range from confusion to coma, the altered mental status resulting from increased ICP. Evaluate and assure a patent airway. Observe the respiratory status in reference to rate and adequacy of oxygenation.

While evaluating the respiratory status, sample the breath for the musty odor of fector hepaticus, which suggests liver failure. If increased ICP has led to herniation of brain tissue, pathological respiratory patterns such as Cheyne-Stokes or central neurogenic hyperventilation may be noted. (This is actually rare in hepatic or uremic encephalopathy.) In kidney failure, ensuing acidosis may cause Kussmaul's respirations as the pulmonary system attempts the mass excretion of carbon dioxide in an attempt to raise the overall pH.

While evaluating the respiratory status, sample the breath for the musty odor of fector hepaticus, which suggests liver failure.

In the early stages of hepatic and uremic encephalopathy, pulses may be normal to slightly elevated. However, in the presence of extreme acidosis from kidney shutdown, or increased ICP from hepatic complications, slower pulse rates may be evident as acidosis depresses brain and heart activity.

In both hepatic and uremic encephalopathy, the skin should be warm and sometimes flushed. Depending on severity and progression, diaphoresis may or may not be present. The presence of jaundice is highly indicative of hepatic difficulties. If uremia is associated with diabetes, signs of poor peripheral perfusion may be apparent.

Physical Exam The physical exam for suspected hepatic or uremic encephalopathy focuses on signs of liver or kidney failure. The following list includes key aspects of the physical exam. Because cerebral herniation presents a potential complication, you should also perform a neurologic exam, as described in Table 7-2:

- ***Head***
  - Pupils (equality, size, and reactivity secondary to potential herniation)
  - Icterus, or jaundice, of the sclera (liver complications)
  - Odor of the oral cavity (musty odor from liver complications)
  - Airway patency
  - Facial *palsy* or droop (secondary to potential herniation)

palsy partial or complete paralysis.

- ***Chest***
  - Breath sounds (possibility of aspiration)
  - Respiratory pattern changes (respirations typical of cerebral edema)
  - Dialysis shunt (kidney failure)
- ***Abdomen***
  - Emaciation
  - Right upper quadrant distention/tenderness (liver damage)
- ***Extremities***
  - Peripheral edema
  - Jaundice
  - Signs of diabetes (amputations, slow-healing wounds, injection sites)
  - Dialysis shunts (upper extremities)
  - Full evaluation of motor, sensory, and perfusion (cerebral edema)
  - Asterixis (rhythmic beating of the hands when wrists are in full extension, a classic indication for hepatic failure)

Vital Signs The vital signs in hepatic and uremic encephalopathy can vary, depending on severity and associated involvement of other body systems. Initially, pulse and blood pressure may be normal to slightly elevated as the sympathetic nervous system attempts compensation. Severe acidosis associated with uremia dilates vessels and decreases cardiac output, thus dropping the overall blood pressure.

Cerebral edema with hepatic encephalopathy can precipitate bradycardia and pathological respiratory patterns such as Cheyne-Stokes or central neurogenic hyperventilation. As stated earlier, Kussmaul's respirations are often associated with moderate to severe kidney failure. The classic response to increased ICP, known as *Cushing's reflex,* consists of increased blood pressure and temperature, and decreased respiratory and pulse rates.

Cushing's reflex a cluster of vital sign changes associated with increased intracranial pressure, consisting of increased blood pressure, increased temperature, decreased respiratory rate, and decreased pulse rate.

Focused History A thorough history is necessary to assist in confirming hepatic or uremic encephalopathy as a possible underlying cause of altered mental status. Also, the history can help ascertain the extent of progression and involvement of other organ systems. Questions posed within the SAMPLE format should address the following.

Signs and Symptoms. Signs and symptoms regarding hepatic or uremic encephalopathy are extremely important in that they illustrate progression of the pathophysiology and involvement of other organ systems. These may include

- Headache (increased ICP)
- Declining or improving mental or neurologic status
- Nausea or vomiting
- *Oliguria* (decreased urinary output)
- Weight loss (liver dysfunction)
- Abdominal pain (liver failure)
- Back and flank pain (kidney involvement)

oliguria decreased urinary output.

Allergies. Note any medical allergies the patient may have.

Medications. All medications that the patient is taking should be documented and relayed to emergency department personnel. Pay special attention to medications that indicate liver, kidney, or diabetic problems.

Past Medical History. Inquire about any and all underlying medical problems. A medical history that relates to liver complication, such as alcoholism, hepatitis, or cirrhosis, is extremely important, as is kidney failure or dialysis use. As diabetics tend to incur renal problems, a history of diabetes should be elicited.

Last Oral Intake. The patient's last ingestion of food will prove important in gauging the possibility of vomiting and in evaluating a recent history of adequate or inadequate nutritional intake.

Events Prior to Illness. The events or behavior of the individual surrounding the onset of hepatic or uremic encephalopathy are important. Ascertain

- Gradual or acute onset
- Time of initial onset
- Improvement or decline in mental status
- Complaints preceding the incident (malaise, dizziness)
- Urinary output
- Acute weight loss
- Diabetic complications
- Last dialysis
- Compliance with medications

Management of the Hepatic or Uremic Encephalopathy Patient

Management of hepatic and uremic encephalopathy focuses on emotional support and the immediate stabilization of life threats. Rapidly direct your attention to establishing and maintaining a patent airway, and adequate ventilation, oxygenation, and circulation. In the event of ventilatory insufficiency, immediately begin positive-pressure ventilation. If the patient presents with coma or becomes comatose, consider tracheal intubation.

Placement of an intravenous line with a crystalloid solution is important because many complications secondary to hepatic and uremic causes exist. For example, patients with liver damage are at increased risk for gastrointestinal hemorrhage; those with poorly controlled hypertension are at increased risk for uremia.

All fluids should be administered in accordance to the hemodynamic status of the patient. Fluid application must be performed judiciously in the patient with renal failure. Because the kidneys have become inefficient at the regulation of body water, excessive administration can create a fluid overload.

Fluid administration must be performed judiciously in the patient with renal failure.

Application of the cardiac monitor is important in that acidosis from renal compromise leaves the heart prone to dysrhythmias. Electrical dysrhythmias should be treated according to your local protocols with the understanding that such disturbances may prove difficult to correct without rectifying the underlying cause of the kidney failure.

Ongoing Assessment

When transporting the patient with possible hepatic or uremic encephalopathy, constantly monitor the patient for changes in mental status and vital function, such as respiratory or cardiac decompensation. Consider positive-pressure ventilation for severe acidosis, and constantly reevaluate the patient with hepatic complications for signs of increased ICP.

Acidosis and Alkalosis

Of the many requirements a cell has for normal function, the maintenance of a normal *pH* is essential. Specific quantities of hydrogen ions produced by the normal processes of metabolism determine the pH of extracellular fluid. Hydrogen ions are produced when carbon dioxide (CO_2) combines with water (H_2O) to produce carbonic acid (H_2CO_3), which dissociates into a bicarbonate ion (HCO_3^-) and a hydrogen ion (H^+). This is expressed in the following equation, which shows how the presence of excess carbon dioxide leads to production of the hydrogen ions that create a reduced pH (increased acidity).

pH literally, "potential of hydrogen." In chemistry, the degree of acidity or alkalinity of a substance is expressed as a pH value. A value of 7.35 to 7.45 is neutral; a value greater than 7.45 expresses alkalinity; a value less than 7.35 expresses acidity.

$$CO_2 + H_2O \rightarrow H_2CO_3 \rightarrow HCO_3^- + H^+$$

A normal concentration of retained hydrogen ions creates a pH range of 7.35 to 7.45, with 7.40 as the average. The body maintains a normal pH through its ability to either excrete or retain hydrogen ions through inherent buffering mechanisms, ventilation, and renal function.

Among many activities, a pH of approximately 7.40 allows for appropriate cellular enzymatic function, electrical transmission, depolarization, and membrane maintenance. If the body fails to regulate the hydrogen ion, the pH will deviate from the acceptable range, with cellular dysfunction soon following. The brain and its activity are particularly susceptible to changes in pH and will exhibit alterations in mental and behavioral capacities if such changes are realized. As a rule, the body tolerates acidemia better than alkalemia (acidemia and alkalemia being the net result of acidosis and alkalosis).

Acidosis

Acidosis is defined as a pH that falls below 7.35 and is caused by either an increase in hydrogen ion production or a decrease in internal HCO_3^- (bicarbonate) reserves. Bicarbonate is used in the buffering of hydrogen. (The chemical reaction expressed previously moves in the reverse direction when bicarbonate ions combine with hydrogen ions, forming carbonic acid, which dissociates into water and carbon dioxide, and can be exhaled.)

As a general rule, acidosis depresses brain function through the alteration of cellular activities, as discussed previously. Without intervention, acidosis will result in death. Acidosis is classified as either respiratory or metabolic.

Respiratory Acidosis Respiratory acidosis is created when the pulmonary system fails to excrete CO_2 as fast as it is produced through cellular metabolism. The retention of carbon dioxide results in hypercapnia as the arterial CO_2 rises above 45 mmHg with an associated decrease in pH below 7.35. (Review the discussion of respiratory acidosis under "Pulmonary Causes.")

Again, brain cells are very sensitive to hypercapnia, and significant increases in CO_2 lead to changes in mental status. Typically, hypercapnia and respiratory acidosis are evidenced by a headache, blurred vision, confusion, somnolence, and fatigue or weakness. As previously stated, the acidotic environment alters normal cellular activity and promotes the depression of cerebral function. In addition, carbon dioxide is a potent vasodilator that serves to create hypoperfusion while increasing ICP. In the absence of intervention, cerebral damage and death will result.

Respiratory acidosis results from any condition that impairs pulmonary ventilation. Table 7-8 lists several causes of respiratory acidosis.

Metabolic Acidosis Acidosis can also have a metabolic origin. In metabolic acidosis, the increase in hydrogen ions is triggered by either an increase in the production of metabolic acids or a decrease in circulating bicarbonate levels below 22 mEq/l that drops the extracellular pH below 7.35.

Again, acidosis depresses normal brain function through changes in enzymatic activity, ion shifts, and electrical transmission deficits. Accordingly, changes in mentation are readily observable as confusion, lethargy, stupor, or coma.

Other signs of metabolic acidosis include Kussmaul's respirations, the deep and rapid ventilations that occur as the body attempts to increase the extracellular pH by excreting tremendous amounts of carbon dioxide. Myocardial depression and ventricular dysrhythmias are also signs of severe acidosis. Table 7-8 lists common causes of metabolic acidosis.

TABLE 7-8 Common Causes of Acid–Base Disturbances

Respiratory Acidosis	COPD Asthma CNS depression Narcotic overdose Hypoventilation
Metabolic Acidosis	Diarrhea Diabetic ketoacidosis Lactic acidosis Renal failure
Respiratory Alkalosis	Anxiety Pulmonary embolus Pregnancy Hyperventilation
Metabolic Alkalosis	Vomiting Gastric fluid loss Alkali ingestion

Alkalosis

Alkalosis occurs when the concentration of hydrogen ions substantially decreases, raising the pH above 7.45. Either a drop in the quantity of hydrogen ions produced during metabolism or an excess of HCO_3^- will drive up extracellular pH and create an alkalotic environment. Alkalosis hyperexcites the nervous tissue of the brain. As with acidosis, alkalosis is categorized as either respiratory or metabolic.

Respiratory Alkalosis When carbon dioxide is excreted faster than it is produced and falls below a $PaCO_2$ of 35 mmHg, respiratory alkalosis is said to occur. Respiratory alkalosis results in the increase of extracellular pH above 7.45 and the exhibition of altered mental status.

Respiratory alkalosis typically arises secondary to any condition that induces hyperventilation and the mass excretion of arterial carbon dioxide with resultant hypocapnia. Hypocapnia leads to electrical hyperexcitation of the brain. Hyperexcitation produces nervousness, irritability, agitation, and even convulsions.

Excessive carbon dioxide is a potent vasodilator; conversely, hypocapnia results in significant vasoconstriction. Within the brain tissue, vasoconstriction decreases cerebral perfusion, causing ischemia with further cellular dysfunction. Table 7-8 itemizes conditions that cause respiratory alkalosis.

Metabolic Alkalosis Metabolic alkalosis results from the loss of hydrogen ions or the presence of excessive circulating reserves of bicarbonate. In either case, H^+ ion concentration falls below normal levels, thereby increasing the extracellular pH above 7.45.

Again, alkalotic conditions cause cerebral hyperactivity leading to apathy, confusion, dizziness, convulsions, and muscle spasticity. A patient with metabolic alkalosis will present with shallow respirations as the body attempts to conserve carbon dioxide to decrease the arterial pH level. Table 7-8 lists causes of metabolic alkalosis.

Assessment of Possible Acidosis or Alkalosis

The following section describes assessment of a patient suffering an acid–base imbalance (Table 7-9)—within the generic framework for assessment that was presented earlier in the chapter. The points raised here may apply to the way you conduct your assessment when you already suspect such an imbalance, or may bring out factors that would point to either acidosis or alkalosis as a cause of the patient's altered mental status.

As with other pathological processes, acidosis or alkalosis often occurs secondary to a specific disease process, so a knowledge of such diseases and their effects is also advantageous (review Table 7-8).

Scene Size-Up In examining the scene for clues to the etiology of the altered mental status, look for items such as cigarettes or medications indicating possible lung problems that could lead to respiratory acidosis. The presence of drug paraphernalia may suggest a toxic ingestion that would cause either a respiratory or a metabolic acid–base disturbance. Look for evidence of diabetes or renal failure, which often underlie metabolic acidosis.

As you approach the patient, quickly form a general impression as to present mental and physical status. Acid–base imbalances can present in a variety of manners, and the initial presentation of the patient can provide important clues as to the type of imbalance. Acidosis tends to depress cerebral activity and therefore

TABLE 7-9 **Acidosis/Alkalosis and Altered Mental Status: Typical Findings**

	Scene Size-up	Initial Assessment	Physical Exam/Vitals	History
Acidosis	Presence of cigarettes or medications indicating possible lung problems; drug paraphernalia indicating possible toxic ingestion; evidence of diabetes or renal failure **Decreased level of consciousness*** Convulsions	**Chief complaint of lethargy, weakness, general malaise, confusion** Hypoventilation (respiratory acidosis) or Kussmaul's respirations (metabolic acidosis) **Normal to slightly elevated pulses early, weaker and slower later**	**Vital signs: normal to slightly elevated pulses early, weaker and slower later** Diaphoresis may or may not be present	Signs/symptoms: chest pain, anxiety or panic, ataxia, **lethargy or weakness** Medications that suggest diabetes, kidney failure, or COPD Diarrhea or vomiting prior to illness, history of kidney dialysis
Alkalosis	Presence of drug paraphernalia indicating possible toxic ingestion **Hyperexcited presentation** Convulsions	**Chief complaint of muscular spasticity, ataxia, inappropriate behavior** Hyperventilation (respiratory alkalosis) or hypoventilation (metabolic alkalosis) **Elevated pulses**	**Vital signs: elevated pulses**	Signs/symptoms: chest pain, anxiety or panic, ataxia, **numbness or tingling in the extremities, dizziness** Medications that suggest diabetes, kidney failure, or COPD Diarrhea or vomiting prior to illness, history of kidney dialysis

*Items in bold type are those that can help distinguish acidosis from alkalosis.

results in a patient with a decreased level of consciousness. Conversely, alkalosis tends to hyperexcite the CNS, presenting with great anxiety or panic. Convulsions may be present with either alkalosis or acidosis.

Initial Assessment Attempt to establish a chief complaint from the onset. A patient will generally not complain of being acidotic or alkalotic but rather will allude to the symptoms of these imbalances. Lethargy, weakness, or general malaise accompanied by confusion may be described in the presence of acidosis. Muscular spasticity, ataxia, and inappropriate behavior may overlie alkalosis.

Evaluate the airway. Any patient with a decreased level of consciousness deserves a thorough evaluation of the oral cavity to assure a clear path for ventilation and oxygenation.

Evaluate the respiratory status in reference to rate and depth. Respiratory patterns are often helpful in determining the type of pH imbalance at play. Recall that hypercapnia and respiratory acidosis occur secondary to hypoventilation, or shallow, inadequate ventilations in which carbon dioxide is retained. Conversely, hyperventilation excretes great amounts of carbon dioxide, thus leading to respiratory alkalosis.

For the patient with metabolic acidosis, Kussmaul's respirations are often evident as the body attempts to compensate for the acidotic internal environment by excreting large amounts of carbon dioxide, as in DKA. Metabolic alkalosis, however, results in the conservation of carbon dioxide and presents with shallow respirations.

Assessment of the circulatory parameters can also yield worthwhile clues. Pulses in the acidotic patient may initially appear normal to slightly elevated; then, as the acidotic environment eventually depresses brain and myocardial activity, pulses will become weaker and slower. With alkalosis, initial pulses will be elevated in response to hyperactivity.

Physical Exam The physical exam can reveal further clues as to the type of imbalance the patient may be suffering from. Important areas in reference to the acidotic or alkalotic patient are listed here. As with any patient exhibiting altered mental status, a neurologic assessment is also encouraged:

- *Airway.* Hydration of the oral mucosa
- *Chest*
  - Adequacy of ventilation
  - Auscultation of breath sounds
  - Kussmaul's respirations (metabolic acidosis)
- *Extremities. Carpopedal spasms* (respiratory alkalosis)

Carpopedal spasms spasms of the wrist or foot.

Vital Signs The respiratory status is most relevant to note. Hypoventilation is the primary cause of respiratory acidosis, while in metabolic acidosis rapid respirations occur as the body attempts to excrete excess CO_2. Alkalosis has the opposite pattern. Hyperventilation is the primary cause of respiratory alkalosis, while shallow respirations may be seen in metabolic alkalosis as the body attempts to conserve CO_2. In the acidotic patient, pulses may initially be normal to slightly elevated but will then become weaker and slower. In the alkalotic patient, pulses will be elevated. Vasoconstriction is often associated with respiratory alkalosis, causing delayed capillary refill. Diaphoresis may or may not be present.

Focused History As stated earlier, certain medical conditions predispose to the creation of pH imbalances, especially acidosis. Additionally, acidosis and alkalosis can have far-reaching effects on other systems of the body. A focused medical history is paramount in assisting the identification of either acidosis or alkalosis and investigating the degree of impact. The SAMPLE method provides a format for the organization of this information.

Signs and Symptoms. Ascertain signs and symptoms, especially those associated with central nervous and cardiovascular system problems:

- Chest pain (hyperventilation and respiratory alkalosis)
- Anxiety or panic (hyperventilation and respiratory alkalosis)
- Lethargy or weakness (respiratory and metabolic acidosis)
- Numbness or tingling in the extremities (alkalosis)
- Dizziness (metabolic alkalosis)
- Ataxia (acidosis or alkalosis)

Allergies. Note any medical allergies the patient may have.

Medications. All medications that the patient is taking should be documented and relayed to emergency department personnel. Medications may help identify underlying medical conditions that predispose the patient to acidosis or alkalosis. Look especially for medications that suggest diabetes, kidney failure, or COPD. Also remember to inquire about use of over-the-counter medications, especially aspirin, and excessive use of antacids.

Past Medical History. Attempt to identify any underlying medical problems. As mentioned previously, patients with diabetes, renal failure, or COPD are particularly prone to acidotic complications. Also note other conditions that impede ventilation or gas exchange at the alveolar–capillary interface.

Last Oral Intake. The patient's last ingestion of food is important in gauging the possibility of vomiting and aspiration and in evaluating adequate or inadequate nutritional intake.

Events Prior to Illness. The events or behavior surrounding the onset of either acidosis or alkalosis should be obtained, especially the following:

- Time of initial onset/gradual or acute onset
- Improvement or decline of mental and neurologic status
- Diarrhea and/or vomiting
- For the renal patient, whether dialysis has occurred
- Complaints preceding the incident (malaise, dizziness)
- Any medications, either prescribed or not prescribed, that have been taken
- Medical complications from diabetes, renal failure, or overdose

Management of the Acidotic or Alkalotic Patient

Definitive treatment of acidosis or alkalosis involves correction of the underlying cause. Occasionally, definitive field treatment can be executed for respiratory acidosis or alkalosis stemming from conditions such as COPD or psychogenic hyperventilation. Acidosis or alkalosis occurring secondary to metabolic complications often require the temporary prehospital stabilization of arterial pH and other complications, with definitive reversal occurring in hospital.

Assurance of a patent airway, ventilation, and maximum oxygenation are paramount in the treatment of both acidosis and alkalosis. Because respiratory acidosis results from hypoventilation, treatment of the underlying causes such as exacerbated COPD or narcotic overdose may be possible by means of bronchodilators and naloxone, respectively.

Having a patient with extensive pulmonary infection sit upright will permit gravity to help drain fluid from the lungs, therein improving gas exchange at the alveolar–capillary interface. In cases of metabolic acidosis where actual reversal is not feasible, assisted ventilation at an accelerated rate will assist with the excretion of accumulated CO_2 and the decreasing of levels of arterial carbon dioxide. The same method is helpful in stabilizing metabolic acidosis, especially if the patient is tracheally intubated.

As respiratory alkalosis can occur secondary to anxiety and hyperventilation, encouragement to the patient to consciously decrease respirations may aid in raising arterial carbon dioxide levels, thereby decreasing the elevated pH. Have the patient close his mouth and breathe through his nose as you coach him to slow his respirations. An older practice of having the patient rebreathe into a paper bag is not recommended. The increased levels of CO_2 may be helpful in restoring arterial carbon dioxide levels, but the decreased levels of O_2 would be dangerous, especially if the patient is already suffering hypoxemia (e.g., from an unsuspected pulmonary embolism). As noted in Chapter 5, never assume that hyperventilation is of psychogenic origin until all other possible causes have been ruled out.

Clinical Insight

Although it is possible that hyperventilation has resulted from anxiety, *do not* assume a psychogenic cause of hyperventilation until all other possible causes have been ruled out.

Because acidosis and alkalosis can disrupt the electrical integrity of the myocardium, evaluation with cardiac monitor is a must. Dysrhythmias should be treated according to your local protocols, with the realization that prehospital correction of the dysrhythmia will be difficult in light of the underlying deviation in pH.

Because acidosis and alkalosis can disrupt the electrical integrity of the myocardium, evaluation with cardiac monitor is a must.

The first-line therapy in metabolic acidosis is intravenous fluids. In severe cases, administration of sodium bicarbonate may occasionally be helpful.

However, the use of sodium bicarbonate can also, paradoxically, worsen intracellular acidosis as increased levels of carbon dioxide return to and accumulate within the cell. Consequently, the assurance of adequate ventilation by mechanical means is highly recommended when sodium bicarbonate is to be administered. The recommended dose for sodium bicarbonate is 1 mEq/kg.

Throughout care for the acidotic or alkalotic patient, note and stabilize any changes in the activity of the pulmonary or cardiovascular systems. Acidosis or alkalosis can precipitate seizure activity, which should be managed as discussed in Chapter 10.

Ongoing Assessment

Conduct ongoing monitoring of the patient en route to the hospital. Repeat the initial assessment, especially with regard to respiratory status. Reassess vital signs, check interventions, and note trends in the patient's condition (e.g., signs of respiratory failure or hypotension).

Electrolyte Imbalances

Electrolytes are substances that dissociate into ions, or electrically charged particles, within the body. Ions with a positive charge are known as cations, while ions with a negative charge are known as anions. They exist in varying concentrations and are predominantly acquired through dietary and fluid intake. Generally regulated by the kidneys, electrolytes are excreted with other waste products in the urine, feces, and perspiration.

Precise concentrations of electrolytes are crucial for the body's numerous regulatory activities. Accordingly, electrolytes exist within narrow ranges from which any significant upward or downward deviation can prove life threatening. Frequently, electrolyte imbalances directly or indirectly upset the working of the CNS, as evidenced by a disturbance in the mental status. Although many electrolytes exist within the body, the remainder of this section focuses on sodium and calcium, two of the most commonly occurring electrolytes. Note that, except for sodium, electrolytes play only an indirect role in altered mental status. For example, decreased potassium causes cardiac dysrhythmias that, in turn, result in altered mental status, but potassium has little direct effect on the brain.

Sodium

Sodium, the primary cation in the extracellular fluid, is instrumental in the overall distribution of body water. In the human body, water is extremely important because it is the medium for reactions, transportation, protection, waste removal, and thermoregulation.

Water has a high affinity for sodium and will move toward an area where it is present. If sodium levels increase, a greater amount of water is drawn toward it. Conversely, as sodium levels decrease, water is less attracted. With the aid of hormones such as aldosterone and ADH, sodium is excreted by the kidney, thus ridding the body of excess water. In summary, the presence of sodium is essential in the control and distribution of water within the body and within the cells themselves. Normal levels of sodium exist within the range of 135 to 145 mEq/l. Quantities of sodium above 145 mEq/l or deficits below 135 mEq/l cause difficulties in water management.

osmolarity ionic concentration. **Plasma osmolarity** is the ionic concentration in plasma.

Hypernatremia Hypernatremia occurs when sodium plasma levels increase above 145 mEq/l. As sodium levels increase, so does the *osmolarity* of the extracellular fluid. The increased osmolarity caused by hypernatremia pulls water from within the cells into the extracellular environment. The resulting cellular dehydration causes the cell to shrink.

Cellular dehydration has a profound effect on the brain. The shrinkage of brain cells amounts to a decrease in overall brain size. A smaller brain mass places tension on the cerebral vessels, predisposing them to tearing and intracranial hemorrhage. Additionally, as water leaves the cells, less of a medium exists for normal metabolic activity. Consequently, cerebral activity is disturbed.

Excessive sodium changes the depolarization characteristics of nerve tissue, producing CNS irritability, evidenced by lethargy, confusion, and delirium. In addition, the hypernatremic individual has a greater propensity for seizure activity. Permanent brain damage and coma are complications associated with severe episodes of hypernatremia.

Causes of hypernatremia are numerous and include any means that increase sodium plasma concentrations to greater than 145 mEq/l. Excessive nonsodium fluid loss, as might occur with excessive diarrhea or polyuria, increases sodium levels by decreasing the fluid medium. Similarly, a decrease in water intake can also result in hypernatremia. Hypernatremia should be considered in any patient who is unable to ingest fresh water, as might be found in the debilitated patient or anyone else with a decreased thirst perception or the physical inability to drink. Additionally, a massive ingestion of sodium through diet, sodium bicarbonate, or hypertonic saline solutions can precipitate hypernatremia.

Hyponatremia Hyponatremia is a sodium plasma deficit of less than 135 mEq/l. As sodium levels decrease, so does the osmolarity of the extracellular fluid. As a consequence, extracellular water shifts into the intracellular space and causes cellular edema.

Again, the cerebral neurons prove sensitive to such changes. As water moves into the cellular environment, cerebral edema occurs. In addition to disrupting neuronal activity, cerebral edema can lead to necrosis as ICP increases and compresses cerebral vessels, thereby decreasing cerebral perfusion.

Initially, the hyponatremic patient will complain of a headache. As ICP increases, stupor and coma may occur. Seizures are a common manifestation of severe hyponatremia. Without treatment, hyponatremia can be fatal.

Calcium

Calcium, another cation, is the most abundant ion in the body. It circulates within the blood plasma and is stored within the bones and teeth. Importantly, calcium promotes cellular membrane stability and regulates the entry of sodium into the cell. Calcium is also used in many other processes, such as the clotting of blood, conduction of nerve and muscular impulses, and contraction of the myocardium.

Measured according to blood plasma levels, normal calcium concentrations exist within the range of 9 to 10 mg/dl. Calcium is one of the most closely regulated ions because any deviation from this normal range can prove fatal. Regulation of calcium involves the kidneys, bone, and skin.

Hypercalcemia If serum calcium rises above 10.5 mg/dl, hypercalcemia is said to exist. Although hypercalcemia promotes changes throughout the body, the brain is particularly sensitive to the elevation. Excessive calcium leaves the cells less permeable to sodium, resulting in a decreased conduction of electrical impulses. As a result, depression of CNS activity is noted. In addition, hypercalcemia decreases the release of neurotransmitters that are used for interneuronal communication.

Seizures, lethargy, and muscular weakness are typical consequences. As with the other electrolytes, failure to lower the elevated calcium level will result in death.

Cardiac effects are the primary manifestation of hypercalcemia, with particular impacts on the conduction system of the heart. The blocking of sodium interferes with the conduction of electricity throughout the myocardium and accounts for a decrease in automaticity. Subsequently, the patient is prone to a variety of dysrhythmias, up to and including a full heart block. An ECG change commonly found in hypercalcemia is the shortening of the QT interval with little to no ST segment. Cardiac complications relate to a decreased cardiac output and decreased cerebral perfusion with associated hypoxia.

Hypercalcemia has many causes. Hyperactivity of the parathyroid gland, which regulates the circulating concentration of calcium, can precipitate hypercalcemia. Other causes include tumors of the bone and excessive calcium ingestion. Thiazide diuretics promote the reabsorption of calcium, resulting in hypercalcemia.

Hypocalcemia Hypocalcemia occurs as calcium falls to levels below 9 mg/dl. As the cellular membrane blocking effect on sodium passage decreases, sodium enters the cells with greater ease, thereby increasing the depolarization of excitable cells. Hypocalcemia affects primarily the peripheral nervous system, observable through tetany (muscle spasms of the extremities), muscular irritability, and hyperreflexion (increased reflex response). Irritability and delusions may be seen. If the deficit is great enough, convulsions may ensue.

Cardiovascular changes are also seen as hypocalcemia elongates the QT interval and the ST segment (Figure 7-9). Also, because calcium is necessary for effective contractility, the deficit of calcium can result in less than optimum contractions

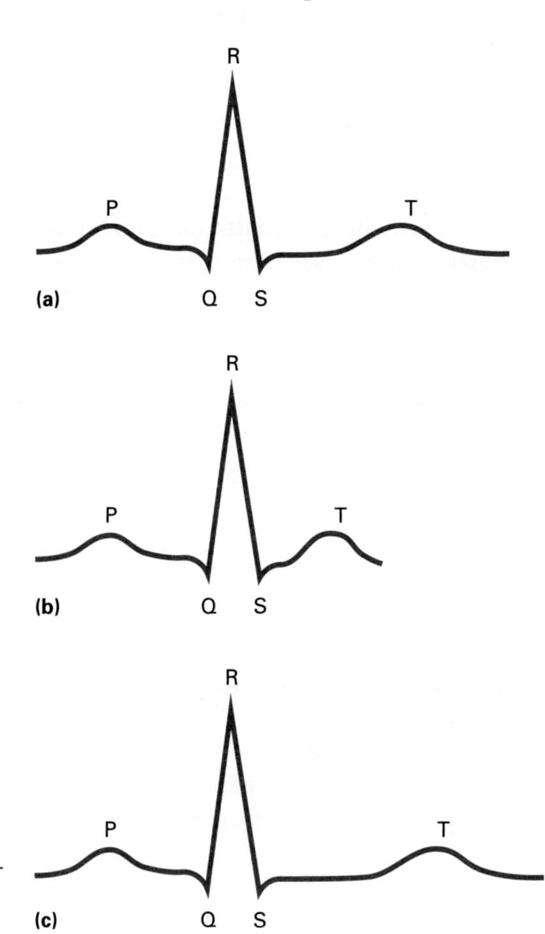

FIGURE 7-9
(a) Normal ECG tracing. (b) Tracing showing shortened QT interval in hypercalcemia. (c) Tracing showing lengthened QT interval in hypocalcemia.

and manifest with pulmonary congestion secondary to CHF. From this perspective, hypocalcemia impacts the brain through a decrease in cerebral perfusion and subsequent hypoxia.

Potassium and Magnesium

Most of the actions of potassium and magnesium affect the peripheral nervous system rather than the CNS. Any alteration of mental status is likely to be secondary to their cardiac effects.

Assessment of Possible Electrolyte Imbalance

The following section details specifics about assessment of a patient suffering an electrolyte imbalance (Table 7-10)—within the generic framework for assessment presented earlier in the chapter. The points raised here may apply to assessment when you already suspect an electrolyte imbalance, or may bring out factors that would point to electrolyte imbalance as a cause of the patient's altered mental status.

Identification of electrolyte imbalances is very difficult and requires a thorough assessment, especially history, and a working knowledge of the electrolytes and their various functions. Remember that frequently, electrolyte imbalances can occur secondary to other medical conditions.

Scene Size-Up Because many electrolytes are obtained through the diet, make a brief note of living conditions. Poor conditions may indicate the inability of the patient to care for himself or to be taken care of, particularly to have a proper diet.

Initial Assessment Typically, chief complaints surrounding electrolyte imbalances revolve around the complaint of altered mental status. Such complaints include confusion, lethargy, weakness, or inappropriate behavior. As certain electrolyte imbalances affect the cardiovascular system, the complaint of chest pain or syncope accompanied by confusion may present.

Provide for airway patency, and evaluate the rate and adequacy of respirations. Although not a direct cause of dyspnea, increases in ICP associated with hyponatremia may present with pathological respiratory patterns, as discussed

TABLE 7-10 Electrolyte Imbalance and Altered Mental Status: Typical Findings

Scene Size-up	Initial Assessment	Physical Exam/Vitals	History
Evidence of poor living conditions, improper diet	Possible pathological respiratory pattern (e.g., with hyponatremia); shallow respirations (e.g., with hypercalcemia) Cardiac dysrhythmias (e.g., bradycardia from infranodal block with hypercalcemia; weak pulse with poor peripheral perfusion with hypocalcemia)	Vision compromise, pupillary dysfunction, facial palsy or droop, tongue deviation, dysphasia or aphasia (from increased intracranial pressure with hyponatremia) Pathological respiratory patterns Distal motor dysfunction, weakness, peripheral edema, weak or unequal distal pulses Vital signs can vary dramatically; however, blood pressure is typically normal to elevated	Signs/symptoms: chest pain, dyspnea, dizziness, palpitations, syncopal episodes (calcium imbalances); headache (sodium imbalances); nausea, vomiting, diarrhea (all electrolytes) Patient taking medications such as diuretics, potassium supplements, digitalis, beta-blockers, thiazides History of electrolyte imbalances, diabetic ketoacidosis, kidney failure, parathyroid hyperactivity associated with hypercalcemia

earlier. Shallow respirations may indicate cerebral depression secondary to hypercalcemia.

Electrolyte imbalances can have a marked impact on the heart and precipitate many types of electrical dysrhythmias. Your first alert to the presence of dysrhythmias will occur when you palpate the radial and/or carotid pulses. A bradycardic pulse may indicate some form of infranodal heart block associated with hypercalcemia, while a weak pulse with poor peripheral perfusion may indicate hypocalcemia.

Physical Exam Key aspects of a physical exam that apply to the patient with possible electrolyte imbalances are itemized here. Secondary to cerebral implications involving sodium imbalances, a neurologic assessment is also warranted:

- ***Head.*** Signs of increased ICP associated with hyponatremia:
  - Pupillary status (gaze, size, equality, reactivity)
  - Vision compromise
  - Facial palsy or droop
  - Tongue deviation
  - Dysphasia or aphasia
- ***Airway***
  - Patency
  - Hydration of the oral cavity
- ***Chest***
  - Respiratory pattern changes (pathological respiratory patterns)
  - Respiratory depression (hypercalcemia)
  - Breath sounds (pulmonary edema, hypocalcemia)
- ***Extremities***
  - Motor ability
  - Grip strength
  - Peripheral edema (hypernatremia)
  - Distal pulses (strength and equality)
  - Carpopedal spasms

Vital Signs In the presence of electrolyte imbalances, vital signs will vary. For this reason, they must be considered in the context of the overall clinical assessment and history.

Focused History A SAMPLE history can help confirm and differentiate electrolyte imbalances. If possible, address the information outlined as follows.

Signs and Symptoms. Signs and symptoms associated with electrolyte disturbances provide evidence of severity. Hypocalcemia and cardiac complications associated with hypercalcemia are particularly important and should be investigated:

- Chest pain, dyspnea, dizziness (calcium)
- Palpitations (calcium)
- Nausea, vomiting, diarrhea (all electrolytes)
- Headache (hypernatremia, hyponatremia)

- Declining or improving mental or neurologic status
- Syncopal episodes (calcium)

Allergies. Note any medical allergies the patient may have.

Medications. Medications may indicate underlying medical problems that leave the patient prone to electrolyte imbalances. Additionally, some medications may themselves produce electrolyte imbalances. Among others, inquire as to the specific medications listed here and determine relative compliancy:

- Loop diuretics
- Potassium supplements
- Digitalis
- Beta-blockers
- Calcium channel blockers
- Steroids (glucocorticoids, mineralocorticoids)
- Thiazide diuretics
- Dietary supplements and vitamins

Past Medical History. Any underlying medical problems should be confirmed. Certain medical conditions may be responsible for the creation of electrolyte imbalances. Important histories as to potentiation of electrolyte imbalances include

- History of electrolyte imbalances
- Diabetic ketoacidosis
- Kidney failure
- Metastatic cancer
- Parathyroid hyperactivity (hypercalcemia)
- Recent thyroid surgery (hypocalcemia secondary to parathyroid damage)

Last Oral Intake. Because many electrolytes are obtained through diet, the patient's last ingestion and recent history of food intake can prove important in gauging the adequate intake of electrolytes. For example, foods such as fruits and juices may be high in potassium, while canned foods tend to contain high quantities of sodium.

Events Prior to Illness. When questioning the patient about events surrounding the onset of electrolyte imbalances, look for sources of fluid and electrolyte loss such as excessive urination or diarrhea, vomiting, or perspiration. Additionally, investigate the following items:

- Gradual versus acute onset
- Time of initial onset
- Improvement or deterioration of mental status
- Complaints preceding the incident (headache, confusion, dizziness, falls)
- Cardiac complaints (chest pain, dyspnea, palpitations, syncope, weakness)

Management of the Patient with Electrolyte Imbalance

Correction of electrolyte disorders is complicated and varies according to the severity and underlying cause. Rapid overcorrection or frank mismanagement can lead to a multitude of adverse side effects affecting vital organs such as the brain, heart, and kidneys. In most situations, field intervention for electrolyte imbalances is limited. Accordingly, prehospital treatment is a function of identification, stabilization of associated life threats, and the conveyance of critical medical information to the hospital staff.

For all patients, secure a patent airway by a means appropriate to the level of consciousness. Ventilation therapy is geared toward maintaining an adequate tidal volume with arterial oxygen saturation (SpO_2) as close to 100 percent as possible.

Carry out intravenous therapy with an isotonic crystalloid such as normal saline solution or lactated Ringer's. Although these solutions do contain electrolytes that can assist in correcting a deficiency, the quantities of these substances are small and will do little harm if electrolytes are elevated. Fluid therapy must be conducted judiciously because excessive fluids can further dilute already scant amounts of liquid-borne electrolytes. Unless the patient is suffering from hypovolemia, intravenous fluids should be run at a TKO rate.

Obtain blood specimens for laboratory analysis. Because fluctuations of potassium can interfere with the storage of glycogen, undertake an evaluation of the blood glucose level.

Significant electrolyte imbalances have particular effects on the electrical and pumping ability of the myocardium. Treat all electrical and hemodynamic aberrations according to your local protocol. However, keep in mind that if a dysrhythmia has been caused by an electrolyte imbalance, correction by conventional methods may not be possible without first restoring the electrolytes to normal parameters.

Some medications do find use in the prehospital environment when a definitive diagnosis has been made. The administration of calcium gluconate or 10 percent calcium chloride may be applicable in the immediate stabilization of acute hyperkalemia. Careful consultation with medical direction is advised prior to these interventions.

Ongoing Assessment

Throughout transport, maintain watchful attention toward changes in mental status, respiratory function, and circulatory function. Note significant changes and stabilize as indicated. Recall that seizure activity can be induced through deviations in electrolytic balances. Be prepared for seizures to occur, and manage them according to the guidelines in Chapter 10.

Thyroid Disorders

The thyroid gland, located just below the larynx, is a component of the endocrine system. Ultimately, the thyroid gland is responsible for the regulation of metabolism, which it accomplishes through the release of bloodborne hormones. Cellular reception of the hormones increases the cell's basal metabolic rate, which is evidenced by an increase in energy expenditure and heat production.

Disturbance of thyroid function can create alteration in mental status ranging from confusion or anxiety to stupor or coma. Thyroid dysfunction is classified into two general categories: hyperthyroidism and hypothyroidism. Keep in mind that, although many effects of hyper- or hypothyroidism take time, usually months, to develop, some conditions (e.g., thyroid storm) may occur suddenly in a patient with underlying thyroid problems..

Hyperthyroidism

Hyperthyroidism results as excessive levels of secreted hormones, primarily thyroxin, induce a hypermetabolic state. The most common cause of hyperthyroidism is overmedication with exogenous thyroid hormones such as levothyroxine. Occasionally, these medications are taken as part of a fad diet in the promotion of weight loss. Additionally, hyperthyroidism may arise secondary to the discontinuation of antithyroid drug treatment. Graves' disease is associated with hyperthyroidism. Thyrotoxicosis is the state produced by excessive endogenous thyroxin secretion, as in Graves' disease, or excessive intake of exogenous insulin. Hyperthyroidism can be transient or permanent and exhibit effects that are mild to severe. A severe and life-threatening form of thyrotoxicosis is called a thyroid storm. A thyroid storm creates an extreme hypermetabolic state with excessive sympathetic nervous system activity.

The presentation of hyperthyroidism revolves around excessive metabolic activity. The mental status of the hyperthyroid patient can range from mild confusion and anxiety to extreme nervousness or paranoia. Frequently, the hyperthyroid patient has a decreased attention span and exhibits dramatic mood changes. The elderly can have a depressed affect in conjunction with hyperthyroidism (apathetic hyperthyroidism).

The hyperthyroid patient is intolerant of heat and is relatively thin with skin that is warm and flushed. Occasionally, a palpable *goiter* in the neck provides a clinical indication of thyroid difficulties. Another clinical indicator of hyperthyroidism is the presence of *exophthalmos,* or protrusion of the eyeballs from the orbital cavities. Caused by inflammatory edema behind the eye, exophthalmos is visually dramatic, making it very difficult to completely close the upper and lower eyelids.

goiter enlarged thyroid gland.

exophthalmos protrusion of the eyeballs from the orbital cavities.

Hypothyroidism

Hypothyroidism results from thyroid hormone deficiency. Hypothyroidism decreases the basal metabolic rate and significantly slows cellular processes. Hypothyroidism occurs more frequently than hyperthyroidism and is considered relatively underdiagnosed among the elderly. In addition to thyroid disorder, other causes of hypothyroidism include hypothalamic dysfunction and pituitary disorders.

Untreated hypothyroidism presents with signs and symptoms indicative of a slow basal metabolic rate. With respect to the CNS, the hypothyroid patient may exhibit a depressed cognitive ability with acute memory deficits. Clumsiness and ataxia may also be noted.

Untreated hypothyroidism presents with signs and symptoms indicative of a slow basal metabolic rate.

The hypothyroid patient is typically heavy and very intolerant of the cold. The patient's skin is generally cool to the touch, and there may be edema to the face, hands, and legs. As with the hyperthyroid patient, there may be a palpable goiter. In addition, a slower heart rate with a subsequent decrease in cardiac output and CHF may be observed.

Myxedema Coma Myxedema coma is a severe complication of hypothyroidism and constitutes a major medical emergency. Myxedema signifies the extreme slowing of cellular processes and is caused by a variety of factors that exacerbate existing hypothyroidism. Specific causes include prolonged exposure to cold temperatures, trauma, infection, stress, or any medication that depresses the CNS.

As the processes within the body progressively slow, the central nervous system becomes severely depressed. This depression affects the vital centers of cardiac, respiratory, vasomotor, and thermoregulatory control. Bradycardia, hypotension, and respiratory inadequacy lead to cerebral hypoxia and respiratory acidosis. The slow, cold, hypoxic brain does not fare well in the acidotic environment. Lethargy leads to coma and coma to death. In the latter stages, the prognosis is quite poor.

Assessment of Possible Thyroid Disorder

The following section describes specifics about assessment of a patient suffering a possible thyroid disorder (Table 7-11)—within the generic framework for assessment presented earlier in the chapter. The points raised here may apply to

TABLE 7-11 Thyroid Disorders and Altered Mental Status: Typical Findings

	Scene Size-up	Initial Assessment	Physical Exam/Vitals	History
Hyperthyroidism	**Hyperactive presentation with anxiety and paranoia***	Chief complaint may reveal patient or family awareness of thyroid condition **Chief complaint of excitation, anxiety, paranoia** **Tachypnea, tachycardia, warm, flushed skin**	Goiter **Exophthalmos** **Warm, flushed skin** **Vital signs: elevated pulse, elevated respirations, elevated blood pressure**	Signs/symptoms: chest pain, dyspnea, dizziness, **fever, agitation/psychosis, hyperactivity/nervousness** **Medications: propylthiouracil (Propacil), methimazole (Tapazole), iodine** Known history of thyroid problems or other endocrine problems (e.g., Cushing's disease, pituitary problems) **Events prior to illness: weight loss, fever, infection, emotional stress**
Hypothyroidism	**Confusion, ataxia, or decreased level of consciousness**	Chief complaint may reveal patient or family awareness of thyroid condition **Chief complaint of confusion, ataxia, or decreased level of consciousness** **Bradypnea, bradycardia, cool skin**	Goiter **Facial edema, jugular vein distention, breath sounds associated with pulmonary edema, edema of the extremities, cool skin** **Vital signs: decreased pulse, decreased respirations, decreased blood pressure**	Signs/symptoms: chest pain, dyspnea, dizziness, hypothermia, lethargy/psychosis, drowsiness/weakness **Medications: levothyroxine (Synthroid), liothyronine (Cytomel), liotrix (Euthroid)** Known history of thyroid problems or other endocrine problems (e.g., Cushing's disease, pituitary problems) **Events prior to illness: cold exposure/hypothermia, uncharacteristic weight gain, infection, drowsiness/weakness**

*Items in bold type are those that can help distinguish hyperthyroidism from hypothyroidism.

assessment when you already suspect that the patient has a thyroid disorder, or may bring out factors that would point to a thyroid-based cause of the patient's altered mental status.

You can readily differentiate the various types of thyroid disorders by a methodic and thorough assessment. Furthermore, an orderly assessment will enable you to determine severity of the current situation and discover complications stemming from the underlying abnormality.

Scene Size-Up As you approach, observing the patient and the patient's activities can be helpful in identifying a thyroid disorder. A hyperthyroid patient is likely to display hyperactivity associated with anxiety and paranoia. A hypothyroid patient or one going into a myxedema coma may present with confusion and ataxia or a decreased level of consciousness.

Initial Assessment Some patients with a known thyroid disorder may be able to relay this information. However, for those who are not aware of the problem or who do not know the implications of thyroid disorders, complaints may revolve around altered mental status exhibited as paranoia with hyperexcitation in hyperthyroidism or as confusion and lethargy in hypothyroidism. If the patient has a sufficiently decreased level of consciousness, the complaint may have to be obtained from other sources or be based on the entire picture of clinical findings.

Evaluate and assure airway patency. The respiratory rate can help differentiate the two thyroid conditions. Tachypnea may be observed in the hyperthyroid patient because increased metabolism demands greater quantities of oxygen and the increased expiration of carbon dioxide. In hypothyroidism, decreased body functions bring about bradypnea. In either case, evaluate the adequacy of oxygenation and ventilation and provide support as needed. Pulse evaluation can also help identify a thyroid problem. Tachycardia with warm, flushed skin suggests hyperthyroidism, while bradycardia and cool skin are typical of hypothyroidism.

Physical Exam A physical exam should be routinely conducted on all patients with suspected thyroid complications associated with the complaint of altered mental status. Clues to thyroid disorder are listed as follows:

- *Head*
  - Exophthalmos, a marked protrusion of the eyeballs (hyperthyroidism)
  - Facial edema or a puffy facial appearance (hypothyroidism)
- *Neck*
  - Goiter in region of the larynx (hyper- or sometimes hypothyroidism)
  - JVD (decreased cardiac activity in hypothyroidism)
- *Chest.* Breath sounds (pulmonary edema in both hyper- and hypothyroidism)
- *Extremities*
  - Edema (hypothyroidism)
  - Skin color and temperature (warm and flushed in hyperthyroidism; cool in hypothyroidism)

Vital Signs Vital signs can also help differentiate thyroid disorders. Elevations of the pulse, respirations, and blood pressure may be associated with hyperthyroidism and an increase in body metabolism. Conversely, hypothyroidism and the associated slowing of body processes is reflected in lower pulses, respirations, and blood pressure.

Focused History A thorough history as applied to thyroid disorders is required to determine the severity of the crisis at hand and further assist in differentiating the two conditions.

Signs and Symptoms. Signs and symptoms surrounding thyroid disorder are important in differentiating hyperthyroidism from hypothyroidism and gauging the severity of either. Remember that lethargy and weakness may be seen in elderly patients with hyperthyroidism (apathetic hyperthyroidism):

Hyperthyroidism

- Chest pain, dyspnea, dizziness
- Fever
- Agitation/psychosis
- Hyperactivity/nervousness

Hypothyroidism

- Chest pain, dyspnea, dizziness
- Hypothermia
- Lethargy/psychosis
- Drowsiness/weakness

Allergies. Note any medical allergies the patient may have.

Medications. Inquire about the use of thyroid medications. Ascertain proper compliance with these medications because inappropriate use may have led to the crisis at hand. Common thyroid medications include

Hyperthyroidism	***Hypothyroidism***
▶ Propylthiouracil (Propacil)	▶ Levothyroxine (Synthroid)
▶ Methimazole (Tapazole)	▶ Liothyronine (Cytomel)
▶ Iodine	▶ Liotrix (Euthroid)

Past Medical History. In addition to general medical problems, inquire about a known history of specific thyroid problems or other endocrine problems such as *Cushing's disease, Graves' disease,* or pituitary problems.

Cushing's disease a syndrome caused by hypersecretion of the adrenal cortex.

Graves' disease a disease complex of unknown etiology characterized by the presence of goiter, eye disorders, and/or skin disorders.

Last Oral Intake. Note and document the patient's last dietary and fluid intake.

Events Prior to Illness. Events leading to the present situation are important in further confirming the diagnosis at hand and/or indicating precipitating factors. Pertinent information would include

Hyperthyroidism	***Hypothyroidism***
▶ Weight loss	▶ Uncharacteristic weight gain
▶ Fever	▶ Cold exposure and hypothermia
▶ Infection	▶ Infection
▶ Emotional stress	▶ Drowsiness/weakness

Management of the Thyroid Disorder Patient

Generally, mild presentations of hyperthyroidism and hypothyroidism do not require extensive intervention, but rather passive support through emotional reassurance and transport to an appropriate facility. However, in situations of clinically significant thyroid disorder, aggressive management is mandated.

With a patent airway established, care must be geared toward oxygenation and ventilatory support. Depending on specific presentation, this therapy will vary. Patients with serious hyperthyroid complications should receive high-flow, high-concentration oxygen secondary to hypermetabolic activity. Severe hypothyroidism and myxedema coma typically present with a greatly decreased respiratory effort, resulting in hypoventilation, hypoxia, and respiratory acidosis. Accordingly, ventilatory support with positive-pressure ventilation may be indicated.

Clinical Insight

Both hyper- and hypothyroid patients are likely to require supplemental oxygen. Hyperthyroid metabolic activity increases oxygen demand. Hypothyroid conditions may lead to reduced respiratory effort, perhaps requiring positive-pressure ventilation.

In both classifications of thyroid disorder, the implementation of IV therapy is important and should be accomplished with an isotonic crystalloid. The excessive metabolic activity commonly associated with hyperthyroidism uses great quantities of water and can precipitate dehydration. If significant dehydration is present, rehydration via intravenous fluids should occur in 20 ml/kg fluid boluses with reevaluation following each administration. Avoid overhydration because a hypermetabolic heart may not tolerate excessive fluids.

Along with drawing blood for laboratory analysis, evaluate the blood glucose level. Hypermetabolic activity can rapidly deplete glucose reserves, leading to hypoglycemia. Decreased blood glucose levels associated with altered mental status have also been found in hypothyroidism and deserve immediate correction with the administration of 50 percent dextrose.

Both hyperthyroidism and hypothyroidism can adversely affect the electrical status of the myocardium. Application of the cardiac monitor may reveal tachydysrhythmias in hyperthyroidism or bradydysrhythmias in hypothyroidism. Treat all dysrhythmias according to your local protocols, while realizing that these dysrhythmias may be quite difficult to correct without first rectifying the underlying metabolic disorder. Additionally, be aware that the cold body temperature induced by myxedema coma can have serious effects on the metabolization of cardiac drugs and lead to a state of toxicity.

Both hyperthyroidism and hypothyroidism can adversely affect the electrical status of the myocardium.

Beta-blockers have application in the treatment of tachydysrhythmias, elevated blood pressure, anxiety, and tremors secondary to severe hyperthyroidism or in a thyroid storm. Consult medical direction prior to such therapy.

Other forms of care for thyroid complications include passive warming of the cold hypothyroid or myxedema patient. Place the patient in a warm environment and cover him with blankets. Cool the critical hyperthyroid by placing cold packs at the neck, wrists, and groin.

Ongoing Assessment

Throughout transport, monitor the patient for changes in hemodynamic, cardiac, or respiratory status. Obtain vital signs every 5 to 10 minutes, and provide continual emotional support.

Wernicke's Encephalopathy and Korsakoff's Syndrome

The metabolization of carbohydrates is necessary for the production of the cellular fuel ATP. However, for this process to be completed, oxygen, glucose, and thiamine must be present in adequate amounts.

As discussed previously, thiamine, or vitamin B_1, is essential for the final transformation of carbohydrates into ATP. Without thiamine, the body has great difficulty in this conversion process, profoundly affecting the brain. Poor cellular nutrition results in the gradual swelling and degeneration of cerebral neurons. In consequence, a disruption occurs in the normal cellular workings and associated activities. Because the body does not readily store thiamine, the vitamin is exclusively obtained through continual dietary intake.

Wernicke's encephalopathy is the disruption of brain activity associated with thiamine deficiency. It results in altered mental status ranging from mild confusion to inappropriate behavior and lethargy. Ataxia may also be present. For Wernicke's encephalopathy, examination of the eyes is particularly informative. The individual with Wernicke's encephalopathy may reveal ocular paralysis or exhibit *nystagmus* and may also exhibit a *dysconjugate gaze* with or without the presence of nystagmus.

As thiamine levels are based purely on diet, Wernicke's encephalopathy should be suspected in anyone with the simultaneous presentation of malnutrition and altered mental status. Individuals prone to the development of Wernicke's include the elderly, alcoholics, the destitute, or anyone else who may be incapable of obtaining an appropriate diet.

Wernicke's encephalopathy is a chronic condition that is unlikely to respond to acute therapy. You should suspect Wernicke's encephalopathy when hypoglycemia fails to respond to the administration of dextrose.

nystagmus rapid and rhythmic movement of both pupils, usually horizontally or vertically.

dysconjugate gaze eyes turned in different directions.

TABLE 7-12 Wernicke's Encephalopathy or Korsakoff's Psychosis and Altered Mental Status: Typical Findings

Scene Size-up	Initial Assessment	Physical Exam/Vitals	History
Signs of alcoholism or improper diet	Chief complaint of confusion, lethargy, ataxia, personality changes, change in cognitive status	Pupillary nystagmus, dysconjugate gaze, oral cavity dehydration, liver distention (hepatic disease with alcoholism), abdominal emaciation or distention (malnutrition)	Signs/symptoms: confusion, amnesia, inappropriate behavior, hallucinations Previous diagnosis of Wernicke's encephalopathy or Korsakoff's psychosis History of chronic alcoholism History of poor dietary intake, malnutrition, progressive mental decline

Over time, the deficiency of thiamine causes continued neuronal damage and can progress to Korsakoff's psychosis. Korsakoff's psychosis expresses itself with major disturbances in cognitive ability and memory retention. Subsequently, Korsakoff's involves amnesia or gaps in memory and a poor attention span. Korsakoff's psychosis is irreversible.

Assessment of Possible Wernicke's Encephalopathy or Korsakoff's Psychosis

The following section describes specifics about assessment of a patient who may be suffering from Wernicke's encephalopathy or Korsakoff's psychosis (Table 7-12)—within the generic framework for assessment presented earlier in the chapter. The points raised here may apply to assessment when you already suspect that the patient has Wernicke's or Korsakoff's disorder, or may bring out factors that would point to such a cause of the patient's altered mental status.

Wernicke's encephalopathy and Korsakoff's psychosis are difficult to distinguish, requiring a knowledge of the disease process and thorough assessment skills.

Scene Size-Up The practice of assuring a safe scene prior to patient contact may prove important if your patient is suffering from Wernicke's encephalopathy or Korsakoff's psychosis. Because these conditions are frequently associated with alcoholism and inadequate diet, be alert to signs of alcoholism or of the patient's inability to obtain a proper diet. Empty alcohol bottles and a residence with little to no food warrants the consideration of Wernicke's encephalopathy or Korsakoff's psychosis.

On approach, observe the patient's general status. Look for signs of malnutrition, such as global wasting, or signs associated with alcoholism. Note if the patient is confused, walking around aimlessly, or exhibiting poor cognition and incoherent speech. Develop an initial impression of the mental status, and approach with caution.

Initial Assessment Patients with Wernicke's encephalopathy or Korsakoff's psychosis generally present with confusion, lethargy, or ataxia. If the complaint is delivered by another source, the concerned party may describe recent personality changes and changes in the patient's cognitive status.

Unless complicated with hypoglycemia or active alcoholic intoxication, patients with isolated Wernicke's encephalopathy or Korsakoff's psychosis generally do not present in an unresponsive state. However, you should still evaluate the airway to ensure full patency. Evaluate respiratory rate and volume. Palpate the pulses and assess skin color and temperature to establish the general status of circulation and perfusion.

Physical Exam The results of a physical exam will also be useful in determining the presence of Wernicke's encephalopathy or Korsakoff's psychosis. Pertinent findings include the following:

- ***Head***
  - Ocular nystagmus
  - Dysconjugate gaze
  - Oral cavity dehydration
- ***Abdomen***
  - Liver distention (hepatic disease associated with alcoholism)
  - Abdominal emaciation or distention (malnutrition)

Focused History Acquiring a medical history is extremely important in identifying the patient with Wernicke's encephalopathy or Korsakoff's psychosis, and in evaluating the progression and severity of the condition. Key aspects of the medical history are outlined in the following SAMPLE format.

Signs and Symptoms. Ascertain any and all signs and symptoms that pertain to cognitive function. Information should include presence or absence of the following:

- Confusion
- Amnesia
- Inappropriate behavior
- Hallucinations

Allergies. Note any medicinal allergies the patient may have.

Medications. Obtain all medications and relay them to hospital personnel.

Past Medical History. Inquire as to any previous diagnosis of Wernicke's encephalopathy or Korsakoff's psychosis. Additionally, a past history of chronic alcoholism is important in establishing Wernicke's encephalopathy or Korsakoff's psychosis as the root of altered mental status.

Last Oral Intake. In addition to the last oral intake, look for a history of poor dietary intake and malnutrition. As thiamine is obtained via diet, nutritional behavior is extremely important in identifying Wernicke's encephalopathy or Korsakoff's psychosis as the possible cause of altered mental status.

Events Prior to Illness. Examine the events surrounding the onset of altered mental status. In relation to Wernicke's encephalopathy or Korsakoff's psychosis, reconfirm the following information:

- Poor dietary intake
- Malnutrition
- Progressive mental decline

Management of the Wernicke's Encephalopathy or Korsakoff's Psychosis Patient

Because Wernicke's encephalopathy occurs secondary to a B-complex vitamin deficiency, field intervention formerly centered on the administration of thiamine. It is now recognized that this is a chronic condition unlikely to be reversed with a single injection of thiamine.

If medical direction or your local protocols call for it, thiamine 100 mg is administered by the intravenous and intramuscular routes, with optimal delivery divided evenly between the two (50 mg IV and 50 mg IM). In this way, rapid delivery is obtained through intravenous administration with a slower, sustained delivery following by way of intramuscular release. Initially, as always, assure an adequate airway and oxygenation. Establish IV access, and draw blood specimens for analysis prior to administering any medication. Then, administer at least 50 mg thiamine for rapid delivery. Inject the remaining 50 mg thiamine in the deltoid muscle or gluteal region. Some protocols allow for all 100 mg to administered intravenously.

In light of the possibility of malnutrition, evaluate blood glucose levels. If hypoglycemia exists, administer 25 grams of 50 percent dextrose after the delivery of thiamine.

Thiamine administration is considered a diagnostic procedure in the confirmation of Wernicke's encephalopathy. In true Wernicke's, the administration of thiamine and, when indicated, 50 percent dextrose, should produce an improvement over a period of several days.

As stated earlier, Korsakoff's psychosis is associated with an irreversible pathology.

Ongoing Assessment

En route to the hospital, perform ongoing assessment. Repeat the initial assessment, reevaluate vital signs, and monitor the patient for any changes in mental status or other parameters.

Toxic Encephalopathies

The human body is a laboratory in which chemical reactions (metabolism) continually occur. For the appropriate chemical reactions to be achieved in the appropriate manners, the body requires a specific chemical composition or makeup.

Metabolically, the central nervous system is very sensitive to changes in the internal chemical environment. Any alteration in the overall chemistry can cause cerebral dysfunction and serve to accelerate, depress, change, or completely halt reactions that occur within the brain. Many times, this alteration of brain function becomes obvious through changes in mental and behavioral presentations.

Ingestion of medications is an effective method of changing the chemical composition of the body. When drugs are taken at medically recommended dosages, the chemical environment and reactions are generally enhanced in a manner that benefits the patient. Excessive ingestion, however, creates a toxic environment that is detrimental to the body's ability to facilitate chemical reactions and organ maintenance. As a result, the body and brain do not operate in typical or optimum fashion.

There exist literally thousands of over-the-counter, prescription, and illicit drugs, all capable of creating a toxic environment with resulting cerebral disturbance. Drugs and toxins that frequently cause altered mental status include alcohol, cocaine, amphetamines, serotoninizing agents (e.g., Prozac), anticholinergics, and benzodiazepines. Among the thousands, a few are encountered more frequently than others. These include barbiturates, antidepressants, phenothiazines, opiates, and salicylates, which, with exposure to carbon monoxide, are discussed in the following sections.

Barbiturates

Barbiturates are prescription drugs. At lower dosages, they have an antianxiety (sedative) effect. Increased dosages of barbiturates have a sleep-inducing (hypnotic) effect. Although falling in popularity in comparison to the more popular benzodiazepines, barbiturates are still used and are the focus of high abuse. Even at prescribed dosages, barbiturates can display side effects that involve the CNS. When taken in excess, toxic levels of barbiturates grossly impair mental function, thereby altering an individual's mental and behavioral presentation and even resulting in death.

Barbiturates function by depressing the activity of the RAS. Decreasing the activity of the RAS results in a decrease in the stimulation of the cerebral cortex. Consequently, a highly anxious or restless individual enjoys a soothing or calming effect. As the dosage is increased, the neurons of the RAS are depressed to the point where sleep ensues. Generally, prescribed dosages prove beneficial to those in need and are not life threatening.

Barbiturates function by depressing the activity of the reticular activating system.

Excessive dosages result in toxicity, grossly disabling the RAS and cerebrum, resulting in a decreased level of responsiveness and alterations in sensory perception. The individual may exhibit ataxia, confusion, hallucinations, and even coma. At higher levels of toxicity, depression of the medullary respiratory, cardiac, and vasomotor centers occurs. This leads to shock as peripheral vasodilation and bradycardia decrease vital perfusion to all tissues, including the brain. In addition, decreased respiratory activity results in hypoxia and hypercapnia. If unchecked, a barbiturate overdose will culminate in death.

Tricyclic Antidepressants

Within the brain, millions of neurons (nerve cells) come together in an organized fashion. Electricity is the major mode of transmission within the neuron, but electricity is unable to bridge the synaptic gap that separates neurons. Instead, chemical neurotransmitters carry messages between neurons and to other target receptors.

On electrical stimulus, the presynaptic neuron releases a chemical neurotransmitter that flows across the synaptic gap until it contacts a target receptor on another neuron or tissue. Once in contact, the chemical neurotransmitter delivers a chemical message that initiates a specific response in the receiving structure. In this manner, neurons communicate by sending and receiving messages throughout the body and within the brain itself.

Within the brain, the limbic system is responsible for the formulation of emotion and emotional response. The limbic system uses several neurotransmitters, including norepinephrine and serotonin. Within the limbic system, norepinephrine produces mania, or good feelings, while deficits of norepinephrine result in depression. The same actions are assumed for serotonin. Consequently, by increasing levels of norepinephrine and serotonin, modification of significant depression can occur.

Tricyclic antidepressants have proven quite useful in the alleviation of certain types of depression. They work in the following manner: After norepinephrine and serotonin are released by the nerve cell, tricyclic antidepressants block the active reuptake of these neurotransmitters. Subsequently, more norepinephrine and serotonin remain within the synaptic gap for stimulation of the limbic system. Because norepinephrine and serotonin are responsible for "feeling good," there is a reversal of the depressive feeling.

Not all of those taking tricyclic antidepressants require the medication for clinical depression. Tricyclic antidepressants are also prescribed in the treatment of chronic pain, insomnia, and migraine headaches.

Unfortunately, tricyclic antidepressants have far-reaching effects that come to the fore in the event of an overdose. Depending on the agent, tricyclic antidepressants exert anticholinergic properties in varying degrees. When the drug is taken in excess, these anticholinergic properties become prominent and manifest themselves through supraventricular tachycardias, respiratory depression, hallucinations, and/or coma.

Unfortunately, tricyclic antidepressants have far-reaching effects that come to the fore in the event of an overdose.

Tricyclic antidepressants also contain properties similar to quinidine. Quinidine is an antidysrhythmic that depresses myocardial automaticity and conduction by impeding ion exchanges across the cellular membrane. In excessive dosages, tricyclic antidepressants exhibit a similar action that results in conduction delays and myocardial depression. Additionally, tricyclic antidepressants induce an alpha-adrenergic blockade that promotes hypotension through vasodilation of the peripheral vasculature.

In response to dysrhythmias and peripheral vasodilation, stubborn hypotension results in decreased perfusion and cerebral hypoxia. The effect on the CNS and outward presentation of mental status correlates closely to the degree of toxicity. Related changes in mental status include, but are not limited to, agitation, restlessness, ataxia, drowsiness, stupor, and coma. In addition, tricyclic antidepressants lower the seizure threshold, resulting in convulsions and the many complications associated with seizure activity.

The establishment of therapeutic plasma levels of a tricyclic antidepressant often takes 1 to 2 weeks. Before the therapeutic level is reached, the patient may feel that he is underdosing and increase intake in an effort to attain the therapeutic benefit more rapidly. Also, many patients on tricyclic antidepressants have a psychiatric history and, consequently, may be more prone to intentional or unintentional overdose.

Phenothiazines

Psychosis is defined as a mental illness in which the afflicted individual suffers gross impairment in the interpretation of reality. Psychosis is a broad umbrella that covers many specific types of mental disorders, including schizophrenia, delusions, hallucinations, paranoia, and Tourette's disorder. When psychosis reaches a stage at which the individual cannot function, pharmacologic therapy is often used to modify and control the adverse behavior.

The central nervous system also uses the chemical neurotransmitters dopamine and acetylcholine. Within the limbic system, dopamine is used for the stimulation of emotion and cognitive function. An increase of dopamine correlates to an increase in the emotional and cognitive responses. Conversely, a decrease in dopamine equates to a decrease in the emotional and cognitive responses. In individuals with psychotic disorders, it is theorized that excessive levels of dopamine are at play. Consequently, decreasing the excessive dopaminergic stimulation can prove successful in the control and modification of the psychotic behavior.

Phenothiazines are classified as antipsychotic drugs. Phenothiazines decrease psychotic behavior by blocking the dopamine receptors in the limbic system. Through antidopaminergic activities, the phenothiazines decrease the rate at which the neurons fire, thus suppressing psychotic behavior.

Phenothiazines are classified as antipsychotic drugs.

Unfortunately, the work of phenothiazines is not confined to the limbic system, and a full understanding of the relationship between the antidopaminergic and anticholinergic properties is extremely important when dealing with phenothiazine overdoses. Motor activity initiated by the cerebral cortex depends on a specific balance between dopamine and acetylcholine. Antidopaminergic properties decrease the stimulatory ability of dopamine, while anticholinergic properties reduce the stimulatory ability of acetylcholine. Because the antidopaminergic property is the dominant effect, phenothiazines do not decrease the stimulatory properties of dopamine and acetylcholine in proportionally equal amounts. Any significant imbalance in the dopamine–acetylcholine relationship can result in both adverse mental and adverse neurologic presentations.

As with tricyclic antidepressants, toxic effects of phenothiazines result in the excessive alpha-adrenergic blockade of the peripheral vasculature. In conjunction with myocardial depression and conduction difficulties, the vasodilation promotes hypoperfusion of the brain and results in cerebral hypoxia evidenced by a decrease in the level of consciousness ranging from confusion to stupor to coma. (Refer to the earlier information on tricyclic antidepressants for discussion of the anticholinergic and quinidine effects.)

Acute Dystonic Reactions Acute dystonic reactions result from the ingestion of phenothiazines and generally occur within 48 to 72 hours of initial ingestion. As dopamine stimulation is blunted, the beneficial effect is seen in the limbic system. However, in the motor aspect of the cerebral cortex, the balance between dopaminergic and cholinergic stimulation is askew. Generally, the anticholinergic activity is less than the antidopaminergic stimulation. Subsequently, the quantity of acetylcholine is greater than the required level of dopamine. Unchecked, the acetylcholine produces unusual motor activity, most notably in the face and upper torso.

Acute dystonic reactions present with facial grimacing, neck twisting to one side (torticollis), facial tics, an upward gaze, and sometimes ocular paralysis. The acute dystonic reaction is reversible with appropriate treatment. Often, the patient is quite panicked by the odd behavior but generally retains a full level of consciousness throughout the event. A common related syndrome is akisthesia, a difficult to describe feeling of discomfort, restlessness, and jitteriness, which may manifest as an altered mental status but not unconsciousness.

Tardive Dyskinesia Tardive dyskinesia is the consequence of long-term antipsychotic drug use. The exact mechanism is unknown, but tardive dyskinesia is represented by continual grimacing, scowling, lip smacking, tongue protrusion, finger rolling, and eyelid spasms. Tardive dyskinesia is an irreversible syndrome. That is, there is no known effective treatment for the condition.

Opiates and Opioids

Derived from naturally occurring opium, opiates are narcotics commonly used in the treatment of moderate to severe pain. Opioids, or synthetic narcotics, closely mimic the actions of natural opiates and are also used in pain management. In addition to analgesia (pain relief), both opiates and opioids produce feelings of euphoria and are consequently drugs with high abuse potential. Excessive ingestion of opiates and opioids adversely affects the central nervous system and serves to change one's mental and behavioral output.

Opiates and opioids depress cerebral function. Although affecting all regions of the brain, the thalamus, cerebral cortex, and medulla prove particularly sensitive.

As the medulla houses the cardiac, vasomotor, and respiratory control centers, medullary depression produces bradycardia, vasodilation, and respiratory hypoventilation. Together, these three factors create an environment of hypoperfusion and cerebral hypoxia.

Decreased perfusion correlates to cerebral dysfunction and further depression of vital functions. Depending on dosage, opiates or opioids generate a variety of mental presentations ranging from confusion and drowsiness to stupor and coma. The individual may present with bradypnea and bradycardia, again depending on the quantity ingested. Noncardiogenic pulmonary edema may also present as dilated capillaries become "leaky" and allow fluid to cross into the interstitial space and alveoli. Pinpoint pupils and hypoventilation (respiratory rate less than 8/minute) are key findings that often indicate narcotic ingestion.

Salicylates

Salicylates are a derivative of salicylic acid, a naturally occurring substance used for its analgesic, antipyretic (antifever), and antiinflammatory properties. Aspirin is a common drug containing salicylate. In therapeutic doses, salicylates prove effective and are even sold over the counter. However, in exorbitant dosages, salicylates induce a chain of events that prove toxic to the tissue of the brain, thus producing adverse changes in mental status.

In exorbitant dosages, salicylates induce a chain of events that prove toxic to the tissue of the brain, thus producing adverse changes in mental status.

Salicylate toxicity progresses in stages and depends on the total amount ingested. Toxicity from salicylate ingestion typically occurs at doses of >150 mg/kg. Initially, overingestion of a salicylate produces a direct stimulatory effect on the CNS. A key is the induction of hyperventilation. Hyperventilation causes an excessive quantity of carbon dioxide to be excreted, thus producing respiratory alkalosis. In itself, respiratory alkalosis leads to hyperexcitation of the cerebral neurons that results in confusion, agitation, *tinnitis,* and muscular twitching.

tinnitis ringing in the ear.

Excessive salicylate ingestion interferes with the processes that produce cellular ATP. This interference greatly increases the amount of generated lactic acid, which precipitates metabolic acidosis. Eventually, the acidotic environment is so significant that it negatively affects many organs, including the heart and the brain. As discussed previously, acidosis depresses the actions of the myocardium and effectively suppresses electrical activity within the cerebral neurons.

With respect to cerebral depression, acidosis produces delirium, hallucinations, convulsions, and stupor. In severe instances of acidosis, coma and death can result as dysfunction occurs in the cardiac, respiratory, thermoregulatory, and vasomotor centers.

Carbon Monoxide

Carbon monoxide is a colorless, odorless gas that results from the incomplete combustion of carbon-containing materials. Sources of carbon monoxide include faulty space heaters or furnaces, house fires, automobile exhaust, and cigarette smoke. Depending on the quantity of exposure and subsequent ingestion, carbon monoxide can manifest in a variety of ways. In large amounts, carbon monoxide is poisonous and will produce death. A toxic level of CO (e.g., 50 ppm) may be revealed by a household CO detector or fire service response to a CO alarm.

Once in the body, carbon monoxide competes with oxygen for the binding sites on the hemoglobin of the red blood cells. In that carbon monoxide has a 200 times greater affinity for the hemoglobin than does oxygen, much of the existing oxygen is readily displaced. In addition, the presence of carbon monoxide impairs the release of whatever oxygen remains on the hemoglobin. Don't be deceived by an extremely high SpO_2 reading in the carbon monoxide-poisoned patient. The SpO_2 monitor is looking for hemoglobin that is red and saturated with oxygen. The carbon monoxide molecule will bind to the hemoglobin and create a red molecule, causing the pulse oximeter to read it as an oxygen-saturated hemoglobin molecule. Thus, severely hypoxic carbon monoxide-poisoned patients may present with SpO_2 readings near or at 100 percent.

Cellular asphyxia and damage occur as anaerobic metabolism and acidosis ensue. Organs with high metabolic rates, such as the heart and brain, are particularly affected. Anaerobic metabolism within the heart and brain lead to dysfunction and depression of activity. In regard to the CNS, cerebral hypoxia leads to the presence of a headache, altered vision, auditory difficulties, cognition deficits, delirium, drowsiness, and/or agitation. At higher dosages, carbon monoxide will manifest through psychotic behavior, seizures, and coma. When greater than 80 percent of the hemoglobin becomes saturated with carbon monoxide, death is almost certain.

Assessment of Possible Toxicologic Encephalopathy

The following section describes specifics about assessment of a patient who is suffering from suspected toxicologic encephalopathy (Table 7-13)—within the generic framework for assessment presented earlier in the chapter. The points raised here may apply to assessment when you already suspect that the patient's problem stems from toxic ingestion, or may bring out factors that would point to a toxic cause of the patient's altered mental status.

In addition to the medications and substances discussed previously, there exist literally thousands of others that can alter mental status. A priority in assessment and management of the patient with toxicologic encephalopathy is to determine what substance was ingested, the quantity ingested, and the time it was ingested. If the substance can be identified, the poison control center should be promptly contacted for further information on the effects and treatment recommendations.

Scene Size-Up At the scene of a patient who is suspected of ingesting a toxicologic substance, look for signs of the type of ingestion that has occurred. Open

TABLE 7-13 Toxicologic Encephalopathy and Altered Mental Status: Typical Findings

Scene Size-up	Initial Assessment	Physical Exam/Vitals	History
Open medication containers, strange odors, unusual patient behavior or presentation	Complaint of suicide attempt or depression (intentional ingestion); complaint consistent with toxic effect of ingested substance (e.g., confusion, ataxia) (unintentional ingestion or overdose) Abnormal respirations, e.g., shallow respirations (barbiturates); rapid, shallow respirations (salicylates); Kussmaul's respirations (massive metabolic acidosis) Abnoramal pulses, e.g., bradycardia (barbiturates, opiates); irregular, weak pulses (tricyclic antidepressants)	Pupillary dysfunction, JVD, abnormal breath sounds, adventitious lung sounds, pathological respiratory patterns, laborious respirations with accessory muscle use, abnormal heart tones, distal pulse abnormalities, poor distal perfusion Injection sites indicating substance abuse; scarring indicating suicide attempts Vital signs: (as listed under "Abnormal respirations" and "Abnormal pulses," at left)	Signs/symptoms: chest pain, shortness of breath, dizziness; nausea or vomiting; syncope; declining or improving mental or neurologic status Thorough assessment of all medications or drugs; note any antidepression or antipsychotic medications History of previous psychiatric illness, suicide attempts, drug or substance abuse, any other medical history

medication bottles can provide invaluable information about an intentional or unintentional ingestion. Strange odors may indicate some sort of vapor poisoning. Always remain aware that a patient who is suicidal and has intentionally ingested medications represents a possible danger to himself and others. Enter the scene cautiously, and only after provider safety has been assured.

Initial Assessment As you approach the patient, quickly form an impression of mental status. Note the patient's behavior and positioning as clues to the level of distress. The patient's actions or lack of actions may provide initial clues as to the type of ingestion that has occurred.

Depending on whether the ingestion or exposure was intentional or unintentional, complaints may vary. Intentional overdoses may provide a complaint of suicide or depression, while the unintentional ingestion may produce a chief complaint in line with the toxic effect of the substance. If EMS was summoned by someone other than the patient, the complaint may center around confusion, ataxia, or other changes in mental and behavioral status. For the comatose patient who cannot relay a chief complaint, look to other sources, such as empty pill bottles or family, friends, or other witnesses.

Fully visualize the airway of any patient with a decreased level of consciousness. Look for pills, vomitus, position of the tongue, or other causes of airway compromise.

Evaluate the respiratory status in reference to rate and adequacy of oxygenation and ventilation. Shallow respirations may suggest an overdose of barbiturates or another CNS depressant. Rapid and shallow ventilation may suggest a salicylate ingestion with a compensatory respiratory alkalosis compounding the situation. As discussed earlier, deep and rapid Kussmaul's respirations may suggest an agent whose ingestion has resulted in significant metabolic acidosis.

Evaluate pulses in terms of rate, regularity, and strength. Barbiturates and opiates tend to depress the overall myocardial activity, resulting in bradycardia. The cardiotoxicity of many tricyclic antidepressants can result in irregular and weak peripheral pulses secondary to hypotension caused by the alpha-adrenergic blockade. Skin color, temperature, and the presence or absence of diaphoresis should also be observed and documented.

Physical Exam A physical exam must be conducted on every patient with suspected toxic encephalopathy. In addition to providing further information as to the type and quantity of agent ingested, the physical exam can reveal the degree of impact on the different organ systems.

Important aspects of the physical exam as it applies to toxicologic-induced encephalopathy include the following:

- ***Head***
  - Pupillary status (gaze, size, equality, reactivity)
  - Oral cavity patency
- ***Neck.*** JVD (depressed pumping of the heart)
- ***Chest***
  - Breath sounds (possibility of aspiration)
  - Adventitious lung sounds (depressed pumping of the heart)
  - Pathological respiratory patterns
  - Auscultation of heart tones
  - Labored respirations with accessory muscle use

- *Extremities*
  - Distal pulses and equality
  - Perfusion parameters
  - Presence of injection sites indicating previous substance abuse
  - Scarring indicating possible previous suicide attempts

Vital Signs Keep in mind that shallow respirations may be associated with barbiturate, opioid, or other CNS depressant overdose; rapid, shallow ventilations with salicylate ingestion. An agent that produces metabolic acidosis may present with Kussmaul's respirations. Bradycardia is associated with barbiturate and opiate overdose. Irregular, weak pulses and hypotension are associated with tricyclic antidepressant overdose.

Focused History If the patient is stable and forthcoming with information, a SAMPLE history can provide valuable information. First and foremost, attempt to identify the agent taken and quantity ingested. Also, the time of ingestion is very helpful. If the patient is a poor historian or cannot respond, look to other sources such as family, friends, or other witnesses.

Signs and Symptoms. Signs and symptoms surrounding the incident are extremely important to ascertain and relay to the hospital staff. Look specifically for symptoms as they relate to the central nervous and cardiovascular systems:

- Declining or improving mental or neurologic status
- Chest pain, shortness of breath, or dizziness
- Nausea or vomiting
- Syncope
- Seizures

Allergies. Note any medical allergies the patient may have.

Medications. Some medications can potentiate the effects of others or create additional side effects and worsen the overall situation. Also, overingestion of prescription medications may have occurred inadvertently. Therefore, a list of all the patient's current medications should be compiled and relayed to hospital staff. In addition, if the patient has ingested a medication, that medication should be taken to the hospital for further evaluation. Also, keep an attentive eye for behavioral medications that may indicate a previous psychiatric history.

Past Medical History. A complete record of the patient's past medical history is important because existing problems may be worsened by the ingestion of certain agents. In particular, pay attention to the following:

- Previous psychiatric history
- Previous suicide attempts
- Previous drug and substance abuse
- Environmental exposures (oil/gas/kerosene/wood heat, etc.)
- Any other medical history available

Last Oral Intake. The patient's last ingestion of food may indicate the potential for significant vomitus. Also, the absorption of some medications into the GI tract may be significantly slowed by the presence of food in the gut.

Events Prior to Illness. The events or behavior of the individual preceding the ingestion may provide important information as to the patient's status. In particular, inquire as to the following:

- When ingestion occurred
- Intentionality of ingestion
- Location where ingestion occurred
- Precipitating depression or suicidal ideation
- Medical complaints prior to ingestion

Management of the Toxicologic Encephalopathy Patient

In addition to the agents discussed previously, a multitude of drugs, organic substances, and chemical substances exist that, when ingested, will alter mental status. In the prehospital environment, treatment of the toxicologic patient will differ depending on presentation and the substance that was actually ingested.

Establish and maintain a patent airway and adequate ventilation, oxygenation, and circulation. If the patient is comatose or has a severely decreased level of consciousness, tracheal intubation should be considered to protect the airway and prevent aspiration. If intubation is not feasible, continuously monitor the airway. If the patient is breathing adequately, provide oxygen via a nonrebreather mask. If the ventilation is inadequate, provide positive-pressure ventilation. If acidosis is a side effect of ingestion, controlled hyperventilation may be considered.

Establish an intravenous line early in the management of any patient with a toxic ingestion. Rapid decompensation is possible, with cardiovascular collapse making intravenous access difficult at a later time. Fluid therapy should proceed according to hemodynamic status. While establishing access, draw blood specimens for rapid analysis once the specimens reach the hospital. Also, be sure to check the blood glucose level in any patient presenting with an altered mental status.

If you know the specific agent involved, contact the poison control center or your local medical direction for further information and advice on continued patient management. The poison control center and local medical direction is an excellent resource for information concerning prognosis, effects, and complications. Often, poison control can also suggest basic treatment; however, the recommendations given do not supersede standing orders and online medical direction.

Several drugs are specific to the emergency treatment of toxicologic emergencies. Table 7-14 lists and describes these agents.

If the drug or substance consumed is on scene, take the container and any remainder of contents to the hospital with the patient. Any vomitus should be packaged and transported to the hospital for analysis.

Ongoing Assessment

Conduct ongoing monitoring of the patient en route to the hospital. Repeat the initial assessment. Reassess vital signs, and note trends in the patient's condition. If there is a decreased level of consciousness, transport the patient in the recovery position to protect the airway in case of vomiting.

Environmental Causes

Metabolic rates are governed by temperature. In the human body, a core temperature of approximately 98°F (37°C) permits reactions to occur at a normal rate. Any

TABLE 7-14 **Drugs for Toxicologic Emergencies**

Agent	Action	Dosage	Route
Activated charcoal	Adsorbant	1–2 g/kg	PO
Magnesium sulfate	Cathartic	30 g	PO
Antidote	**Agent**	**Dosage**	**Route**
Acetylcysteine	Acetaminophen	140 mg/kg	PO
Glucagon	Beta-blocker	3–10 mg	IV
Atropine	Cholinergic	2 mg	IV
Naloxone	Opiates	2 mg	IV, IM, SQ, SL, IL, ET, or IN
Diphenhydramine	Dystonic reaction	25–50 mg	IV or IM
Flumazenil	Benzodiazepine	For mixed ingestion: 0.2 mg IVP over 30 sec; add'l doses of 0.3 to 0.5 mg each minute to max 3 mg	IV
Calcium chloride or glucagon	Calcium channel blocker	Calcium chloride 1–4 g slow IVP of 10 percent solution; glucagon 5–15 mg IV or IM (for hypotension)	
Oxygen	Carbon monoxide poisoning	100 percent by nonrebreather mask	

increase in core temperature serves to increase reaction rates, while a decrease in temperature results in a slower rate of reaction. Small increases in temperature are tolerated and often serve as a protective mechanism (fever) to destroy invading pathogens. However, if the body temperature rises above 105°F (40°C), reaction rates accelerate to a danger point. Conversely, a core temperature significantly below 94°F (34°C) will slow reaction rates to the point of detriment.

The human body has inherent mechanisms geared toward the maintenance of an optimal temperature. In times of excessive heat production or gain, vasodilation occurs, sending warm blood to the periphery for heat radiation into the environment. Sweating serves to rid the body of excess heat through evaporation. When additional heat is needed, the body attempts to generate heat through muscular shivering or increases in the basal metabolic rate. Failure of these corrective actions will produce changes in reaction rates that directly affect the central nervous system and overt mental and behavioral status.

Heat Exhaustion

Heat exhaustion is a complication of heat gain and increase in body temperature. Generally, heat exhaustion produces massive sodium and fluid loss as an individual experiences profuse sweating in a hot environment. Dehydration, hyponatremia, and overall increased metabolic reaction rates occur but, by the definition of heat exhaustion, not at the extremes necessary to cause altered mental status. An altered mental status should lead to suspicion of heat stroke.

Outside the central nervous system, the patient may exhibit tachycardia as the body attempts to push warm blood to the periphery for heat radiation. In addition, the skin may be diaphoretic, with progressive drying as the condition progresses. A dramatic increase in respiratory rate and acute hypotension may be observed as the body continues to sustain fluid and sodium loss. At this juncture, progression from heat exhaustion to heat stroke is a distinct possibility.

Heat Stroke

Heat stroke constitutes a dire medical emergency. As the body's mechanisms for heat dissipation become exhausted, extreme elevation of the core temperature ensues. At temperatures greater than 105°F (40°C), damage occurs to the hypothalamus. Because the hypothalamus is the center responsible for temperature maintenance, the body loses all ability to rid itself of the excess heat. Also, high temperatures directly damage brain tissue, resulting in cerebral edema and dysfunction.

Initially, the patient with heat stroke will exhibit confusion, agitation, and irrationality. As the core temperature rises, seizures and coma will ensue. As the body's normal compensatory mechanisms for heat dissipation become depleted, hot, flushed, dry skin will present. (In exertional heat stroke, the skin will usually be hot but wet.) In the early stages of heat stroke, elevated vital signs may be observed as the cerebral neurons dysfunction. However, this stage is short lived as decompensation begins, giving way to circulatory shock, coma, and eventual cardiopulmonary arrest.

Hypothermia

Hypothermia is a decrease in body temperature, which correlates to a decrease in metabolic reaction rates. Because cold effectively depresses the brain as a whole, slowing of the cardiac, respiratory, and vasomotor centers occurs. Below 94°F (34°C), the ability of temperature regulation is impaired as the ability to generate heat by muscular shivering is severely impeded. A temperature under 86°F (30°C) results in total hypothalamic dysfunction and complete loss of temperature maintenance. Eventually, the outcome is cardiac and pulmonary arrest and death.

As cerebral function becomes impaired, the mental status of a hypothermic patient can range from drowsiness to stupor to coma. The patient may present with cool to cold, dry skin and exhibit depressed vital signs. In colder temperatures, the hemoglobin is more resistant to the off-loading of oxygen at the cellular level. Therefore, the signs and symptoms of hypoxia may also be present. Through decreased central nervous stimulation, acidotic blood, and the direct effect of the cold internal temperature, the heart may become irritable and exhibit bradycardia with a variety of ectopic beats. Often, a "J", or Osborne, wave may be observable immediately following the QRS complex (Figure 7-10). Immediate intervention is needed to prevent death.

As cerebral function becomes impaired, the mental status of a hypothermic patient can range from drowsiness to stupor to coma.

Assessment of Possible Environmentally Caused Altered Mental Status

The following section describes specifics about assessment of a patient who is suffering from altered mental status with a possible environmental cause

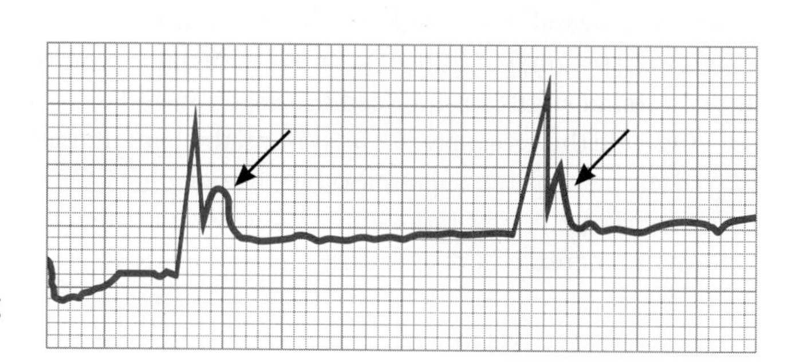

FIGURE 7-10
ECG tracing showing "J" wave (Osborne wave) following the QRS complex as seen in hypothermia.

TABLE 7-15 Environmental Causes and Altered Mental Status: Typical Findings

Scene Size-up	Initial Assessment	Physical Exam/Vitals	History
Hot, warm, cool, or cold ambient temperature	Chief complaint of confusion, agitation, delirium, decreased level of consciousness Bradypnea (hypothermia, end-stage respiratory failure in heat stroke); tachypnea (heat exhaustion, early heat stroke) Tachycardia (heat exhaustion, moderate heat stroke); bradycardia (advanced heat stroke, hypothermia) Warm to hot skin with or without diaphoresis (heat emergency); cool or cold skin (cold emergency)	Pupillary dysfunction, oral cavity dehydration, respiratory and pulse parameters, skin temperature and perfusion Vital signs: respiratory and pulse parameters as listed at left; elevated blood pressure (early heat emergency); decreased blood pressure (advanced heat stroke, hypothermia)	Signs/symptoms: pain or cramps, chest pain, dyspnea, dizziness, syncope, ataxia or confusion, weakness, nausea or vomiting History of diabetes, heart condition, thyroid condition (can complicate or be complicated by heat or cold effects); history of prior thermoregulatory disturbance Exposure to heat or cold prior to illness

(Table 7-15)—within the generic framework for assessment presented earlier in the chapter. The points raised here may apply to assessment when you already suspect that the patient has an environmentally caused condition, or may bring out factors that would point to an environmental cause of the patient's altered mental status.

Through a systematic assessment, the type of thermoregulatory dysfunction at play can readily be identified and treated.

Scene Size-Up As you enter the scene, note the ambient temperature. An extremely hot environment may be the initial clue to heat exhaustion or heat stroke, whereas a cool to cold setting may relate to hypothermia. The elderly and extremely young do not have the thermoregulatory compensatory capacity that young and middle-age adults possess. Therefore, even a slightly cool or warm environment is capable of inducing a thermoregulatory emergency in these patients.

Initial Assessment The chief complaint surrounding a thermoregulatory disturbance may involve confusion, agitation, delirium, or a decreased level of consciousness. If the patient is unresponsive and no other sources of information exist, the chief complaint must be derived from scene information and assessment findings.

As always, ensure a patent airway. For the conscious patient in early stages of heat exhaustion or hypothermia, the ability to communicate illustrates an open airway. However, as the impact of internal temperatures intensifies, a decreased level of consciousness may occur, and along with it the loss of airway control. In such situations, full airway evaluation and protective measures are warranted.

The respiratory status can provide important clues. Bradypnea may indicate hypothermia or end-stage respiratory failure found in advanced heat stroke. Tachypnea suggests heat exhaustion or early heat stroke as the body attempts compensation by expelling heat.

Evaluation of the circulatory system can also provide clues to the type and degree of thermoregulatory disturbance. Tachycardia commonly occurs in heat exhaustion and continues into moderate heat stroke. However, as heat stroke progresses, the pulse rate will eventually become slower and weaker as cardiovascular collapse ensues. The skin in heat-related emergencies tends to be warm to hot. Diaphoresis is found in heat exhaustion but is often absent in heat stroke because massive volume depletion and loss of nervous system control take their toll.

Hypothermic patients exhibit a decreased-to-bradycardic pulse rate. In severe cases of hypothermia, significant bradycardia may occur. It may be difficult to establish whether a pulse is present; thus, it is appropriate to assess the pulse for 30 to 45 seconds. If no pulse is found, or if you are unsure whether a pulse is present, begin chest compressions and ventilation. Skin in the hypothermic patient tends to be cool or cold to the touch. In the extremely hypothermic patient, assess for pulse rates carefully because the cardiac output may be so decreased that the patient is mistakenly believed to be pulseless.

Physical Exam Key points to address in the physical exam of the patient with possible environmentally induced altered mental status include the following:

- ***Head***
  - Pupils (size, reactivity, equality)
  - Oral cavity hydration
  - Reassure patency
- ***Chest***
  - Auscultate breath sounds
  - Auscultate an apical pulse—a pulse over the apex of the heart (hypothermia)
- ***Extremities***
  - Skin temperature
  - Peripheral perfusion

Vital Signs Vital signs will vary, depending on the type and severity of disturbance. When heat- or cold-related altered mental status is suspected, a rectal temperature must be obtained.

As discussed previously, tachycardia commonly occurs in heat exhaustion and continues into moderate heat stroke. However, as heat stroke progresses, the pulse rate will eventually become slower and weaker as cardiovascular collapse ensues. Again, slower pulse rates are the general rule in hypothermia.

Respiratory rates will also vary. Heat exhaustion and early heat stroke generally produce tachypnea. As with the pulse rate in heat stroke, however, the respiratory rate will decrease as compensatory mechanisms are depleted and systemwide failure occurs. Bradypnea is generally found in hypothermia.

Blood pressure will also vary according to the type of disturbance present. Although elevations in cardiac output relate to an increased blood pressure in heat exhaustion, cardiovascular collapse in the end stage of heat stroke leads to profound hypotension. In hypothermia, decreased cardiac output produces hypotension. If the hypotension is severe, you may have a difficult time obtaining a blood pressure.

Focused History If obtainable, a focused medical history can be helpful in attributing a specific thermoregulator.y cause to the altered mental status. Using the SAMPLE format, consider the points as itemized in the following sections.

Signs and Symptoms. Inquire as to signs or symptoms that indicate the extent of impact of the thermoregulatory disturbance on other organ systems, especially the cardiac system and the CNS. Such inquiries should include, but are not limited to, the following:

- Pain or cramps
- Cardiac symptoms (chest pain, dyspnea, dizziness, syncope)
- Ataxia or confusion
- Weakness (dehydration or electrolyte imbalances)
- Nausea or vomiting

Allergies. Note any medical allergies that the patient may have.

Medications. Obtaining all medications that a patient is currently taking will provide insight into existing medical problems. In addition, keep in mind that the disruption of internal temperatures can alter the metabolization of some medications, leading to ineffectiveness or relative toxicity at normal dosages.

Other medications may actually contribute to or potentiate thermoregulatory disturbances. For example, barbiturates tend to decrease the internal temperature while anticholinergic-type medications may increase body temperature. Alcohol is a vasodilating agent that makes hypothermia more likely to occur in cold environments.

Past Medical History. Existing medical problems may be complicated by a thermoregulatory disturbance. For example, administered insulin tends to lose effectiveness as the body gets colder. The strain that heat compensatory mechanisms place on a damaged heart may lead to a myocardial infarction. Thyroid complications can be precipitated by exposure to a cold or hot environment.

Ascertain any previous history of thermoregulatory disturbance because those with such a history are predisposed to future occurrences.

Last Oral Intake. Inquire as to the last oral and fluid intake. With heat-related disturbances, recent fluid intake is a concern in estimating the need to replenish lost reserves.

Events Prior to Illness. Events surrounding onset are important to determine in assessing thermoregulatory disturbances. Ask about exposure to a hot or cold environment and the duration of the exposure. Also find out about activity or exertion, especially in a hot environment.

Management of the Environmental Disorder Patient

Restoring normal internal temperatures, thus preventing further injury, is the cornerstone of prehospital care of thermoregulatory disturbances. Associated life threats and complications should be addressed as encountered, as discussed later in this section. Throughout assessment and care of the hypothermic patient, keep in mind that gentle handling is critical because rough manipulation can precipitate ventricular fibrillation. Measures to assure adequate airway, breathing, and circulation must occur prior to any other intervention. All patients with thermoregulatory disturbances must receive high-flow, high-concentration oxygen by nonrebreather mask or tracheal tube, as appropriate.

Remove the heat exhaustion or heat stroke patient from the hot environment and initiate rapid cooling. Conversely, of course, the hypothermic patient requires rewarming.

Remove the heat exhaustion or heat stroke patient from the hot environment and initiate rapid cooling in order to prevent additional damage to vital organs. After placing the patient in a cool environment, remove the patient's clothing and apply ice packs to the forehead, neck, axillary region, groin, and ankles. In addition, apply a wet sheet or cool mist to the patient and use a fan to direct a wind current over the patient, creating convection currents to remove radiated heat. Do not immerse the patient in an ice bath because this will promote shivering, thereby producing more internal heat. Consult local protocols or medical direction regarding possible administration of diazepam or another benzodiazepine to control shivering if it occurs during your cooling process.

Conversely, of course, the hypothermic patient requires rewarming. Rewarming should be gradual, not abrupt. Perform passive rewarming by placing the patient in a warm, draftfree enclosed space and covering the patient with warm blankets. If the patient is responsive, proceed with active rewarming, which includes application of hot packs to the forehead, neck, axillary region, groin, and ankles to help rewarm the blood as it passes near the surface of the skin. Oxygen and IV fluids should be warmed before they are administered to the hypothermic patient. If the patient has an altered mental status, continue with passive rewarming.

Cardiac dysrhythmias are common in thermoregulatory disturbances and deserve special mention. In the hypothermic patient, an initial attempt at dysrhythmia correction can be made according to American Heart Association guidelines. Bradycardia is thought to be a physiological response to the hypothermia; thus, pacing is not recommended. If these attempts are unsuccessful, additional attempts should be delayed until substantial rewarming has resulted in a body core temperature up at least 86 degrees Fahrenheit or 30 degrees Celsius.

In the hypothermic patient, defibrillation of ventricular fibrillation should be limited to one shock. If conversion is not achieved, additional shocks should be withheld until the core temperature is raised to 86 degrees Fahrenheit or 30 degrees Celsius, making the myocardium more receptive to electrical and pharmacologic therapy. Regardless of temperature, CPR should be performed continuously throughout the management of cardiac arrest associated with hypothermia.

In heat exhaustion and heat stroke, clinically significant cardiac dysrhythmias should be treated according to your local protocols. As the body cools, dysrhythmias should decrease in frequency or become more responsive to conventional pharmacologic therapy.

Do not allow warming or cooling procedures to delay transport to a hospital. Advanced procedures such as a warmed gastric peritoneal lavage or an iced saline peritoneal lavage—effective countermeasures for hypothermia and hyperthermia, respectively—must be carried out in a hospital setting.

Ongoing Assessment

Conduct ongoing monitoring of the patient en route to the hospital. Repeat the initial assessment, reassess vital signs, and note trends in the patient's condition. Be especially alert to manage any changes in the patient's cardiac function.

Shock

Cellular survival and normal metabolic activity depend on adequate perfusion. Perfusion is the delivery of oxygen and other nutrients to the tissues of the body and the removal of waste products. Perfusion is the result of constant and adequate circulation of blood, which in turn depends on the presence of proper fluid volumes and pressures. Hypoperfusion, or shock, is defined as inadequate tissue perfusion, and results in abnormal cellular metabolic activity.

Loss of adequate tissue perfusion has several etiologies related to either loss of fluid or inadequate systemic vascular resistance. Shock is broadly classified into several categories as follows:

- Hypovolemic shock (resulting from a loss of fluid volume: blood, plasma, or body water)
- Obstructive shock (resulting from a mechanical obstruction, such as tension pneumothorax, cardiac tamponade, or pulmonary embolus)
- Distributive shock (resulting from an abnormality in vasodilation, vasopermeability, or both)
- Cardiogenic shock (resulting from abnormal heart function, such as failure of the heart muscle, valvular insufficiency, or rhythm disturbance)

Cerebral neurons are quite sensitive to hypoperfusion, regardless of its cause. Brain dysfunction will result from the associated hypoxia, anaerobic metabolism, and ensuing acidosis, and will present with an altered mental status that may progress from confusion to lethargy to stupor to coma and death. Sepsis and septic shock (a form of distributive shock) is an especially common cause of altered mental status among elderly and debilitated patients. For a detailed discussion of the pathophysiology, assessment, and management of shock, review Chapter 4, Hypoperfusion.

SUMMARY

Altered mental status is a frequently encountered complaint in the out-of-hospital setting. Encompassing a multitude of varied behavioral presentations, altered mental status occurs secondary to a wide variety of underlying disease processes. Consequently, altered mental status is one of the most challenging presentations faced by the health care provider.

Effective prehospital management of altered mental status depends on the ability of the health care provider to think multidimensionally. This open-mindedness is necessary because many of the possible causes of altered mental status are elusive and difficult to recognize. The health care provider must keep in mind that altered mental status is not a disease in itself but rather is a symptom of an underlying abnormality in need of correction.

Proper identification and management depend on a working knowledge of individual disease processes coupled with strong assessment skills (Table 7-16). When these abilities are developed and applied, effective identification of the etiology of altered mental status is often possible, with appropriate management of the underlying cause (Figure 7-11) making a critical contribution to a positive outcome for the patient.

TABLE 7-16 **Hallmarks for Differential Diagnosis of Altered Mental Status**

Patient History

Patient history, if available, is the most important element of differential diagnosis for altered mental status. Key information would include a history of diseases such as cardiovascular or pulmonary disease, diabetes, alcoholism, thyroid condition, liver or kidney disorder, infection, nutritional problem, or psychiatric problem, as well as any medications the patient is taking and the patient's compliance with prescribed medications. In addition to history, the following are some of the hallmark findings that can help differentiate the underlying cause of altered mental status. For more complete information, review the tables throughout this chapter and in Chapters 4 (Hypoperfusion), 5 (Dyspnea), 6 (Chest Discomfort or Pain), 10 (Seizures), and 11 (Syncope).

Findings	Possible Etiology
Hot/warm/cool/cold environment	Heat- or cold-related emergency (heat exhaustion, heat stroke, hypothermia)
Syringes	Diabetic emergency, toxic overdose
Drug paraphernalia, open medication containers	Toxic ingestion/overdose, metabolic acidosis or alkalosis
Poor living conditions, poor nutrition, alcoholism	Electrolyte imbalance, Wernicke's syndrome/Korsakoff's psychosis
Pathological breathing patterns	Stroke, cranial infection, intracranial tumor, hepatic/uremic encephalopathy, electrolyte imbalance, toxicologic encephalopathy
Kussmaul's respirations	Metabolic acidosis, diabetic ketoacidosis
Hypoventilation	Respiratory acidosis, metabolic alkalosis, opiate or barbiturate overdose
Hyperventilation	Respiratory alkalosis, metabolic acidosis
Flexion/extension posturing	Stroke, intracranial tumor
Facial droop, swallowing difficulty, tongue deviation, weakness or paralysis to one side	Stroke, cranial infection, intracranial tumor, hepatic/uremic encephalopathy, electrolyte imbalance
Lethargy, malaise, confusion, decreased level of consciousness	Diabetic emergency, hepatic/uremic encephalopathy, acidosis, hypothyroidism
Hyperexcited/hyperactive	Alkalosis, hyperthyroidism
Bizarre behavior	Seizure, stroke, cranial infection, intracranial tumor, diabetes/hypoglycemia, alkalosis, Wernicke's syndrome/Korsakoff's psychosis
Ataxia, distal motor dysfunction	Stroke, cranial infection, acidosis/alkalosis, electrolyte imbalance, hypothyroidism, Wernicke's syndrome/Korsakoff's psychosis, toxic encephalopathy, hypothermia
Jaundice	Liver disease/hepatic encephalopathy
Breath odors	
Fruity/ketone	Diabetes/diabetic ketoacidosis
Musty	Liver failure/hepatic encephalopathy
Fever	Cranial infection (meningitis, encephalitis), hyperthyroidism
Diaphoresis	Diabetes/hypoglycemia, heat emergency
Injection sites	Diabetes, toxic overdose
Scarred fingers, slow-healing wounds, distal prostheses	Diabetes
Dialysis shunt	Renal failure/uremic encephalopathy
Chest pain	Cardiac disease, diabetes/hypoglycemia/hyperglycemia, acidosis/alkalosis, electrolyte imbalance, hyperthyroidism/hypothyroidism, toxicologic encephalopathy, hypothermia/hyperthermia
Peripheral edema	Hepatic/uremic encephalopathy, electrolyte imbalance, hypothyroidism
Neck pain or rigidity	Cranial infection (meningitis, encephalitis)
Poor skin turgor/dehydration	Diabetes/hyperglycemia
Visual disturbances	Stroke, cranial infection intracranial tumor, electrolyte imbalance
Polyuria, polyphagia, polydipsia	Undiagnosed diabetes
Blood glucose < 40 mg/dl	Diabetes/hypoglycemia
Blood glucose > 300 mg/dl	Diabetes/hyperglycemia
Cardiac dysrhythmia	Cardiac disease, stroke, intracranial tumor, electrolyte imbalance, environmental disorder

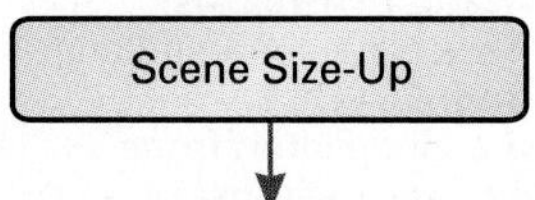

ALTERED MENTAL STATUS TREATMENT PATHWAY

Scene Size-Up

Observe patient presentation and clues such as medications, glucometer, home oxygen.

Initial Assessment

Assess chief complaint, AVPU level of consciousness, airway, breathing, and circulatory status. Note any pathological respiratory pattern. Assure patent airway; support respirations, oxygenation, and circulation as needed.

Focused History and Physical Exam

For all patients with altered level of consciousness:
Support airway patency, ventilation, and oxygenation. Perform endotracheal intubation if needed. Apply a cardiac monitor and treat any dysrhythmias according to AHA guidelines. Establish an IV line with an isotonic crystalloid. Draw blood and analyze for glucose level. If blood glucose is low, administer dextrose. Provide judicious fluid therapy as dictated by the patient's hemodynamic status; avoid fluid overload. Consult standing orders and medical direction regarding specific drugs and treatments. Transport.

Assess for underlying etiology (see "Typical Findings" tables throughout this chapter). For a specific etiology, provide the care listed above "for all patients with altered level of consciousness." Additionally, provide the care listed below for the specific etiology.

Stroke/TIA: Judicious hyperventilation; avoid dextrose; follow local protocols for reduction of hypertension; prompt transport.

Cardiac Cause: See the Treatment Pathway in Chapter 6.

Thyroid Disorder: Emotional support. For severe hyperthyroidism: beta-blockers (consult medical direction), cool the patient. For severe hypothyroidism: warm the patient.

Cranial Infection: Judicious hyperventilation; avoid dextrose; transport in semi-Fowler's position.

Diabetes Mellitus: For hypoglycemia, IV dextrose with thiamine if patient is malnourished. For hyperglycemia, judicious fluid therapy.

Wernicke's Encephalopathy: Administer thiamine after glucose.

Seizures: See the Treatment Pathway in Chapter 10.

Hepatic or Uremic Encephalopathy: Provide supportive care.

Toxic Encephalopathy: Contact poison control center, but standing orders and medication direction take priority.

FIGURE 7-11
Altered mental status treatment pathway.

Continued on the next page

FIGURE 7-11
Altered mental status treatment pathway. *(continued)*

Intracranial Tumor: Judicious hyperventilation; transport in semi-Fowler's position.

Acidosis/Alkalosis: Acidosis: hyperventilate; from COPD: bronchodilator; from narcotic overdose: naloxone. Metabolic acidosis: judicious sodium bicarbonate with mechanical ventilation. Respiratory alkalosis: coach patient to decrease respirations.

Environmental Cause: For hypothermia: handle gently; warm the patient. Limit defibrillation to 3 shocks until patient is warmed. For hyperthermia: cool the patient.

Pulmonary Cause: See the Treatment Pathways in Chapters 2 and 5.

Electrolyte Imbalance: For hypocalcemia, 10% calcium chloride or calcium gluconate (consult medical direction).

Shock: See the Treatment Pathway in Chapter 4.

SCENARIO FOLLOW-UP

Early in your shift, you are called to a neighborhood residence for a male patient exhibiting altered mental status. You find the 68-year-old patient on a bed, making loud gurgling noises. As you pass a nightstand, you note cigarette-filled ashtrays and medicine containers labeled Lovastatin and Vasotec. The patient displays flexion to painful stimuli.

As your partner aggressively suctions pooling vomitus from the hypopharynx, you note Cheyne-Stokes respirations and a pulse oximetry reading of 78 percent. Your partner places an oropharyngeal airway and begins high-flow, high-concentration oxygen therapy with tracheal intubation to follow. Continuing the initial assessment, you note a slow radial pulse accompanied by cool, slightly diaphoretic skin with a capillary refill of 2 seconds.

Because the patient is critical, you call dispatch to request additional paramedics and proceed to conduct a physical and neurologic exam. During the physical and neurologic exam you note the following information:

Fixed and dilated right pupil
Right-sided facial droop
Tongue deviation to the right side
Pulmonary rhonchi secondary to the aspiration of vomitus
Musculature flaccidity to the left arm and leg
No motor ability
Urinary incontinence

As your partner correctly places a tracheal tube, the paramedic backup arrives. You instruct the crew to obtain vital signs and place an IV of 0.9 percent normal saline solution, draw blood specimens, and evaluate the blood glucose level.

You remove yourself from the bedroom to address the family and obtain a SAMPLE history. Family members tell you that the patient was raking leaves when he suddenly complained of a tremendous headache. They say that after coming into the house, he began vomiting and "acting funny" and that his speech became slurred. After a family member called 911, the patient suddenly went unresponsive.

You are told that the patient has a medical history of hypertension, high cholesterol, and cigarette smoking. As far as the family is aware, the patient is only on the two medications you found and is not allergic to anything. His last oral intake was 2 hours earlier at breakfast.

You return to the patient's side and are informed that the vital signs are blood pressure 240/158 mmHg, heart rate of 56 beats per minute, and positive-pressure ventilation being delivered at 10 to 12 breaths per minute. The cardiac monitor reveals sinus bradycardia with no ectopic beats. Recognizing a possible hemorrhagic stroke with increased ICP and cerebral herniation, you instruct your partner to hyperventilate at a rate of 20 breaths per minute. With the IV line in place and a blood glucose level of 88 mg/dl, you order the isotonic crystalloid to be administered at a TKO rate. The patient is placed in the semi-Fowler's position on the cot for expedient transport to the hospital.

Early in the transport, you notify the receiving facility of the appropriate information. Even though the patient is severely hypertensive, you realize that attempting to lower his blood pressure with beta-blockers is unacceptable in light of the bradycardic rhythm. You continue to monitor and manage the patient until you arrive at the hospital and transfer care to the emergency department physician.

Later in the day, you ask about your patient and learn that he suffered a massive intracerebral hemorrhage of the frontal and right parietal lobe. Hospital staff was able to significantly lower the blood pressure, and the patient was taken for surgical evaluation. At the present time, the prognosis for recovery is poor.

FURTHER READING

1. Bates, B., L.S. Bickley, and R.A. Hoekelman. *A Guide to Physical Examination and History Taking.* 7th ed. Philadelphia: Lippincott, 1999.
2. Bledsoe, B., R. Porter, and R. Cherry. *Paramedic Care: Principles and Practice.* Vols 1-5. Upper Saddle River, NJ: Pearson/Prentice Hall, 2006.
3. Bullock, Barbara L. *Pathophysiology: Adaptations and Alterations in Function.* 4th ed. Philadelphia: Lippincott-Raven, 1996.
4. Guyton, A.C., and J.E. Hall. *Textbook of Medical Physiology.* 10th ed. Philadelphia: W.B. Saunders, 2001.
5. Marieb, E.N., and K. Hoen. *Human Anatomy and Physiology.* 7th ed. Benjamin-Cummings, 2007.
6. Marx, J.A., R.S. Hockberger, and R.M. Walls. *Rosen's Emergency Medicine: Concepts and Clinical Practice.* 5th ed. St. Louis: Mosby, 2002.
7. Mistovich, J.J., R.W. Benner, and G.S. Margolis. "Acute stroke," in *Prehospital Advanced Cardiac Life Support.* Upper Saddle River, NJ: Pearson/Prentice Hall, 2004.
8. Salmeraeo, E., E. Salerno, and L.M. McKenry. *Pharmacology in Nursing.* 21st ed. St. Louis: Mosby, 2001.

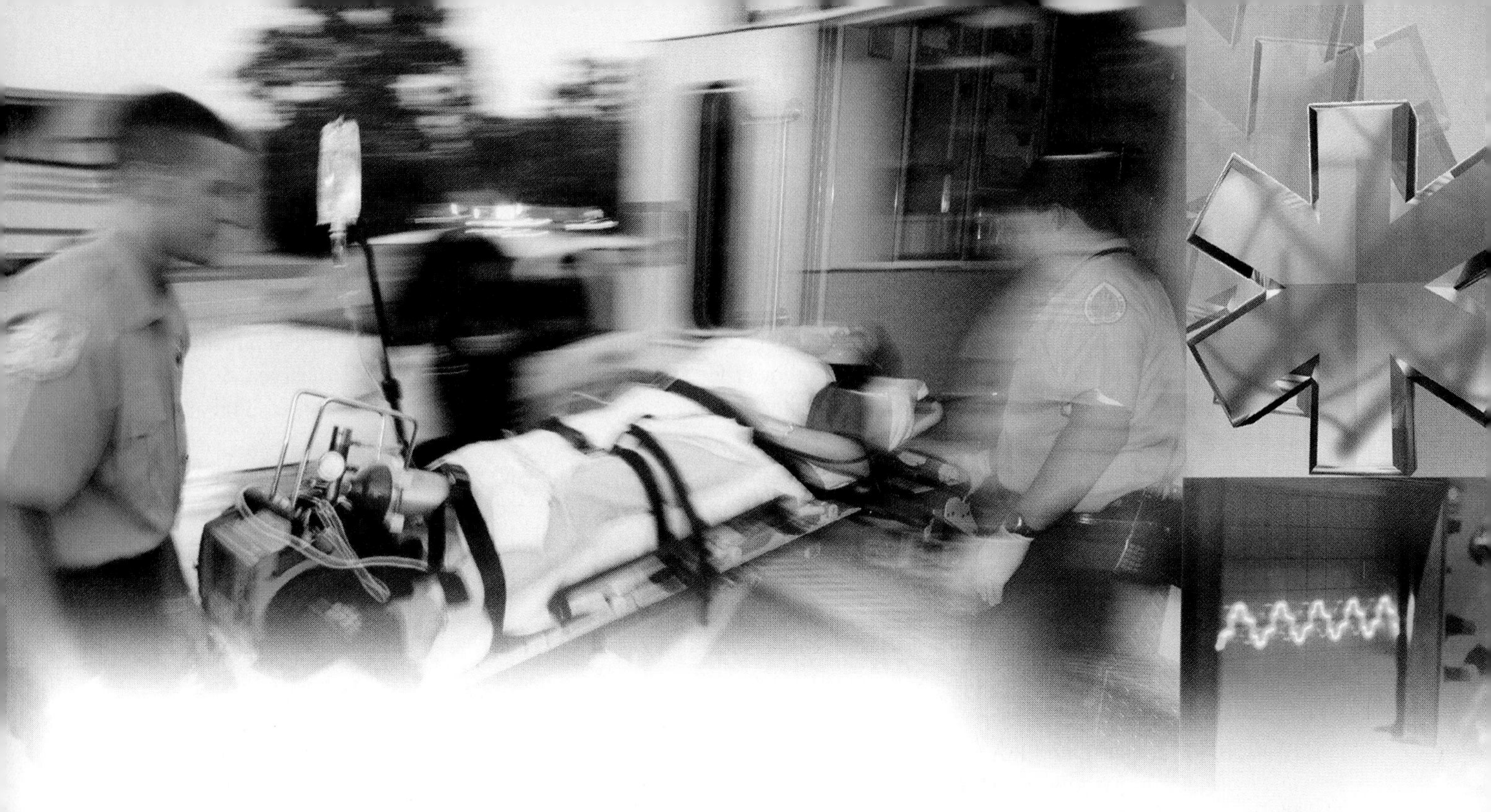

ACUTE ABDOMINAL PAIN

8

Abdominal pain is a common chief complaint and the presenting symptom for a number of diseases. Despite a wide variety of causes, sudden and severe pain is nearly always a symptom of intraabdominal pathology. Although a definitive diagnosis cannot generally be reached at the emergency scene, it is critical for the care provider to be able to determine whether the condition is life threatening, potentially life threatening, or non-life threatening. Treatment for abdominal pain is primarily aimed at supporting vital functions, making the patient as comfortable as possible, and transporting him to the hospital.

Topics that are covered in this chapter are

- When the Chief Complaint Is Abdominal Pain
- Anatomy, Physiology, and Pathophysiology
- Differential Diagnosis
- Assessment
- Treatment

SCENARIO

You are called to the scene of a 35-year-old female with syncope. You find her lying on her side on the living room couch. She appears pale but is awake and alert. She tells you that she was lying down reading a book when she began to feel sick. She got up to go to the bathroom and became so dizzy she had to lie down again. She is talking to you in complete sentences and is oriented. Her skin is cool and dry.

During history taking, you discover that your patient is a marathon bike rider who decided to skip an important race 2 days ago because "I kept getting this pain, off and on, here." She points to the lower left quadrant of her abdomen. You ask what the pain was like. "It started as cramps that just kept getting worse and worse. And then by today it got to be just a constant pain, and now it's spread all across my whole lower abdomen." She states that her menses has always been irregular, and although this one is late, it is not unusually so. She is sexually active but has had a tubal ligation. She denies vaginal drainage.

As she turns onto her back for your physical exam, your patient complains of a sudden, sharp pain in her left neck and shoulder but denies any trauma. As she tries to get comfortable, she remarks, "The pain gets better when I bend my knees." Her vital signs are pulse 90, respirations 18, and blood pressure 110/86.

How would you proceed with the assessment and care of this patient?

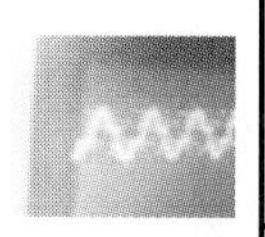

WHEN THE CHIEF COMPLAINT IS ABDOMINAL PAIN

When the chief complaint is abdominal pain, its location and characteristics may indicate the possible origin. Textbook descriptions of abdominal pain, however, have severe limitations. Each individual reacts differently according to a variety of factors:

- *Age*—Infants and children may be unable to localize their discomfort, and they have diseases not seen in adults.
- *Tolerance*—Obese or elderly patients tend to tolerate pain better.
- *Preexisting Conditions*—Neuropathy, such as that which occurs with diabetes, can mask intraabdominal pathology, as can alcohol and certain medications, especially steroids.
- *Perception*—What is perceived as severe pain to one person may not be to another.
- *Mental State*—Hysteria tends to exaggerate pain, and emotional pain tends to worsen physical pain.

For most patients with acute or chronic abdominal pain, narrowing the possible cause to a given organ may be impossible outside a hospital environment. Determining whether an actual or potential life-threatening condition exists may be established by a careful history, a focused physical examination, and the limited number of diagnostic tests (e.g., blood sugar values, 12-lead ECG, and orthostatic blood pressure checks) done in the field.

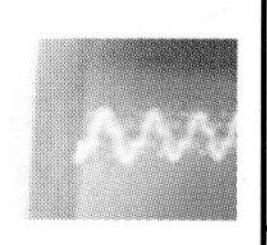

ANATOMY, PHYSIOLOGY, AND PATHOPHYSIOLOGY

A review of abdominal anatomy and physiology, followed by the pathophysiology of abdominal pain, will set the basis for understanding the characteristics of abdominal pain.

Anatomy and Physiology of the Abdomen

Abdominal organs are suspended within the abdominal cavity (Figure 8-1). This cavity has two essential functions: 1) protection of organs from the accidental bumping and jostling that occurs during daily activity, such as walking, jumping,

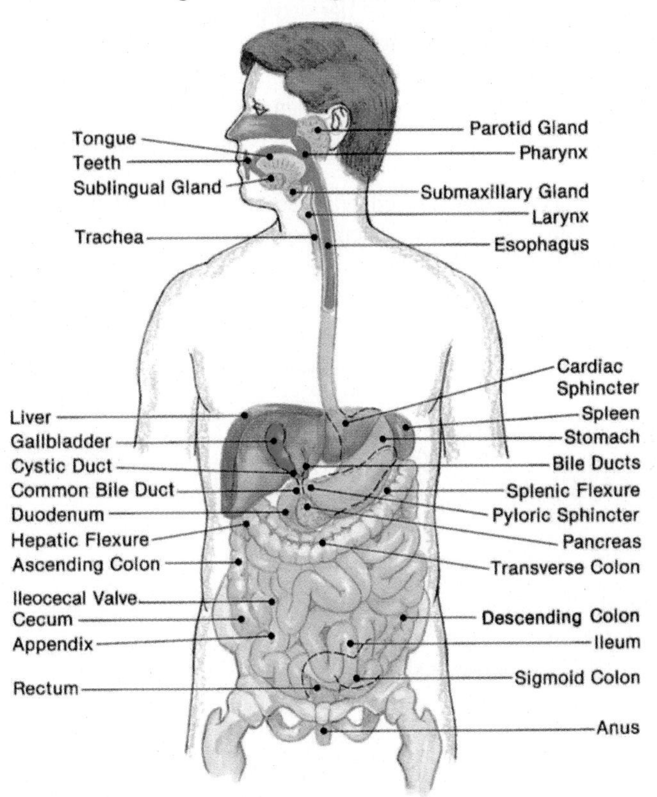

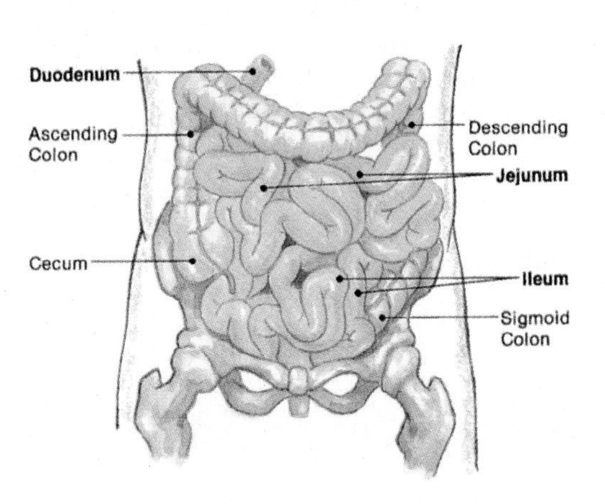

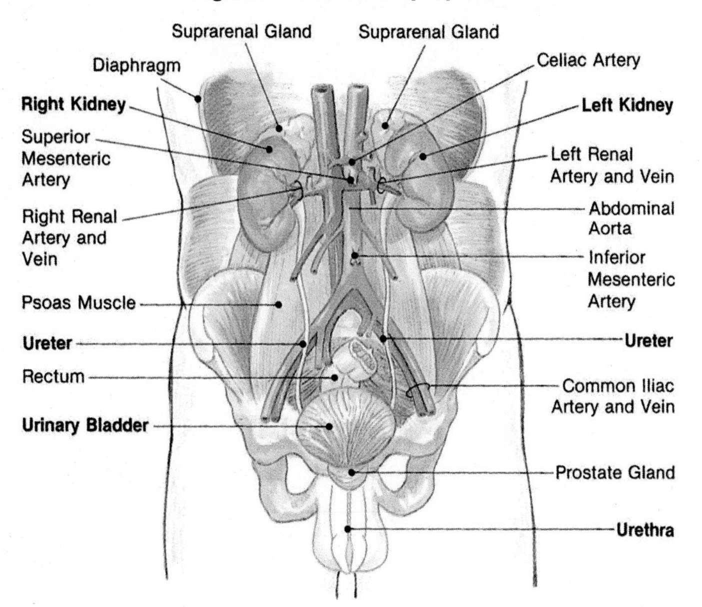

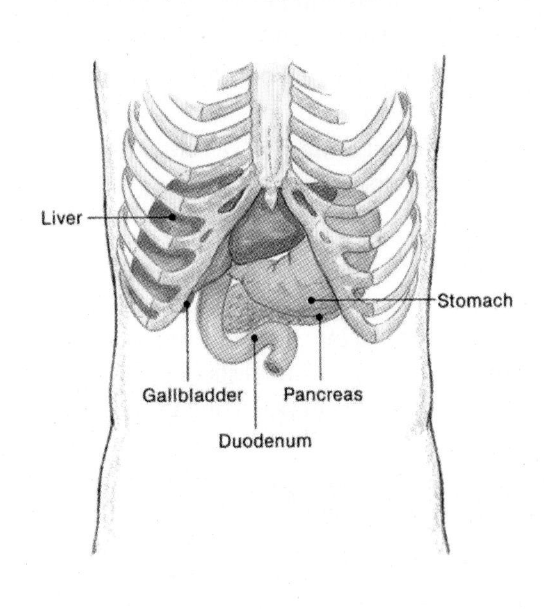

FIGURE 8-1
Abdominal organs.

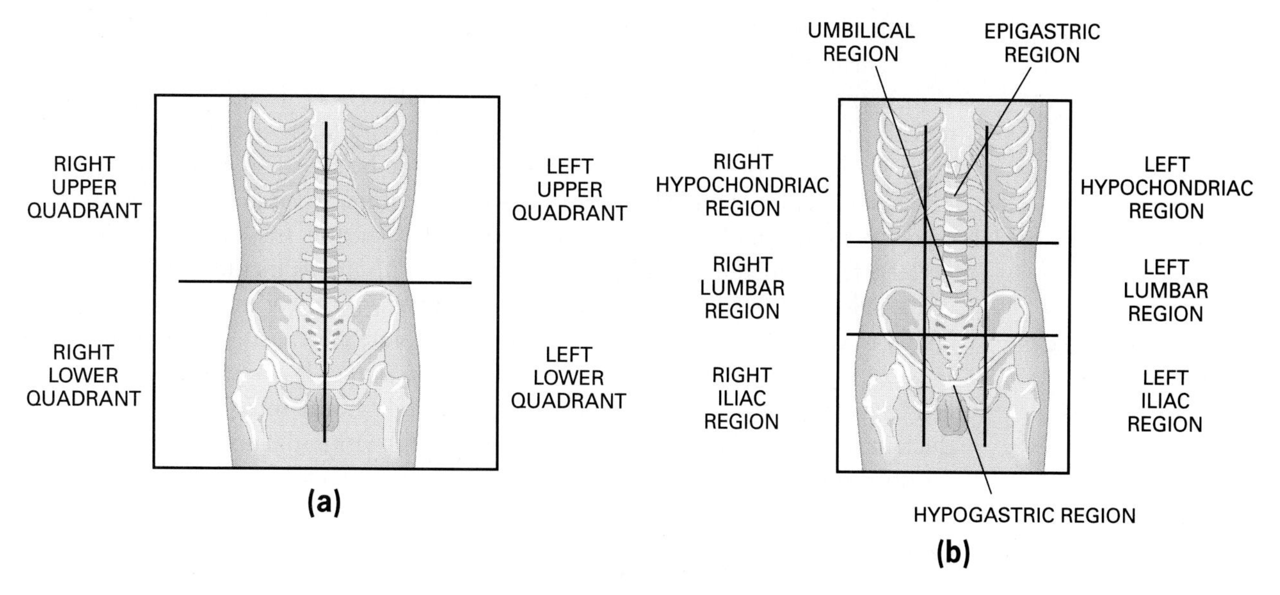

FIGURE 8-2
(a) Abdominal quadrants and (b) abdominal regions.

and running; and 2) permitting organs to expand and contract without disrupting surrounding tissues or organ functions.

The diaphragm forms the superior dome of the abdominal cavity and the floor of the chest cavity. To help describe the location of findings, the abdominal area is divided into four *quadrants:* the right upper quadrant (RUQ), the left upper quadrant (LUQ), the right lower quadrant (RLQ), and the left lower quadrant (LLQ) (Figure 8-2a). These terms and their abbreviations are commonly used in clinical discussions. However, more precise *regions* are also described. They include the right hypochondriac region, epigastric region, left hypochondriac region, right lumbar region, umbilical region, left lumbar region, right iliac region, hypogastric region, and left iliac region (Figure 8-2b). Quadrants and regions are useful because there is a known relationship between superficial anatomical landmarks and the locations of underlying organs.

The abdominopelvic cavity contains spaces lined by a delicate serous membrane called the *peritoneum.* The *parietal* portion of the peritoneum forms the inner surface of the outer wall of the body cavity and lines the muscle wall. The *visceral* portion of the peritoneum covers the surfaces of the internal organs, or *viscera,* where they project into the body cavity.

Many organs undergo changes in size and shape. For instance, the stomach expands to accommodate the meals we eat, and the diaphragm constantly expands and contracts as we breathe, thus moving underlying organs. The serous membrane prevents friction between adjacent viscera and between the visceral organs and the body wall. The spaces between opposing membranes are very small, but they are filled with a thin layer of fluid. If, for some reason, the thin layer of fluid is absent in a particular area, or tension is produced when the peritoneum moves, pain results and is related to movement of organs in that particular area.

The peritoneum helps further subdivide the abdomen vertically, into the *peritoneal space,* which is anterior, and the *retroperitoneal space,* which is posterior. Most of the organs in the abdominopelvic cavity project into the peritoneal space, which is also referred to as the peritoneal cavity. Organs such as the stomach, small intestine, appendix, and portions of the large intestine are suspended within the peritoneal cavity by double sheets of peritoneum, called *mesenteries.* Mesenteries

peritoneum the serous membrane that lines the abdominopelvic cavity. The **parietal peritoneum** covers the outer wall. The **visceral peritoneum** covers internal organs.

viscera the internal organs.

peritoneal space anterior portion of the abdomen.

retroperitoneal space posterior portion of the abdomen.

mesenteries double sheets of peritoneum that support the intestines and contain the blood vessels that supply the intestines.

contain blood vessels supplying the intestines and provide support and stability while permitting limited movement.

Some organs, such as the kidneys, ureters, and aorta, are located in the retroperitoneal space. Other organs, such as the pancreas and aorta, share both spaces.

The organs of the abdominopelvic cavity can be classified as hollow or solid. The *hollow organs* include the stomach, small intestine, appendix, large intestine or colon, rectum, gallbladder, and connecting tubes such as the common bile duct, ureters, fallopian tubes, uterus, and bladder. *Solid organs* include the liver, pancreas, spleen, kidneys, and ovaries. Hollow organs, with few exceptions, have the ability to contract and/or have the ability to generate *peristalsis,* a rhythmic movement of contraction that moves substances either within the organ (e.g., the stomach or gallbladder) or along the length of a tube (e.g., the intestine, common bile duct, or ureter). This contraction and flow of fluid within the hollow viscera of the intestine generates the bowel sounds heard when the abdomen is auscultated.

peristalsis rhythmic contractions that move substances through hollow organs or tubes.

Pathophysiology of Abdominal Pain

There are three mechanisms for abdominal pain: mechanical, inflammatory, and ischemic. Abdominal organs, with the exception of the aorta, are not sensitive to mechanical stimuli such as cutting or tearing. However, abdominal organs and membranes are sensitive to stretching and distention, which activate nerve endings in both hollow and solid structures. The capsules that surround organs such as the liver, spleen, and gallbladder also contain pain fibers that are stimulated by stretching if these organs swell.

Onset of pain is associated with rapid distention, while gradual distention causes little pain. An example is when gas builds up in the stomach, rapidly distending that organ, causing pain and discomfort. When belching occurs, the pain is relieved because the distention is relieved. In contrast, cirrhosis of the liver is a gradual process that can cause the liver to swell to as much as twice its normal size. However, because the process is gradual, pain is not an early symptom.

Traction, or tension, on the peritoneum caused by adhesions, distention of the common bile duct, or forceful peristalsis resulting from intestinal obstruction, generally causes pain.

An exception to this rule is pregnancy. The peritoneum is considerably stretched by the slow growth of the uterus. By the third trimester, the peritoneum is no longer as sensitive to stretching; therefore, the response to stimuli that would normally produce pain is blunted. This helps explain why conditions such as cholelithiasis (gallstones) and appendicitis in a pregnant woman have the potential

Clinical Insight

Abdominal pain in a pregnant patient, other than the pain caused by contractions, is usually considered serious, until proven otherwise.

Hollow Organs	
Aorta	Large intestine or colon
Appendix	Rectum
Bladder	Small intestine
Common bile duct	Stomach
Fallopian tubes	Ureters
Gallbladder	Uterus
Solid Organs	
Kidneys	Pancreas
Liver	Spleen
Ovaries	

to be so serious. They can go for long periods without pain being perceived. Once recognized, the problem is usually far advanced.

Biochemical mediators of the inflammatory response, such as histamine, prostaglandins, bradykinin, and serotonin, stimulate organ nerve endings and produce abdominal pain. The edema and vascular congestion that accompany chemical, bacterial, or viral inflammation also cause painful stretching of organs and organ walls.

In solid organs, pain from stretching the organs and organ capsules is a steady pain. In hollow organs, however, edema and vascular congestion from inflammation may also cause an obstruction or contribute to further irritation of the membranes lining the walls. Obstruction or irritation of the lining of hollow organs frequently stimulates contractions and peristalsis. The resulting pain is often described as *crampy* or *colicky*. In gastroenteritis, increased peristalsis of the small or large intestine may also trigger diarrhea. If the obstruction is not relieved, intermittent pain may become constant.

crampy, colicky intermittent or spasmodic pain.

Clinical Insight

The description of pain is important for determining hollow versus solid organ cause, or aortic cause versus other causes of abdominal pain, as is the progression of the pain (e.g., intermittent progressing to steady or generalized to specific).

Obstruction of blood flow caused by the distention of bowel or mesenteric vessel occlusion produces the pain of ischemia. This process results in increased concentrations of tissue metabolites and waste products, which stimulate pain receptors. This pain is steady but severe, worsening as the ischemia increases.

Descriptions of abdominal pain can be identified as visceral, parietal (somatic), or referred:

- *Visceral pain* arises from an abdominal organ. It is usually felt near the midline in the epigastrium or umbilical region. Visceral pain is *poorly localized* and is dull rather than sharp.

  Visceral pain is diffuse and vague because nerve endings within the abdominal organs are sparse and multisegmented. As explained earlier, visceral pain involving hollow organs may be described as crampy or colicky and tends to be dull and intermittent. In contrast, visceral pain involving solid organs tends to be dull and constant.

- *Parietal pain* arises from the parietal peritoneum. This pain is more *localized* and intense than visceral pain. Nerve fibers from the parietal peritoneum travel with associated peripheral nerves to the spinal cord, and the sensation of pain most frequently corresponds to skin *dermatomes* T6 and L1 (Figure 8-3) that are innervated by those segments of the spinal cord. Parietal pain is localized to one side or the other because, at any particular point, the parietal peritoneum is innervated from only one side of the nervous system.

  Parietal pain is often described as sharp and constant. Patients often feel better lying in the fetal position with their knees drawn up. This relaxes the parietal peritoneum and helps reduce the pain. Any activity that moves the peritoneum, such as coughing, deep breathing, or lying flat with legs outstretched, will often produce pain. The characteristics of parietal pain are sometimes seen as signs of peritoneal irritation. Parietal pain frequently occurs after visceral pain.

  Pain arising from the appendix is an example. At first, it may be described as intermittent and dull, arising from the umbilical region. (*Note:* This is visceral pain from distention of the appendix.) As time goes on and bacteria penetrate the wall of the appendix, the pain described more closely resembles parietal pain. The pain gradually becomes sharper, constant, and localized to the right lower quadrant with the patient more comfortable if the knees are drawn up. (The localization of pain then reflects dermatome distribution.)

- *Referred pain* is visceral pain felt at some distance from a diseased or affected organ. The site of referred pain is usually well localized and felt in skin or

visceral pain pain arising from a visceral organ, usually dull and poorly localized.

localized/poorly localized localized pain is limited to a definite area; poorly localized pain is diffuse or may be felt in a somewhat different location than the affected organ.

parietal pain pain that arises from the parietal peritoneum, usually sharp, intense, and localized.

dermatomes areas of the skin innervated by specific spinal cord segments.

referred pain visceral pain felt at some distance from a diseased or affected organ (e.g., pain from an ovarian cyst felt in the shoulder or neck). This occurs when the brain misinterprets the pain as originating from a cutaneous nerve that innervates an area that is, in fact, at a site other than the affected organ.

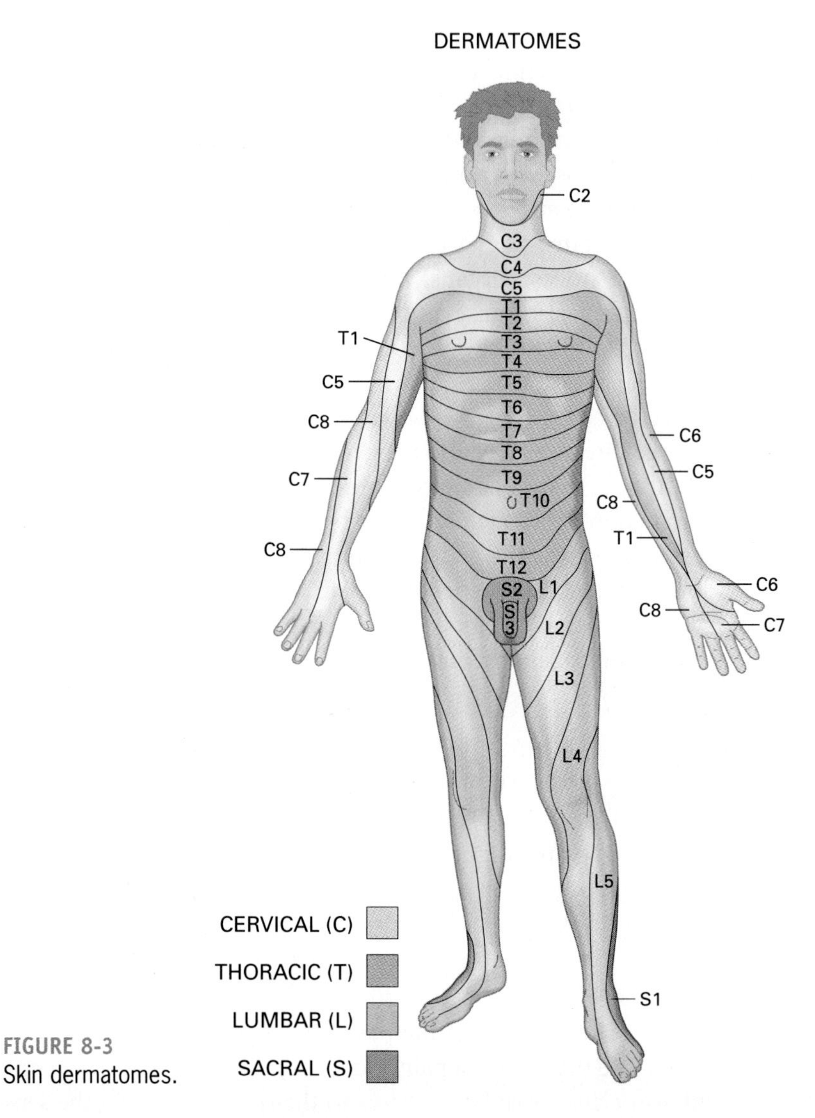

FIGURE 8-3
Skin dermatomes.

deeper tissues that share a central afferent nerve pathway (toward the spinal cord) with the affected organ. Referred pain generally develops as the intensity of a visceral pain stimulus increases. For instance, intense gallbladder pain is referred to a scapula or to the back between the scapulae. The pain may begin as a crampy discomfort in the right upper quadrant and then, as inflammation worsens, progress to a sharp, localized, referred pain to the right scapula or between the shoulder blades. See Figure 8-4 for common areas of referred pain for given organs.

Just as abdominal pathology may refer pain to areas away from the abdomen, extraabdominal problems may refer pain to the abdomen. Examples are given here and in Table 8-1.

Extraabdominal Problems That May Refer Pain to the Abdomen

- AMI may be accompanied by diffuse abdominal pain, or more commonly, indigestion. Palpation may worsen indigestion due to an ulcer but usually has no effect on the indigestion due to AMI.
- Pneumonia can lead to diffuse abdominal pain, but there is no localized abdominal tenderness. A productive cough and fever may also be present.
- Diabetes (in particular, diabetic ketoacidosis) can lead to diffuse abdominal pain with vomiting, probably caused by high potassium levels.

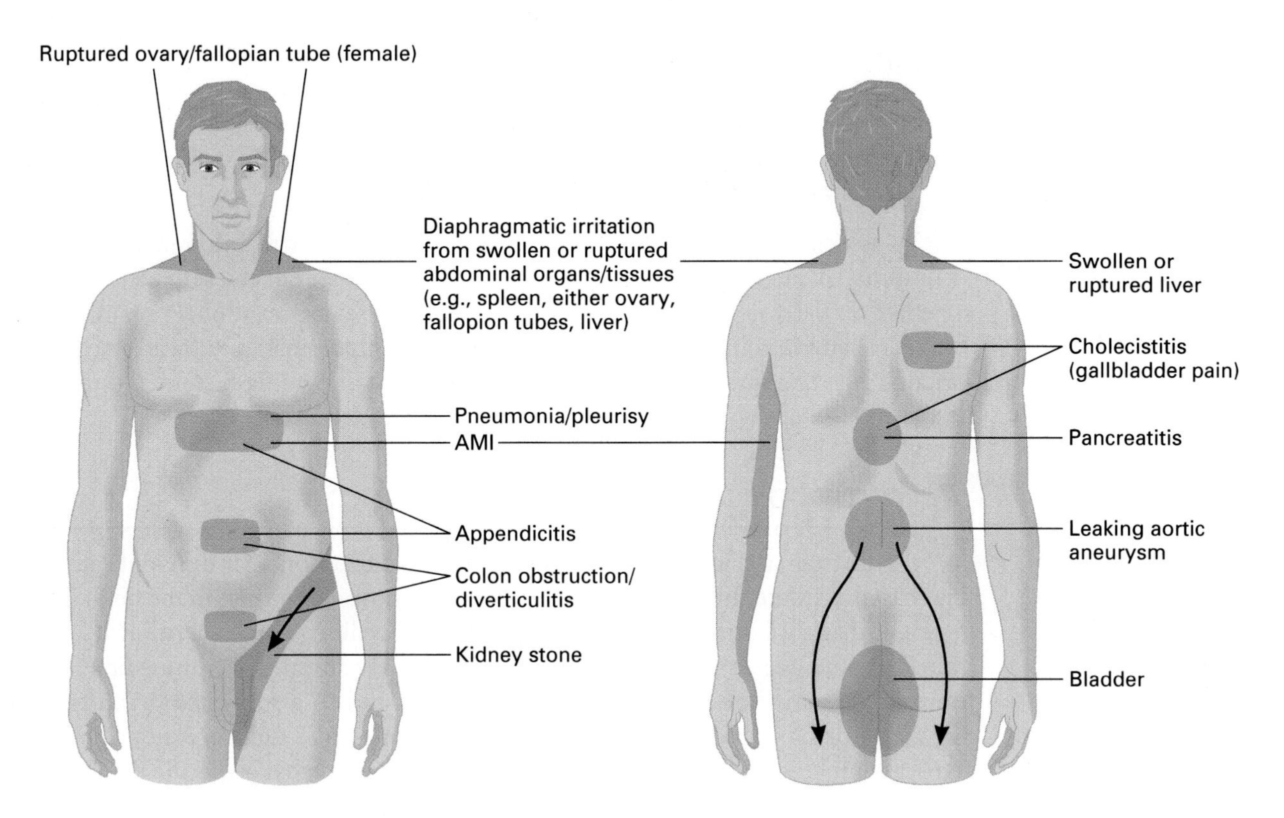

FIGURE 8-4
Common areas of referred pain.

Widespread smooth muscle contractions affecting the small intestine have been blamed.

- Drug addicts suffering withdrawal symptoms may have severe colicky pains that suggest intestinal obstruction.
- Sickle cell disease may be associated with attacks of severe abdominal pain, which may be due to infarction of capillary beds in organs such as the spleen.

TABLE 8-1 Abdominal Pain from Extraabdominal Causes: Signs and Symptoms

These signs or symptoms associated with abdominal pain . . .	. . . may indicate these extraabdominal causes.
Chest pain with "indigestion"	Acute myocardial infarction (apply ECG monitor)
Dyspnea with "indigestion"	Acute myocardial infarction (apply ECG monitor)
Productive cough and fever with diffuse abdominal pain but no localized abdominal tenderness	Pneumonia
Vomiting with diffuse abdominal pain	Diabetes (check blood glucose level)
Severe, collicky pains that suggest intestinal obstruction	Addictive drug use
Attacks of severe abdominal pain	Sickle cell disease, systemic lupus erythmatosis (SLE)
Chronic abdominal pain	Spinal or central nervous system disease (commonly caused by radiculitis, e.g., herpes zoster/shingles)

- Spinal or CNS disease can produce pain referred to the abdomen. The most common cause is radiculitis (inflammation of spinal nerve roots), of which herpes zoster, or shingles, is the best-known example. This pain is usually chronic rather than acute. In the case of shingles, pain may precede the appearance of the rash.

If associated signs and symptoms indicate a possible extraabdominal cause of abdominal pain, ask questions or look for environmental clues to determine whether the patient has any known or suspected disease or condition. Previous history is usually very important. Although it may be impossible to know exactly the origin of the abdominal pain, a thorough assessment, including history and physical exam, will always be the best basis for treatment decisions.

DIFFERENTIAL DIAGNOSIS

A differential diagnosis determined in the field takes on a far different meaning than the differential diagnosis determined in a hospital setting. In the field, differential diagnosis for abdominal pain is frequently limited to determining two things: 1) the degree of threat to life (i.e., if the condition is an immediate life threat, a potential life threat, or not a life threat), and 2) a suggested organ type (i.e., if the pain is typical of a hollow organ or a solid organ). Only occasionally will a disease process exhibit such classic signs and symptoms that a specific diagnosis will be unmistakable. In most cases, a careful history and complete physical may narrow the problem to suspected bleeding, obstruction, sepsis, or an irritant isolated to a particular area or organ type. It is these determinations, along with the mental status, cardiovascular status, and respiratory status, that will determine probability for immediate, potential, or no life threat and the determination of whether the patient is critical, unstable, potentially unstable, or stable (CUPS).

In the field, differential diagnosis for abdominal pain is frequently limited to determining the degree of threat to life and whether the patient is critical, unstable, potentially unstable, or stable (CUPS).

To begin to recognize and differentiate between these levels of severity, a knowledge of the organs and disease states associated with a particular location of pain is required (Tables 8-2 and 8-3). To help simplify this process, reference will be made to the nine abdominal regions outlined in Figure 8-2b.

Right Hypochondriac Region

Underlying organs in this region include the liver and the gallbladder. Pain may be referred to this area from the lungs (as in pleuritis or pneumonia).

Liver

The liver is the largest abdominal organ. The left lobe extends to the midclavicular line of the left hypochondriac region. Normally, the liver in an adult is not palpable in the field.

The liver is surrounded by a capsule that allows the organ to swell and expand. Pain from sudden swelling and expansion is described as steady and dull. When the capsule is irritated, either from swelling, chemical irritation, or infection, it rarely swells enough to break. However, on the rare occasion that the capsule does break, its close proximity to the diaphragm results in irritation extending to the right phrenic nerve with referred pain to the right neck and shoulder.

hepatitis inflammation of the liver that can have a variety of causes, including viruses, bacteria, drugs, and toxic agents.

Hepatitis is an inflammation of the liver that can have a variety of causes, including viruses, bacteria, drugs, and toxic agents. Enlargement of the liver may be

TABLE 8-2 Patterns of Findings for Specific Abdominal Organs

Affected Organ	Pattern of Findings
Liver	*Any liver disease:* Steady, dull pain. Possible bleeding tendencies, noticed as bruising; jaundice to skin or sclera. *Inflamed (hepatitis):* Enlarged with mild pain and tenderness in right hypochondriac region, jaundice of the sclera, preceded by flu-like symptoms (e.g., vomiting, diarrhea, chills, fever). *Chronic liver disease (cirrhosis):* Dyspnea rather than pain, ascites. *Ruptured capsule:* Pain referred to right neck and shoulder.
Gallbladder	*Gallstone obstructing common bile duct:* Intermittent, crampy or collicky pain occurring 30-60 minutes after eating. Can radiate left to right or be localized at gallbladder or anywhere along length of bile duct. If localized, radiates to right scapula or to the back between the scapulae. Patient cannot get comfortable, may pace. *If inflammation of gallbladder (cholecystitis) results:* Pain in upper abdomen or radiating to the back or right shoulder with possible nausea, vomiting, jaundice, fever.
Stomach	*Inflammation of stomach lining (gastritis) and stomach ulcers (peptic ulcer disease):* Both cause localized, steady, burning pain in epigastric region. Vomiting may be bloody. *Perforated ulcers:* Bleeding and spillage of stomach contents with signs of peritoneal irritation. Pain may be pronounced on the left or right (side where perforation occurs).
Pancreas	*Pancreatic inflammation (pancreatitis):* Usually causes peritoneal irritation resulting in sudden, constant, severe pain. Patient feels more comfortable lying still with knees drawn up.
Spleen	*Enlarged or irritated:* Steady, dull pain. May radiate to left neck and shoulder. *Ruptured:* Sharp, intense pain, lets up, then recurs, increases in intensity, radiates to left neck and shoulder; syncope, postural hypotension.
Small Intestine and Large Intestine	*Inflammation of gastrointestinal tract (gastroenteritis), may be specified as inflammation of the intestine (enteritis or inflammatory bowel disease), also known by its location along the intestinal tract (ileitis, colitis):* Intermittent, crampy or colicky pain, possibly with diarrhea and vomiting resulting in dehydration. *Food poisoning:* Sudden onset within 2-8 hours of ingesting contaminated food. Usually begins with nausea, vomiting, cramping, colicky, intermittent pain, followed by diarrhea, possibly bloody. Resultant blood loss, dehydration, electrolyte imbalance. *Bowel obstruction:* Begins with intermittent, crampy or colicky pain. If unrelieved, distention and peritoneal irritation with increasingly intense, steady, poorly localized pain. Patient may lie in fetal position. Shallow respirations; pain worsened by coughing or deep breathing. *Inflamed pockets in colon wall (diverticulitis):* Dull pain, tenderness on palpation. If perforated, spillage of contents into peritoneal space, causing steady, sharp pain and signs of peritoneal irritation. Early pain is poorly localized and referred to hypogastric region; later pain becomes localized, commonly to lower left quadrant. Diarrhea, fever, bleeding (from occult to massive) may be present.
Aorta	*Weakened, dilated area (aneurysm):* May present with syncope with or without pain. Usually presents with steady, deep, boring or tearing visceral pain in lower back, radiating to lower abdomen or vice versa. Pain may also radiate to one flank or the other or down either leg or both legs. May be felt on palpation as a pulsating mass and may be tender to palpation. May leak, then rupture, causing severe pain. A serious threat to life.
Kidneys and Ureters	*Inflammation of kidney:* Dull, steady pain localized to the affected side, posterior. Difficult or painful urination may or may not be present (especially in the elderly) if infection involves bladder. *Kidney stone obstruction of ureter:* Sharp, intermittent, crampy or colicky pain localized to one side, intensifying if not relieved. May radiate the length of the ureter or to the groin. Blood may be present in the urine.
Appendix	*Inflammation (appendicitis):* May begin with intermittent, dull pain in umbilical region, becoming more localized and intense with possible signs of peritoneal irritation. Nausea, vomiting, anorexia, and fever may be present. *Ruptured appendix:* Possible sudden relief of pain, soon followed by sharp, severe, constant pain worsened by any movement.
Ovaries and Fallopian Tubes	*Ovarian inflammation or cyst:* Dull, constant pain localized to one side. *Ruptured ovarian cyst:* Pain may lessen, then become severe, poorly localized, with signs of peritoneal irritation. May radiate to either side of neck or shoulder. *Fallopian tube blockage or rupture (due to ovum growing in tube):* Intermittent, crampy, colicky pain, recurring as severe, intense, and constant after rupture, with radiation to either side of neck or shoulder.

TABLE 8-3 Pain Referred to Abdominal Regions

Pain occurring in these regions	. . . may be caused by/referred from . . .
Right hypochondriac region	Pleuritis or pneumonia in the right pleural cavity
Epigastric region	Cardiac condition; appendicitis
Left hypochondriac region	Pleuritis or pneumonia in the left pleural cavity
Umbilical and hypogastric regions	Obstruction of the intestine

rapid, resulting in mild pain in the right hypochondriac region with tenderness on palpation. Jaundice of the skin may not be as readily apparent as jaundice of the sclera. The appearance of jaundice is generally preceded by flu-like symptoms, which may include nasal discharge, nausea, vomiting, diarrhea, chills, fever, and fatigue.

cirrhosis chronic liver disease that can have a variety of causes, including nutritional deficiencies, alcohol ingestion, or prior viral or bacterial inflammation.

ascites accumulation of serous fluid from the liver that accumulates in the abdominal cavity.

Fibrotic changes of the liver, known as *cirrhosis,* cause gradual swelling of the liver. This gradual swelling does not cause liver pain; instead, it frequently results in dyspnea. The formation of *ascites* (a result of cirrhosis that is an accumulation of fluid from the liver that collects in the peritoneal space) can be enormous. The extremely distended abdomen can compromise movement of the diaphragm, resulting in difficult or even painful breathing.

Because normal functions of the liver include production of clotting factors and clearing the blood of bilirubin (a byproduct of the destruction of aged red blood cells), any disease of the liver may result in bleeding tendencies, noticed as bruising, and/or jaundice to the skin and sclera.

Gallbladder

Located under the right lobe of the liver, the gallbladder is also surrounded by the liver capsule. The gallbladder stores and concentrates bile necessary for digestion of fat. The bile is collected by a tube-like structure called the cystic duct. The cystic duct joins the hepatic duct, which collects bile from the liver, to form the common bile duct. The common bile duct then extends from the gallbladder across the abdomen to the left side, passing through the pancreas, and connecting with the pancreatic duct at the sphincter of Oddi (Figure 8-5). If a stone has formed (due to excess concentration of bile), contractions and peristalsis will attempt to move it along with the rest of the bile. If the stone becomes lodged anywhere along these ducts, an obstruction will occur and pain will result. Initial pain is often described as intermittent, crampy or colicky, and dull. Pain can occur any time from 30 to 60 minutes after ingestion of food, particularly food with a high fat content.

An obstruction can occur anywhere along the cystic duct, the hepatic duct, the common bile duct, or at the sphincter of Oddi. The resulting pain can radiate along the entire length of the bile duct, from right to left, or be localized at the gallbladder itself or at any one spot along the entire length of the duct. If localized at the gallbladder or within the hepatic duct, radiating pain is to the right scapula or to the back between the scapulae. The patient cannot get comfortable. Because the pain is unrelated to movement, the patient may pace. If unrelieved, contractions of the bile duct may put traction on the peritoneum, causing the pain to become more parietal in character, constant and sharp.

cholecystitis inflammation of the gallbladder.

In some patients with gallstone obstruction, the back-up of bile may cause chemical irritation and inflammation of the gallbladder (*cholecystitis*), with associated pain in the upper abdomen or referred to the back or right shoulder, with nausea and vomiting. Fever and jaundice may occur if the condition is acute. If the obstruction occurs at the sphincter of Oddi, the pancreas may also become obstructed and inflamed.

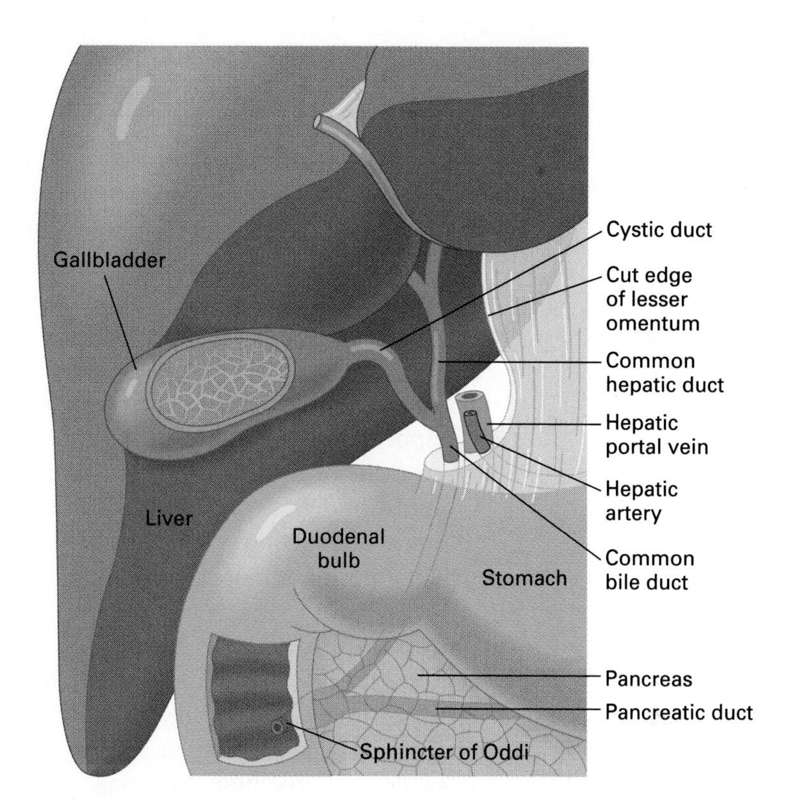

FIGURE 8-5
The gallbladder, cystic duct, common hepatic duct, common bile duct, and pancreatic duct.

Pain Referred to the Right Hypochondriac Region

Right hypochondriac pain may also result from referred pain associated with pleuritis or pneumonia in the right pleural cavity. Pain in this area, in the presence of localized wheezes or rhonchi, warrants further history taking and pulmonary assessment. A thorough assessment, including auscultation of lung sounds, will help distinguish between referred pain and pain from underlying organs. For a discussion of respiratory diseases and difficulty breathing, see Chapter 5, Dyspnea, Respiratory Distress, or Respiratory Failure.

Epigastric Region

Organs in this region include the stomach and pancreas, with referred pain from the heart and the appendix.

Stomach

The stomach is a muscular, sac-like organ, shaped like an expanded J. It is located primarily in the epigastric region of the abdominopelvic cavity. The outer surface of the stomach is covered by the peritoneum, which is continuous with a pair of mesenteries, the greater omentum (a site for fat deposit that protects the abdominal organs), and the lesser omentum.

The stomach is lined with mucous cells that secrete mucus to help protect the stomach lining from the acids, enzymes, and abrasive materials it contains. Gastric glands secrete hydrochloric acid, enzymes, and intrinsic factor (a substance that makes possible the absorption of vitamin B12). If, for some reason, the mucous protection is insufficient or absent, inflammation of the gastric mucosa, called *gastritis,* occurs. When stomach acids and enzymes actually erode through the stomach lining or proximal portions of the small intestine, a small crater is formed.

gastritis inflammation of the gastric mucosa.

Once the normal gastric defenses have been breached, a normal resident bacterium called *Helicobacter pylori* is responsible for ulcer formation at the site of the

peptic ulcer disease formation of a disruption in the mucosa of the stomach or proximal portion of the small intestine.

crater (*peptic ulcer disease*). Both gastritis and stomach ulcers are painful, with localized, steady, burning pain in the epigastric region. When severe, ulcers may perforate the stomach wall, causing bleeding or spillage of stomach contents into the peritoneal space, resulting in signs of peritoneal irritation. Peritoneal pain may be especially pronounced on the side of the perforation. Thus, pain in the epigastric or the right or left hypochondriac region may be evident.

Chemical or mechanical irritation of the stomach and proximal portions of the small intestine commonly result in vomiting. The presence of vomiting is nonspecific for any one disease entity. However, repeated and persistent vomiting is indicative of obstruction, spreading peritonitis, or severe, continuing irritation of the gastric mucosa such as that seen with gastritis or toxins from food poisoning. It is important to ask about the character of emesis. Stomach contents and the bilious green color of duodenal contents are considered "normal." Bright red or "coffee grounds" of digested blood or the dirty yellow prelude to the foul, feculent emesis of bowel obstruction is abnormal with a high probability for immediate or potential life threat. For more information, see Chapter 9, Gastrointestinal Bleeding.

Pancreas

The pancreas is a tadpole-shaped solid organ approximately 20 cm long. It lies parallel to and beneath the stomach with its head tucked into the curve of the duodenum and its tail touching the spleen. A swollen, irritated pancreas usually results in peritoneal irritation. The resulting pain may develop suddenly and is constant and severe. Because the pancreas lies in both the peritoneal and the retroperitoneal spaces, it is associated with radiating pain often described as "boring through to the back." The patient feels more comfortable when lying still and with knees drawn up.

When large quantities of digestive enzymes pool within the pancreas, the pancreatic secretions begin, literally, to digest the pancreas itself.

The pancreas secretes digestive enzymes and controls blood sugar levels through the production of insulin. The digestive enzymes are normally inactive until secreted into the intestine. However, when a blockage occurs, and large quantities of digestive enzymes pool within the pancreas, the pancreatic secretions rapidly become activated and begin, literally, to digest the pancreas itself.

In most cases, only a portion of the pancreas is affected and the process is self-limiting. In 10 to 15 percent of cases, however, the process does not subside and severe necrosis and hemorrhage result. These patients "look toxic" and are extremely ill. Because the pancreas lies in both the peritoneal and the retroperitoneal spaces, pancreatic exudate-containing toxins and activated pancreatic enzymes permeate the retroperitoneum, often including the anterior or peritoneal cavity. These toxins and enzymes induce a chemical burn and increase the permeability of blood vessels. This leads to the phenomenon of *third spacing*, producing hypovolemia and shock. Circulating activated enzymes may damage tissue directly, causing hemorrhage, respiratory failure (from injury to alveolar membranes of the lungs), and/or cardiac failure (e.g., from circulating myocardial depressant factor). When tissue damage is extensive, the endocrine function is also affected, causing hyperglycemia.

third spacing leakage of fluid from the vascular and/or intracellular space into the interstitial space.

Clinical Insight

Because injury to alveolar membranes of the lungs (usually on the left side) may occur with pancreatic disease, lung sounds may include wheezing or crackles.

Pain Referred to the Epigastric Region

Referred pain from the heart is another cause of epigastric pain. The vagus nerve bundle and the position of the heart "sitting" on the dome of the diaphragm above the stomach have been implicated in this pattern of referred pain. The vagus nerve innervates the atrial conductive tissue at the sinoatrial and atrioventricular nodes, then continues down behind the heart and through the diaphragm to innervate the stomach and small intestine. Close proximity of infarcted myocardial tissue to vagus nerve fibers stimulates vasovagal reflexes, causing indigestion, nausea, and vomiting.

In its early stages, the pain of appendicitis is visceral and poorly localized. Pain is referred to the epigastric or umbilical regions. It is typically dull and vague and, in some, intermittent. The pain typically becomes more acute and distinct in cases where there is considerable obstruction. As the process of inflammation and/or obstruction continues and bacteria penetrate the wall of the appendix, the pain will eventually become more localized and constant. This may take several hours or as much as a day. (See the further discussion of the appendix and appendicitis later in this chapter.)

Left Hypochondriac Region

The left hypochondriac region contains the pancreas (discussed previously) and the spleen, with referred pain from the left pleural space.

Spleen

The spleen is a solid organ located between the stomach and the left kidney with the diaphragm on top. The adult spleen is rather flat, about 1 to $1^1/_2$ inches thick, and about the circumference of an adult's hand. It is surrounded by a capsule and is suspended on a stalk of blood vessels. The capsule allows the spleen to swell and expand. When the capsule is irritated—from swelling, chemical irritation, or infection—pain is often perceived as being steady and dull. The spleen's close proximity to the diaphragm results in the irritation frequently extending to the distribution of the left phrenic nerve. This causes referred pain, usually to the left neck and shoulder.

Normally, the spleen cannot be palpated due to its posterior location, surrounded by the stomach and the ribs.

The work of the spleen is to remove abnormal blood cells and other components of blood from the circulation. It is also important in preventing infection and helping with immune responses. The spleen has a tremendous blood supply and is permeated with capillaries that are highly porous and lined with vast numbers of macrophages. This enables the spleen to work very efficiently and thoroughly in "cleansing" the blood of old or damaged red blood cells, bacteria, or shreds of virus.

On rare occasions, certain conditions or infections (e.g., mononucleosis) can cause the spleen to swell, resulting in dull pain, usually on palpation. The swelling may be so pronounced that relatively slight body contact or vigorous coughing will cause the splenic capsule to rupture. Rupture of the capsule is commonly perceived as a sharp, intense pain that then lets up, only to recur more intensely later. Because of its extensive blood supply, bleeding from a ruptured spleen can be profuse. The abdominal pain will steadily increase in intensity and be accompanied by syncope, postural hypotension, referred pain to the left neck/shoulder, and signs of peritoneal irritation. If the splenic capsule is leaking, signs and symptoms of shock may not be readily apparent, especially if the patient is lying down. Orthostatic blood pressure checks should be done as a field test for volume loss.

The spleen is not necessary for survival; however, it takes the liver time to pick up the extra load. During that time the body is vulnerable to infection, and *sepsis* is one potential consequence. Sepsis is most commonly seen within the first year of removal of the spleen and commonly presents with the history of an upper respiratory infection that "just didn't get better."

Clinical Insight

If swelling of the spleen has been gradual, there may not be a classic complaint of "pain"; rather, the description will be an "ache" or a "stitch" in the side.

Clinical Insight

The presence of postural hypotension in the presence of an abdominal complaint (which may *not* be described as "pain") is highly suggestive of acute blood loss from a ruptured organ such as the liver or spleen, a tubal pregnancy, or a leaking aortic aneurysm.

sepsis infection that is spread from its initial location to the bloodstream.

Pain Referred to the Left Hypochondriac Region

Left hypochondriac pain may also result from referred pain associated with pleuritis or pneumonia in the left pleural cavity, much like the referred pain to the right hypochondriac area from pleuritis or pneumonia in the right pleural cavity. Pain in this area, in the presence of localized wheezes or rhonchi, warrants further history taking and pulmonary assessment. A thorough assessment, including auscultation of lung sounds, will help distinguish between referred pain and pain from underlying organs. For a discussion of respiratory diseases and difficulty breathing, see Chapter 5.

Umbilical and Hypogastric Regions

The umbilical region contains the small intestine, large intestine, and aorta with referred pain from the appendix, as described previously. The hypogastric region contains the bladder and aorta with referred pain from intestinal obstruction. Together, these regions are often referred to as the central abdomen, with several disease states manifesting pain in this area.

enteritis inflammation of the intestine.

ileitis inflammation of the ileum.

colitis inflammation of the colon (large intestine).

gastroenteritis inflammation of the gastrointestinal tract.

inflammatory bowel disease disease complex causing chronic inflammation of the small or large intestine; colitis.

Crohn's disease a chronic inflammatory disease that can occur anywhere in the digestive tract, usually in the small or large intestine.

epithelium cells that form the outer surface of the body and the lining of the body cavity and principal tubes and passageways leading to the exterior.

Clinical Insight

An important part of history taking is determining where the patient has been within the last several days prior to onset of nausea/vomiting and diarrhea.

Small Intestine

The small intestine, also called the small bowel, is a muscular, hollow tube lined with a series of finger-like projections called villi, which, in turn, are covered with microvilli that absorb nutrients. The small intestine has a diameter ranging from 4 cm at the stomach to about 2.5 cm at the junction with the large intestine (colon). From stomach to large intestine, the small intestine has three segments: the duodenum, the jejunum, and the ileum.

Inflammation of the intestine (*enteritis*) may be localized in the ileum (*ileitis*) or in the colon (*colitis*). *Gastroenteritis* is a general term that refers to inflammation of the entire gastrointestinal tract and is characterized by vomiting followed by diarrhea. *Inflammatory bowel disease* is a blanket term that refers to both ulcerative colitis and *Crohn's disease.* These are chronic disorders that primarily affect both the small and the large intestines. Because the intestine is a hollow organ, capable of peristalsis, irritation of the lining will often trigger hyperperistalsis. The resulting pain is described as intermittent, crampy or colicky, and dull. It also frequently results in diarrhea. Bacterial, viral, or protozoan infection, such as *Giardia,* of the small intestine or colon may cause acute bouts of diarrhea lasting several days or longer.

A side effect of frequent diarrhea is dehydration and electrolyte imbalance. In conditions such as cholera, bacteria bound to the intestinal lining release toxins that stimulate a massive fluid secretion across the intestinal *epithelium.* Without treatment, the victim may die of acute dehydration in a matter of hours.

In conditions such as food poisoning, bacteria such as salmonella, *Shigella,* or staphylococcal enterotoxin rapidly affect the intestinal lining, causing an abrupt onset of nausea and vomiting followed by watery diarrhea. It is believed that the benefit of the watery diarrhea is to "wash out" the toxin or irritant. Again, the risk is dehydration with electrolyte imbalance. Onset is usually sudden, within 2 to 8 hours of ingesting contaminated food. Symptoms usually begin with nausea, vomiting, and abdominal pain described as crampy or colicky and intermittent, followed by diarrhea.

In some cases, the irritation to the epithelial lining is extreme, causing sloughing of the villi and bloody diarrhea with a particularly foul odor. Blood loss, body water loss, and electrolyte imbalance are the main problems.

Important elements of the patient history include determining a possible relationship between onset of symptoms and intake of food or water, the progression of symptoms, and the frequency of stools within a given time period.

Occasionally, the small bowel may become obstructed, resulting in distention of the bowel itself. Pain may begin as intermittent and crampy or colicky, as peristalsis increases to try to bypass the obstruction. Eventually, if the obstruction is not relieved, distention of the bowel will cause peritoneal irritation, resulting in steady, poorly localized pain that increases in intensity. Signs of peritoneal irritation include the patient lying in the fetal position, a side-lying position with knees drawn up, which reduces movement of the peritoneum. Shallow respirations and complaints that coughing worsen the pain are also characteristics of peritoneal irritation.

If ischemia or infarction of the bowel occurs, as a consequence of vascular obstruction or mesenteric interruption, pain is severe and steady and increases in intensity over a short period of time. There may be some widespread abdominal tenderness to palpation, but the pain described is usually out of proportion to the tenderness felt on palpation and poorly localized. Patients with this condition have a variable presentation: Some may be in extremis, complain of terrible pain, and often writhe in agony. Others, particularly the elderly, may have only mild symptoms despite a devastating underlying disease. Vomiting is common, and diarrhea may occur early on. Eventually stools, with necrosis of the bowel, become frankly bloody.

Patients with bowel ischemia or infarction may be in extremis, complain of terrible pain, and often writhe in agony.

Large Intestine

The horseshoe-shaped large intestine, also called the colon or the large bowel, begins at the end of the ileum and ends at the anus. The large intestine lies below the stomach and liver, and almost completely frames the small intestine.

Irritation in the large intestine has many of the same characteristics as irritation in the small intestine, such as increased peristalsis with pain described as intermittent, crampy, and colicky. This pain may or may not be accompanied by diarrhea. Bloody diarrhea is more common with inflammatory bowel disease. Vomiting is not as common.

Obstruction results in distention that, if unrelieved over time, is often observable. Causes can range from the relatively benign, such as constipation, to the serious, such as complete bowel obstruction. Resultant pain begins as intermittent, crampy, colicky pain; if the obstruction is not relieved, the parietal peritoneum becomes inflamed, with pain described as steady and localized as the result of peritoneal irritation becoming more obvious.

Diverticula are formed when various areas of the muscular wall of the colon are weakened and develop little pockets in the mucosa that get forced outward, a condition known as *diverticulosis*. When the diverticula become inflamed (*diverticulitis*), the pain is very similar to the pain of appendicitis. Early in the process the pain is visceral and poorly localized, with referred pain to the hypogastric region (as compared to the epigastric or umbilical region with appendicitis). Later in the process, the pain becomes more localized to the region of the inflamed diverticuli, most commonly, the left lower quadrant. Another characteristic is the pronounced change in bowel habit, most often diarrhea, with the presence of fever. Bleeding may be present but not always obvious. Bleeding may also be massive.

diverticula pockets in the walls of an organ.

diverticulosis the presence of diverticula.

diverticulitis inflammation of diverticula. Inflamed diverticula of the colon may perforate, causing spillage into the peritoneal space.

The danger of diverticulitis, similar to the danger of appendicitis, is perforation of the diverticula. Spilling of bacteria into the peritoneal space will cause signs of peritoneal irritation with steady, sharp pain and eventually a tense, rigid abdomen. The patient may be acutely ill.

Diverticulitis is more common in older adults; however, it can occur in those younger than 50 years of age.

Aorta

The abdominal aorta is considered a hollow organ that protrudes primarily into the retroperitoneal space. It does not have peristaltic movement but does have the ability to contract. Its three layers contain nerve fibers that are sensitive to both stretching and tearing. The most common problem causing abdominal pain from the aorta is an *aneurysm.*

aneurysm a weakened, dilated area of the wall of a vessel.

Aortic aneurysms are pathological dilations of the aorta. They typically occur in one of two types: fusiform, which is a symmetric dilation of the aorta, and saccular, in which the dilation involves mainly one wall. Because they generally form gradually, aneurysms are notorious for often causing no pain during the process of formation and enlargement until the aneurysm actually ruptures or leaks enough blood to result in symptoms. Syncope may be the first presenting sign.

A third type of aneurysm, a dissecting aneurysm, occurs when a tear in the aortic intima exposes a diseased medial layer to the systemic pressure of blood. The blood, under higher arterial pressure, forces the two layers apart. This forced cleaving may cause intense pain. Dissections typically occur in the thoracic portion of the aorta and may extend to the abdomen, producing both chest and abdominal pain.

When present, abdominal aortic aneurysm pain may be described as pulsating or steady, deep, boring, or tearing (depending on the type and location of the aneurysm) and is visceral in quality. Occasionally, the pain may begin as low abdominal pain and radiate to the back. However, it usually occurs in the lumbosacral area of the back and may radiate around to the front as low abdominal pain or may radiate along the aorta, distally. For example, if the aneurysm is located at the renal arteries, pain may be described as radiating to the affected side. If the aneurysm is located above the iliac bifurcation, pain may be described as radiating down one leg or both or into the groin. If the legs are affected, alterations in their skin color and diminished or absent pedal pulses may be detected.

Ordinarily, the aorta cannot be palpated; however, sometimes the aneurysm can be felt as a pulsating mass.

Ordinarily, the aorta cannot be palpated; however, sometimes the aneurysm can be felt as a pulsating mass, when it exceeds 5 to 6 cm in diameter, depending on the type of aneurysm that has formed, the systolic pressure, and the patient's body habitus. Gentle palpation may reveal an abnormally wide pulsation felt on both sides of the midline; however, in heavyset individuals, this may be very difficult to detect. Aneurysms may be tender to palpation. Aneurysms also frequently leak, prior to rupturing, and may rupture without warning, causing severe, constant pain. Blood most frequently collects in the retroperitoneal space; thus, little abdominal distention may be noted until complete rupture occurs.

An aneurysm is a serious threat to life, requiring immediate care and transport.

Pain Referred to the Umbilical and Hypogastric Regions

Referred pain to the umbilical and hypogastric regions is usually due to intestinal obstruction. The abdomen may be distended and tender to palpation proximal to the obstruction.

Right and Left Lumbar Regions

Organs in these regions include the kidneys and their associated ureters.

Kidneys and Ureters

The kidney is a solid organ surrounded by a capsule. Its work is to filter blood and remove waste products and excess body water, forming urine. The urine is collected in the pelvis of the kidney where it then spills into the ureter to travel to the bladder.

Because the kidney is surrounded by a capsule, swelling and inflammation of the kidney itself will result in stretching of the capsule and pain. Pain is localized to the affected side and posterior because of its retroperitoneal location. The pain is described as dull and steady. If the swelling and inflammation are due to an infective process involving the urine and bladder, *dysuria* may also be present.

dysuria painful or difficult urination.

The ureter is a hollow organ capable of peristaltic movement. If the ureter is obstructed, hyperperistalsis occurs to try to overcome the obstruction. The most common cause of an obstruction is a kidney stone. Kidney stones are rough and irregularly shaped crystals. Pain is caused when hyperperistalsis forces the crystal down the ureter. The sharp edges of the crystal will actually lacerate the sides of the ureter, causing radiating pain and blood in the urine. Pain is localized to one side and is perceived as intermittent and crampy or colicky, and may radiate the length of the ureter. The patient may state that the pain radiates to the groin.

The pain is not affected by movement. The patient cannot get comfortable and may be unable to sit still. If the obstruction is not relieved, the pain will intensify. This condition is rarely life threatening. However, the pain is extreme.

Right Iliac Region

The right iliac region contains the ascending colon and the appendix and, in the female, a right ovary and fallopian tube.

Appendix

The vermiform appendix attaches to the cecum of the large intestine along its posteromedial surface. The average appendix is almost 9 cm (3.5 in) long in the adult. Its walls are dominated by lymphoid tissue. It is not firmly attached to the surrounding mesenteries, and it often wriggles and twists as its muscular walls contract.

Inflammation of the appendix (*appendicitis*) usually results in relative or absolute obstruction by a concretion, kink, or swollen mucous membrane. Bacterial infection causes accumulation of irritating products, which erode the epithelial lining of the appendix. Bacteria that normally inhabit the lumen of the large intestine then cross the epithelium and enter the underlying tissues. Inflammation occurs, and the opening between the appendix and the rest of the intestinal tract may become constricted. Mucus secretion accelerates, and the organ becomes increasingly distended.

appendicitis inflammation of the appendix.

Clinical Insight

Because of its ability to wriggle and twist, an inflamed appendix may be located more to the posterior or more to the left than normal. This may cause atypical descriptions of appendicitis.

The stretching of the appendix, like other parts of the bowel, causes pain. Early in the process, the pain may be perceived around the epigastric or umbilical region as intermittent and dull. As the inflammation continues, the pain becomes more localized and, depending on whether tension is applied to the peritoneum, signs of peritoneal irritation may occur, particularly in the right lower quadrant. The location of the pain, in most cases, is so typical that it has been given a name, McBurney's point. Depending on the location of the swollen appendix, pain may extend to the low pelvis, to the back, or even higher in the right abdomen. Nausea, vomiting, *anorexia,* and fever are also frequently present.

anorexia loss of appetite.

Eventually, the swollen and inflamed appendix may rupture or perforate. If this occurs, bacteria and toxins will be released into the peritoneal space, where widespread infection may cause a threat to life. A perforated appendix may cause a sudden release of abdominal pain. However, this is soon followed by parietal pain described as sharp, severe, and constant, accentuated by any movement of the peritoneum, such as deep breathing, coughing, or lying flat with legs extended. Peritonitis is considered a serious consequence with the possibility of sepsis leading to septic shock.

Ovaries and Fallopian Tubes

The ovaries and fallopian tubes, one of each on the right and the left, are part of the female reproductive system. For ease of discussion, both right and left ovaries and fallopian tubes are described in this section.

Each ovary is a solid organ surrounded by a capsule, located in the peritoneal space. Each is connected to the uterus by a fallopian tube. As with all other capsules, stretching of the ovarian capsules causes pain. Inflammation, infection, and swelling of the ovaries is perceived as pain, located on one side or the other, often described as dull and constant. In cases of widespread infection of the female reproductive organs, pain is felt on both sides of the pelvis.

The ovaries are also vulnerable to formation of cysts, which can rupture. The typical pattern of pain is a gradual onset of dull, constant pain that gradually intensifies. At the time of rupture, the pain may suddenly lessen, only to return as more severe, poorly localized, and with signs of peritoneal irritation.

Radiating pain can also occur. Ruptured capsules release chemicals of inflammation that irritate the peritoneum and, in turn, the diaphragm and phrenic nerves. This leads to radiating pain to either side of the neck or either shoulder. It is not dependent on body position and can occur without warning.

The fallopian tubes are hollow and are capable of peristaltic waves to move a fertilized ovum to the fundus of the uterus. If the fallopian tube is too narrow for the ovum, the fertilized egg will become stuck. The ovum, however, will continue to grow (resulting in one type of *ectopic pregnancy*, or *tubal pregnancy*). This stretches the fallopian tube. The stretching is perceived as intermittent, crampy, or colicky pain.

ectopic pregnancy a pregnancy in which the ovum is implanted in an area outside the uterus, usually in a fallopian tube (**tubal pregnancy**).

Eventually, the fallopian tube ruptures from the growth of the ovum and the ruptured tube bleeds. (Ruptured ectopics typically occur between 6 and 12 weeks, far before fetal viability.) Bleeding will enter the peritoneal space and may also enter the uterus, where it sometimes drains from the vaginal vault. The uterine lining may also bleed because it now lacks hormonal support. Because her menses is late, the patient may assume her period has started and may describe it as the "worst period I've ever had." If she knows she is pregnant, she may assume she is miscarrying. It is common, however, for the patient to be unaware that she is pregnant.

Clinical Insight

The presence of shoulder/neck pain, in the presence of syncope and absence of trauma, is highly suggestive of a hemorrhagic capsule rupture, with or without any other complaint of pain.

Pain will commonly begin as intermittent and crampy. There may be a short time of relief when the tube ruptures, only to have the pain recur as more severe, intense, and constant. Signs of peritoneal irritation are also present. Radiating pain to either side of the neck or either shoulder is common. The presence or absence of pain is not related to the amount of blood present.

Because of the close proximity of the right ovary and fallopian tube to the appendix, appendicitis and a swollen, inflamed ovary or right-sided tubal pregnancy have often been confused. It is not the intent of this text to enable the care provider to discriminate between the two. However, it is very important to assess for signs of peritoneal irritation and shock. Assume the worst—and the worst is shock from hemorrhage or peritonitis from sepsis.

Left Iliac Region

Organs in this region include the descending colon (large intestine) and, in the female, the left ovary and fallopian tube. (See the previous discussion of ovaries and fallopian tubes.)

Most of the pain from diseases affecting the large intestine is referred to the umbilical or hypogastric region. However, certain specific conditions may localize pain in either the right or the left iliac region, such as diverticulitis, which localizes pain in the left iliac region. (See the discussion of diverticulitis under "Large Intestine," earlier in this chapter.)

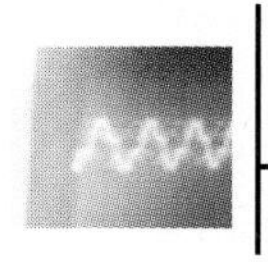

ASSESSMENT

Scene Size-Up and Initial Assessment

As you approach the scene, the patient's position can give clues to the type of pain. A patient lying in the fetal position may be suffering from parietal pain, while a patient who is lying supine may be feeling visceral pain. A patient up and walking around, or pacing because he can't get comfortable, is typical of a patient suffering a hollow organ obstruction such as a kidney stone or gallstone.

Clinical Insight

The action of being up and walking around suggests that a perfusing blood pressure is present.

Mental status is usually determined by talking to the patient. If, on approach, the patient has spontaneous eye opening and makes eye contact, assume a state of alertness, which you will confirm by verbal communication. Follow verbal communication with an assessment of the quality of mental status. Determine orientation, confusion, or disorientation. Keep in mind that an altered mental status will be one of the early indicators of internal hemorrhage and shock.

The patient who has complained of abdominal pain and then progresses to unresponsiveness must be considered to have a threat to life until proven otherwise.

If the patient is talking, a patent airway is demonstrated. If the patient is not talking and is unresponsive, inspect the airway manually for any foreign body, secretions, bruises, or abrasions to the tongue. Presence of vomit is often associated with a problem with the stomach, liver, gallbladder, or appendix. The presence of bright red or coffee ground-like blood indicates a problem with the stomach or esophagus.

Respiratory rate and depth is another important observation. Tachypnea may be a result of compensatory mechanisms for loss of blood or body fluid, loss of tidal volume, or a reaction to pain. Loss of tidal volume is most often noticed as shallow respirations. Shallow respirations may be the result of pain, peritoneal irritation, or compression of the diaphragm.

A greatly enlarged abdomen may be a sign of an obstruction, ascites, or both. Distention of the abdomen also compresses the diaphragm, affecting tidal volume. If you observe this condition, adequacy of respirations should be an immediate concern.

Quickly check the pulse during the initial assessment. A rapid pulse, one of the signs of shock, may indicate internal hemorrhage.

Observing the patient's skin color is also important. Pale skin may indicate vasoconstriction, which occurs with a sympathetic response. A sympathetic response can be triggered by extreme pain or by compensatory mechanisms for hypoperfusion (shock). Pale skin may also occur with an infective process. The net effect of chemicals can cause either shunting, resulting in pale skin, or dilation of capillary beds, resulting in flushing. In any case, the presence of pallor warrants further thorough assessment of the cardiovascular system.

Cyanosis or a gray cast to the skin, especially of the circumoral area, is also an indication of lack of perfusion and is a serious sign of respiratory and/or cardiovascular compromise. Administration of high-flow, high-concentration oxygen, either by nonrebreather mask at 15 lpm or assisted with a bag-valve-mask (depending on the patient's mental status), should be an immediate consideration. In the unconscious patient, consider tracheal intubation.

Mottled skin is caused by blood pooling in capillary beds. This most commonly occurs with blood loss. In the case of abdominal complaints, mottled skin in the abdomen may be due to ruptured aortic aneurysms or extensive internal bleeding. In an adult, this is usually a sign of an actual life threat.

Skin temperature often corresponds to skin color. Pale skin due to sympathetic response is usually cool, mottled skin is usually cold or clammy, and flushed skin is usually warm or hot. Warm, pale skin suggests fever with vasodilation and settling of blood.

Focused History and Physical Exam

Because of the many problems that can occur with the various organs in the abdomen, the focused history and focused physical exam do not try to discriminate between an appendicitis attack and severe constipation, or between an aortic aneurysm and hemorrhagic pancreatitis. Rather, the focus is to determine the probabilities of an immediate threat to life, a potential threat to life, or no threat to life—recognition of the CUPS patient—and then to treat appropriately. Your knowledge of the characteristics of certain organ systems, the location of pain, the patient's descriptions of pain and order of symptoms, and the physical exam you perform will help guide your thinking process as you determine the probabilities and will be important information for the hospital staff.

The focus of assessment is not to discriminate between possible causes of abdominal pain. Rather, the focus is to determine the probability of a life threat.

Focused History

A focused history helps clarify the potential for threat to life and helps identify the organ system that is probably involved. Pain is a subjective complaint. To qualify and quantify that complaint, you can use mnemonics such as OPQRST (Onset, Palliation/Provocation, Quality, Radiation, Severity, and Time) and rate the pain from 1 to 10, 10 being the worst. These categories are very helpful in addition to more specific questions, as summarized here:

1. Onset
   - *Was the onset sudden?* A sudden pain severe enough to cause fainting suggests a perforated viscus or ruptured aneurysm. Similar symptoms in a woman of childbearing age may be due to a ruptured ectopic pregnancy or an ovarian cyst.
   - *What were you doing when it started?* If the patient was engaged in physical activity or was coughing when sudden abdominal pain started, something may have torn (e.g., a hernia) or a muscle may have been pulled. If the patient also has a history of mononucleosis, consider a ruptured splenic capsule, especially if syncope or orthostatic hypotension is also present.
   - *Has this pain happened before?* If so, how has it changed to require calling EMS? Pain that has been chronic may be subject to complication, such as a perforated ulcer, perforated diverticulitis, or perforation from inflammatory bowel disease.
2. Palliation/Provocation
   - *What makes the pain better? What makes it worse?* Answers to these questions may tell you if the pain is peritoneal, for instance, whether the pain is better when lying on the side with knees drawn up or worsens with coughing. If the patient is walking in an attempt to relieve the pain, an obstruction such as a kidney stone or gallstone is more likely. If antacids give relief, a peptic ulcer may be suspected. If symptoms sound like indigestion but there is no relief from antacids, suspect the problem may be cardiac in nature.

3. Quality
   - *Can you describe the pain.* A severe, knife-like pain, especially if associated with shock, indicates a potential life threat. Burning pain is often associated with ulcers. Tearing pain is characteristic of a dissecting aneurysm. Colicky pain that becomes steady can indicate a worsening obstruction of a hollow viscus. Dull pain is often associated with a solid organ. Intermittent, crampy, or colicky pain is often associated with a hollow organ.
4. Radiation
   - *Does the pain go anywhere?* Radiation often occurs along the distribution of the nerves of the same spinal segment. Gallbladder pain is often felt beneath the right scapula. Diaphragmatic irritation from blood or pus can be felt in the region of either shoulder or both shoulders. Renal pain radiates to the region of the groin. In an older patient, severe pain beginning in the midback and rapidly spreading to the abdomen is characteristic of an aortic aneurysm.
5. Severity
   - *On a scale of 1 to 10, 10 being the worst, how bad is the pain?* This attempts to quantify the severity of the pain in objective terms. Sudden pain that is severe and steady tends to be more serious, especially when associated with syncope or hypotension.
6. Time
   - *How long ago did this pain start?* Time is essential in determining the pattern of symptoms.
   - *How long did the attack last?* An attack of pain that suddenly lets up may be the calm before the storm. A patient with a perforated appendix or perforated ulcer may experience temporary relief prior to the severe, intense pain of peritonitis.
7. Associated Symptoms or Pattern of Onset
   - *What other problems or complaints have you also noticed?* Asking this question may help narrow the problem. Symptoms that occurred prior to the pain or in association with it are important. When vomiting precedes pain, especially if it is followed shortly by diarrhea, gastroenteritis is probable. Pallor, sweating, or fainting are rough guides to the severity of the pathological process. The presence of shock is an ABSOLUTE indicator of severity. When these are present, assume a life threat. Associated shoulder and/or neck pain suggests perforation of a viscus with bleeding or infection. Presence of jaundice indicates a liver obstruction and should be considered infectious until proven otherwise. If a rash is present, assume an infectious disease is present. Onset of severe pain followed by vomiting that has lasted 5 to 6 hours or longer is most likely a problem that will require surgery and should be considered a potential life threat. If fever is present, ask "When did the fever start—before or after the pain began?" Fever indicates possible inflammation or infection. Fever in the presence of hypotension indicates sepsis or septic shock.

Focused Physical Exam

The physical exam should accomplish three things:

- First, confirm whether the patient is critical or unstable with an immediate threat to life, potentially unstable or with a potential threat to life, or stable with a low probability of threat to life (Table 8-4).

TABLE 8-4 Abdominal Pain: Clues to the Severity of the Patient's Condition

The following characteristics of abdominal pain and associated signs/symptoms indicate a serious condition and potential threat to life—a critical, unstable, or potentially unstable condition—warranting expeditious care and transport:

- Sudden onset (*potentially unstable*)
- Severe pain (may be described as "knife-like") (*potentially unstable*)
- Pulsating mass present (*unstable or potentially unstable*)
- Fainting; loss of consciousness (*critical or unstable*)
- Any signs of shock or internal blood loss (e.g., diminished mental status; pale, moist skin; mottled skin; rapid, shallow respirations; rapid pulse; falling blood pressure) (*critical or unstable*)
- Orthostatic hypotension or positive tilt test (*critical or unstable*)

- Second, determine a high or low probability for the involvement of a specific organ or the presence of a specific condition, such as bleeding, infection, or obstruction (Table 8-5).
- Third, determine what treatment is appropriate.

A thorough physical exam, including the heart and respiratory system, together with a good history, should also indicate the likelihood that the abdominal pain the patient feels is radiated from another site. (Review Figure 8-4 and Tables 8-1 and 8-3.)

The focused physical exam includes inspection, auscultation, and palpation:

1. *Inspection.* When you inspect the abdomen, note the presence or absence of distention and the skin color. Distention is something that family members or the patient himself may be more accurate in determining. Distention may be due to an obstruction or from a collection of gas resulting from significantly decreased or absent peristaltic movement or from ascites.

   Observe for abnormal color, such as jaundice or discolorations. Jaundice suggests liver dysfunction that may or may not be infectious. Assume the disease process is infectious, and maintain body substance isolation.

   Bluish to purple discolorations in the navel and/or the same discoloration in the flank area may be a sign of bleeding in the retroperitoneal space. It takes time for the blood to seep through the tissues in the flank and along the connective tissue to the navel. Bleeding in the retroperitoneal space is more typical of leaking aneurysms or hemorrhagic pancreatitis.

   As previously discussed, mottling indicates pooling of blood in the capillary beds, usually from blood or fluid loss, and is a sign of severe distress.

2. *Auscultation.* Auscultation of the abdomen, although commonly done in the hospital setting, is not recommended for short transport times in the field for several reasons. To accurately assess bowel sounds, the environment must be relatively quiet, and 3 to 5 minutes in each quadrant is recommended. Although a quiet environment may be managed, the time frame is too long for most prehospital situations. Another and perhaps more important reason is that treatment isn't based on the presence or absence of bowel sounds.

   Auscultation of the chest, however, is recommended. The presence of wheezing, crackles or rales, and rhonchi in a patient complaining of abdominal pain may indicate that the primary problem might be outside of the abdomen, as in pneumonia or pleuritis, with the abdomen being the site of radiating pain. Presence of wheezing or crackles may also be a result of sepsis

TABLE 8-5 Abdominal Pain: Clues to Underlying Cause

Findings	Typically Associated With . . .
SCENE SIZE-UP AND INITIAL ASSESSMENT	
Patient's position: ■ Fetal position (curled up on side) ■ Supine ■ Up, pacing, can't get comfortable	 ■ Parietal pain ■ Visceral pain ■ Hollow organ obstruction (e.g., kidney stone, gallstone)
Patient's color: ■ Pale ■ Cyanotic ■ Mottled ■ Jaundiced	 ■ Extreme pain and/or internal bleeding (shock) ■ Respiratory or cardiovascular compromise (shock) ■ Blood pooling (shock) ■ Liver abnormality
Enlarged abdomen	Obstruction or fluid collection (ascites or blood)
FOCUSED HISTORY	
Pain present	Rapid onset (distention of an abdominal organ)
No or little pain present	Gradual onset (distention of an abdominal organ)
Steady pain	Solid organs (liver, pancreas, spleen, kidneys, ovaries)
Intermittent (crampy, colicky) pain	Hollow organs (stomach, small intestine, large intestine, appendix, rectum, gallbladder, uterus, bladder, common bile duct, ureters, fallopian tubes, aorta)
Poorly localized, diffuse pain (generally felt near the midline in the epigastric, umbilical, or hypogastric region)	Visceral organs (hollow or solid)
Localized, intense pain (localized to one side)	Parietal peritoneum, generally corresponds to the associated dermatomes
Pain felt at some distance from the affected organ or from the location of abdominal tenderness	Referred pain (originating in visceral organs but felt in another area)—see Figure 8-5
Abdominal pain with signs/symptoms commonly associated with extraabdominal causes (e.g., chest pain, dyspnea)	Referred pain (originating outside the abdomen but felt as abdominal pain)—see Table 8-1
Sudden onset of pain (severe enough to cause fainting)	Perforated visceral organ, ruptured aneurysm
Onset during or caused by physical activity or coughing	Hernia; pulled muscle; ruptured spleen (especially with history of mononucleosis)
This pain has happened before	Complication of chronic condition (e.g., perforated ulcer, diverticulitis)
FOCUSED PHYSICAL EXAM	
Inspection: ■ Distention ■ Bluish discoloration at naval or flank	 ■ Obstruction; collection of gas, fluid ■ Bleeding in retroperitoneal space
Auscultation of chest: ■ Abnormal breath sounds (wheezing, crackles or rales, rhonchi) with abdominal pain ■ Wheezing with abdominal distention	 ■ Primary problem outside the abdomen (e.g., pneumonia) ■ Abdominal distention exerting pressure on diaphragm and lungs
Palpation: ■ Softness ■ Rigidity ■ Localized tenderness ■ Pulsating mass	 ■ Lesser severity (softness is normal) ■ Greater severity (inflammation; internal bleeding) ■ Involvement of underlying organ ■ Aortic aneurysm

Continued on the next page

TABLE 8-5 Abdominal Pain: Clues to Underlying Cause *(continued)*

VITAL SIGNS	
Respirations: ■ Rapid ■ Shallow	 ■ Blood or fluid loss or low tidal volume (shock) ■ Pain, peritoneal irritation, or compression of diaphragm
Pulse and blood pressure—Orthostatic hypotension or tilt test—Rising from a supine position causes dizziness and/or nausea, rapid change in skin color, disappearance of radial pulse, increase in pulse 20 bpm, drop in systolic BP 10 mmHg	■ Hypotension (shock); blood loss

or pancreatitis, where the primary problem is in the abdomen but with secondary effects on other organs. Wheezing may also occur when distention of the abdomen has exerted so much pressure on the lungs that terminal bronchioles suffer bronchospasm. In any case, if the lungs are affected in the presence of a chief complaint of abdominal pain, assume the problem is more serious.

3. *Palpation.* Palpation of the abdomen is a part of the physical assessment that can give important information. Consider the complaint of abdominal pain and the principle of care "first, do no harm." Increasing pain may or may not be considered "harm," but we should not be increasing the discomfort of our patients if we can help it. Therefore, ask the patient to point with one finger to where it hurts the most. This will help determine whether the pain is localized or is diffuse and nonlocalized.

   When you begin palpation, start at the point farthest away from the location of the pain. Use gentle, fingertip pressure. Assess the general "feel" of the abdomen for softness, the firmness of muscle guarding, or the rigidity of peritonitis. Then assess each quadrant for masses, degree of tenderness, pulsations, or the feel of the organs themselves. If you are not familiar with what a specific organ feels like, you can note its presence as a "mass."

   Remember that localized tenderness is often directly related to the underlying organ or organ system and is a valuable clue that should be documented (Figure 8-6). Direct assessment for rebound tenderness, an increase of pain on sudden release of the palpator's hand, is not generally done in the field. Indirect assessment, such as an increase of pain on coughing or straightening the legs when supine, will give the same information and should be documented.

   Spontaneous complaints of shoulder or lateral neck pain, or movement of the patient that precipitates complaints of shoulder or lateral neck pain, should alert you to the presence of peritoneal or diaphragmatic irritation, usually from a ruptured capsule or ruptured viscus. Frequently, this involves bleeding into the peritoneal space. This may be accompanied by complaints of syncope when the patient changes position from lying to sitting or sitting to standing.

Vital Signs

Baseline measurements of respiration, pulse, and blood pressure should be taken, with additional measurements taken at intervals and compared to the baseline readings. Vital signs help determine possible blood loss and hypoperfusion, severity of pain, and physical changes within the abdominal cavity:

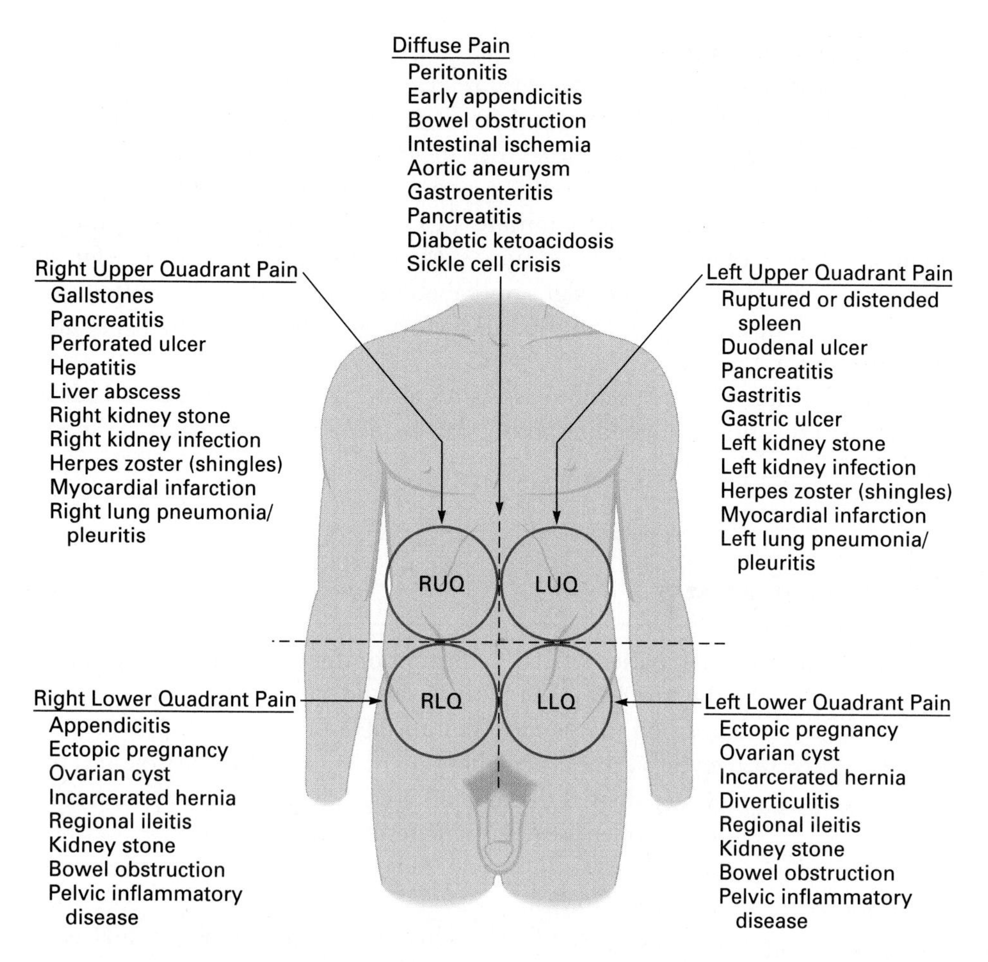

FIGURE 8-6
Locations of abdominal pain and possible causes.

1. *Respirations.* As discussed earlier, rapid respirations may be present as a compensatory mechanism for blood or body fluid loss. Shallow respirations may result from pain, peritoneal irritation, or compression of the diaphragm from swelling or distention within the abdomen.
2. *Pulse and Blood Pressure.* Tachycardia in the presence of pain can be due to the pain or due to a compensatory mechanism. Tachycardia in the presence of hypotension is a serious sign of shock. However, certain medications may affect the body's ability to produce a tachycardic response to shock.

    Pulse rates and blood pressure measured when a patient is at rest should serve as baseline measurements and should be reassessed after a patient has moved.

    One diagnostic test that should be performed on every patient who exhibits signs of peritoneal irritation or who has indicated the presence of dizziness or faintness is an evaluation of orthostatic vital signs. This is also known as the *tilt test* or test for *orthostatic* (or *postural*) *hypotension.* Take the pulse and blood pressure when the patient is placed in the sitting or standing position and compare the readings with those that were taken when the patient was supine. Sometimes the rapid change in skin color, immediate complaints of dizziness and/or nausea, and a disappearance of the radial pulse are enough to suggest internal bleeding. In general, if the pulse increases 20 beats/min and the systolic pressure drops 10 mmHg from the baseline vital signs, then the test is positive for orthostatic hypotension or is defined as a positive tilt test, indicating significant blood or fluid loss.

Clinical Insight

Dizziness or weakness when getting up suggests that orthostatic hypotension is present.

tilt test test for **orthostatic** or **postural hypotension.** Pulse and blood pressure taken when the patient is supine are compared with measurements when the patient rises to a sitting or standing position. Internal bleeding or severe fluid loss is indicated by a rapid change in skin color, dizziness or nausea, disappearance of the radial pulse, an increase in pulse of 20 beats, or a drop in blood pressure of 10 mmHg.

Special Considerations

Because the abdomen tends to be a site for referred pain, the ECG should be monitored in older patients and diabetic patients. An AMI may be in progress and, due to peripheral neuropathies common to both groups, indigestion or epigastric pain may be the chief complaint. Look for associated weakness and/or breathlessness, especially on exertion, and initiate ECG monitoring. Diabetic patients should also have a blood sugar evaluation. If the abdomen is the site for referred pain in a diabetic, look for other signs of diabetic ketoacidosis, such as rapid respirations with an acetone or fruity odor, history of polyuria, tachycardia, and poor skin turgor.

Pulse oximetry can be useful to assess respiratory function; however, it does not serve as a substitute for good respiratory assessment and is inaccurate in shock states.

TREATMENT

Treatment for the patient with acute abdominal pain is symptomatic. Treat for possible shock, place the patient in a position of comfort, apply oxygen or assisted ventilations as needed, and IV therapy per local protocols. Expedite transport.

Treatment for the patient with acute abdominal pain is symptomatic (Figure 8-7). The patient should be allowed to assume the position that is most comfortable. If factors are present that reveal a critical/unstable patient or the probability of an actual or potential threat to life (e.g., signs of shock; positive tilt test; sudden, severe pain; respiratory compromise; mottled face, chest, and/or abdomen), provide high-flow, high-concentration oxygen.

For patients who have complained of abdominal pain and who are now unresponsive, assist ventilations with a bag-valve-mask and a reservoir at 15 lpm, and tracheally intubate the patient if appropriate. If the patient is awake, apply a nonrebreather mask with a flow rate of 15 lpm.

Depending on the problem, IV access may be appropriate, but do not delay transport to get a line. IV access can be obtained en route. If internal bleeding is a high probability, ensure that administration of IV fluids does not cause disruption of clot formation. This has a high probability of occurring when the systolic pressure is above 100. In the case of an abdominal aortic aneurysm, high systolic pressures may increase the likelihood of complete rupture. Suggested guidelines include keeping the systolic pressure between 70 and 100 mmHg, using mental status as a guide.

The pneumatic antishock garment (PASG) has been suggested for treatment of abdominal bleeding, especially for an abdominal aortic aneurysm. The garment helps stabilize the aneurysm by exerting circumferential pressure. Use of this device is highly controversial, however, and local medical direction is required.

When dehydration is suspected, such as when prolonged diarrhea or vomiting has occurred, IV access and administration of a fluid bolus of 250 to 500 ml may be sufficient. A fluid bolus may also help manage an elevated temperature.

Crystalloids, such as normal saline (0.9 percent NaCl) and lactated Ringer's, are recommended. When hypotension is severe and uncorrected by crystalloid administration, and sepsis is suspected, treatment may include pharmacologic

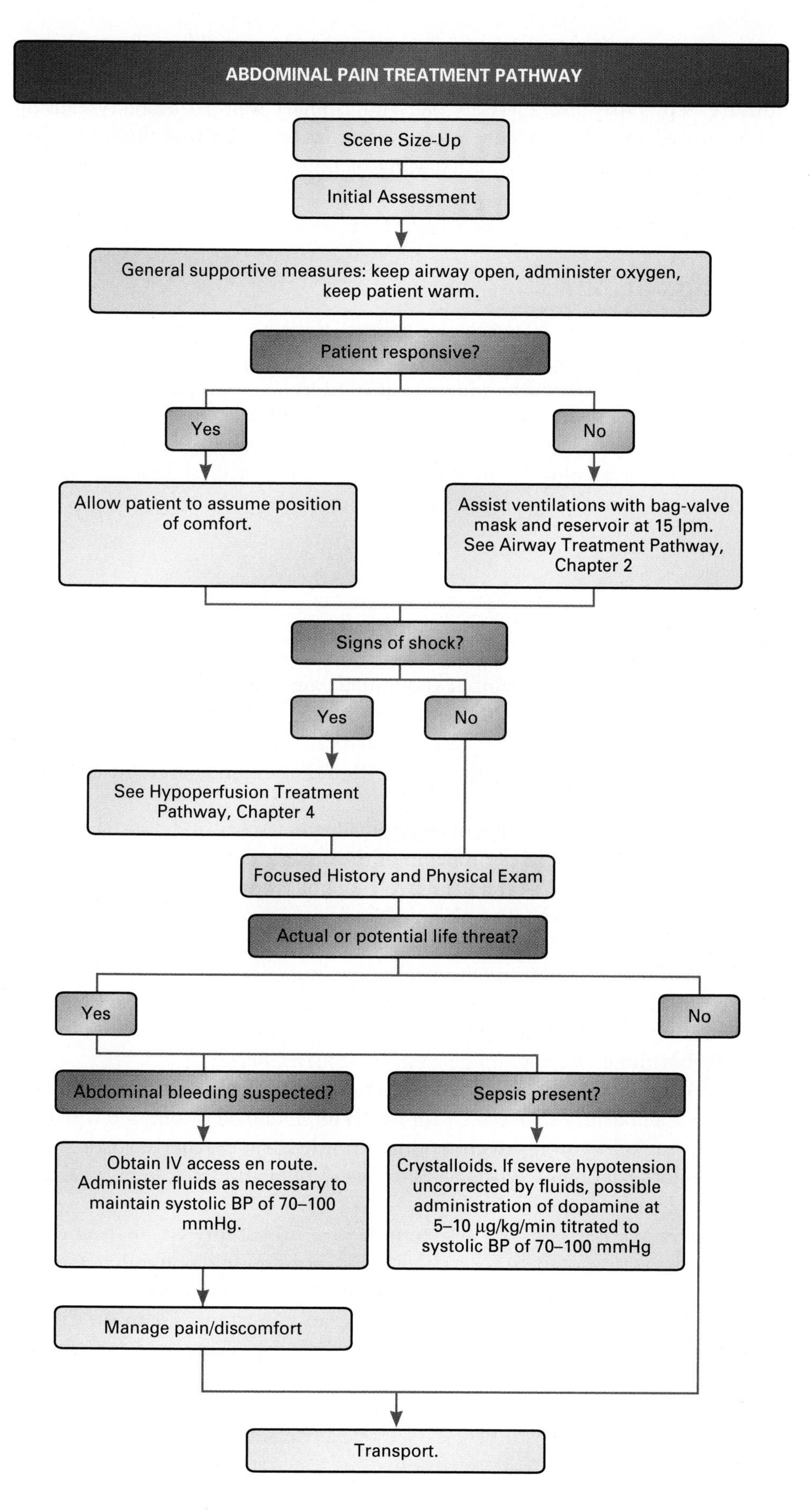

FIGURE 8-7
Abdominal pain treatment pathway.

therapy. The drug of choice in the field is dopamine. The dosage is based on μg/kg/min with 5 to 10 μg/kg/min as a usual starting dose, titrated to systolic pressure. Sepsis may also affect alveolar and capillary wall permeability, causing pulmonary edema. Thus, positive-pressure ventilations along with fluids are often necessary. Dehydration with third spacing of fluid is a significant finding with sepsis.

Palliation of Pain

Many systems are using pharmacologic pain relief methods, such as nitrous oxide, morphine, or fentanyl, if pain is present. Midazolam (Versed) does not relieve pain but does relieve anxiety. Promoting patient comfort is important and plays a role in the success of further treatments. However, use of such pain relief measures mandates complete assessments and thorough study of the pharmacologic agents used. Use of pharmacologic pain management is up to medical direction and the availability of CT scanning. Follow local protocols.

SUMMARY

Patients with the complaint of abdominal pain may suffer from a wide variety of diseases and conditions. Basically, there are three mechanisms that may result in abdominal pain; they are mechanical, inflammatory, and ischemic processes. A fourth is referred pain either within the abdomen or to the abdomen from outside causes.

There are two general types of abdominal pain, visceral and parietal. Visceral pain arises from the visceral peritoneum or the organs themselves and tends to be more diffuse and vague. Visceral pain involving hollow organs tends to be crampy and colicky, dull and intermittent. Visceral pain involving solid organs tends to be dull and constant.

Parietal pain arises from the parietal peritoneum and is more localized, intense, and constant. Signs of peritoneal irritation include lying in the fetal position and increased pain with activities that move the peritoneum, such as coughing, deep breathing, or lying supine with legs outstretched.

Referred pain *to* the abdomen is common with conditions such as AMI, pneumonia, and diabetes. Referred pain *within* the abdomen is common with conditions such as kidney stones or aneurysms. Knowledge of the characteristics of the various abdominal organs, especially in terms of referred pain, can be a valuable assessment tool.

Assessment is based on determining the probability of an immediate threat to life or the potential for a threat to life, or no life threat and determining the condition of the patient as CUPS. During the scene size-up and initial assessment, observation of patient position is an important clue to the type of pain suffered. The description of pain during history taking, and the physical exam and vital signs measurements, provide additional information. Treatment is symptomatic, with patient positioning an important part of treatment. Oxygen and IV fluids may be necessary, especially if shock is present. In the case of septic shock with severe hypotension, dopamine may be a necessary adjunct to treatment. Use of palliative measures is up to medical direction and local protocol.

SCENARIO FOLLOW-UP

Your patient is a 35-year-old female marathon biker who has suffered a bout of syncope at home. You find her lying on her side on a couch, alert and oriented. She is speaking in complete sentences. She is pale with cool, dry skin. She says she got dizzy and passed out when she tried to get up to go to the bathroom. She reports intermittent, crampy abdominal pain for the past 2 days, worsening until today. The pain is now constant and spread across the entire lower abdomen. Her menses is late, but not unusually so. She is sexually active but has had a tubal ligation. She denies vaginal drainage. As she turns onto her back, she reports a sudden, sharp pain in her left neck and shoulder and says that the pain is better if her knees are bent. Her vital signs are pulse 90, respirations 18, and blood pressure 110/86.

Your patient confirms that her abdomen is distended. You see no sign of skin discoloration or rash. You ask her to point to where it hurts most and she indicates the lower left quadrant. You then start gentle palpation at the most distant quadrant. You note guarding with diffuse tenderness to palpation, more so as you approach the lower left quadrant. Her lungs are clear, but she complains of increased pain when she takes a deep breath.

Because your patient has signs of peritoneal irritation (knees bent to decrease abdominal pain, deep breaths increase abdominal pain) and radiating pain to her neck and shoulder, you place her on oxygen by nonrebreather mask and start an IV of normal saline. You suspect a ruptured viscus with associated fluid or blood loss, but her vital signs appear to be within normal limits. However, even though her pulse would be considered normal for most patients, you recall that she is a marathon bike rider and estimate that her pulse most likely has a much lower resting rate than 90.

To confirm your suspicion of compensated shock, you assess for orthostatic hypotension. With you and your partner on either side, holding onto her, you place your hand on the patient's radial pulse and help her stand up. Immediately, she complains of nausea and dizziness. Her color pales, she breaks out in a sweat, and you lose her radial pulse. Your suspicions confirmed, you quickly lay her down flat and elevate her legs. While your partner takes a second set of vital signs, you administer a fluid bolus of 300 ml. Vital signs are now pulse 96, respirations 20 and shallow, and blood pressure 80/62. After the fluid bolus, her vital signs are pulse 82, respirations 16, and blood pressure 100/82. She continues to be alert and oriented, although she does continue to complain intermittently about left neck and shoulder pain.

On admission to the emergency department, lab work is drawn and an ultrasound done. A ruptured ectopic pregnancy in the fallopian tube is suspected. The emergency department physician tells you that a tubal ligation is one of the risk factors for a tubal pregnancy. The patient is taken to surgery where a liter of blood is removed, along with her left fallopian tube and ovary. She recovers well, as you note when you open the newspaper a few months later and find your patient's picture with the caption "Local Athlete Wins Blue Mountain Bike Marathon."

FURTHER READING

1. Alexander, D. "New concepts in shock management," *Air Medical Journal,* 1996;15(2):85–91.
2. Berkow, R, M.H. Beers, and M. Burs, eds. *The Merck Manual of Diagnosis and Therapy.* 17th ed. Rahway, NJ: Merck & Company, 1999.
3. Bickell, W.H., M.J. Wall, P.E. Pepe, R.R. Martin, V.F. Ginger, M.K. Allen, and K.L. Mattox. "Immediate versus delayed fluid resuscitation for hypotensive patients with penetrating torso injuries," *New England Journal of Medicine,* 1994;331(17): 1105–1109.
4. Bledsoe, B.E., R.S. Porter, and R.A. Cherry. "Gastroenterology," in *Essentials of Paramedic Care.* 2nd ed. Upper Saddle River, NJ: Pearson/Prentice Hall, 2006.
5. Capone, A.C., P. Safar, W. Stezoski, S. Tisherman, and A.B. Peitzman. "Improved outcome with fluid restriction in treatment of uncontrolled hemorrhagic shock," *Journal of the American College of Surgeons,* 1995;180:49–56.
6. Cope, Sir Zachary (original author, 1921), Silen, W., ed. *Cope's Early Diagnosis of the Acute Abdomen.* 20th ed. New York: Oxford University Press, 2000.
7. Fontanarosa, P.B. "Abdominal, genitourinary, and back pain," in P.T. Pons and D. Cason, eds., *Paramedic Field Care: A Complaint-Based Approach.* St. Louis: American College of Emergency Physicians, Mosby –Year Book, 1997.
8. Goldman, L., and D. Ausiello, eds. *Cecil Textbook of Medicine.* 22nd ed. St. Louis: Saunders, 2004.
9. Guyton, A.C., and J.E. Hall, "Gastrointestinal physiology," in *Textbook of Medical Physiology.* 10th ed. Philadelphia: Saunders, 2001.

10. HEUTHER, S.E. "Structure and function of the digestive system," in K.L. McCance and S.E. Heuther, eds., *Pathophysiology: The Biologic Basis for Disease in Adults and Children.* 4th ed. St. Louis: Mosby, 2002.
11. HEUTHER, S.E. AND K.L. MCCANCE. "Alterations of digestive function," in K.L. McCance and S.E. Heuther, eds., *Pathophysiology: The Biologic Basis for Disease in Adults and Children.* 4th ed. St. Louis: Mosby, 2002.
12. KAWESKI, S.M., ET AL. "The effect of prehospital fluids on survival in trauma patients," *Journal of Trauma,* 1990;30(10):1215.
13. LINGAPPA, V.R. "Gastrointestinal disease," in S.J. McPhee, V.R. Lingappa, and W.F. Ganong, eds., *Pathophysiology of Disease: An Introduction to Clinical Medicine.* 4th ed. Chicago: McGraw-Hill, 2003.
14. MARTINI, F.H., AND E.F. BARTHOLOMEW. "The digestive system," in F.H. Martini and E.F. Bartholomew, eds., *Essentials of Anatomy and Physiology.* Upper Saddle River, NJ: Pearson/Prentice Hall, 2000.
15. MCQUAID, K.R. "Alimentary tract," in L.M. Tierney, S.J. McPhee, and M.A. Papadakis, eds., *Current Medical Diagnosis and Treatment.* Norwalk, CT: Appleton & Lange, 1997.
16. VAN ZILE, J. AND M.L. EMERICK. "Acute abdominal pain," in G.C. Hamilton, A.B. Sanders, G.R. Strange, and A.T. Trott, eds., *Emergency Medicine: An Approach to Clinical Problem Solving.* 2nd ed. Philadelphia: Saunders, 2003.

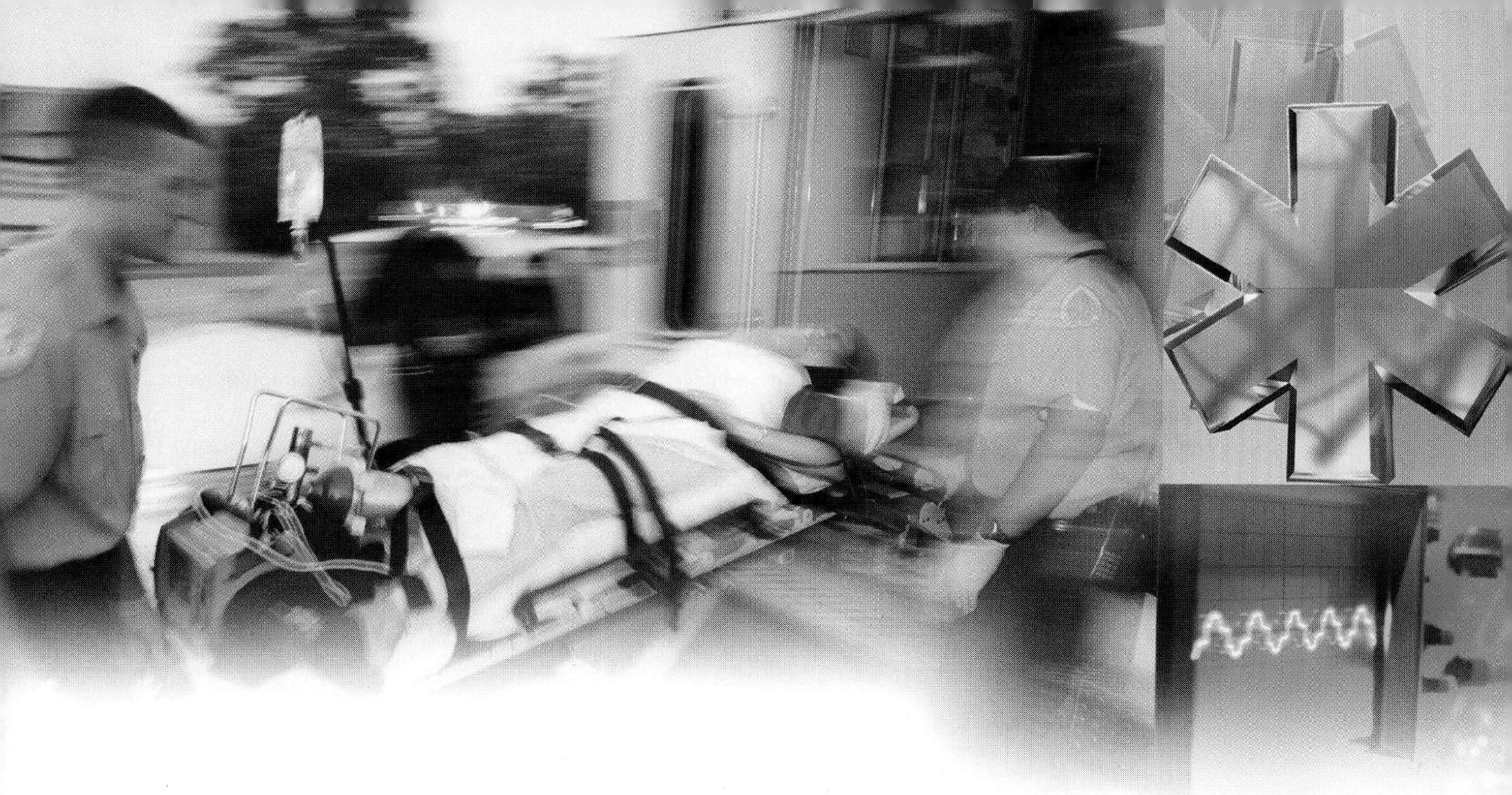

GASTROINTESTINAL BLEEDING

9

The severity of gastrointestinal (GI) bleeding may range from the relatively insignificant (e.g., hemorrhoidal bleeding) to an immediate threat to life (e.g., a major arterial bleed). Bleeding may be overt or occult, and abdominal pain may or may not be present. The origin of bleeding may be located anywhere from the mouth to the anus. The patient's presentation may vary as widely as the causes of bleeding. Because of this variety in patient presentation, GI bleeding may be missed. This chapter acquaints you with the tools necessary to develop a high index of suspicion when bleeding is not immediately obvious and reviews treatment once it is suspected.

Topics that are covered in this chapter are

- Anatomy, Physiology, and Pathophysiology
- Characteristics of Blood in the GI Tract
- Assessment
- Treatment

SCENARIO

You are called to the scene of a 68-year-old female who has experienced an episode of dizziness. On arrival, you find your patient sitting in the hallway of her high-rise apartment building. The manager and a friend are with her. They explain that the patient had just arrived home from her weekly dialysis treatment when this event occurred. She tells you that she became dizzy when walking to her apartment and eased herself to the floor. She is awake, oriented, and alert, is talking in complete sentences, has an intact radial pulse, and is in no apparent distress.

Her skin is cool and dry. Her dialysis fistula is in her left arm, so you take vital signs in her right arm. Her vital signs are pulse 82, respirations 16, and blood pressure 110/80, and her lung sounds are clear. She denies any pain. A general palpation of all extremities, pelvis, abdomen, and chest wall is negative for pain or crepitation. She tells you that she is on nitroglycerin for angina and is on dialysis three times a week for kidney failure.

How would you proceed with the assessment and care of this patient?

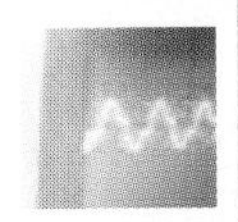

ANATOMY, PHYSIOLOGY, AND PATHOPHYSIOLOGY

The GI tract is essentially a tube that passes through the body, extending from the mouth to the anus. Depending on where you are along the length of the tube, characteristics of the mucosa vary along with the function. To visualize the anatomy of the digestive system, as discussed in this section—esophagus, stomach, small and large intestines, rectum, and anus—you may want to review Figure 8-1 in Chapter 8, Acute Abdominal Pain. See also Table 9-1.

The esophagus is a thin-walled, hollow, muscular tube designed to propel swallowed food to the stomach. It lies posterior to the trachea and the heart. When not in use, the esophagus is normally flattened. The blood vessels of the esophagus drain into the portal vein of the liver. When the liver swells, as in cirrhosis, blood backs up into the portal system, causing the phenomenon of portal hypertension. Portal hypertension leads to swollen, distended vessels in the esophagus, known as *esophageal varices.* Suspect the presence of esophageal varices when there is a history of cirrhosis (common causes include alcoholism and hepatitis) or when ascites is present (accumulation of fluid from the liver in the peritoneal cavity that results in abdominal distention) or when surface varicosities are noted on the abdomen (Figure 9-1). The act of swallowing or vomiting may easily irritate these fragile esophageal vessels, predisposing to leakage of blood, which drains into the stomach.

esophageal varices swollen, distended veins in the esophagus resulting from any condition that causes obstruction of venous drainage into the portal vein of the liver, often associated with chronic alcoholism or cirrhosis of the liver.

At the junction of the esophagus and stomach is the esophagogastric, or cardiac, sphincter. This is composed of an upper and a lower esophageal sphincter,

TABLE 9-1 Locations of GI Bleeding

Locations	Cause
Esophagus	Esophageal varices leak or tear
Esophagogastric (cardiac) sphincter	Vomiting tears sphincters (Mallory-Weiss syndrome) or esophageal varices extend to the sphincter
Stomach	Gastritis, ulcers erode blood vessels
Intestines	Polyps, ulcers, diverticulitis, tumors, radiation therapy may cause bleeding, AV malformations
Rectoanal area	Hemorrhoids form and bleed as a result of straining

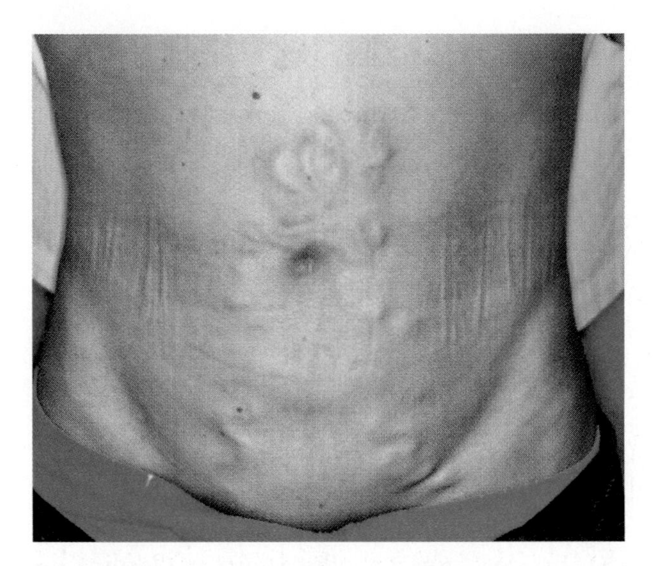

FIGURE 9-1
Dilated cutaneous veins around the umbilicus that may develop with cirrhosis of the liver; termed *caput medusae (medusa head)* because the veins resemble the head of the snake-haired Medusa of myth. (© 2005 Massachusetts Medical Society. All Rights Reserved.)

which generally perform as one sphincter, except during the process of vomiting. When vomiting occurs, the alternating constriction and relaxation of the esophageal sphincters, along with the dilation of the esophagus and the extreme force of reverse stomach contractions, propels contents back up the esophagus. If the esophageal sphincter(s) have weakened or esophageal varices extend to the sphincters, tearing may occur. If an arterial site is involved, massive bleeding can result. Forceful vomiting or retching can also cause tears to the distal esophagus or proximal stomach. This is called *Mallory-Weiss syndrome.* Usually the bleeding is self-limiting, but, again, if an artery is involved, massive bleeding can occur.

Mallory-Weiss syndrome hemorrhage from the distal esophagus or proximal stomach resulting from tearing caused by forceful vomiting or retching.

The pair of esophageal sphincters protects the esophagus from the acidic gastric secretions, except under abnormal conditions. Two common abnormal conditions are gastric-esophageal reflux disease (GERD) and hiatal hernia. GERD occurs when the cardiac sphincter is abnormally relaxed or stretched, resulting in reflux of gastric secretions into the esophagus. Fatty foods, alcohol, and chocolate are known to react with gastric secretions to form mediators that relax the sphincter. Additional factors, such as large meals, obesity, and lying down immediately after eating, cause increased pressure, which also contributes to reflux. The contact of gastric secretions with the unprotected tissue of the esophagus causes spasms and pain, often described as "burning" and "indigestion."

The stomach is a hollow, muscular organ that secretes pepsin and hydrochloric acid. It is lined with a protective mucous membrane. Substances such as alcohol, aspirin, or nonsteroidal antiinflammatory drugs (NSAIDs) may cause the mucous membrane to erode or become less effective. Resulting inflammation of the mucosa (gastritis) may allow the action of naturally occurring bacteria, *H. pylori,* to irritate the stomach wall. This may lead to ulcer formation. If the irritation is sufficient, small capillaries located in the mucosa of the stomach will be eroded and may cause bleeding. If the erosion occurs next to a vein or an artery, the bleeding may be extensive.

At the point where the stomach attaches to the duodenum, there is another sphincter called the pyloric sphincter. It regulates when and how much of the stomach contents will enter the small intestine. The area including the pylorus and duodenum is where the highly acidic stomach contents meet the highly alkaline intestinal environment. This area is also a frequent site for erosions, ulcer formation, and resultant bleeding.

The intestines are muscular, hollow tubes designed to absorb nutrients from the food we eat. Polyps, cancer, and ulcerations from irritants or diseases (e.g., typhoid, inflammatory bowel disease, infectious diarrhea) are causes of bleeding

occult bleeding obscure or hidden bleeding; bleeding in minute quantities that can only be detected by microscopic or chemical tests.

from this area. Bleeding may be obvious or occult. Causes of *occult bleeding* include polyps, cancer, vascular malformations, and previous radiation therapy.

The large intestine, or colon, is the site of water reabsorption along with production of certain vitamins. Ulcerations of the mucosa, or ulcerative colitis, cancerous tumors, and diverticulitis may result in bleeding from this area. Bloody diarrhea with abdominal pain may occur with any of these conditions. Bleeding from the colon usually has not had time to "digest" (turn black or dark brown through interaction with intestinal secretions) and will be dark red or maroon in color or may appear bright red, depending on the rapidity of the bleeding or how fast the blood is propelled to the rectum.

hemorrhoids swollen, distended veins in the rectoanal area, usually caused by muscle straining. Bleeding may occur, especially after bowel movements.

The descending colon terminates in the rectum and anus. A common cause of bleeding in this area is *hemorrhoids.* Hemorrhoids usually form during episodes of constipation, when muscle straining has forced blood to dilate surrounding veins, causing varicosities. Bleeding usually occurs during or after bowel movements. This type of bleeding seldom leads to anemia or shock-producing hemorrhage. If either anemia or shock is present, suspect another source of bleeding.

Another cause of bleeding in the GI tract is arteriovenous (AV) malformations. Bleeding from these lesions can range in severity from minor, subacute anemia to major, life-threatening blood loss. The locations include upper GI (stomach and duodenum) and lower GI (small bowel or colon) sources.

An often unsuspected cause of bleeding in the GI tract is kidney failure. The kidneys are responsible for the production of erythropoietin, a hormone that stimulates the red bone marrow to produce red blood cells and platelets. Patients with kidney failure are often anemic due to poor red cell production and may have decreased platelet counts. Chronic stress often leads to small gastric ulcerations, and occult blood loss can occur, especially in the presence of a decreased platelet count. Problems with anemia and occult blood loss in the kidney failure patient are multifactorial and can be confusing. Close monitoring of hemoglobin and hematocrit alerts staff to the need to prescribe iron and erythropoietin supplements.

Clinical Insight

Syncope in an elderly patient who is also on nonsteroidal antiinflammatory agents—aspirin, ibuprofen (Motrin), naproxen (Naprosyn), celecoxib (Celebrex), etc.—suggests a GI bleed until proven otherwise.

Heparin is given during kidney hemodialysis treatment to prevent clotting of blood while it is flowing through the filter. Heparin is stopped about 20 minutes prior to the end of the treatment to minimize bleeding tendencies. If bleeding is already a problem, it will be exacerbated by the heparin. Common problems associated with dialysis include hypovolemia, hypoglycemia, anemia, electrolyte imbalances (e.g., of potassium and calcium), and fragile bones. These associated problems may further complicate the picture of any dialysis patient with a suspected GI bleed.

Some conditions that commonly predispose to GI bleeding are summarized in Table 9-2.

TABLE 9-2 Conditions Predisposing to GI Bleeding

Conditions	Examples and Descriptions
Medications	Aspirin (for arthritis, prevention of stroke, or AMI), warfarin (Coumadin), NSAIDs (nonsteroidal antiinflammatory drugs) such as ibuprofen (Motrin), celecoxib (Celebrex), indomethacin (Indocin), naproxen (Naprosyn), or prednisone
Diseases/toxins	Crohn's disease, ulcerative colitis, cirrhosis of the liver, diverticulitis, tumors, irritants such as arsenic, typhoid, shigella
Dialysis	For kidney failure, procedure of passing the blood through a membrane to cleanse and maintain fluid, electrolyte, and acid–base balance; process involves heparin administration
Radiation of the GI tract	In treatment of cancers; long-term effects may include occult loss of blood.

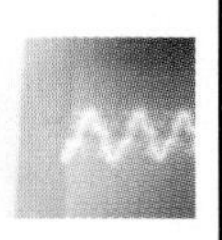

CHARACTERISTICS OF BLOOD IN THE GI TRACT

Blood originating in the GI tract—as present in emesis or stools—may be occult or may have a characteristic color and appearance (Table 9-3).

Hematemesis is the vomiting of blood. The blood that is mixed with the emesis may be bright red, or it may have a "coffee ground" or dark, grainy appearance, indicating an upper GI source of the bleeding, which is almost always above the ligament of Treitz. This ligament is located a short distance from the pyloric sphincter that separates the stomach from the duodenum. Bright red blood indicates brisk bleeding, usually from an arterial source or varicosity, while coffee ground emesis results from bleeding that has stopped or slowed enough for gastric acid to convert red hemoglobin to brown hematin. This is commonly referred to as "digested" blood.

hematemesis vomiting of blood.

Blood in the GI tract is irritating and increases peristalsis, causing diarrhea. If bleeding is from the lower GI tract, the result is frankly bloody diarrhea called *hematochezia.* Hematochezia may also result from vigorous upper GI bleeding with rapid transit of blood through the intestines. If the stool is black and tarry, it is termed *melena*, which is stool containing dark-colored, truly digested blood. The presence of melena typically indicates upper GI bleeding with digestion of blood components. A small bowel or right colon bleeding source with slow transit time can also present with melena. About 100 to 200 ml of blood in the GI tract are required to produce melena. Melena may continue for several days after a severe hemorrhage and does not necessarily indicate continued bleeding. The presence of melena may be detected prior to visualizing by its distinctive foul odor.

hematochezia passage of stools containing red blood.

melena passage of dark, tarry stools.

Black stool that is negative for occult blood may result from ingestion of iron, bismuth, or a variety of foods and should not be mistaken for melena. Usually, the difference is the presence of loose stools when the condition is due to blood.

Clinical Insight

Products that have bismuth include Pepto-Bismol, a common over-the-counter medication for indigestion or an "upset" stomach. The reason that such a product has been ingested may be the clue to the problem.

Chronic occult bleeding—less than 100 ml of blood—is not easily detected by the naked eye and typically does not cause melena or loose stools. However, the loss of oxygen-carrying capacity of the blood that is due to chronic red blood cell loss may leave the patient tachycardic and dyspneic on exertion.

In response to the decrease in oxygen-carrying capacity of the blood, metabolic acidosis occurs as body cells switch to anaerobic metabolism. As a result, heart rate and stroke volume increase, increasing the cardiac workload. Anemia

TABLE 9-3 Presentations of GI Bleeding

Presentations	Descriptions
Hematemesis	Bloody vomitus with either bright red- or maroon-colored blood or dark, grainy, digested blood with "coffee ground" appearance
Hematochezia	Bright red or darker maroon-colored stool caused by frank bleeding or quick passage of blood before it can be digested
Melena	Black, tarry, sticky, foul-smelling stool caused by digestion of blood in the GI tract
Occult bleeding	Trace amounts (usually less than 100 ml of blood) detectable only by testing; suspect chronic occult bleeding if the patient exhibits signs of pitting edema or pulmonary edema in the presence of extreme pallor of the mucosa

also lessens the viscosity (thickness) of the blood, causing the heart to have to pump harder to move the same volume of blood. The older the patient, the less likely the heart will be able to tolerate the increase in workload. Left ventricular failure has been known to occur, resulting in pulmonary edema.

ASSESSMENT

The manifestations of GI bleeding depend on the source, rate of bleeding, and the underlying or coexistent diseases; for example, the patient with underlying ischemic heart disease may present after brisk GI bleeding with angina or signs of an acute myocardial infarction (AMI). Other important coexistent diseases—including heart failure, hypotension, pulmonary disease, renal failure, or DM—may be aggravated by severe GI bleeding. History will be extremely important, depending on thorough questioning to include any change in bowel or bladder habits. A high index of suspicion should be confirmed by your physical exam.

Because of the variety in patient presentation, GI bleeding may be missed, so it is important to maintain a high index of suspicion, even when bleeding is not immediately obvious.

Massive bleeding may present as shock (see Chapter 4, Hypoperfusion). Lesser degrees of bleeding may be manifested as orthostatic changes in pulse and blood pressure. Orthostatic changes must be interpreted with caution in patients with underlying heart disease or peripheral vascular disease or those taking drugs known to influence peripheral vascular resistance, such as nitroglycerin preparations, ACE inhibitors, or calcium channel blockers. In patients with hematemesis, signs and symptoms of cirrhosis and portal hypertension may be evident. Along with history, signs and symptoms include ascites and enlarged liver or abdominal varicosities.

Clinical Insight

Chronic blood loss may not result in apparent diaphoresis.

Chronic occult bleeding may be detected by chemical testing of a stool specimen. If the amount of blood is scant, there may not be enough to be detected by chemical testing. If occult bleeding is allowed to continue, this patient may lose enough red blood cell content to result in tachycardia, tachypnea, and dyspnea on exertion. In older patients with chronic, occult bleeding, high-output failure may result.

You may be called to treat a patient in respiratory distress. History may not indicate a GI bleed because it is chronic and not manifested by black, tarry stools. Signs and symptoms of congestive failure may be pronounced. However, while the high-output failure patient may have pallor, a thorough assessment of the patient with a chronic GI bleed, including observation of mucous membranes, will reveal extreme pallor, with the cotton-white mucous membranes of chronic blood loss. If that is present in the patient with dyspnea, suspect a chronic GI bleed as the precipitating factor. Also remember that anemia without heart failure can present with dyspnea.

Clinical Insight

Discriminating between cardiogenic shock from AMI and CHF from anemia is vitally important. Obtaining a 12-lead ECG may be required.

It is also critical to differentiate this patient from the AMI patient in cardiogenic shock (see Chapter 5, Dyspnea, Respiratory Distress, or Respiratory Failure). The biggest differences will be that the chronic GI bleed patient will not have the associated complaints that would be consistent with AMI, and the color of the mucous membranes will be different. Cardiogenic shock patients have dusky or cyanotic mucous membranes as contrasted to the distinctly pale mucous membranes of anemic patients. Signs of pulmonary edema are more common in patients with cardiogenic shock, although they may also be seen in high-output heart failure.

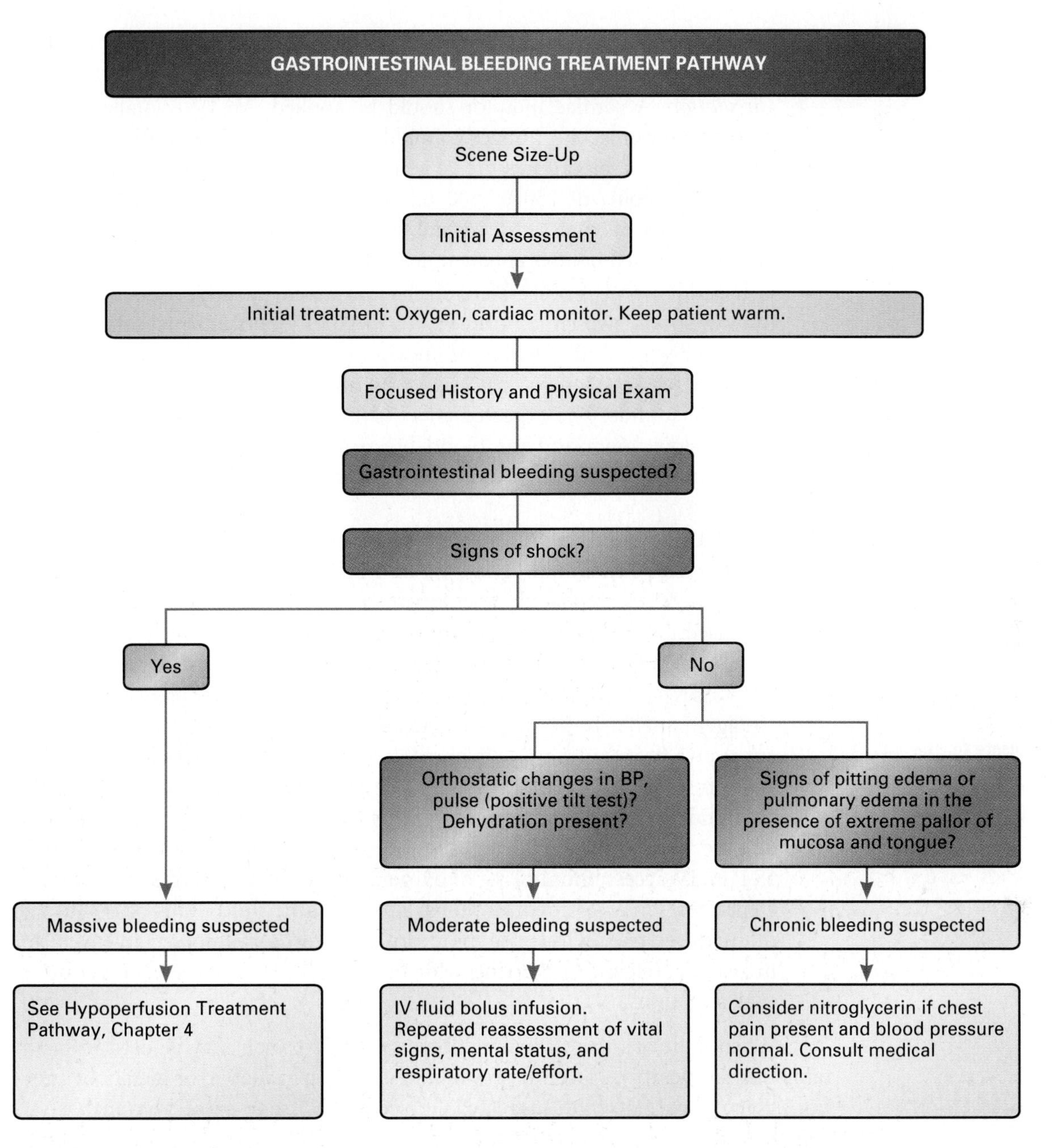

FIGURE 9-2
Gastrointestinal bleeding treatment pathway.

TREATMENT

When GI bleeding is suspected or evident, treatment involves supporting the ABCs (Figure 9-2):

When GI bleeding is suspected or evident, treatment involves supporting the ABCs.

- ***Airway and Breathing:*** Treatment begins with oxygen administration. Depending on the degree of respiratory dyspnea, pallor, and/or obvious bleeding, you should apply a nasal cannula or a nonrebreather mask with reservoir at 15 lpm. The goal is to provide maximum oxygen content for the hemoglobin that remains and to supersaturate the plasma to preserve the brain and other cellular function as much as possible in the presence of anaerobic metabolism. If breathing is inadequate, positive-pressure ventilation is required.

- *Circulation.* A cardiac monitor should be applied. An IV crystalloid, either normal saline or lactated Ringer's, should be started. Fluid therapy is usually dictated by systolic blood pressure. When orthostatic hypotension is present, an initial fluid bolus of 250 to 500 ml should be administered with repeated reassessments of vital signs, mental status, respiratory rate/effort, and lung sounds. Repeated boluses are often needed.

  If sudden and profuse bleeding has occurred, causing signs and symptoms of shock, two large-bore IVs (16 to 14 gauge) of normal saline should be started with rapid infusion of multiple boluses (250-500 ml), followed by repeated reassessment of vital signs, mental status, respiratory rate/effort, and lung sounds. The expected effect is that the pulse and respiratory rates should slow down and the blood pressure should stabilize to at least 70 to 100 mmHg. Mental status should also improve as perfusion to the CNS improves.

  If chronic bleeding is suspected and signs of dehydration are present, an IV of crystalloid should be started and bolus infusion given as needed. In older patients, repeated assessment of cardiopulmonary tolerance to increased preload is necessary. Continuous infusion rates such as 200 ml/hr allow their bodies to adjust gradually and are usually tolerated well.

  In cases of steady, mild, chronic bleeding, resulting anemia may present in younger patients as dizziness or syncope but may present in older patients as congestive heart failure, as explained earlier. If GI bleeding as a precipitating factor is suspected, the CHF patient is best managed in an ICU where cardiac and fluid status can be measured, using invasive monitors. Field treatment is delicate and should include oxygen by nonrebreather mask with reservoir at 15 lpm, IV access, monitoring of oxygen saturation, and cardiac monitoring. Depending on assessment findings, a low-volume fluid bolus of 200 to 250 ml might be tried with close monitoring for cardiopulmonary tolerance for increased preload. Conferring with medical direction may be advisable in such situations.

Clinical Insight

Most patients with chronic blood loss demonstrate no significant findings because the body has had time to compensate for the blood loss.

When there is a loss of hemoglobin, available oxygen may be used to maintain body temperature. This may result in less oxygen available for metabolic functions. Keep all patients with suspected GI bleeding warm to preserve available oxygen for normal cellular metabolism.

SUMMARY

The patient with a GI bleed can be challenging and requires thorough assessment, including history and physical examination. Determination of immediate life threat, potential life threat, or no life threat is at the core of treatment decisions. The occult GI bleed is the most difficult to determine. A high index of suspicion for the older patient with a history of radiation therapy on the GI tract and pulmonary edema, use of diagnostic tests (e.g., the tilt test for orthostatic hypotension), and observation for signs of portal hypertension can be extremely useful. Noting pertinent negatives, such as absence of dyspnea, is as important as noting pertinent positives. Reassessment is the guide to further treatment.

SCENARIO FOLLOW-UP

You find your 68-year-old female patient sitting on the floor of her apartment hallway with the apartment manager and a friend hovering over her. She is awake, oriented, and alert; talks in complete sentences; and is in no apparent distress. Her skin is cool and dry. Because her dialysis fistula is in her left arm, you take vital signs in her right arm. Vital signs are pulse 82, respirations 16, and blood pressure 110/80, and her lung sounds are clear. Palpation of extremities, pelvis, abdomen, and chest wall is negative for pain or crepitation. She tells you that she is on nitroglycerin for angina and is on dialysis three times a week for treatment of kidney failure. She had just returned from a dialysis treatment when she became dizzy.

You know that episodes of dizziness and syncope in dialysis patients can include hypoglycemia, cardiac dysrhythmias, electrolyte imbalances, and hypovolemia, so you start by testing her blood sugar. After getting a blood sugar result of 90, you assess her rhythm by putting her on the cardiac monitor. After you see a regular sinus rhythm that matches her pulse, with no ectopy and no sign of potassium or calcium imbalance, you decide to perform a tilt test. With your hand on her pulse, you and your partner help her to a standing position. She immediately exclaims that she is going to "pass out," and her radial pulse weakens and increases its rate substantially.

Your suspicion is heightened for hypovolemia, so you lay her on your cot and elevate her feet. Repeat vital signs show a pulse of 110, respirations 20, and a blood pressure of 82 systolic. You start an IV of normal saline in her right arm and, because of her history of dialysis, you deliver a low-volume bolus of 200 ml. On further questioning, she reveals that her stools have been "red jelly" for the last 2 days. She did not want to go to the hospital, she confides, so she did not tell the dialysis nurse. Her history and description of the bleeding lead you to suspect that the origin of the bleeding is most likely the colon and that the process of administering heparin during hemodialysis exacerbated her GI bleed, resulting in the episode of dizziness.

Further assessment shows cotton-white mucous membranes and clear lung sounds. She continues to deny all pain or discomfort. Because she is a dialysis patient, you choose to administer a second 100-ml fluid bolus. Reassessment of vital signs reveals a blood pressure of 100/78, pulse 96, and respirations 18. Because of her age and history of kidney failure, you closely monitor her respiratory rate and effort for tolerance to preload and volume. There are no changes en route to the hospital.

On arrival, your patient informs the emergency department physician that she is ready to go home. However, a blood count shows evidence of chronic bleeding and anemia. She is started on 1 unit of packed red blood cells and admitted so the staff can rule out cancer, polyps, ulcers, or diverticulitis.

Several days later, you ask the emergency department physician about your patient. He tells you they weren't able to find a source of bleeding and she was dismissed. After emphasizing that GI bleeding sometimes happens with dialysis patients, he adds, "You'll probably see her again. Let's hope next time turns out as well."

FURTHER READING

1. ALEXANDER, D. "New concepts in shock management," *Air Medical Journal*, 1996;15(2):85–91.
2. BERKOW, R., M.H. BEERS, and M. BURS, eds. *The Merck Manual of Diagnosis and Therapy*. 17th ed. Rahway, NJ: Merck & Company, 1999.
3. BLEDSOE, B.E., R.S. PORTER, and R.A. CHERRY. "Gastroenterology," in *Essentials of Paramedic Care*. 2nd ed. Upper Saddle River, NJ: Pearson/Prentice Hall, 2006.
4. CAPONE, A.C., P. SAFAR, W. STEZOSKI, S. TISHERMAN, and A.B. PEITZMAN. "Improved outcome with fluid restriction in treatment of uncontrolled hemorrhagic shock," *Journal of the American College of Surgeons*, 1995;180:49–56.
5. COPE, SIR ZACHARY (original author, 1921), Silen, W., ed. *Cope's Early Diagnosis of the Acute Abdomen*. 20th ed. New York: Oxford University Press, 2000.
6. FONTANAROSA, P.B. "Abdominal, genitourinary, and back pain," in P.T. Pons and D. Cason, eds, *Paramedic Field Care: A Complaint-Based Approach*. St. Louis: American College of Emergency Physicians, Mosby–Year Book, 1997.
7. GOLDMAN, L., and D. AUSIELLO, eds. *Cecil Textbook of Medicine*. 22nd ed. St. Louis. Saunders, 2004.
8. GUYTON, A.C., and J.E. HALL, "Gastrointestinal physiology," in *Textbook of Medical Physiology*. 10th ed. Philadelphia: W.B. Saunders, 2001.

9. HEUTHER, S.E. "Structure and function of the digestive system," in K.L. McCance and S.E. Heuther, eds., *Pathophysiology: The Biologic Basis for Disease in Adults and Children.* 4th ed. St. Louis: Mosby, 2002.
10. HEUTHER, S.E., and K.L. MCCANCE. "Alterations of digestive function," in K.L. McCance and S.E. Heuther, eds., *Pathophysiology: The Biologic Basis for Disease in Adults and Children.* 4th ed. St. Louis: Mosby, 2002.
11. LINGAPPA, V.R. "Gastrointestinal disease," in S.J. McPhee, V.R. Lingappa, and W.F. Ganong, eds, *Pathophysiology of Disease: An Introduction to Clinical Medicine.* 4th ed. Chicago: McGraw-Hill, 2003.
12. MARTINI, F.H., and E.F. BARTHOLOMEW. "The digestive system," in F.H. Martini and E.F. Bartholomew, eds., *Essentials of Anatomy and Physiology.* Upper Saddle River, NJ: Pearson/Prentice Hall, 2000.
13. MCQUAID, K.R. "Alimentary tract," in L.M. Tierney, S.J. McPhee, and M.A. Papadakis, eds., *Current Medical Diagnosis and Treatment.* Norwalk, CT: Appleton & Lange, 1997.
14. VAN ZILE, J., and M.L. EMERICK. "Acute abdominal pain," in G. C. Hamilton, A.B. Sanders, G.R. Strange, and A.T. Trott, eds., *Emergency Medicine: An Approach to Clinical Problem Solving.* 2nd ed. Philadelphia: W.B. Saunders, 2003.

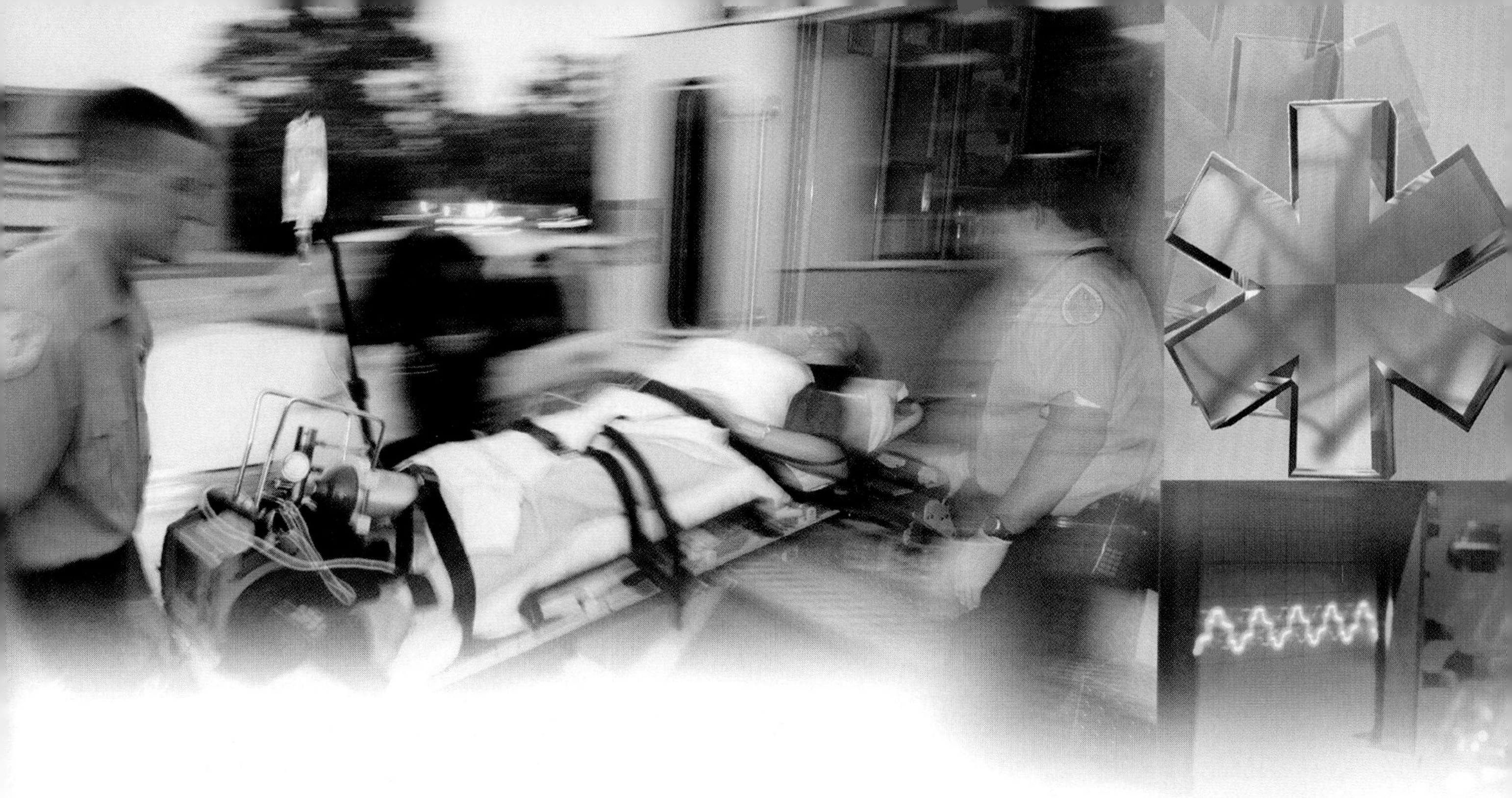

SEIZURES AND SEIZURE DISORDERS

10

Seizures and seizure disorders are among the oldest recorded diseases. A seizure is defined as a recurrent paroxysmal disorder of cerebral function characterized by sudden brief attacks of altered consciousness, motor activity, sensory phenomena, or inappropriate behavior, and caused by abnormal excessive discharge of cerebral neurons. People used to think that those afflicted with these "attacks" were possessed by demons. The fears reached a climax when it was believed that the attacks could be transferred as easily as the common cold. Even today, the more the research reveals to the medical community, the more we realize how little we still know about this disease.

Topics that are covered in this chapter are

- Anatomy and Physiology of the Brain
- Classification and Terminology
- Pathophysiology
- Differential Diagnosis
- Assessment and Management Priorities

SCENARIO

You and your partner are performing a stand-by at a local high school football game on a cool fall evening. Your partner has just brought back a fresh supply of hot coffee when a police officer rushes over to your ambulance. The officer reports that there is a fan down on the other side of the stadium, apparently having a seizure. You immediately dump your coffee, grab your jump kit and oxygen, and head over.

As you and your partner round the fence, you notice a crowd of people standing around something or someone on the ground. As you make your way through the crowd, you can see a 30- to 35-year-old male apparently having a seizure.

What would you do next for this patient?

INTRODUCTION

seizures abnormal neurologic function caused by the abnormal electrical discharges of neurons within the brain.

Seizures may be defined as abnormal neurologic function caused by the abnormal electrical discharges of neurons within the brain. Seizures, although originating within the neurons of the brain, are primarily a clinical event, and how they manifest themselves largely depends on where in the brain they occur. In terms of medical events, seizures occur with relative frequency. It is estimated that approximately 10 percent of individuals will experience a seizure in their lifetime. About 1 to 2 percent will have recurrent seizure activity. Under the appropriate conditions, anyone can have a seizure.

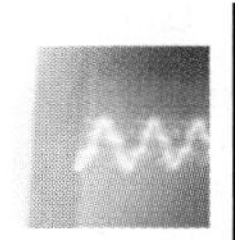

ANATOMY AND PHYSIOLOGY OF THE BRAIN

To fully understand seizures, you must understand the anatomy and physiology of the central nervous system (CNS), which consists of the spinal cord and the brain (Figure 10-1).

Anatomy and Physiology

The brain lies in the cranial cavity and is continuous with the spinal cord through the large opening at the base of the skull called the foramen magnum.

The brain weighs approximately 3 pounds, receives 30 percent of the cardiac output, accounts for 20 percent of the body's oxygen consumption, and requires the most energy per gram of tissue of all the tissues in the body. As these requirements evidence, the brain is demanding and does not cope well with deficiencies in oxygen, glucose, blood flow, or energy. (Brain cells do not store energy internally like other cells.) Alterations in any of these areas can cause a disturbance in cerebral function.

The brain is enveloped by three coverings, or *meninges,* inside the cranium, which provide protection for the brain. The names of the meninges from outermost to innermost are the *dura mater,* the *arachnoid membrane,* and, finally, the *pia mater.* The dura mater, which literally means "tough mother," is a thick, fibrous tissue that lines the inside of the cranium. The arachnoid layer separates the dura and pia maters. It contains the cerebrospinal fluid, which cushions and supports the brain and the spinal cord. Finally, the pia mater covers the brain and spinal cord tissue.

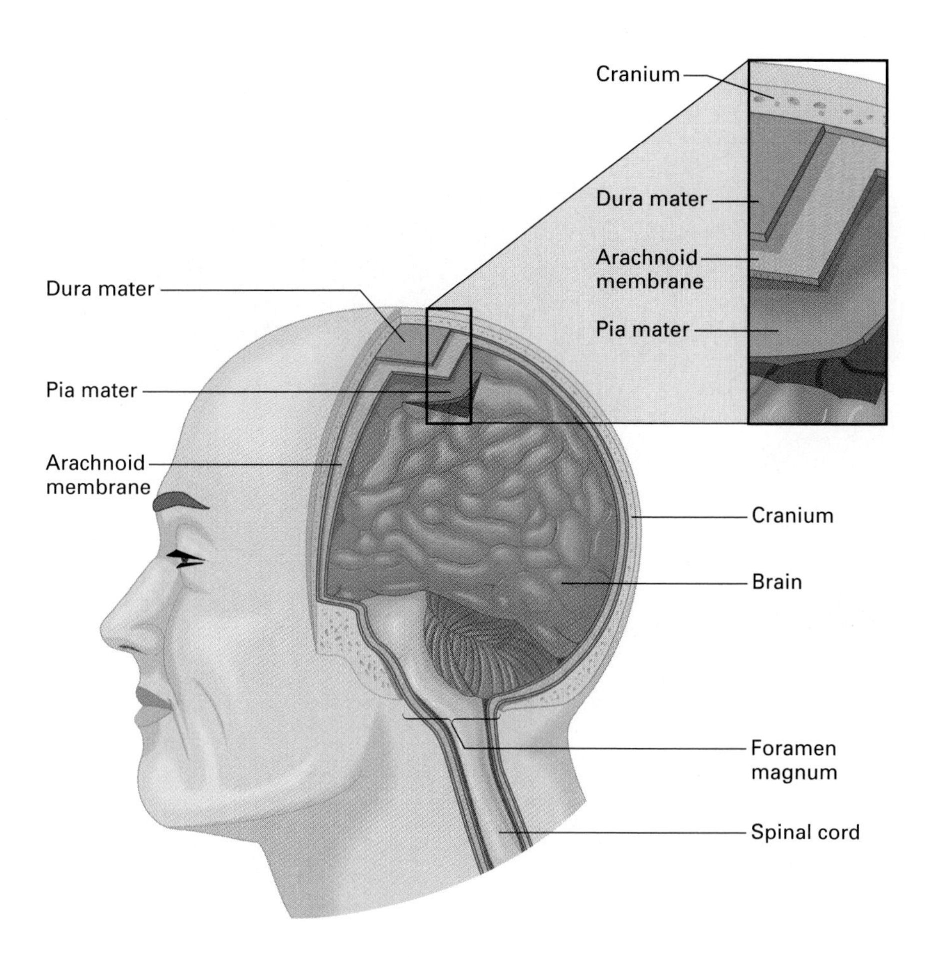

FIGURE 10-1
The brain in the cranial cavity.

It is a thin, delicate membrane that overlies and encloses the arterial circulation of the brain. The meninges, along with the cranial vault, provide protection for the delicate structures of the brain.

Seizures are primarily caused by excitation of the neurons in a specific area of the brain. Although the exact cause of seizures at the neuronal level remains unclear despite extensive research, how the seizure presents and evolves is fairly well understood. Knowing the functional anatomy of the brain will help you understand how to correlate the signs and symptoms associated with seizure activity with the probable location in the brain in which the seizure originates.

Arrangement of structures inside the cranium is not as complex as it may appear. The architecture of the brain is derived from its embryological development. As the brain develops during fetal growth, sections of the brain evolve to form various permanent structures (Figure 10-2). The general organization is such that two symmetric sections (the telencephalon) divide to form the cerebral hemispheres; a large, central portion (the diencephalon) forms the familiar thalamus and hypothalamus; a smaller segment (the mesencephalon) forms the midbrain; a projection of neural tissue (the metencephalon) evolves into the cerebellum and the pons; and a thickened segment (the myelencephalon) results in the medulla. In general, the organization of the brain is such that the more primitive functioning structures reside lower and within the core of the brain, and the more sophisticated components exist outward, nearer the surface. This is known as a rostral-caudal organization.

A standard method of categorizing brain structures is to divide the brain into four sections (inferior to superior): the brainstem, the cerebellum, the diencephalon (the only section that retains the embryological name), and the cerebrum.

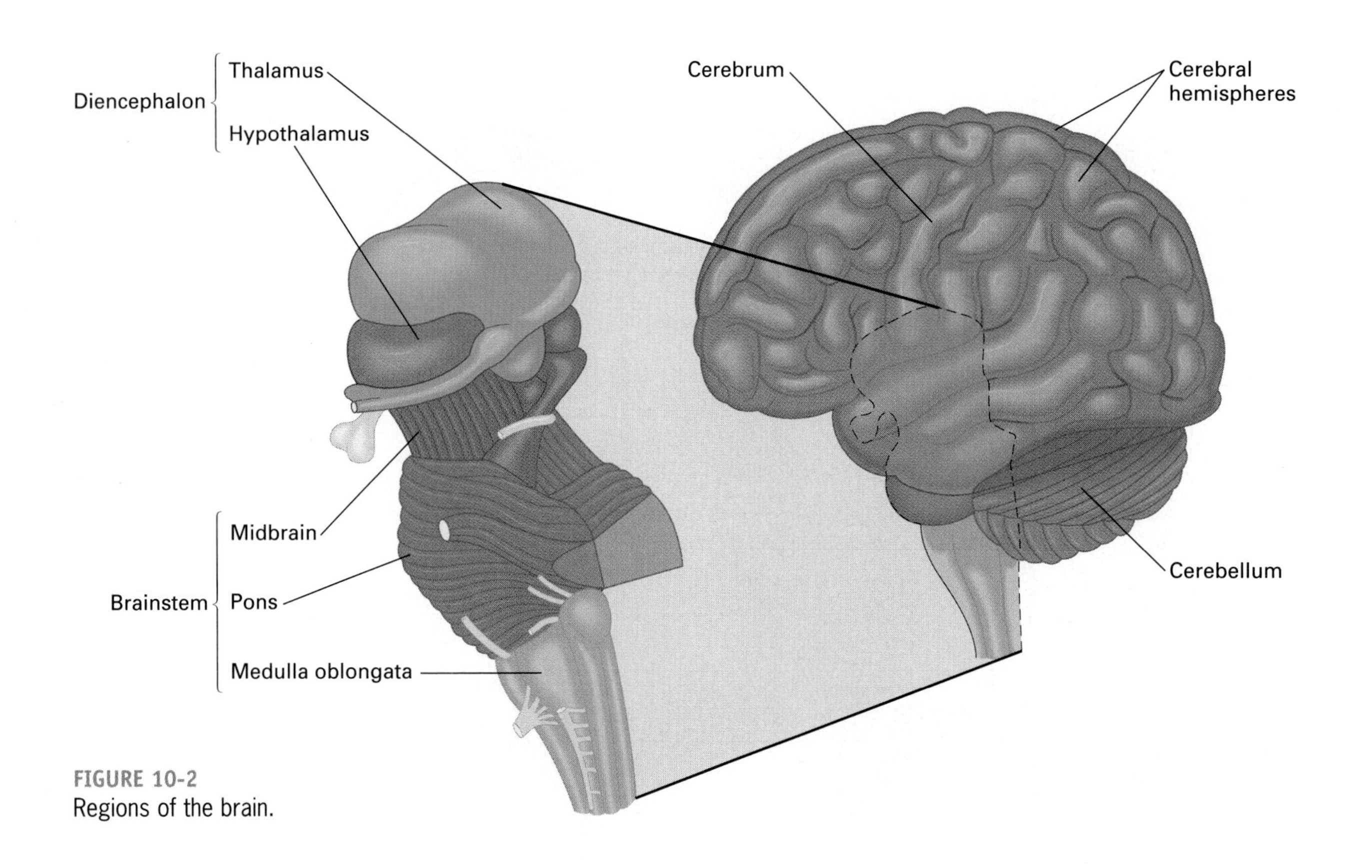

FIGURE 10-2
Regions of the brain.

Brainstem

The *brainstem* is the oldest and smallest functional region of the brain. The divisions of the brainstem are the *midbrain*, the *pons*, and the *medulla oblongata*. These structures together provide unconscious control of the basics of respiration, circulation, and digestion. These are commonly referred to as "vegetative functions." That is, these life-sustaining functions can be carried on even if the cerebral cortex is severely damaged.

Cerebellum

The *cerebellum* is attached to the posterior surface of the brainstem and is separated from the cerebrum by the portion of the dura mater known as the tentorium. The cerebellum is responsible for spatial relationships (how the body maintains proper positioning in space), coordination, and refinement of motor movements. A seizure may cause abnormalities in any of these functions. For example, repetitive motor movements during a seizure indicate that the cerebellum is involved or is possibly the site of origin.

Diencephalon

homeostasis equilibrium of the body's internal environment, including water balance; temperature regulation; and sugar, fat, and electrolyte balances.

The *diencephalon* consists of the hypothalamus and the thalamus. The *hypothalamus* is the internal regulator for *homeostasis* (equilibrium of the body's internal environment, including water balance; temperature regulation; and sugar, fat, and electrolyte balances). It regulates peripheral nervous system discharges associated with behavioral and emotional expressions. The hypothalamus also plays an integral role in the regulation of hormones in the body. Superior and slightly posterior to the hypothalamus lies the *thalamus*. Its main function is as the primary relay station for impulses reaching the cerebral cortex from the spinal cord, brainstem, cerebellum, and other parts of the cerebrum.

Cerebrum

The major divisions of the *cerebrum* are the *right* and *left cerebral hemispheres,* which comprise approximately 80 percent of the total weight of the brain. The cerebrum is highly developed in an adult and is responsible for many higher functions, including most of our conscious and sensory functions. In general, each cerebral hemisphere is responsible for the control of actions on the contralateral side of the body. The left cerebral hemisphere is dominant in approximately 98 percent of all individuals.

Consciousness

The brain is the seat of *consciousness*—but what is consciousness? Full consciousness is a state of awareness of oneself and one's environment, complete with response to that environment. Any decrease in the state of awareness and response to the environment is termed an "altered level of consciousness" or "altered mental status."

consciousness a state of awareness of oneself and one's environment with response to that environment.

Consciousness has two distinct components: arousal and awareness. Arousal is the state of awakeness. The level of arousal is mediated by the reticular activating system (RAS) that extends from the midpons to the diencephalon and provides arousal to the cerebral hemispheres. When stimulated by the RAS, the cerebral hemispheres provide a level of awareness. When cerebral function is lost, the RAS and brainstem can maintain a crude waking state (the vegetative state mentioned earlier), where there is a degree of arousal but no awareness.

Seizures, depending on the type, do not affect consciousness uniformly. Some seizures affect the cerebral cortex, while others affect both the cortex and the RAS. This is why, in some seizures, the patient appears to be awake but with neither intact awareness of the environment nor normal responses. It also explains why some seizures are confused with mental illness or the "high" brought on by illicit drugs. Understanding this aspect of cerebral physiology may help you identify the true nature of the problem and determine the appropriate approach and treatment. For more on the RAS and consciousness, review Chapter 7, Altered Mental Status.

Clinical Insight

If the apparently awake patient is without awareness of the environment or normal responses, keep in mind that the patient may be experiencing a type of seizure rather than mental illness or a drug "high."

CLASSIFICATION AND TERMINOLOGY

In 1981, the International League against Epilepsy developed a new classification system for seizure disorders. The rationale was the need for a universal system and terminology for the identification of seizures. This system permits more precise localization of specific areas of the brain responsible for seizure activity, the use of more specific antiseizure medications for different types of seizures, and, finally, more appropriate identification by health care providers. The system also allows improved communication between prehospital and hospital personnel.

Under this system (Table 10-1), the two main classes of seizures are generalized seizures and partial seizures. Each classification is subdivided into additional classes.

Generalized Seizures

generalized seizure a seizure that involves both cerebral hemispheres and produces loss of consciousness.

The classification *generalized seizure* encompasses older descriptive classes that included grand mal, petit mal, minor motor, limited grand mal, and drop attack seizures. Generalized seizures are usually bilaterally symmetric, involving both

TABLE 10-1 Classification of Seizures

Generalized seizures
Absence seizures
Tonic-clonic seizures
Partial seizures
Simple partial seizures
Complex partial seizures

cerebral hemispheres. These seizures involve uncontrolled neural activity from both cerebral cortexes, producing a loss of consciousness. Generalized seizures are subdivided into a number of categories, depending on the type of muscle movement involved with the seizure. We will not attempt to teach recognition of all generalized seizures but will identify the two major divisions, which are the absence seizure and the tonic-clonic seizure.

Absence Seizures

absence seizure a type of generalized seizure characterized by a brief loss of awareness (possible manifestations: a blank stare, a brief cessation of activity), sudden onset, and rapid recovery.

Absence seizures are primarily seen in children and adolescents and rarely after the age of 20. A sudden onset and brief loss of awareness characterize this type of seizure. During the seizure, the patient might develop a blank stare and stop whatever activity he was performing before the onset. The patient usually recovers rapidly and remembers nothing of the seizure. The seizure generally does not last more then a few seconds. Patients subject to absence seizures may experience one or two a month up to a few hundred seizures a day. Absence seizures are commonly misdiagnosed as inattentiveness or daydreaming. Seizure activity may gradually decline and eventually disappear as the patient gets older or may develop into tonic-clonic seizure activity.

Tonic-Clonic Seizures

tonic-clonic seizure a type of generalized seizure characterized by rapid loss of consciousness and motor coordination, muscle spasms, and jerking motions. Recovery is slow and characterized by exhaustion and confusion that gradually improves.

tonic spasm persistent involuntary contraction of the muscles.

The second major classification of generalized seizures is the *tonic-clonic seizure.* Just as the term "absence seizure" describes the absent look the patient may exhibit during the seizure, "tonic-clonic" describes the motor activity seen with this type of seizure.

Tonic-clonic seizures are among the most dramatic medical events seen in the field. There is a rapid loss of consciousness because of the involvement of both cerebral hemispheres. Following this, the patient may produce a loud cry. This cry often scares bystanders because they think the patient is experiencing pain. In reality, the cry results from a forceful expiration caused by abdominal and thoracic spasms. The patient will fall to the ground because of loss of motor coordination and consciousness. At this time, the patient's muscles will develop *tonic spasms* lasting for 10 to 30 seconds.

All muscles of the body can be affected during this period. Respiratory muscles, neck and facial muscles, and the muscles of the upper and lower extremities produce some of the most visible signs of this phase. The respiratory muscles will become paralyzed, and the patient may develop peripheral cyanosis. Facial and neck muscles can flex to one side and become fixed in that position. The extremities can become fixed in an extended position. The degree of extension and length of the tonic period depend on the intensity of the seizure. The tonic stage will give way to the clonic phase of a generalized seizure.

clonic activity alternative contraction and relaxation of the muscles resulting in jerking movements.

Clonic activity will produce violent jerking of the head, thorax, and extremities. This phase involves contraction and relaxation of opposing muscle groups, resulting in the characteristic jerking movements of the thorax, extremities, and muscles of the face. The contractions gradually decrease in number, but not in strength. Clonic movements can injure the patient from the rapid and powerful alteration of contraction and relaxation. Injuries to the tongue, long bones, and muscles are commonly seen after a tonic-clonic seizure. These seizures usually last from 3 to 5 minutes but can last as long as 30 minutes.

The *postictal phase* is the period of time following a seizure in which the patient regains consciousness. During this phase, the patient will experience a period of extreme tiredness. The length of the postictal phase depends on the length and intensity of the seizure. The patient will regain consciousness slowly, often remaining sluggish for hours to days. This is partially due to the extreme exertion during the seizure activity and the increased use of adenosine triphosphate (ATP). ATP is a compound present in all cells, especially muscle cells, that produces energy when split by an enzyme. So much ATP is used during a seizure, and the body's fuel storage is so drastically reduced, that the seizure patient may exhibit signs and symptoms that mimic hypoglycemia or possibly a stroke.

postictal phase the period of time following a seizure in which the patient regains consciousness. The postictal phase may last from hours to days, depending on the length and intensity of the preceding seizure.

The patient usually has retrograde amnesia (no recollection of the seizure or seizure activity). This period after the seizure is often mistaken for an altered level of consciousness, diabetic emergency, or a stroke if the EMS provider arrives after the seizure activity has stopped and there are no eyewitnesses to the seizure. Additionally, some patients suffer hemiparesis or monoparesis for a few minutes, hours, or even days after an epileptic seizure (called Todd's paralysis or postepileptic paralysis), which can further complicate the assessment of seizure versus stroke.

The most severe manifestation of seizure activity is *status epilepticus.* Status epilepticus is a prolonged seizure or multiple (two or more) seizures where the patient does not regain consciousness between seizures. The seizure duration that traditionally defined status epilepticus was 30 minutes or longer. However, it has now been determined that motor seizures of 5 minutes or longer may cause damage, which has changed the definition of status epilepticus for generalized motor seizures. It is believed that the uncontrolled seizing that occurs in the patient with status epilepticus results from high levels of catecholamines that are released during generalized seizure activity. The problem with persistent seizures is that there is a marked increase in metabolic rate, which leads to several physiological changes that produce greater physiological stress. The physiological stressors that require immediate intervention include hypoxia, hypercapnia, hypoglycemia, metabolic acidosis, and electrolyte disturbances. Patients will usually recover from a seizure of limited duration, no matter how dramatic its presentation, but status epilepticus can have severe consequences as a result of the depletion of oxygen and glucose stores from the prolonged neuronal activity. This state of persistent hypoxia and/or hypoglycemia may result in permanent brain damage or even death. Although there exist many possible causes of status epilepticus, including hypoglycemia, hyponatremia, hepatic failure, meningitis, strokes, and poisons, the most common cause is a failure of the patient to take prescribed antiseizure medication (often accompanied by withdrawal).

status epilepticus a prolonged seizure, lasting 30 minutes or more, or multiple seizures in which the patient does not regain consciousness between seizures. It is a life-threatening emergency.

Partial Seizures

The other main class of seizures, besides the generalized seizure, is the *partial seizure.* This classification encompasses older descriptive classes that included focal motor seizures, Jacksonian seizures, temporal lobe seizures, and psychomotor seizures. Partial seizures involve neurons from only one cerebral hemisphere, often have only a local onset, and usually originate from superficial foci. A partial seizure may progress to involve neurons from both cerebral hemispheres, producing a loss

partial seizure a seizure that involves only one cerebral hemisphere and may have only a local onset.

of consciousness. When this occurs, the seizure is classified as a secondarily generalized seizure.

Partial seizures are further divided into simple and complex seizures.

Simple Partial Seizures

simple partial seizure a partial seizure that involves local motor, sensory, or autonomic signs such as contraction of specific muscle group, auditory or visual deficits or hallucinations, or vertigo. There is no loss of consciousness or alteration of mental status.

Simple partial seizures can occur with motor, sensory, and autonomic signs. For example, a simple seizure that involves motor signs can present with recurrent contraction of a specific muscle group (e.g., a finger, hand, arm, leg, or face). Sensory symptoms that can manifest include auditory and visual deficits, hallucinations, and vertigo. Simple seizures involve no loss of consciousness and have little to no postictal phase. Simple seizures can start in one part of the body and then transfer or progress to another area of the body. This type of seizure was formerly known as a Jacksonian seizure.

A key difference between simple partial seizures and complex partial seizures is that complex seizures result in an altered level of consciousness, while simple seizures do not affect or alter a patient's level of consciousness.

Complex Partial Seizures

complex partial seizure a partial seizure with behavioral manifestations and an altered level of consciousness, which may be mistaken for a psychiatric emergency or drug intoxication. It usually begins with an aura and proceeds to physical presentations such as twitching, lip smacking, or repetitive movements.

aura a subjective sensation, such as a smell, taste, visual or auditory hallucination, or psychic experience, that precedes some types of seizures.

Complex partial seizures are episodic changes in behavior in which an individual loses conscious contact with the environment. This type of seizure can easily be mistaken for a psychiatric emergency. As mentioned previously, altered level of consciousness in the complex partial seizure is an important difference from the simple partial seizure, which does not affect the patient's mental status.

The complex partial seizure usually begins with some type of *aura* (a subjective sensation) ranging from the smell of burning rubber, to a feeling of déjà vu, to visual disturbances, to hallucinations. After the aura, the patient may have minor muscle tremors resulting in lip smacking, nervous twitches, or repetitive movements. A patient suffering one of these seizures may sometimes unconsciously perform a highly technical skill such as walking or running, driving a car, or playing a musical instrument. The patient may also experience an emotional disturbance such as fear, sadness, or laughter.

Some seizures cannot be classified because of incomplete or inadequate information and/or bizarre actions during the seizure. Unidentifiable seizures are common in the realm of neonatology, where the population of patients is relatively small, ordinary classifications do not apply to the underdeveloped neonatal brain, and the long-term survival rate for studying disease pathology is short.

PATHOPHYSIOLOGY

As defined at the beginning of this chapter, a seizure is a recurrent paroxysmal disorder of cerebral function, characterized by brief sudden attacks of altered levels of consciousness, motor activity, sensory phenomena, or inappropriate behavior, caused by abnormal excessive discharges of cerebral neurons. Simply stated, the neurons in an area of the brain began to fire uncontrollably, without any purpose. If the firing of the neurons is uninhibited, as in a generalized seizure, the electrical conduction of the brain will allow the impulse to spread to the opposite side, so that the seizure now involves both hemispheres.

During a seizure, the body will require 250 times the normal amount of ATP to provide the energy needed to sustain the seizure. Along with the increase in ATP production, cerebral blood flow is increased by 250 percent, and cerebral oxygen consumption is increased by approximately 60 percent. Even these drastic increases, however, are not enough to supply the brain's requirements for ATP, oxygen, and glucose. When respiration fails to supply sufficient oxygen, the cells will switch from aerobic metabolism to anaerobic metabolism. This is true in the brain and in the rest of the body. The switch to anaerobic metabolism increases the production of lactic acid by 20 percent. Lactic acid builds up in the brain, leading to cellular acidosis, hypoxia, and, ultimately, necrosis of the brain. If the seizure is stopped early and not allowed to progress to the anaerobic stage, cerebral damage can be limited.

DIFFERENTIAL DIAGNOSIS

Seizures are either *idiopathic* (spontaneous, or without an identifiable cause) or secondary to another injury, disorder, or disease that predisposes the patient to seizure activity. The known causes of seizures can be organized into three categories: CNS injury or dysfunction, metabolic disorder, or infectious disease (Table 10-2).

idiopathic seizure a seizure that has no identifiable cause.

Central Nervous System Injury or Dysfunction

CNS injury or dysfunction is the leading cause of nonidiopathic seizures and seizure disorders. Leading this category is trauma, especially blunt or penetrating injury to the cranium. The brain is a sophisticated and integral organ and operates in a delicate environment that can be easily disrupted.

Clinical Insight

When assessing the patient experiencing a seizure, remember that the cause may be traumatic or medical.

Traumatic Injury

Trauma to the CNS, particularly the brain, can cause a range of events from a decreased level of consciousness to seizures to death. Patients who suffer brain trauma usually have signs and symptoms that are clues to the cause.

The cranial vault is very dense, and thus it can withstand a significant amount of trauma. Outward signs of trauma include hematomas, lacerations, and a mechanism of injury. Trauma can manifest itself by changes in level of consciousness, pupil size and reactivity, and respiratory patterns. As a result of the trauma, edema will develop and push on the brain, forcing it against other brain tissue and downward through the foramen magnum. This results in pupillary

TABLE 10-2 Causes of Seizures: Typical Findings

Causes	Examples	Typical Findings
CNS injury or disorder	Trauma, brain tumor, brain lesion, stroke	History (of recent head injury, stroke or TIA, diagnosed brain tumor or disorder); signs of head injury; signs of medical dysfunction: changes in mental status, pupil size/reactivity/orientation, respiratory pattern; facial droop, hemiparesis
Metabolic disorder	Hypoxia, hyponatremia, hypocalcemia, hypomagnesemia, hypokalemia, hypoglycemia, hypercapnia, hypernatremia, hypercalcemia, hyperglycemia; hepatic or renal failure; drug side effect; failure to take antiseizure medication	Low blood oxygen level (pulse oximetry); low blood sugar level (blood glucose test); history of liver or kidney disease; history of diabetes; history of seizure disorder; medication containers; headache, visual disturbances, altered respiratory pattern
Infectious disease	Meningitis, encephalitis	Elevated temperature; headache; stiff neck; photophobia; dehydration; confusion or unconsciousness; history of infection

changes caused by compression of nerve tracts, decreasing level of consciousness, and increased respirations. Initially, the respirations increase in an attempt to remove CO_2 in order to decrease the swelling. Then, they will become irregular and decrease in depth and rate until they completely stop.

Medical Dysfunction

When we talk of trauma to the brain, there are four main "traumas" that can be considered: structural damage, free blood, scar tissue formation, and hypoxia. These can all occur from medical causes (e.g., structural lesions, tumors, and strokes—especially hemorrhagic strokes) and from classic trauma (a blow to the head), as discussed previously.

Tumors and lesions are generally slow growing and present few or no outward signs or symptoms. They are usually diagnosed with the use of CT and MRI scans. Strokes, however, do result in noticeable symptoms (see Chapter 7). The level of consciousness is not usually affected unless there is a massive stroke, but there may be facial drooping, pupillary constriction or dilation, a dysconjugate gaze (failure for both eyes to move in unison toward a central, parallel gaze), hemiparesis, or hemiplegia (weakness or paralysis on one side).

The incidence of seizures resulting from brain tumors is higher in the population between 35 and 55 years of age. Slow-growing tumors involving the cerebrum result in seizure activity more often then any other type of tumor. Strokes cause a lack of oxygen to the brain, resulting in cerebral hypoxia. The same hypoxia that causes tissue necrosis can also stimulate or cause irritable foci/neurons to fire, thus causing a seizure. Hemorrhagic strokes cause neurons to fire as a result of the irritating effects of the vessel break and free blood. Lesions of the CNS involve destruction of nervous tissue, which can cause seizure activity. The lesion can be caused by pathological changes or by trauma.

Slow-growing tumors involving the cerebrum result in seizure activity more often than any other type of tumor.

Seizures that occur directly after the initial insult and/or within 24 hours of the injury (whether traumatic or medical in origin) do not indicate a grim prognosis; however, seizures that occur 2 or more weeks after the initial event indicate a high likelihood of severe brain injury or damage. The extent and type of seizure has been shown to have a direct correlation with the extent of damage to the brain.

The mainstay prehospital treatment for CNS injuries includes the following:

- Administer high-flow, high-concentration oxygen by nonrebreather mask.
- Assure adequate ventilations (with tracheal intubation, if necessary).
- If intubation is required, end-tidal CO_2 should be monitored.
- Limit intravenous fluids except as indicated by signs of hypovolemia.
- Provide rapid transport to the nearest appropriate facility.

Keep in mind that the newest treatments for stroke patients include fibrinolytic therapy and the use of neuroprotective medications. These treatments, if initiated in a timely manner, may be able to reverse most or all of the damage, so prompt prehospital identification and transportation to a facility that can perform these treatments are of the utmost importance.

hypoperfusion inadequate delivery of oxygen and other nutrients to the tissues resulting from interrupted or inadequate circulation of blood.

hypoxia inadequate oxygenation.

Metabolic Disorders

Metabolic disorders can cause alterations in the normal homeostasis of the body, with the result being seizure activity. Inadequacies in the cardiovascular or respiratory system can cause inadequate blood flow (*hypoperfusion*) and inadequate oxygenation (*hypoxia*) to the brain. In addition, although hypoperfusion interferes with removal of cellular byproducts, including carbon dioxide, compensatory mechanisms will cause a patient with metabolic acidosis to have a low blood level of carbon dioxide (*hypocapnia*). The increased levels of CO_2 remaining in the tissues foster the edema, or swelling, that commonly accompanies head injuries. Hypoperfusion and disturbances in CO_2 levels in the blood and tissues, regardless of the cause, can lead to a number of serious consequences, ranging from seizures to strokes and even to death.

hypocapnia a decreased level of carbon dioxide in the blood.

Besides these somewhat obvious causes, deficient or excessive levels of electrolytes can cause seizures. Electrolytes play a key role in maintaining homeostasis. They control or play a part in almost every function of the body, including cardiac conduction, sensory and nerve impulse transmission and reception, stimulation of cerebral activity, and the list goes on indefinitely. Deficiencies in the electrolytes sodium (*hyponatremia*), calcium (*hypocalcemia*), magnesium (*hypomagnesemia*), and, rarely, potassium (*hypokalemia*) and the nutrient glucose (*hypoglycemia*) have all been known to play a key role in the stimulation of seizure activity.

hyponatremia a decreased level of sodium in the blood.

hypocalcemia a decreased level of calcium in the blood.

hypomagnesemia a decreased level of magnesium in the blood.

hypokalemia a decreased level of potassium in the blood.

hypoglycemia a decreased level of glucose in the blood.

Probably the most common serum deficiency encountered in the prehospital setting is hypoglycemia. As discussed earlier, the brain is highly dependent on glucose as a fuel. A low level of glucose causes the neurons of the brain to become very irritable, which can stimulate seizure activity.

Excessive levels of sodium (*hypernatremia*), glucose (*hyperglycemia*), and calcium (*hypercalcemia*) can occasionally produce seizures, just as low levels do. As you can guess, maintaining a perfect chemical balance is difficult, but the consequences involved with fluctuations are very serious.

hypernatremia an increased level of sodium in the blood.

hyperglycemia an increased level of glucose in the blood.

hypercalcemia an increased level of calcium in the blood.

Additionally, failure of the liver (hepatic failure) or kidney (renal failure or nephritis) can produce damaging byproducts that may stimulate seizure activity. When the kidneys begin to fail, urea, a nitrogenous waste product normally excreted by the kidneys, builds up in the blood. The high levels of nitrogen can cause symptoms from nausea and vomiting to seizures to death. With failure of the liver, the major cleansing system for circulating blood is disrupted. Venous blood bypasses the liver, allowing a build-up of toxic byproducts, including ammonia. High levels of ammonia, to which the CNS is especially sensitive, can depress the CNS, causing seizures, coma, increased intracranial pressure (ICP), and death.

The brain responds poorly to deficiencies of oxygen or glucose, excesses of waste products, and electrolyte imbalances, as well as to insults resulting in edema or hemorrhage. Deficiencies of oxygen and glucose alter the brain metabolism, which causes a hyperexcitation of the neurons. Potent vasoconstriction of cerebral vasculature can occur as a result of oxygen deficiency.

These deficiencies can manifest as altered levels of consciousness, severe headaches, visual disturbances such as diplopia (double vision), and altered breathing patterns. The patient's level of consciousness can range from completely unarousable to an agitated state. Headaches or visual disturbances signify an alteration of metabolism or a structural injury. Breathing patterns can vary in depth, rate, and pauses between respirations. (See Chapters 5 and 7 for discussions of abnormal breathing patterns.)

Many drugs, both legal and illegal, are known to produce seizures (Table 10-3). With some therapeutic medications, seizures may manifest as a toxic effect. Therapeutic medications that commonly have this side effect include aminophylline, lidocaine, phenothiazines, physostigmine, tricyclic antidepressants, and certain antihypertensive medications. Illicit substances such as cocaine and hallucinogenic drugs such as PCP have been known to cause seizures.

TABLE 10-3 Drugs That May Produce Seizures

Therapeutic Drugs	Illegal Drugs
Aminophylline	Amphetamines
Antibiotics (e.g., penicillin)	Cocaine
Lidocaine	Hallucinogens (e.g., PCP)
Phenothiazines	
Physostigmine	
Tricyclic antidepressants	
Some antihypertensives	

One of the most common causes of seizure activity is the sudden withdrawal from alcohol, an illicit drug, a medication, or other substance. A sudden halt or decrease in dose of an antiseizure medication (Table 10-4) is one of the most common causes of seizure activity, especially status epilepticus. If the dose is too rapidly decreased, or the patient forgets or stops taking the medication altogether, there will be a decrease in the therapeutic level of the drug in the blood. When that occurs, the chance of breakthrough seizure activity jumps drastically. Barbiturates, alcohol, and benzodiazepines can all cause a physical dependence that can lead to seizure activity if the medication or drug is abruptly stopped.

Patients who take diuretics to manage hypertension and congestive heart failure (CHF) can develop severe electrolyte imbalances. Hyponatremia can cause decreased levels of consciousness and muscle weakness. Hypocalcemia's effects are principally neurologic, with depression, muscle spasms, and laryngospasms. Hypomagnesemia causes lethargy, nausea and vomiting, and tremors. Hypokalemia initially causes muscle weakness, which can lead to respiratory failure. A build-up of a waste product such as urea can cause seizures. Renal failure (inability to remove the urea that has built up in the blood) will cause an increase in serum potassium leading to muscle weakness, cardiac dysrhythmias, nervous system hyperactivity, coma, and death.

Misuse of many types of illegal drugs, as well as prescription and over-the-counter drugs, can also have observable consequences. A number of illegal drugs, such as crack cocaine, PCP, amphetamines, and others, lead to a generalized hyperactive state that can cause neurons to fire rapidly. The hyperactive state can present as agitation, hypertension, pupil constriction, cardiac dysrhythmia, increased diaphoresis, and an altered level of consciousness. Often, multiple drugs are used, rather than just one drug, and this can mask signs and symptoms and make it very difficult to determine etiology.

TABLE 10-4 Common Antiseizure Medications

Common Antiseizure Medications
Phenytoin (Dilantin)
Phenobarbital
Ethosuximide (Zarontin)
Carbamazepine (Tegretol)
Valporic acid (Depakene or Depakote)
Primidone (Mysoline)
Clonazepam (Clonopin)
Clorazepate (Traxene)
Felbamate (Felbatol)
Fosphenytoin (Cerebryx)
Gabapentin (Neurontin)
Lamotrigine (Lamictal)

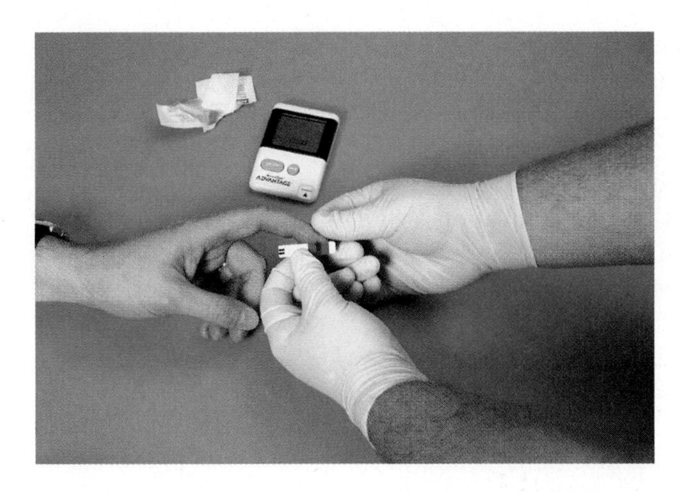

FIGURE 10-3
Monitor the blood glucose level of any seizure patient with a suspected metabolic etiology.

Look for evidence such as medical alert tags, pill bottles, or syringes, and ask family or friends about a history of seizure disorder. If you suspect an overdose or medication withdrawal, bring all pill bottles, pills, syringes, or other forms of drugs that the patient is known to have taken or that were found at the scene to the hospital to help the staff determine the cause of the patient's condition.

The general treatment for a patient with a suspected metabolic etiology of seizure is as follows. (*Note*: This treatment is for the patient who is not actively seizing!)

- Obtain a complete SAMPLE history. It is very important to find and bring any medications or other drugs that the patient may have taken to the emergency department for further evaluation.
- Use pulse oximetry, cardiac monitoring, and glucose monitoring (Figure 10-3) as part of the physical examination.
- Provide treatment to correct the underlying cause, including the following:
  - Administer high-flow, high-concentration oxygen by nonrebreather mask and support ventilations (to increase PaO_2 and decrease $PaCO_2$).
  - Initiate an IV line for medication administration, if the IV has not already been started.
  - If the patient is hypoglycemic, administer 25 g of D_{50} and possibly thiamine, depending on local protocol.
  - Consider the use of naloxone (Narcan) 2.0 mg if the patient has a decreased level of consciousness from possible opiate overdose. Narcan is administered by a variety of routes, including intravenous, intramuscular, subcutaneous, sublingual, intralingual, and tracheal. Intranasal (IN) administration is an alternative route that avoids the use of needles and can be delivered quickly because establishment of an intravenous line is not necessary. The Narcan is administered in a 2.0-mg dose using a 3-ml syringe and a mucosal atomizer device (MAD). The onset of action and plasma levels when administered via IN are almost identical to that of IV administration. The primary benefit is quick and easy administration with the avoidance of potential needlestick injury.

Infectious Diseases

Infection is another common cause of seizures. Many different infectious diseases can cause seizures, but two that are commonly associated with seizures are meningitis and encephalitis.

meningitis inflammation of the meninges, the coverings of the spinal cord and brain.

encephalitis inflammation of the brain tissue.

Meningitis is an inflammation of the meninges that cover the spinal cord and brain, most commonly caused by bacteria or by viral infection. Bacterial meningitis is the most severe form. The inflammatory process associated with meningitis can have several effects (e.g., fever, irritation from chemicals of inflammation, increased ICP) that all predispose to seizure activity.

Although meningitis is an inflammation of the meninges, *encephalitis* is an inflammation of the actual brain tissue. Encephalitis can be caused by a variety of pathogens or can be secondary to another disease. Just as with meningitis, the inflammation can stimulate seizures.

The study of and treatment for infectious diseases has progressed very rapidly. Today, infectious diseases are not as life threatening or debilitating as they once were. However, infectious conditions such as meningitis and encephalitis can still be very serious. Meningitis is most often found in children but can also occur in adults, and up to 60 percent of untreated bacterial meningitis cases are fatal. However, the vast majority of meningitis is caused by viruses, which have a low mortality.

Patients with meningitis and encephalitis present with the same array of possible symptoms, including elevated temperatures, headaches, decreasing levels of consciousness (leading to coma), signs of irritation of the meninges including a stiff neck, photophobia (aversion to light), and dehydration.

The general treatment for a patient with a suspected infectious etiology of seizure is as follows. (*Note:* This treatment is for the patient who is not actively seizing!)

- Take appropriate body substance isolation precautions to protect yourself and the patient.
- Administer high-flow, high-concentration oxygen by nonrebreather mask.
- Initiate appropriate monitoring, including pulse oximetry and cardiac monitoring.
- Initiate IV access for possible medication administration, if not already started.

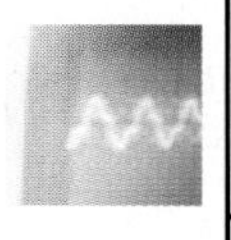

ASSESSMENT AND MANAGEMENT PRIORITIES

Scene Size-Up

Begin your size-up for scene hazards before you even leave the safety of the ambulance, and continue it as you approach the scene. From the preceding discussion of differential diagnosis, you know that there are many possible causes of seizure activity. Look around for mechanisms of injury that would suggest trauma as a cause for the seizure. Observe the scene for prescription pill bottles, evidence of alcohol and other drug abuse, or anything that may indicate a pharmacologic etiology for the seizure. Be sure you have taken adequate body substance isolation precautions.

Move furniture and objects to prevent the patient from striking them. Place nothing in the patient's mouth.

As you approach the patient who is actively seizing, immediately remove any furniture or objects that could cause harm if the patient comes into contact with them while seizing (Figure 10-4). In fact, you should do this even if the patient is in the postictal phase because repeat seizures are common.

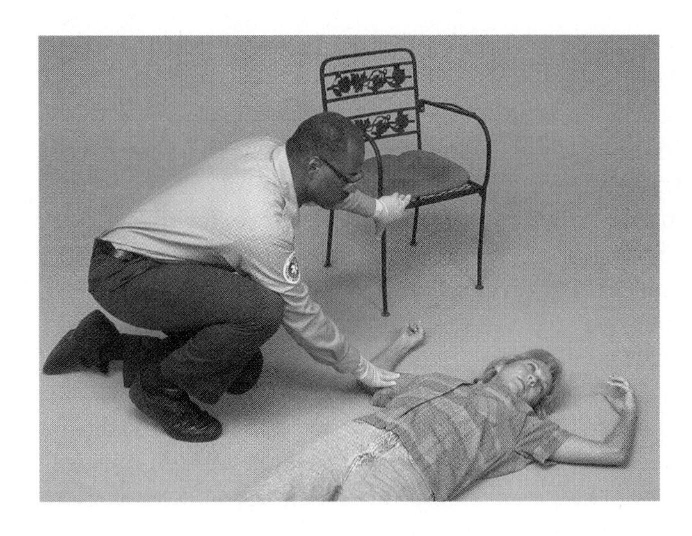

FIGURE 10-4
Move objects to prevent injury to the seizing patient.

Initial Assessment

The goals of your initial assessment are the same regardless of whether your patient is actively seizing or postictal when you arrive at his side: Life-threatening conditions must be uncovered and treated appropriately.

The goals of initial assessment are the same whether the patient is actively seizing or is postictal: Protect the airway, support respirations as needed, and assess the pulse.

The first priority is to assure that the patient has a clear airway. The patient does not need to be actively seizing to have a potential airway problem. The patient who is postictal is commonly unable to completely control his own airway. This patient may have blood or vomitus in the oral pharynx that needs to be suctioned out. To help manage the airway, place the patient in the recovery position if trauma is not suspected (left lateral recumbent position) (Figure 10-5). This allows secretions and/or vomitus to drain or to be rapidly removed from the oropharynx.

If the patient is actively seizing, make sure that no well-meaning citizen has placed anything inside the patient's mouth. Items that are commonly placed inside the mouth include spoons, wallets, and other hard items, supposedly to prevent the

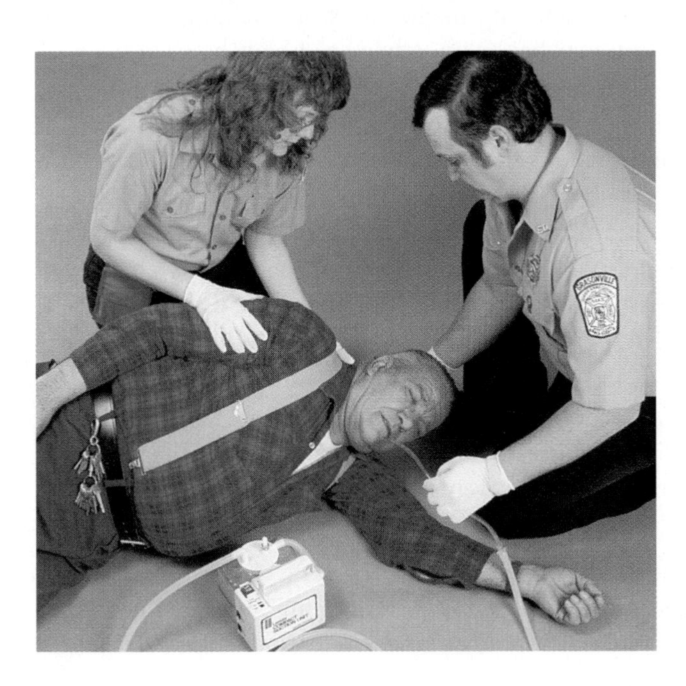

FIGURE 10-5
If trauma is not suspected, place the postictal patient in the recovery position to help maintain a clear airway.

victim from swallowing or biting his tongue. In reality, such an item can break teeth and/or cause an airway obstruction.

The airway of choice for an actively seizing or postictal patient is the nasopharyngeal airway. This airway is usually easily inserted and well tolerated by the patient. Very rarely, the postictal patient who cannot control his airway may require intubation. Ordinarily, however, airway maintenance for the seizure patient consists of a nasopharyngeal airway and suctioning for secretions until the patient is alert enough to maintain his own airway.

Next, assess the patient's respiratory status. Patients who are postictal usually appear very fatigued and can have shallow respirations. During the seizure, the patient can actually become apneic as a consequence of the extreme muscle contractions. The apnea is usually self-limited to the time of the seizure. All seizure patients should be placed on a nonrebreather mask with 100 percent supplemental oxygen at 15 lpm. Monitor the patients' respirations closely and be ready to assist them with positive-pressure ventilation if needed.

Finally, check to determine whether a pulse is present and the pulse rate. Seizure activity is common before cardiac arrest due to hypoxia from hypoperfusion. Thus, be sure to monitor the patient's pulse.

Clinical Insight

Seizure activity is common prior to cardiac arrest due to hypoxia. This is a key reason why pulse checks are critical in a seizing patient.

Focused History and Physical Exam

Postictal Patient

If your patient is not actively seizing, the initial assessment is complete, and life threats are under control, you can proceed to the focused history and physical exam. Your patient may seem confused and tired after the seizure activity. Attempt to gather as much information about the incident as possible from the patient and from bystanders, if necessary, by using the SAMPLE mnemonic:

- *Signs and symptoms* can range from the confusion associated with the postictal period, to a bleeding tongue that was bitten during the seizure, to bystander and eyewitness reports of the seizure, to mechanisms of injury if trauma is suspected. Keep in mind that bystanders tend to be inaccurate in their description of the length and severity of the seizure.
- *Allergies* to any substance, including medications, foods, animals, dyes, or other. An allergic reaction may be the underlying cause of the seizure.
- *Medications* the patient is taking. Remember, one of the most common causes of seizure activity is incomplete compliance or abrupt withdrawal from an antiseizure medication (review Table 10-4). Also remember that seizures can be a toxic effect of some therapeutic medications and illegal drugs (review Table 10-3).
- *Past medical history* can usually shed some light if the patient has a history of seizures, brain injury, hypoglycemia, diabetes, or any of the diseases or problems discussed earlier in the "Differential Diagnosis" section.
- *Last oral intake* to assess the likelihood of vomiting and aspiration.
- *Events leading up to the incident* are very important. Have the patient describe to the best of his ability what occurred before, during, or after the seizure. If the patient cannot remember these events, family or bystanders may provide useful information.

Perform a rapid head-to-toe physical exam to check for any injuries the patient may have sustained during the seizure. Manage any injuries found, and continue to monitor the patient's airway, breathing, circulation, and vital signs.

Pulse oximetry can provide valuable information concerning the postictal patient's respiratory status. You will already have placed the patient on high-flow, high-concentration oxygen, which should increase the reading, and oximetry will allow you to assess the results of this intervention. (Pulse oximetry is usually of no value while the patient is seizing because the seizure activity will generally prevent an accurate reading.)

Provide reassurance and general supportive measures, and prepare the postictal patient for transport to the hospital.

Actively Seizing Patient

The chief goal of management of the actively seizing patient is to stop the seizure activity as rapidly as possible.

The chief goal of management of the actively seizing patient is to stop the seizure activity as rapidly as possible.

Benzodiazepines have been a cornerstone of the emergency management of seizures for years. The pharmacologic mechanism of action of benzodiazepines involves the stimulation of gamma-aminobutyric acid (GABA) neurotransmitters. GABA decreases presynaptic stimulation of neurons. By decreasing stimulation of the neurons, the seizure activity can be decreased or stopped altogether. Diazepam, more commonly known by the brand name Valium, is the most popular drug of this class. Diazepam can be administered by both IV bolus and IV piggyback infusion. The dosage for IV bolus is 2 to 5 mg slowly over 3 to 5 minutes. Diazepam can be readministered every 5 minutes up to a total of 20 mg. The effective duration of action for diazepam is 30 to 40 minutes, so careful observation of the patient, in case of recurrent seizures, is warranted. Be careful to watch for respiratory depression following the administration of a benzodiazepine. One drawback to the use of diazepam is that it has poor absorption and is often unreliable if given intramuscularly. In addition, diazepam has long-acting byproducts of metabolism. As a result, many systems have shifted to other agents, such as lorazepam.

Lorazepam is also a benzodiazepine, having a similar chemical structure to diazepam and the same mechanism of action. Lorazepam is commonly known by the brand name Ativan. Like diazepam/Valium, it is a commonly prescribed antianxiety medication. The main advantage of lorazepam in seizure management is its duration of action, which is much longer than that of diazepam. The effective action of lorazepam has been reported to last up to 90 minutes. For this reason, many clinicians believe that it is the drug of choice not only for stopping status epilepticus, but also for preventing it. The dosage for seizure control is 2 mg every 3 to 5 minutes slow IV push, not to exceed a total of 0.1 mg/kg. Again, start with a low dose of 2 mg and titrate the dose upward until the seizure activity has stopped or the maximum dose has been given. Lorazepam may be more difficult to maintain for field use because of the need for refrigeration if kept on the shelf for long periods.

Diazepam and lorazepam are the first-line medications for emergency treatment of an actively seizing patient. Other drugs that are sometimes used include the benzodiazepines midazolam (Versed) and clonazepam, but these have not been as thoroughly researched or proven to be as effective as diazepam and lorazepam. One important caution: Remember that not all seizures require a benzodiazepine. Most seizures are self-limiting, with the "cure" being worse than the disease. Keep in mind that these drugs can produce hypotension and respiratory depression.

After a seizure has been stopped, depending on the cause, it is not uncommon for a patient to lapse back into seizure activity if there is a long transport. Monitor the patient closely, and be prepared to administer another dose of medication if seizure activity resumes.

Clinical Insight

It is not uncommon for a patient to lapse back into seizure activity after it has been stopped. Monitor the patient closely.

When a patient presents as a new-onset seizure patient (i.e., the patient has not been subject to seizures in the past), you must consider all the possible causes for the seizure. As discussed earlier, metabolic etiologies are very common causes of seizure activity. Hypoglycemia is one potential, but treatable, problem that should be investigated. If the seizing patient has a history of diabetes, then the administration of 25 g of D_{50} (dextrose) is reasonable. However, there is controversy about when to give the D_{50}. If a patient is actively seizing, it will be very difficult to start an IV to administer D_{50}. The better option is first to wait for the seizure to stop (or, if necessary, to stop the seizure activity with an anticonvulsant given intramuscularly), and then check the blood sugar. If the blood sugar is below 40 mg/dl and the patient has a history of diabetes, then administer 25 g of D_{50}. Do *not* administer D_{50} to any patient who is either actively seizing or has a head injury *and* is normoglycemic.

Be especially cautious when administering dextrose to the malnourished or alcoholic patient with seizures and hypoglycemia. They often have a deficit of thiamine, or vitamin B_1, simply because these are individuals who don't eat right. (The body does not produce thiamine, but instead depends on the intake and metabolization of thiamine from food.) Thiamine is essential to metabolic processes and the liberation of energy. If the body is thiamine deficient, then a significant amount of glucose will not be able to be used.

As discussed in Chapter 7, Wernicke's encephalopathy is a brain dysfunction caused by thiamine deficiency. Administering dextrose to a thiamine-deficient patient may actually trigger Wernicke's encephalopathy or, if it is already present, may make it worse. Wernicke's can progress to Korsakoff's psychosis, which is irreversible. Thus, thiamine is commonly administered with D_{50}.

However, a controversy has arisen around the administration of thiamine in the prehospital setting. Research has shown no benefit of prehospital administration of thiamine to patients receiving dextrose. Instead, the patient needs a monitored replacement of thiamine in the hospital. However, many local protocols still call for administration of thiamine as part of the prehospital management of seizures, and you should follow your local protocols in this regard.

One pharmacologic approach that can be used is as follows:

1. If the patient has prolonged seizures, administer an appropriate antiseizure medication (diazepam or lorazepam) to stop the seizure activity.
2. After the seizure has stopped, check the patient's blood glucose level and inquire about past medical history, especially the possibility of diabetes. If the patient has a low blood sugar level, administer 25 g of D_{50} slow IV push.
3. Follow local protocol as to the administration of IV thiamine.

Once the seizure has stopped, turn your attention to maintaining the seizure-free state. The etiology of the seizure should be investigated before determining how best to prevent any further seizure activity. If you suspect the seizure was associated with hypoxia, apply pulse oximetry to confirm. The treatment of choice is maintaining an open airway, an adequate respiratory exchange, and high-flow, high-concentration oxygen supplementation. If the patient is found to have a low blood sugar, then the treatment is 25 g of D_{50}. The treatment of febrile seizures is to cool the patient or administer antipyretics and treat the source of infection. For an overdose, treat with the appropriate antidote or to support body systems as indicated.

After the seizure has been stopped, management is aimed at treating the underlying cause.

As you can see, the initial management of the actively seizing patient is to support the airway and respiration, and then to stop the seizure. Further management is aimed at treating the underlying cause.

Within the last few years, an innovative new therapy has been introduced to mitigate seizures in the epileptic population. This device is the vagus nerve stimulator (VNS). A VNS is a device that employs nonpharmacologic measures to control seizure activity. They are implanted in the subcutaneous tissues of the chest with a wire lead inserted into the vagus nerve that delivers regularly timed cycles of electrical impulses to suppress epileptic foci.

There have been several cases in the recent past where vagal stimulators have been linked to vagally mediated nonadrenergic, noncholinergic, allergen-induced bronchoconstriction. For this reason, the device is not inserted into patients with chronic respiratory conditions. Additionally, a patient with a vagal stimualtor may present with acute bronchospasm of an unknown etiology. In light of the fact that the bronchospasm is nonadreneergic and noncholinergic, it is unlikely that ipratropium bromide or albuterol will effectively mitigate the bronchospasm. It is recommended that in the event of VNS-mediated bronchospasm the device be turned off.

One of the drugs most commonly used to treat and prevent further seizures in patients who have suffered status epilepticus or seizure(s) of unknown etiology is phenytoin (Dilantin). Introduced in 1938, it is the oldest nonsedative antiepileptic drug still in use. However, phenytoin is appropriately administered in the hospital rather than in the prehospital setting. Remember not to administer phenytoin via a solution of 5 percent dextrose and water because the two are incompatible. Fosphenytoin is a newer agent that has the antiseizure activity of phenytoin but can be administered as an intravenous or intramuscular medication.

Status epilepticus, as discussed previously, is one continuous seizure lasting 30 minutes or longer, or two or more seizures without full recovery (without regaining consciousness) between the two attacks. The repetitive seizure activity puts the patient at high risk for hypoxia, cardiovascular collapse, or other injuries. The patient's prognosis is directly related to the time spent actively seizing. As the seizure time increases, the patient's chances of survival decrease. Convulsive status epilepticus has an overall mortality of 30 percent. It is very important that these patients be managed aggressively to prevent further injury.

The status epilepticus patient requires aggressive airway management to decrease associated hypoxia and use of antiseizure medications, including diazepam and lorazepam. High doses of each drug may need to be used. If the seizure is not stopped with conventional pharmacology in the field, the patient may need to receive phenytoin (or fosphenytoin), phenobarbital, or general anesthesia on arrival at the hospital. If these treatments are ineffective, the patient may be placed in a barbiturate coma to break the seizure activity. The primary goal is to rapidly stop the seizure activity and maintain the patient seizure free.

The last treatment we will mention is aimed at the patient with a complex partial seizure. As discussed previously, this patient will not be convulsing on the ground but rather will be experiencing sensory, motor, and behavioral disturbances that can make him appear to have a psychiatric problem or to be under the influence of a mind-altering drug. In complex partial seizures, the patient may stare; fail to respond or respond inappropriately to questions; sit, stand, or move aimlessly; smack the lips; chew; pick at clothing; pull hair; or show other purposeless behavior. The key in distinguishing this from a psychiatric or drug problem is in the nondirected nature of partial complex seizure behavior, as contrasted with the directed behavior in

In complex partial seizures, the patient may stare; fail to respond or respond inappropriately to questions; sit, stand, or move aimlessly; smack the lips; chew; pick at clothing; pull hair; or show other purposeless behavior.

the violent patient or the total loss of contact with the environment in a patient on mind-altering drugs. It is also important to know if the patient has a history of partial complex seizures. (Family or bystanders may provide this information.)

Your initial actions and approach to this patient can determine how the patient responds to you. If your observations and the information you gather indicate that this is a patient suffering a complex partial seizure, you should approach the patient as follows:

1. Approach the patient slowly from the rear or the side.
2. Speak calmly to the patient, advising him of your actions.
3. Avoid physical contact with the patient because violation of space can upset the patient to the degree that he will refuse all your gestures or offers and may even become violent.
4. Gently guide the patient away from any potential dangers.
5. Stay with the patient until he regains a normal mental status (is alert and oriented).

The patient will have no recollection of the incident and may refuse transport. Follow local protocols concerning refusals and sign-offs. Transport to a medical facility is important for all seizure patients. Some may refuse it, especially if they are accustomed to having seizures, but you should attempt to persuade the patient that he needs to be checked out at the hospital.

Ongoing Assessment

Perform ongoing assessment en route to the hospital. Monitor the patient's airway, respirations, and vital signs. Be prepared to manage any additional seizures.

SUMMARY

Possible causes of seizures include trauma, hypoxia, CNS injuries, metabolic disorders, electrolyte imbalances, infections, overdose, and many others.

Assessment and treatment of the seizure patient are summarized in Figure 10-6. The initial approach to this type of patient is the same as the initial approach to any patient. Scene safety is the main priority. If the patient is actively seizing, your next priority is to protect the patient from harming himself.

Next, address the airway. Usually, the seizure patient requires simple airway maneuvers to open the airway, application of a nasopharyngeal airway, and suctioning to remove secretions until the patient is alert enough to maintain his own airway. Administer high-flow, high-concentration oxygen as the seizure permits.

If the seizure persists, begin advanced life support, including IV diazepam or lorazepam. After the seizure stops, measure the blood glucose level and, depending on the reading, administer D_{50} as needed. (Follow local protocols regarding administration of thiamine with the D_{50}.)

After the seizure activity has been stopped, you should begin to investigate and treat the underlying cause.

The goals of seizure management are stopping the seizure, supportive care, and searching for and treating the possible cause.

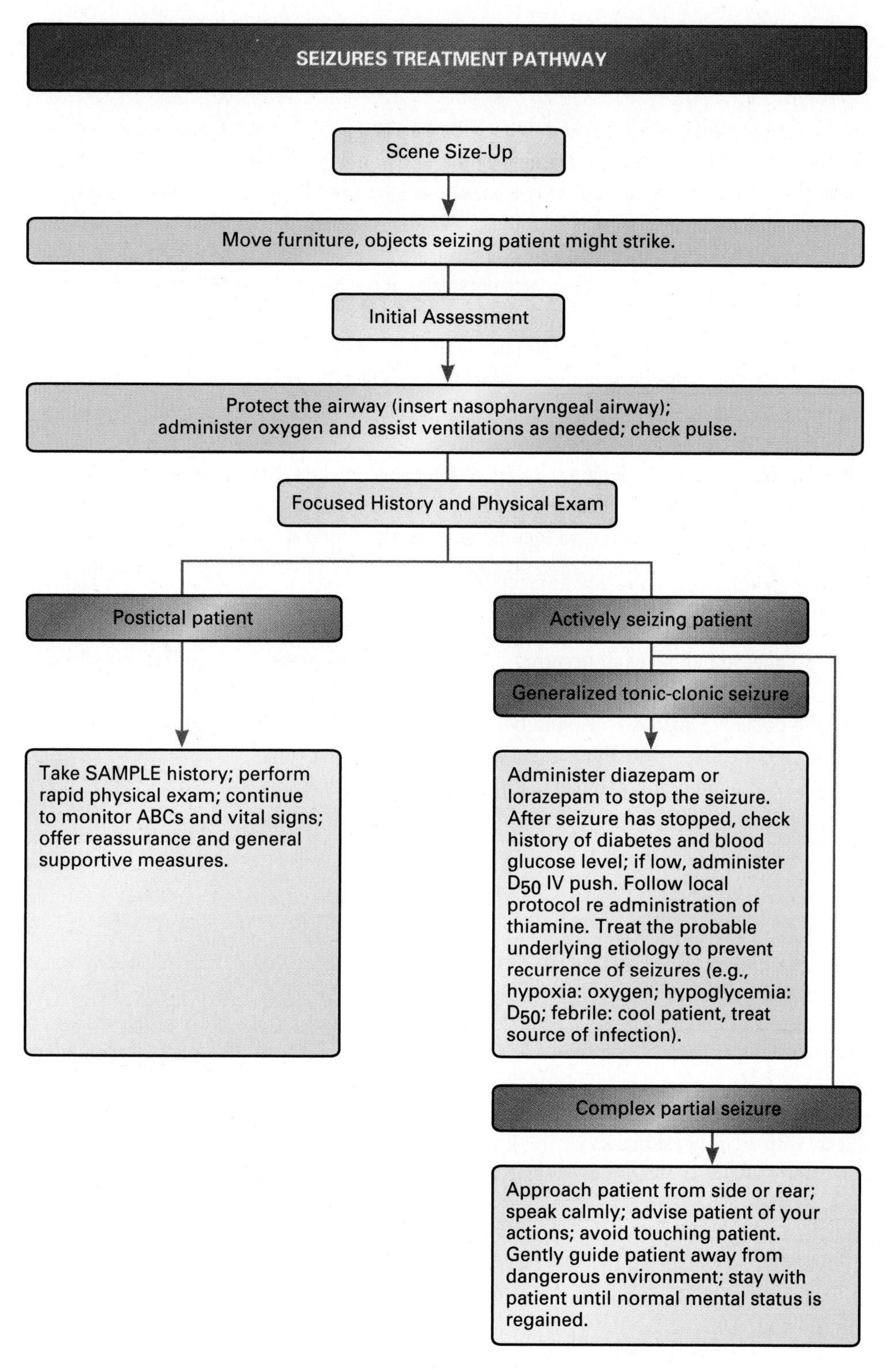

FIGURE 10-6 Seizures treatment pathway.

SCENARIO FOLLOW-UP

You and your partner are performing a stand-by at a local high school football game on a cool fall evening when you are called to the other side of the field for a 30- to 35-year-old male who is apparently having a seizure on the ground.

Your first priority is to move the crowd back and protect your patient, who is exhibiting tonic-clonic movements. You insert a nasopharyngeal airway and are able to safely place the patient on a nonrebreather mask at 100 percent oxygen. The patient's wife comes over and tells you the patient has a seizure disorder but has been seizure free for more than 2 months. You determine that your patient has been actively seizing for approximately 10 minutes and does not appear to be stopping.

You are able to gain IV access in the forearm and administer lorazepam 2 mg slow IV push. The patient stops seizing after the lorazepam administration. You reevaluate his vital signs, finding pulse 96 and bounding (normal sinus rhythm on the monitor), respirations 14 and shallow, and blood pressure 132/60. You suction the patient's oral pharynx and maintain the high-flow, high-concentration oxygen. You evaluate his blood glucose level, which is 142 mg/dl.

In talking further with his wife, you find out that the patient has just been weaned off Dilantin by his neurologist. He was feeling fine when they came to the game, but just as they started walking over to the hot dog stand at halftime, he began to feel "funny," sat down on the ground, and then began to seize. Your patient is still very groggy but alert to voice. You complete the rest of the assessment, finding no signs of trauma or other injuries. You package the patient and prepare for transport.

The transport is uneventful, with the patient regaining full consciousness. He states that he has felt great since he was weaned off his Dilantin and does not know what occurred tonight. You provide emotional reassurance to your patient and monitor his vitals throughout the trip.

On arrival, you are met by the patient's anxious wife, who beat you to the hospital. You give your report to the nursing staff and go to find a hot cup of coffee—which hopefully you'll get to drink this time.

Later, you encounter your patient at another football game. He tells you that his doctor readjusted his medication and that he has had no seizures for several weeks.

FURTHER READING

1. Barton E., J. Ramos, C. Colwell, J. Benson, J. Baily, and W. Dunn. "Intranasal administration of naloxone by paramedics," *Prehospital Emergency Care,* 2002;6(1):54–58.
2. Bernards, C.M. "An unusual cause of airway obstruction during general anesthesia with a laryngeal mask airway," *Anesthesiology,* 2004; 100(4):1017–1018.
3. Boss, B. "Concepts of neurologic dysfunction," in K.L. McCance and S.E. Huether, eds., *Pathophysiology: The Biological Basis for Disease in Adults and Children.* 3rd ed. St. Louis: Mosby, 1998.
4. Bijwadia, J.S., R.C. Hoch, and D.D. Dexter. "Identification and treatment of bronchoconstriction induced by vagus nerve stimulator employed for management of seizure disorder," *Chest,* 2005;127(1):401–402.
5. Chipps, E., N. Clanin, and V. Campbell. "Seizure disorder (convulsions and epilepsy)," in E. Chipps, N. Clanin, and V. Campbell, eds., *Neurologic Disorders.* St. Louis: Mosby, 1992.
6. Guyton, A.C., and J.E. Hall, "States of brain activity: sleep, brain waves, epilepsy, psychoses," in *Textbook of Medical Physiology.* 10th ed. Philadelphia: Saunders, 2001.
7. Henze, R. "Common adaptations and alterations in higher neurologic function," in B. Bullock, ed., *Pathophysiology: Adaptations and Alterations in Function.* Philadelphia: Lippincott-Raven, 1996:1000–1006.
8. Paradiso, C. *Fluids and Electrolytes.* 2nd ed. Philadelphia: Lippincott Williams & Wilkins, 1999.
9. Pellegrino, T. "Seizures and status epilepticus in adults," in D.M. Cline, G. Kelen, S. Stapczynski, J. Tintinalli, and J. Ma, eds., *Emergency Medicine: A Comprehensive Study Guide.* 5th ed. New York: McGraw-Hill, 1999.
10. Schachter, S.C. "Vagus nerve stimulation therapy summary: five years after FDA approval," *Neurology,* 2002;59(6), supplement 4.

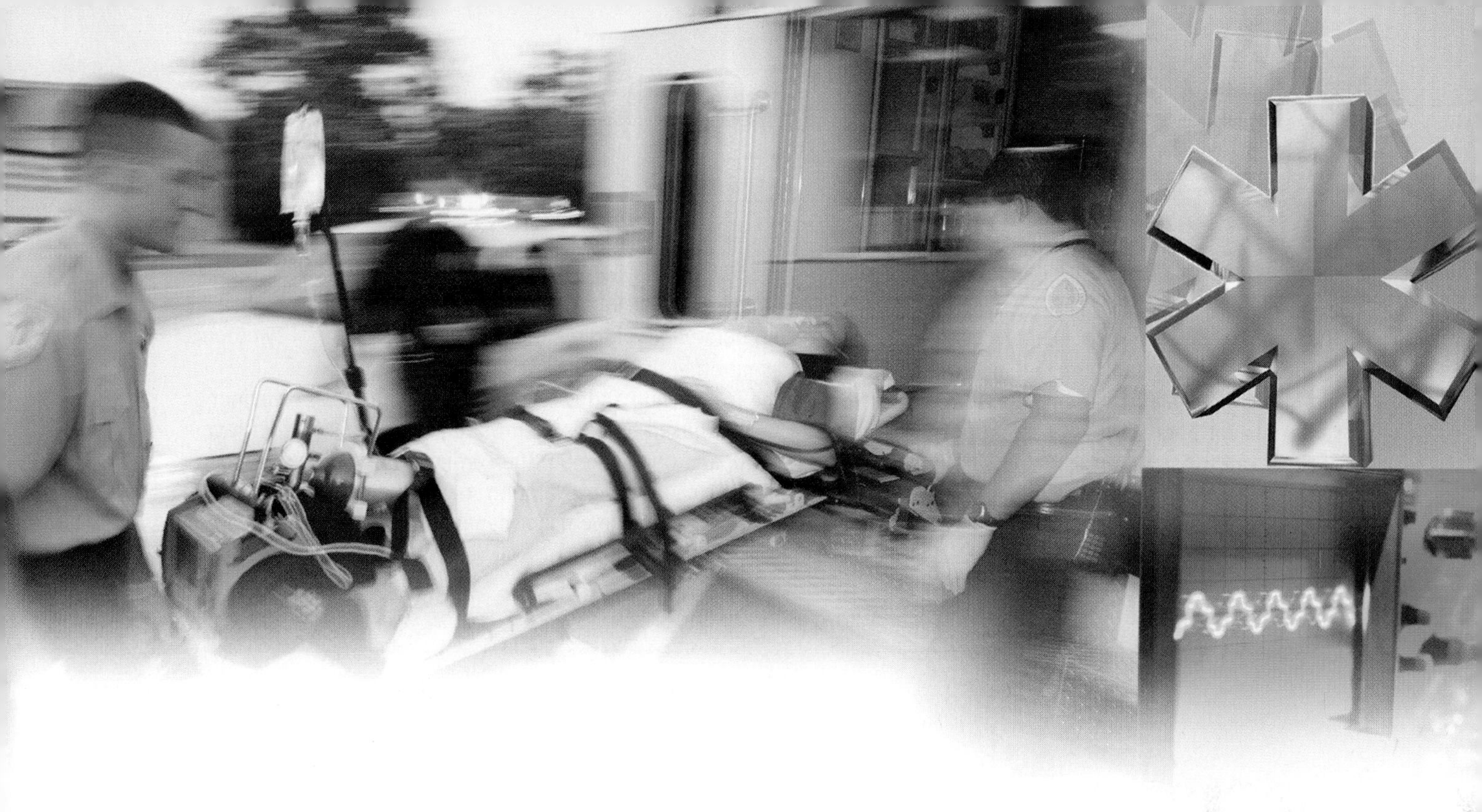

11 SYNCOPE

Syncope (the Greek word for fainting) is the medical term for a transient loss of consciousness. Syncope is self-correcting. The period of unresponsiveness is brief, and the patient will quickly regain consciousness without medical intervention. The cause of a syncopal episode is usually benign and often cannot be diagnosed; however, the EMS provider must evaluate for serious causes of syncope, such as cardiac dysrhythmias, and must be able to distinguish true syncope from other conditions that mimic syncope. If a serious causative pathology is suspected, treatment will be focused on the suspected underlying condition. If the patient who has apparently recovered from a syncopal episode refuses transport, it is important to ensure that the patient is not left alone and that arrangements will be made for follow-up care.

Topics that are covered in this chapter are

- Pathophysiology
- Mechanisms of Syncope
- Patient Assessment and Differential Diagnosis
- Prehospital Management

SCENARIO

You and your partner have just arrived at the home of 48-year-old Margaret Beale. Margaret's sister called for EMS after Margaret "fainted" at her niece's bridal shower. Margaret tells you she felt "a little flutter" in her chest while sitting on the sofa and then "blacked out." Other than taking hormone replacement therapy for menopausal symptoms, Margaret has no significant past medical history and takes no other medications.

Margaret is somewhat embarrassed at the attention she is receiving and is reluctant to submit to an examination and transportation to the emergency department. After being coaxed by her sister, Margaret is compliant with your assessment. Her blood pressure is 132/90, respiratory rate 20, and pulse rate 96. The cardiac monitor shows an occasional PVC. After you explain to Margaret your concern about the cause of her "fainting spell," she agrees to treatment and transport. You establish venous access, and then transport her to the emergency department without recurrence of syncope.

What is the likely outcome of this patient's syncopal episode?

INTRODUCTION

syncope a transient loss of consciousness with loss of postural tone.

Syncope is defined as a transient loss of consciousness with loss of postural tone, generally of less than 5 minutes' duration. The immediate cause of syncope is sudden, temporary hypoperfusion of the cerebrum. There are a number of underlying pathophysiological mechanisms that may lead to the interruption of cerebral perfusion. True syncope is self-limited. Syncope resolves when the patient assumes a recumbent position, thereby restoring cerebral circulation (Figure 11-1). Syncope related to paroxysmal cardiac dysrhythmia resolves on spontaneous termination of the dysrhythmia. Although many cases of syncope are preceded by *prodromal* symptoms, syncope is at times of such acute onset that injury is sustained from resulting falls.

prodrome a set of warning symptoms.

Advanced medical life support for the patient with syncope follows the three phases of care involved in the assessment and management of all patients with a medical emergency. The first phase is the scene size-up and initial assessment to identify and correct immediate threats to life. The next phase is an investigatory phase to help determine the cause of syncope, as well as to detect any injuries possibly sustained during the episode, through a focused history and physical exam. The final phase is aimed at management of any treatable cause of syncope that was discovered, including measures to prevent recurrence.

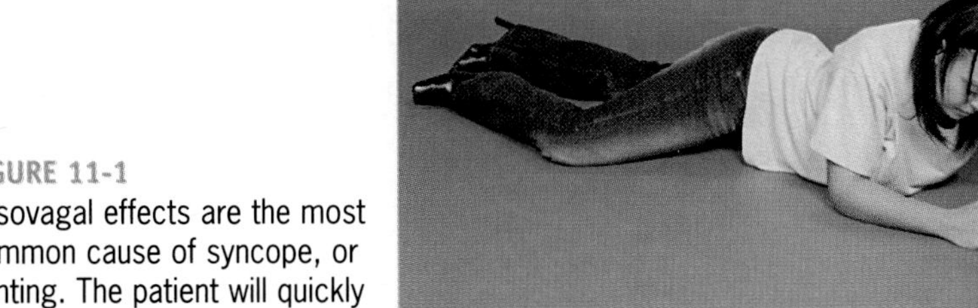

FIGURE 11-1
Vasovagal effects are the most common cause of syncope, or fainting. The patient will quickly regain consciousness after assuming a recumbent position.

Most cases of syncope are relatively benign. In fact, as many as 50 percent of patients visiting the emergency department for syncope do not receive a definitive diagnosis of the etiology of the episode prior to discharge. The transient nature of syncope makes definitive diagnosis elusive because even the most advanced diagnostic tests cannot detect signs that have resolved. Fortunately, most occurrences of syncope, except those related to more ominous causes, require minimal intervention.

The EMS provider has an advantage over the emergency department staff in evaluation of the syncope patient. Because EMS often arrives on the scene within minutes of the onset of the syncopal episode, it is possible to make observations, obtain information, and note patient assessment findings that may not be available at the emergency department. This information may provide the most conclusive information about the cause of syncope.

Information gathered by EMS at the scene may provide the most conclusive information about the cause of syncope.

PATHOPHYSIOLOGY

Syncope occurs when, for any reason, there is a temporary interruption in cerebral circulation resulting in cerebral hypoperfusion. The brain, unlike some body tissues, cannot use proteins or fats for energy. There is limited carbohydrate storage in the brain, so the brain requires a constant supply of glucose for cellular metabolism. The brain does not engage in anaerobic metabolism and therefore requires an uninterrupted supply of oxygen and nutrients for energy metabolism. The brain accounts for about 20 percent of oxygen consumption when the body is at rest. As neuronal activity increases, so does cerebral oxygen consumption.

When there is no energy production in cerebral cells, the cells cease to carry out their functions. The cerebrum is responsible for higher functions (i.e., those functions not related to vegetative existence). Therefore, dysfunction of the cerebrum disrupts consciousness.

Prolonged hypoxia results in breakdown of cerebral neuronal lysosomes, which release enzymes that destroy brain cells. Note that any physiological derangement that leads to cerebral anoxia or prolonged hypoxia, thereby causing prolonged unresponsiveness and requiring resuscitative measures, is by definition *not* syncope. (Syncope, as noted earlier, is self-limited and resolves itself once the patient is recumbent and blood flow to the brain is restored.)

Clinical Insight

If unresponsiveness is prolonged and requires resuscitative measures, the condition is, by definition, *not* syncope. Assessment and treatment should be focused on a more serious etiology.

Interruption of cerebral perfusion can be brought about by hypovolemia, anemia, vasodilation, mechanical obstruction of cerebral blood flow, or anything leading to reduced cardiac output—including cardiac dysrhythmias, valvular insufficiency, pulmonary hypertension, and decreased myocardial contractility.

Often, it is the interaction of multiple factors that brings about an episode of syncope. For example, medications that interfere with vasoconstriction may pose little problem for a patient until he has suffered a bout of severe vomiting and diarrhea, resulting in decreased circulatory volume. The combination of decreased peripheral vascular resistance (PVR) and hypovolemia may result in postural hypotension and syncope.

Often, it is the interaction of multiple factors that brings about an episode of syncope.

MECHANISMS OF SYNCOPE

The most common general mechanisms of syncope (Table 11-1) include vasovagal syncope (which accounts for approximately 55 percent of syncopal episodes), vasodepressor syncope, cardiac syncope, orthostatic hypotension, neurologic causes,

TABLE 11-1 Mechanisms of Syncope: Typical Findings

Mechanisms	Typical Findings
Vasovagal/Vasodepressor Causes	Classic prodrome: dimming of vision, roaring in ears, sighing or yawning, weakness, diaphoresis, pallor, nausea Possible history of stress, such as pain, bad news, sight of blood
Orthostatic Hypotension	Possible history of hypotension, hypovolemia from blood loss, protracted vomiting or diarrhea, use of diuretics, or inadequate fluid intake Possible use of nitrates, vasodilators, beta-blockers, calcium channel blockers, neuroleptic drugs that interfere with compensatory reflexes Possible autonomic nervous system impairment (e.g., diabetic neuropathy or age-related changes resulting in orthostatic hypotension)
Cardiac Causes/Outflow Obstruction	May occur while recumbent; may be accompanied by chest pain, palpitations Tachycardias: ventricular or PSVT (often associated with preexisting heart disease or rates > 180/min) Bradycardia/tachycardia syndrome following termination of PSVT Transient episodes of reduced cardiac output (e.g., bow hunter's stroke, Stokes-Adams attacks) Exertional onset associated with mechanical conditions that limit cardiac output (e.g., aortic stenosis, pulmonary hypertension)
Carotid Sinus Stimulation	Stimulation of oversensitive carotid sinus (e.g., by tight collar, shaving, rapid head turning) History of similar episodes
Metabolic Causes	Typically presents with gradual onset/resolution Possible history of hyperventilation, diabetes, alcohol ingestion, hypokalemia, or adrenal cortical insufficiency
Neurologic Causes	Possible history of diabetic neuropathy, syphilis, alcoholic neuropathy, other disease-related neuropathies, spinal cord lesions, surgical sympathectomy, standing still for a long period
Miscellaneous Causes	Possible history of coughing, pregnancy, gastric distension in the elderly Possible use of any of a variety of pharmacologic substances (e.g., tricyclic antidepressants, quinidine, beta-blockers, diuretics, antihypertensives, neuroleptics, nitrates, ACE inhibitors, sympatholytics, phenothiazines)

metabolic causes, and drug-induced causes. There are some causes of syncope that, although less frequently encountered, should be considered as part of the EMS provider's differential diagnosis.

The complex neuroendocrine regulation of cardiovascular function makes it difficult to discretely categorize the causes of syncope. Because the common factor in all syncope is cerebral hypoperfusion, there is some overlap in the classification of syncope.

vasovagal referring to action on the blood vessels caused by stimulation of the vagal nerve.

vasodepressor having the effect of depressing circulation; lowering blood pressure by dilating the blood vessels.

Cardiocirculatory Syncope

Vasovagal and Vasodepressor Syncope

Vasovagal and *vasodepressor* syncope are common and tend to be familial. A familiar (perhaps more in prehospital legend than in the literature) form of vasovagal syncope occurs when a susceptible individual strains against a closed glottis, such as during a bowel movement or, in individuals with urinary obstruction, on micturition (urination). Swallowing syncope, a condition seen in patients with esophageal disease, is generally caused by vasovagal reflex mechanisms. It is believed that syncope associated with swallowing is likely related to mechanical irritation from esophageal distention or spasm, or from stimulation of associated esophageal structures such as the heart.

Stimulation of the vagus nerve, which, among other functions, is responsible for slowing the heart rate, results in a bradycardia, reducing cardiac output and causing cerebral hypoperfusion. Vasovagal, or neurocardiogenic, syncope and vasodepressor syncope, which is related to decreased PVR, typically occur in susceptible individuals in response to a stressful situation. The stressful stimuli may include pain, hearing bad news, the sight of blood, and similar situations.

These types of syncope are accompanied by prodromal symptoms that may include a dimming or "whiting out" of the vision, a roaring noise in the ears, sighing or yawning, weakness, diaphoresis, pallor, or nausea. At times, these prodromal symptoms may resolve without subsequent syncope, a condition known as near-syncope. Some individuals may experience brief myoclonic activity (muscle twitching or spasm) at the onset of syncope. In these cases, EMS may be called for a "seizure" because the lay public cannot generally differentiate between this phenomenon and a true seizure. Vasovagal and vasodepressor syncope are brief in duration. Recumbency increases cerebral perfusion and restores neurologic function.

Orthostatic Hypotension

Orthostatic hypotension is another form of cardiocirculatory syncope. Orthostatic hypotension occurs when the patient moves from a recumbent or sitting position to an upright position (Figure 11-2). Although cerebral perfusion may have been adequate prior to changing positions, gravitational forces result in dependent venous pooling, thus decreasing preload and cardiac output, with resultant hypotension that is not corrected by normal compensatory mechanisms. As explained here, orthostatic hypotension may arise from hypovolemia, from interference with compensatory reflexes, from autonomic nervous system failure, or from a combination of these factors. The effect of venous pooling is exaggerated in individuals with extensive varicosities of the lower extremities.

orthostatic hypotension a decrease in the blood pressure or an increase in heart rate or a sensation of light-headedness when a patient moves to an upright posture from a sitting or reclining position (or after standing still for a long time); also called **postural hypotension.**

Hypovolemia may be a result of obvious or occult blood loss, protracted vomiting and diarrhea, and the use of diuretics. Hypovolemia due to diuretic use is not limited to patients who have been prescribed diuretics for fluid retention.

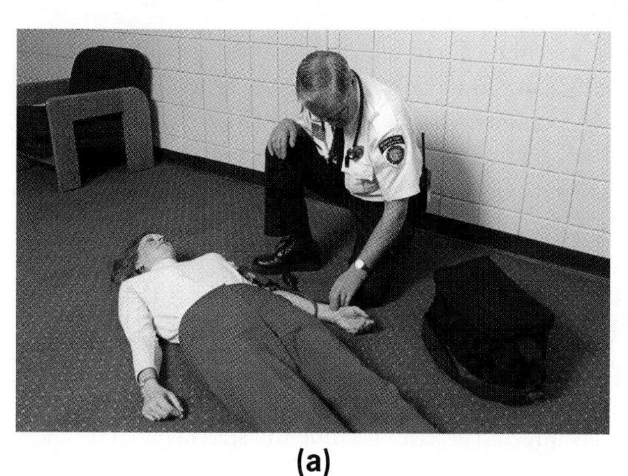

(a)

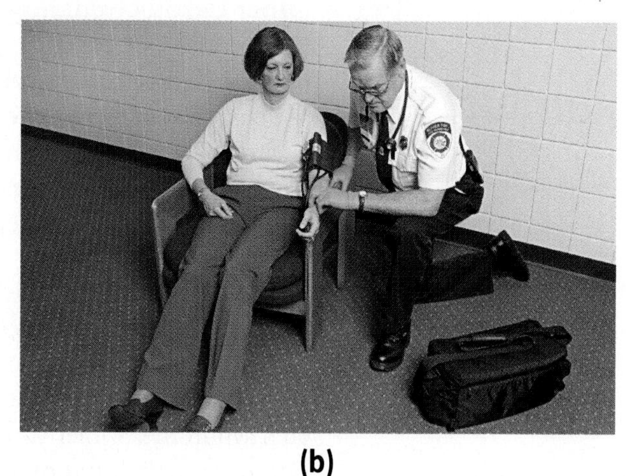

(b)

FIGURE 11-2

(a) While the patient is lying supine, assess the heart rate and blood pressure. (b) Place the patient in a standing or seated position and reassess the heart rate and blood pressure. An increase in the heart rate and/or a decrease in the systolic blood pressure while obtaining orthostatic vital signs may indicate volume depletion.

Diuretics, including over-the-counter medications with diuretic effects, may be used by some as an adjunct to dieting. Other misguided attempts to lose weight, such as body wraps, can also lead to dehydration. Inadequate fluid intake, even without any of the previous factors, may also lead to hypovolemia, particularly in an overly warm environment.

Baroreceptor-mediated reflexes normally stimulate vasoconstriction and increased cardiac output on rising to an upright position. Arterial pressure-sensitive or stretch-sensitive nerves (e.g., those in the *carotid sinuses*) detect less pressure or stretch on rising to an upright position because gravity pools blood in the lower extremities. This, in turn, normally triggers the compensatory mechanisms that maintain cardiac output and cerebral perfusion. However, nitrates, vasodilators, beta-blockers, calcium channel blockers, and neuroleptic drugs interfere with reflex vasoconstriction and/or cardioacceleration.

carotid sinus dilated area at the point where the common carotid artery bifurcates. It is densely supplied with sensory nerve endings that are stimulated in response to changes in pressure.

Autonomic nervous system impairment may be either primary or secondary. Diabetic neuropathy is the most common form of secondary autonomic failure, while age-related changes are the most common form of primary autonomic failure. In either situation, lack of autonomic regulation of vasoconstriction leads to orthostatic hypotension. Shy-Drager syndrome is a chronic form of orthostatic hypotension caused by autonomic failure in which plasma levels of norepinephrine do not increase on standing.

Outflow Obstruction

Outflow obstruction is another cardiocirculatory classification of syncope, referring to decreased cardiac output resulting from mechanical obstruction. Underlying causes include aortic stenosis, mitral or pulmonic valve stenosis, and failure of mechanical heart valves. Circulatory obstruction may also occur as a result of pulmonary embolism, pulmonary hypertension, or pericardial tamponade. These patients often present with exertional syncope when there is an inability to meet the increased demand for cardiac output. Subclavian steal syndrome may occur during arm exercise as blood flow is diverted from the cerebral circulation to the upper extremity. An unusual cause of outflow obstruction is a pedunculated atrial myxoma—a tumor attached to the atrium by a stalk-like structure whose position may intermittently cause outflow obstruction.

Other Cardiocirculatory Causes

Bow hunter's stroke is a type of mechanical circulatory obstruction characterized by transitory vertebrobasilar insufficiency induced by turning the head in the presence of structural abnormalities at the craniocervical junction. This most commonly occurs in the elderly as a result of cervical spondylosis, but it has been reported to have occurred due to lateral herniation of cervical intervertebral discs as well as idiopathically. Not surprisingly, bow hunter's stroke may be implicated in motor vehicle crashes.

Takayasu's arteritis is an inflammatory disease of large arteries that leads to arterial stenosis and reduced blood flow through the affected arteries. Although it is a rare disease, it is more common in adolescent and young adult females and in Asia. The aorta is the most commonly affected site, thus the alternative term "aortic arch syndrome." Other commonly affected arteries include the subclavian, common carotid, vertebral, and pulmonary arteries.

Idiopathic hypertrophic subaortic stenosis (IHSS) is a chronic condition that causes progressive thickening of the left ventricle of the heart. IHSS has not been definitively linked to any specific etiology, but those affected by it are believed to have a genetic predisposition. The severity of the presentation is directly related to the degree of stenosis. If there is enough stenosis, obstruction of oxygenated blood flow may be seen, and the heart will be incapable of pumping enough blood to meet the body's metabolic demands. It is important to note that IHSS generally affects the ventricular septum rather than the free wall of the ventricle, which is why outflow obstruction is relatively common. The exacerbation of IHSS is almost always seen during exertion and is most commonly seen in adolescents or young adults. In the past, IHSS was often called hypertrophic cardiomyopathy (HCM).

Also in the classification of cardiocirculatory syncope, both tachydysrhythmias and bradydysrhythmias can lead to decreased cardiac output and resultant syncope. Dysrhythmia-induced syncope generally occurs at heart rates less than 35 and greater than 150. Some specific conditions implicated include Stokes-Adams attacks, sick sinus syndrome and A-V node blocks, long Q-T syndrome, paroxysmal supraventricular tachycardia (PSVT), Wolf-Parkinson-White syndrome, and ventricular tachycardia. In dysrhythmia-induced syncope, the dysrhythmia is paroxysmal. A sustained dysrhythmia resulting in an altered mental status requires intervention to terminate the dysrhythmia. By definition, this is not syncope. Dysrhythmia-induced syncope may occur in a recumbent position and may be accompanied by chest pain and/or palpitations.

Carotid sinus hypersensitivity is the final cardiocirculatory type of syncope discussed here. In individuals with a hypersensitive carotid sinus baroreceptive mechanism, hyperextension of the head, such as is common with shaving or tight collars, may induce vasodilation and bradycardia resulting in syncope. In such individuals, there is most likely a history of similar incidents.

In individuals with a hypersensitive carotid sinus, hyperextension of the head, such as with shaving or tight collars, may result in syncope.

Metabolic Syncope

The most common type of metabolic syncope is caused by hyperventilation syndrome. After a period of hyperventilation, hypocapnia leads to cerebral vasoconstriction, resulting in hypoperfusion of the brain. Weight lifter's syncope occurs as a result of intentional preexertional hyperventilation in combination with straining against a closed glottis during exertion.

Complications of diabetes mellitus may lead to syncope, either secondary to osmotic diuresis due to hyperglycemia, or due to hypoglycemia. Alcohol ingestion can also lead to metabolic syncope because alcohol has an inhibitory effect on the vasomotor center and inhibits antidiuretic hormone, leading to hypotension. Hypokalemia limits an increase in PVR on standing and can lead to orthostatic hypotension. Similarly, adrenal cortical insufficiency, as in Addison's disease, limits both an increase in PVR and heart rate.

Neurologic Syncope

Neurologic causes of syncope include diabetic neuropathy, neurologic sequelae of syphilis, alcoholic neuropathy, spinal cord lesions, postinfectious neuropathy of Guillain-Barré syndrome, Parkinson's disease, and Riley-Day syndrome (dysautonomia, a rare hereditary diseases characterized by mental retardation, incoordination, and convulsions, among other effects). Patients having undergone surgical sympathectomy (removal of a portion of the sympathetic nervous system) also fall into this category. In these situations, the underlying cause of syncope is failure of vasoconstriction, resulting in peripheral venous pooling. Parkinson's disease results in a decrease of dopamine and norepinephrine, resulting in postural hypotension.

TABLE 11-2 Medications Commonly Associated with Syncope

Tricyclic antidepressants
Quinidine
Beta-blockers
Diruetics
Antihypertensives
Neuroleptics
Nitrates
ACE inhibitors
Sympatholytics
Phenothiazones

In so-called "parade square" faints, an individual standing still for a long period of time faints because of venous pooling in the lower extremities.

Among patients with spinal cord injury, failure of the skeletal muscle pump (along with unopposed parasympathetic tone) enhances venous pooling. Inadequate skeletal muscle action to assist in venous return to the heart is also implicated in so-called "parade square" faints, where an individual standing still for a long period of time faints because of venous pooling in the lower extremities. This, of course, can be exacerbated by an overly warm environment, preexisting dehydration, effects of medications, and other contributory causes of syncope.

TIAs are rarely implicated in syncope. When a TIA results in syncope, the mechanism by which it occurs is ischemia of the reticular activating system (RAS). Migraine headaches may be preceded by a syncopal episode, particularly in adolescents.

Miscellaneous Causes of Syncope

Other causes of syncope relate to the previously described mechanisms. Many pharmacologic substances (Table 11-2) can result in syncope through a variety of mechanisms, including cardiovascular and neurologic effects. Cough syncope occurs due to increased intrathoracic pressure on coughing, which reduces preload and thus cardiac output. Preload is also reduced by the weight of a pregnant uterus on the inferior vena cava and may occur in a recumbent or semirecumbent position. Pregnancy also results in production of hormones that lead to peripheral vasodilation, which may also be a cause of syncope. More prevalent among the elderly, postprandial syncope is syncope occurring after meals due to gastric distension.

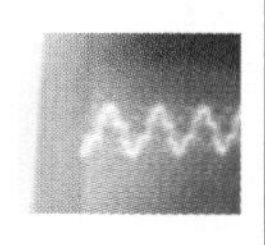

PATIENT ASSESSMENT AND DIFFERENTIAL DIAGNOSIS

Scene Size-Up and Initial Assessment

The scene size-up and initial assessment for syncope are essentially the same as for other medical emergencies. In the case of syncope, depending on your response time, you may find the patient unresponsive. Because of the self-correcting nature of a true syncopal episode, however, the patient is likely to have already regained consciousness by the time you arrive. As noted earlier, if the patient remains unresponsive for a prolonged time or requires resuscitation, the patient's condition, by definition, is not simple syncope, and a more critical pathology should be considered as the cause for the unresponsiveness.

The scene size-up provides important safety information. A report of syncope may actually be a situation in which the patient is unresponsive for another reason, possibly a scene hazard. The scene size-up may also provide clues to the patient's actions prior to the episode, environmental conditions, medications, and other information that can help the EMS provider establish the cause of the syncopal episode. Statements from bystanders or family members who witnessed the episode may also be helpful in narrowing down the circumstances surrounding the syncopal event.

Initial assessment, as always, focuses on airway, breathing, and circulation. If the possibility of cervical spine injury exists, or the episode was unwitnessed and the potential for injury is unknown, immediate manual stabilization of the cervical spine is indicated.

The patient who experiences a true syncopal episode will regain consciousness within a relatively short time, generally 5 minutes or less. The recovery may be more rapid if the patient lands in or is placed in a recumbent position. Although some types of syncope, particularly those from metabolic causes, are associated with a more gradual onset and resolution, persistent altered mental status should steer the investigatory phase toward conditions other than syncope.

In the absence of spinal injury, elevating the legs may be beneficial in correcting venous pooling and increasing the level of responsiveness. As stated previously, the need for resuscitation rules out simple syncope and indicates a more serious underlying pathology.

Focused History and Physical Exam

The common pathophysiological processes resulting in syncope have already been discussed. Physical examination and collection of the patient history in the context of this knowledge of pathophysiology guides the EMS provider in differential diagnosis, which in turn guides prehospital patient management. Although it may not be possible to determine the cause of syncope, it is important to look for findings that differentiate syncope from other conditions, particularly those that indicate a potentially life-threatening underlying cause such as occult bleeding or cardiac dysrhythmia.

History

Obtain the patient history (Figure 11-3) efficiently and in an organized manner through the application of the SAMPLE format, as described here:

1. Signs and Symptoms
   - *How did you feel prior to fainting?*
   - *Did you have any pain or unusual sensations?*
   - *Did you have any warning that you were going to faint?*
   - *Did you fall or injure yourself when you fainted?*
   - *How do you feel now?* (If the patient complains of "dizziness," be sure to explore further, as the lightheadedness associated with syncope is often described as "dizziness." It is helpful to ask, "When you say you felt dizzy, do you mean you it felt as though things were spinning around, or that you felt as if you were going to black out?" Vertigo is indicative of different pathophysiology than syncope, making it important to clarify the patient's complaint before proceeding.)
2. Allergies
   - *Are you allergic to any medications, foods, or other substances?*
   - *Have you come into contact with anything you are allergic to?*

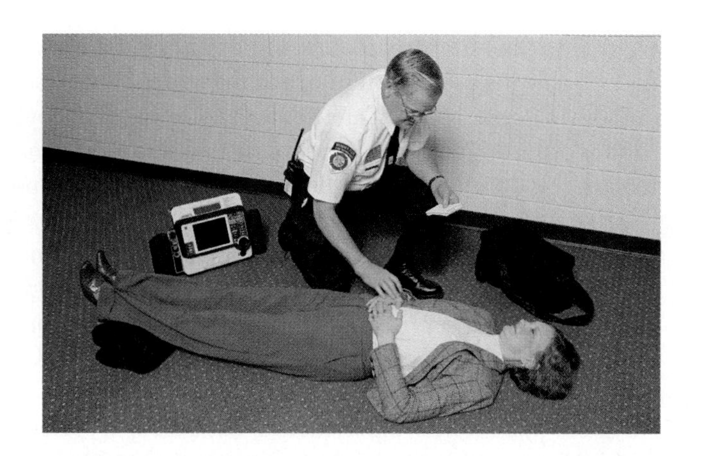

FIGURE 11-3
Obtain a SAMPLE history and perform a physical exam.

3. Medications
   - *Do you take any medications? What medications do you take?*
   - *Have you taken your medications today?*
   - *Have you recently changed dosages of medication or started or stopped taking a medication?*
   - *Do you take any medications other than those prescribed by your doctor, such as over-the-counter cold or allergy medications or diet pills?*
4. Past Medical History
   - *Have you ever had an episode similar to this before? If so, did you seek medical attention? Did your doctor tell you what might have caused you to faint?*
   - *Do you have any medical problems such as seizures, diabetes, high blood pressure, a stroke, or heart disease?*
   - *Have you been ill recently, had a fever, or had any vomiting or diarrhea?*
5. Last Oral Intake
   - *When was the last time you had anything to eat or drink?* (Remember that insufficient oral intake of fluids can contribute to syncope, particularly in warm conditions. Hypoglycemia may also be a contributing factor.)
6. Events Prior to Illness
   - *What were you doing (or what happened) just before you fainted?* (Remember that some forms of syncope occur on exertion, while others occur at rest or when standing for a long period of time. Yet, other types of syncope are brought about by turning or hyperextending the head or straining against a closed glottis.)

Physical Examination

Physical examination begins with the scene size-up and initial assessment and continues with observations made during the patient interview. The physical examination will proceed with particular attention to relevant findings of the history and initial assessment. The following methods of physical examination may yield important information:

- ***Cardiac Monitoring.*** Cardiac monitoring (Figure 11-4) is especially important in circumstances indicative of cardiac syncope. Syncope accompanied by chest pain or palpitations and syncope occurring in a recumbent position are significant findings. Although it may not be possible to capture the dysrhythmia that induced the syncopal episode, the dysrhythmia may recur. Where available, diagnostic-quality 12-lead ECG tracings may indicate acute (AMI) or ischemia.

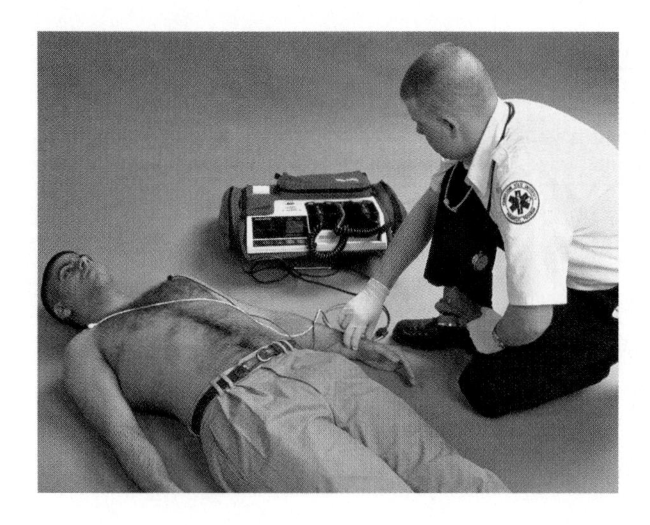

FIGURE 11-4
Cardiac monitoring may detect borderline bradycardias or tachycardias that are still present after an episode of cardiac syncope or the onset of further dysrhythmic episodes.

- *Orthostatic Vital Signs.* A 10 mmHg or greater decrease in blood pressure and a 20 bpm or greater increase in the heart rate when changing from a supine to a standing position are diagnostic of orthostatic hypotension. This is best assessed in the hospital with the use of a tilt table and pharmacologic intervention. Additionally, orthostatic changes are best assessed if the patient has been supine for a period of at least 10 minutes. Orthostatic changes may not occur for up to 2 minutes after the patient assumes a standing position. Therefore, orthostatic hypotension may be significant when noted in the prehospital setting, but its absence does not rule out orthostasis as the cause of the syncopal episode. Any changes in the patient's condition on standing, such as pallor, faintness, or other premonitory symptoms of syncope, should be considered a positive tilt test for the purposes of prehospital care.
- *Others.* Other tests that may be indicated, based on the history and initial assessment, include neurologic assessment for signs of stroke, such as slurred speech, unilateral weakness, or facial droop. Blood glucose testing may be useful if the history and other physical exam findings support its use.

PREHOSPITAL MANAGEMENT

The dilemma in the management of syncope is determining how to treat a condition that now appears to have resolved. General management includes keeping the patient in a supine or semirecumbent position to prevent recurrence of the episode and potential subsequent injury (Figure 11-5).

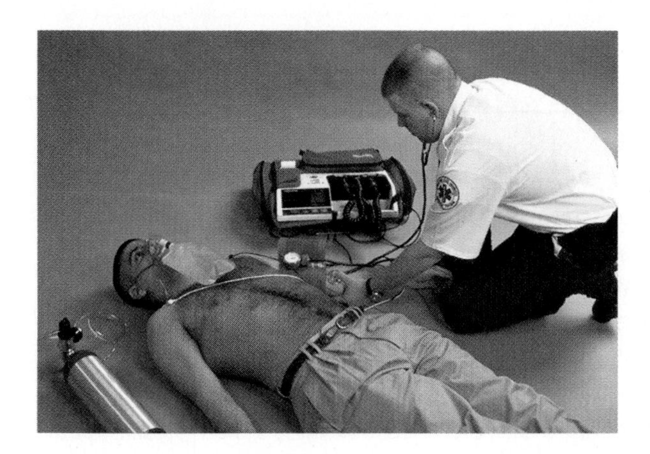

FIGURE 11-5
Keep the syncopal patient in a recumbent position and provide oxygen, especially if the patient shows persisting signs of instability.

TABLE 11-3 **Conditions That Mimic Syncope: Differential Findings**

Conditions	Differential Findings
Stroke	Neurologic signs and symptoms present, including slurred speech, hemiparesis, unilateral numbness, motor deficits
Hypoglycemia	Gradual onset History of diabetes Unusual behavior Not transient/self-correcting
Seizure	Patient may experience an aura prior to the seizure Seizure activity Postictal period History of seizures Greater incidence of injury from falls than in syncope

For patients with a suspected serious underlying pathology, such as hypovolemia or AMI, oxygen administration is indicated. Patients suspected of having a hypovolemic component to their episode should receive intravenous fluids. Venous access is also indicated if there is a potential need to administer antidysrhythmic medications, antiseizure medications, or 50 percent dextrose. Other causes of unconsciousness that can mimic syncope, such as stroke, hypoglycemia, or seizure, may be revealed during your assessment. Table 11-3 lists differential findings for these conditions. Their assessment and treatment are discussed in other chapters, particularly Chapter 7, Altered Mental Status, and Chapter 10, Seizures and Seizure Disorders. As always, adhere to your system's applicable protocols when treating any patient.

The transient nature of syncope, and sometimes the patient's feelings of embarrassment, may lead to the patient's refusal to be transported to the emergency department. Make every effort to explain to the patient that the underlying cause of the episode needs to be investigated by a physician, and that some underlying causes, such as cardiac dysrhythmias, may recur and result in death. Even with relatively benign underlying causes, the episode may recur, resulting in injury.

Clinical Insight

After an episode of syncope, a patient will often refuse transport. Never leave such a patient alone. Always enlist someone to stay with the patient, and emphasize the importance of scheduling follow-up care.

If the patient still refuses care, enlist the aid of family members, coworkers, or friends who are present and make sure the patient is not left alone. Ensure that arrangements for follow-up care are made immediately. The patient should be instructed to recognize the prodromal symptoms of syncope and to assume a supine or head-down position if the symptoms occur. Because of the potential for liability inherent in all patient refusals, accurate and comprehensive documentation is critical. Always follow your protocols regarding patient refusal.

SUMMARY

Syncope is a transient loss of consciousness with a loss of postural tone. Syncope is self-limited because, when the temporary state of cerebral hypoperfusion is corrected, consciousness returns. Most underlying causes of syncope are benign, although more ominous causes of syncope and conditions that mimic syncope should be kept in mind when determining a differential diagnosis and plan of prehospital management. A critical comparison of your findings with the pathophysiological bases of syncope will assist in establishing potential causes of syncope and tentatively ruling out other causes. Care of the patient with a syncopal episode is largely supportive and aimed at preventing recurrence of the episode (Figure 11-6).

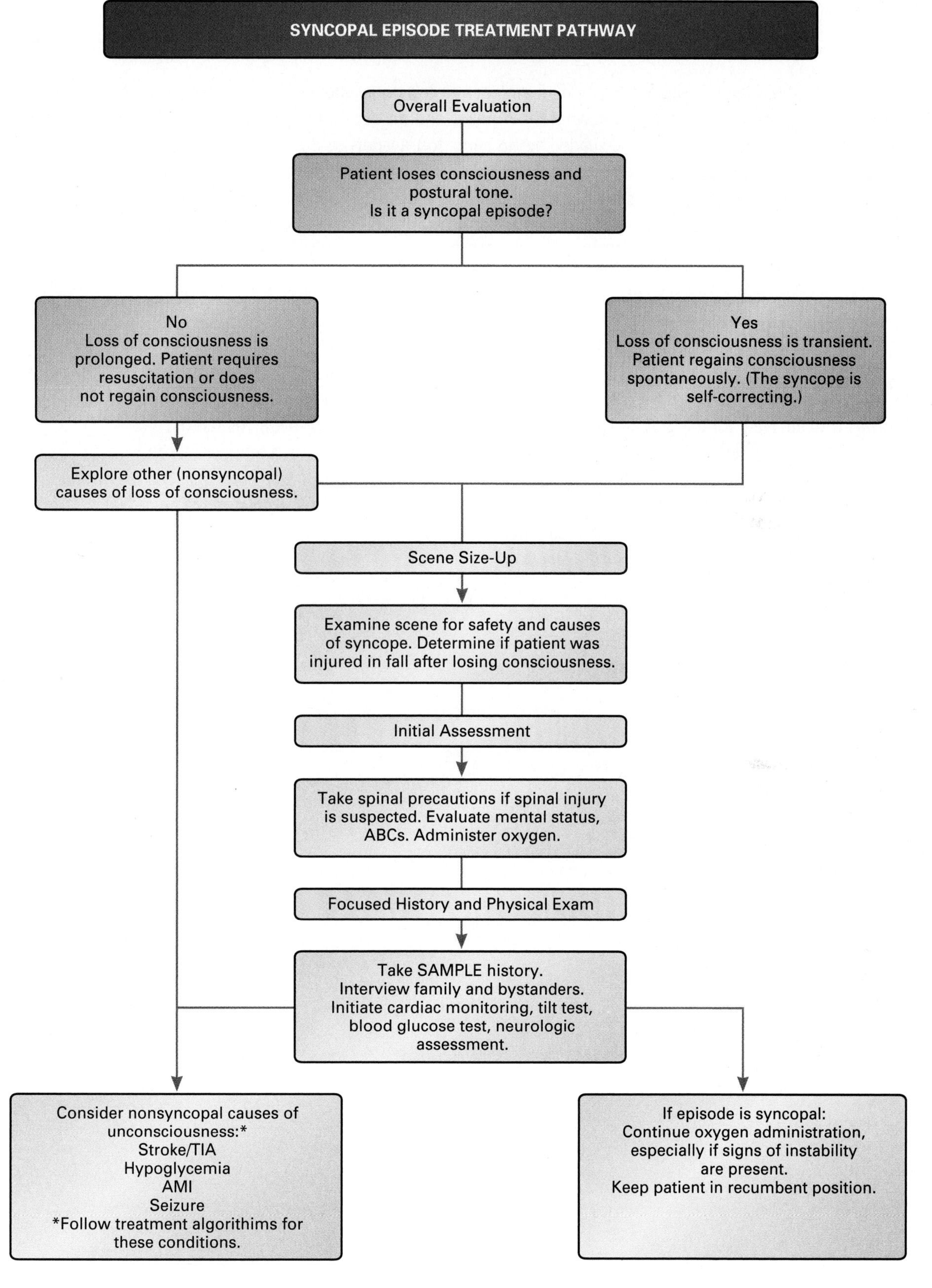

FIGURE 11-6
Syncopal episode treatment pathway.

SCENARIO FOLLOW-UP

Forty-eight-year-old Margaret Beale has "fainted" during her niece's bridal shower. Your assessment reveals a normal blood pressure and respiratory rate, a somewhat rapid pulse, and an occasional premature ventricular contraction (PVC) on the cardiac monitor. You have persuaded her to agree to transport to the hospital for evaluation.

Following an inconclusive cardiac workup in the emergency department, Margaret is admitted to a telemetry unit for cardiac monitoring. During her stay, she experiences an episode of ventricular tachycardia resulting in another syncopal episode. After implantation of a cardioverter-defibrillator, Margaret is released from the hospital.

FURTHER READING

1. Braunwald, E., D.L. Longo, J.L. Jameson, A.S. Fauci, and D.L. Kasper, eds. *Harrison's Principles of Internal Medicine.* 15th ed. New York: McGraw-Hill, 2001.
2. Guyton, A.C., and J.E. Hall., "Nervous regulation of the circulation," in *Textbook of Medical Physiology.* 10th ed. Philadelphia: Saunders, 2001.
3. Kapoor, W.N. "Work-up and management of patients with syncope," *Medical Clinics of North America,* 1995;79:1153.
4. Olshansky, B. "Is syncope the same thing as sudden death except that you wake up?" *J. Cardiovasc Electrophysiol,* 1997; 8:1098-1101.
5. Tierney, L.M., S.J. McPhee, and M.J. Chatton, eds. *Current Medical Diagnosis and Treatment 2002.* 41st ed. Stamford, CT: Appleton & Lange, 2002.

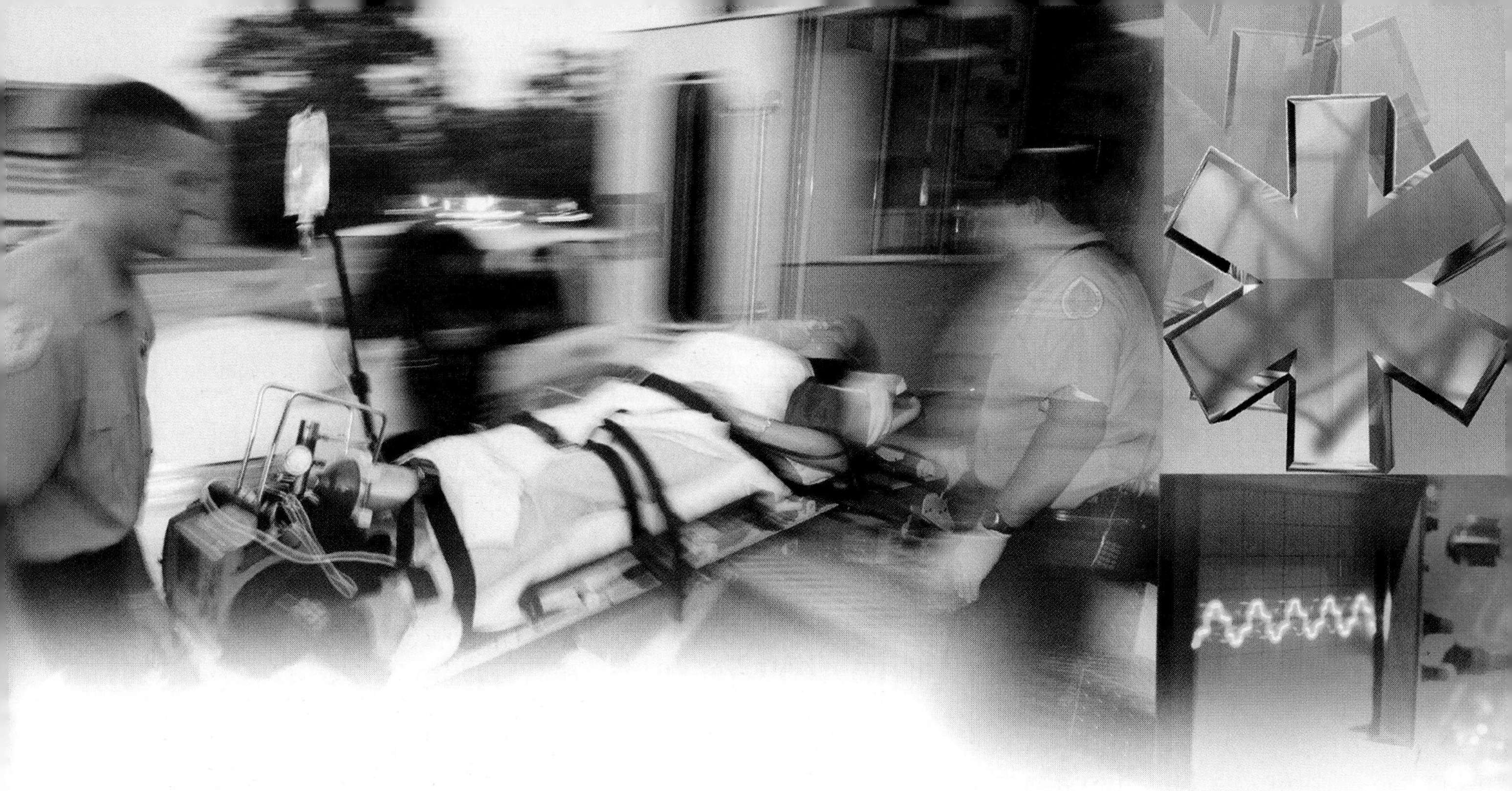

HEADACHE, NAUSEA, AND VOMITING

12

Headache is one of the most common conditions that people suffer. Headaches may be experienced as isolated attacks or as chronic, recurring attacks. A headache may be a benign phenomenon or an indication of serious illness, such as intracranial tumor, meningitis, or stroke, to name a few. Nausea and vomiting frequently accompany headache; however, either may be a sign or symptom of another underlying condition, such as toxic ingestion, myocardial ischemia, or pregnancy. When a serious underlying condition is suspected, it is important always to treat that condition. Specific management of headache, nausea, or vomiting that is not associated with a serious underlying condition often requires only supportive care in the prehospital setting.

Topics that are covered in this chapter are

- Headache
- Nausea and Vomiting

SCENARIO

You are called to the scene for a patient who has "passed out" while playing basketball at the local high school gymnasium. Upon arrival, you find a 39-year-old male patient lying supine on the basketball court in a pool of vomitus. The patient's body and extremities are extended in a rigid posture. He is not responding to verbal stimuli.

The bystanders at the scene state that the man was playing basketball when he suddenly stopped and began to complain about a severe headache. He was heard to say, "This is the worst headache I've ever had in my life." He sat down on the floor, complained of feeling nauseated, and slowly became unresponsive. He has thrown up twice—"like a fire hose" says one of his teammates—before your arrival.

How would you proceed with the immediate care of this patient?

INTRODUCTION

The most common complaints of medical patients have been addressed in the previous chapters. This chapter deals with three other complaints that are often encountered: headache, nausea, and vomiting. Although these complaints often present together, they also exist independently of each other. All may be chronic or episodic, subtle or severe, not associated with any serious underlying condition, or an indication of a life-threatening injury or illness.

Headache, nausea, and vomiting must never be treated lightly just because they are common.

Headache, nausea, and vomiting must never be treated lightly just because they are so common. As with any other presenting complaint, these complaints must be systematically assessed, with any life-threatening conditions identified and managed before you attempt to determine the etiology and establish a differential field diagnosis.

HEADACHE

Almost everyone has suffered a headache at some point in life; only a few people claim never to have had one. Headache is one of the most common complaints and, although not typically associated with serious illness, may be a symptom of a more serious condition. People who seek medical care with a chief complaint of headache are usually those who have never suffered a headache before, patients who experience a change in the typical characteristics of their recurring headaches, and those with chronic headaches who seek medical care for pain control. Not many people who complain of headache have a serious illness; however, a few will require immediate intervention because of a significant etiology of the head pain.

Every patient complaining of headache should be carefully assessed for alterations in mental status, cognitive deficits, and neurologic dysfunction and monitored closely for evidence of deterioration, any of which would indicate a more serious etiology.

The quality and intensity of headache pain is very subjective; thus, it is not a reliable indicator for further evaluation and in forming a differential field diagnosis. The intensity of a headache does not always indicate the severity of the condition. It is more important to consider all of the signs and symptoms as a whole and the evolution of the signs and symptoms in gauging the seriousness of the condition. Every patient complaining of headache should be carefully assessed for alterations in mental status, cognitive deficits, and neurologic dysfunction and monitored closely for evidence of deterioration, any of which would indicate a more serious etiology.

Headaches are classified as primary or secondary. Primary headaches include tension-type, migraine, and cluster headaches. These types of headaches account for approximately 90 percent of the patients seen by physicians for the complaint of headache. A secondary headache is a result of an underlying disease or process with one of the symptoms of the condition being head pain or a headache. Secondary headaches are more serious because they could be an indication of an underlying condition.

Anatomy and Physiology

The brain tissue itself does not have any sensory pain fibers and cannot sense pain itself. Likewise, the pia mater, arachnoid, skull, or mass of tiny blood vessels contained in the ventricles of the brain (choroid plexus) are not sensitive to pain. The structures that are sensitive to pain include the scalp; components of the dura mater; dural arteries; intracerebral arteries; cranial nerves V, VI, and VII; and the cervical nerves. Thus, a headache results from activation of peripheral pain receptors in surrounding tissue within the cranium and other structures. Headache pain is transmitted along unmyelinated nerve fibers, which provide the slowest nerve transmission. That could explain why headaches typically develop slowly over a period of minutes to hours and are rarely well localized. Headache may result from any of the following mechanisms:

- Contraction of extracranial muscles of the neck and scalp
- Dilatation and distention of intracranial vessels
- Inflammation of peripheral vessels and nerves of the head and neck and the meninges at the base of the brain
- Traction due to stress on intracranial structures from meningeal irritation and increased intracranial pressure (ICP)

The International Headache Society (IHS) has developed a classification system for headaches that includes categorization by etiology or mechanism. These mechanisms, or a combination of these mechanisms, result in three main types of headaches:

- ***Tension-Type Headaches.*** A tension-type headache is believed to be caused by contraction of the muscles of the neck and scalp; however, there is no research that supports muscular contraction as the sole etiology of the pain. This type of headache is usually generalized in location and often described as "tight" or "vise-like."
- ***Vascular Headaches/Migraines.*** Dilatation or distention of vessels and inflammation result in a vascular headache. Severe hypertension headaches and vasodilator headaches from drugs and other toxic substances are types of vascular headaches. Migraines are believed to be caused by vascular spasm, followed by vasodilatation of the cerebral arteries, coupled with changes in the neurotransmitters in the brain. Migraines are sometimes, but not always, preceded by an "aura" that may include visual disturbances, numbness, or other symptoms. Migraines are often described as throbbing and may be generalized or localized to one side. A hypertension headache usually requires a diastolic blood pressure of at least 120 mmHg to elicit head pain.
- ***Cluster Headaches.*** Cluster headaches are similar to migraines and are sometimes classified as a migraine variant because they are believed to be vascular

in origin. Cluster headaches are also known as histamine headaches, because histamine is believed to play a role in precipitating the headache. The headache is typically characterized by excruciating pain to one side of the face or head, usually periorbital or in the temporal region. The patient may also complain of excessive tear production (lacrimation) on the side of the pain, nasal congestion or rhinorrhea (runny nose), and nausea.

Physical assessment findings may include conjunctival congestion, facial sweating, restlessness or agitation, facial flushing or pallor, scalp or facial tenderness, pupil contraction (miosis), or eyelid edema and drooping (ptosis). The lacrimation, rhinorrhea, and nasal congestion are effects of parasympathetic nervous system innervation, whereas facial sweating results from the sympathetic discharge. During the initial assessment, you may find the patient pacing or sitting with his head lowered, pressing on the site of pain. The patient may be crying or screaming.

The headache may be very brief in duration and usually will last no more than 2 hours. The headaches will occur several times a day for weeks or months followed by a headache-free period. Some proposed pathophysiological etiologies of cluster headaches include vascular dilatation, neuronal discharge from the trigeminal nerve, hypothalamus origination associated with the circadian rhythm, serotonin, and histamine. Attacks commonly follow ingestion of alcohol, nitroglycerin, or substances containing histamine. The headaches may also be related to stress, changes in the climate, or allergens.

Clinical Insight

Oxygen may relieve a cluster headache.

Cluster headaches occur more often in males, as much as 10 times more often. The headaches normally begin in midlife with a peak onset age of 30 years. Oxygen therapy, as near 100 percent as possible, may eliminate the headache if used early. The exact mechanism of action of oxygen related to headache reduction is not understood.

Tension type and migraine are the most common types of headache.

Of the headaches mentioned previously, tension and migraine are the most common types. As noted, cluster headaches are often classified as a type of migraine. Etiologies of tension-type headache and migraine are discussed in more detail in the following sections.

Other etiologies of headache include fever, hypoxemia, anemia, tumors, intracranial hemorrhages, or the weight of the brain following removal of cerebrospinal fluid. Toxic substances such as carbon monoxide, cyanide, and solvents, as well as certain medications such as oral contraceptives and nitrates, are common producers of headache. A commonly overlooked cause of headache is depression.

Tension-Type Headache

Tension-type headache is the most common type of recurring headache occurring in children, adolescents, and adults. Sustained muscular contraction of the muscles of the neck and scalp from stress and emotional experiences was once believed to be the causative factor; however, research has shown that these factors may contribute to the pain but are not the sole etiology of the pain. Most recent evidence suggests that tension-type headaches result from an imbalance in the neurotransmitters (dopamine, serotonin, norepinephrine, and enkephalins) within the central nervous system (CNS), leading to an increased sensitivity of nerves and pain. Depression and some sleep disorders have been linked to alterations in serotonin levels; thus, chronic tension-type headaches may be a result of depression. A theory that is not supported by clinical evidence suggests that contraction of the muscles of the neck and scalp causes pressure on the nerves, resulting in pain. Also, vessels at the base of the neck may be constricted, causing an increase in pressure and a build-up of lactic acid and other waste products, contributing to the pain. Therefore, muscle factors may be associated with tension-type headaches, but the evidence is not conclusive.

Tension-type headaches are more prevalent in females and predominate in patients older than 20 years of age. Close to two-thirds of the patients with new onset of tension-type headache are older than 20 years of age. Onset of tension-type headaches is unusual for patients older than the age of 50 years. This should be a major consideration during the physical assessment and as an indication to look for another organic cause of headache in patients older than 50. New headache onset in an elderly patient is suggestive of an etiology other than a primary headache and is cause for concern. Most frequently, new-onset headache in the elderly is of a secondary nature and is associated with more serious pathology.

Clinical Insight

New headache onset in the elderly patient is suggestive of a secondary etiology with a more serious pathology.

The headaches are recurrent and typically last anywhere from 30 minutes to 7 days. The IHS further classifies tension-type headache into episodic or chronic. Episodic tension-type headache patients have a history of at least 10 previous headache episodes that last from 30 minutes to 7 days and do not occur more than 180 days out of the year. Also, for the headache to be classified as an episodic tension-type headache, the patient must present with at least two of the following signs or symptoms:

- No nausea or vomiting
- Vise-like, pressing, tightening-type pain that doesn't pulsate and is located bilaterally
- Intensity that is mild to moderate
- Sensitivity to light or sound but not to both light and sound
- The head pain is not aggravated by physical activity

Chronic tension-type headaches occur on average 15 days per month for at least 6 months. Also, chronic tension-type headache must meet the previously mentioned signs and symptoms associated with episodic tension-type headaches.

The pain associated with tension-type headache is usually bilateral and may be described as aching, squeezing, pressure, or vise-like. The pain is usually located in the frontal, temporal, and occipital regions of the head. The pain will often radiate to the neck and shoulders. There is no nausea or vomiting associated with the headache; however, the patient may complain of anorexia (absence of appetite). The pain is more throbbing in nature and the onset is more gradual as compared to a migraine. Also, the tension-type headache has more variability in the duration of the pain, has a more consistent quality, and is normally less severe when compared to a migraine.

History findings may include a variable duration, no nausea or vomiting, avoidance of light (photophobia), insomnia, commonly present on rising or shortly thereafter, no aggravation by physical activity, difficulty in concentrating, no warning symptoms, and history of similar headaches. The pain is frequently described as "fullness," "a band around my head," "tight or squeezing," "pressure," or "vise-like." Physical examination may reveal normal vital signs, tenderness in the cervical area, trapezius muscle spasm, tenderness to the scalp, and pain on flexion of the paracervical muscles. This must be distinguished from pain associated with nuchal rigidity found in meningitis. Assessing for meningeal nuchal rigidity will be discussed in more detail later in the chapter.

When conducting the scene size-up, be cognizant of medications the patient may be taking to treat the headaches. Nonsteroidal antiinflammatory drugs (NSAIDs) may be used to alleviate headache pain by inhibiting prostaglandin synthesis, reducing the release of serotonin, and blocking platelet aggregation. The following NSAIDs may be prescribed to manage headaches in these patients:

- Ibuprofen (Ibuprin, Advil, Motrin)
- Naproxen (Naprosyn)
- Ketoprofen (Oruvail, Orudis, Actron)
- Ketorolac (Toradol)

Acetylsalicylic acid (aspirin) is also used for management of headaches in these patients. Acetylsalicylic acid relieves the headache by inhibiting prostaglandin production. Common trade names of aspirin you might find the patient taking include Anacin, Ascriptin, Bayer Aspirin, and Bufferin.

Other agents, such as barbiturates and narcotic analgesics, may be prescribed to control headache pain. Fioricet is a combination of acetaminophen, butalbital, and caffeine. Fiorinal is a combination of aspirin, butalbital, and caffeine. The combination of the acetaminophen or aspirin and a barbiturate is to relieve pain and to induce sleep. The caffeine is used to increase gastrointestinal absorption of the drugs. Analgesics may include Percocet (acetaminophen and oxycodone) and simple acetaminophen (Tylenol, Panadol, Aspirin-Free Anacin). Preventative therapy drugs might include antidepressants, beta-blockers, and anticonvulsants.

Migraine

Migraine headaches are recurrent headaches that affect primarily females (in a 3:1 female-to-male ratio) and typically begin during childhood; however, they may occur during or after puberty. In childhood, migraines are more common in boys than in girls. Almost all patients will have an onset of migraines before the age of 30, even though the headaches will continue to recur at any age. It is very unusual for the initial migraine headache onset to occur after age 50. Migraines typically decrease in frequency and intensity as the patient ages. Migraines present with variable severity and an inconsistent duration. The pain is normally (60 to 70 percent) unilateral. Unilateral headache pain is also known as hemicrania. Additionally, the patient may complain of nausea and may report vomiting. Some migraines are preceded by or associated with neurologic or mood disturbances.

Almost all patients with migraines will have an onset before the age of 30, even though the headaches will continue to recur at any age.

The IHS classifies migraines as 1) migraine without aura, once known as a common migraine; and 2) migraine with aura, previously termed a classic migraine. The migraine without aura (common migraine) accounts for approximately 80 percent of all migraine headaches. The prodrome (early symptoms of disease or condition) is normally vague and varies in duration. The patient typically presents with anorexia, nausea, vomiting, malaise, light sensitivity (photophobia), and sound sensitivity (sonophobia). Common migraines are not normally associated with visual changes or defects.

The migraine with aura, or classic migraine, has a much lower incidence, accounting for approximately only 12 percent of all migraine headaches. The migraine with aura has a well-defined prodromal phase that lasts up to 1 hour prior to the onset of the headache itself. There are a number of different auras that may occur in the prodromal phase (Table 12-1). The most common is a temporary condition described as a localized area of blindness edged by brilliantly colored shimmering lights (scintillating scotoma) or blindness or a defect in the right or left halves of the visual fields of both eyes (homonymous hemianopia), which may progress from the ventral visual fields to the periphery.

TABLE 12-1 Other Auras Associated with Migraine

Other Auras Associated with Migraine
Negative scotoma (blind spots)
Positive scotoma (bright shimmering lights)
Luminous appearance before the eyes
Unilateral weakness
Unilateral numbness or tingling (paresthesias)
Aphasia or other speech difficulty
Visual or auditory hallucinations
Double vision (diplopia)
Ataxia (uncoordination)
Syncope

A migraine is primarily associated with a vasodilatory problem, but also involves a significant inflammation response. Historically, migraines are believed to occur from a phase in which the intracranial arteries constrict, causing ischemia. This ischemia produces the typical prodromal symptoms such as lights, haze, and zig-zag lines. Subsequently, a vasodilatation phase occurs that affects primarily the extracranial arteries and causes a "steal syndrome," where blood is shunted away from the cortical brain areas and into the dilated extracranial arteries, which leads to some of the characteristic signs and symptoms of a migraine. The other signs and symptoms are believed to occur as a result of neuroactive substances that are released as the migraine progresses.

More recent migraine theories are based on serotonergic transmission abnormalities, trigeminovascular neuronal transmission dysfunction, vascular structures, neurogenic inflammation, and platelet aggregation. Serotonin and dopamine are believed to play a major role in migraine pathophysiology. Dopamine receptor stimulation is associated with some of the signs and symptoms of migraine such as nausea, vomiting, yawning, irritability, and hyperactivity. Dopamine is believed to be the migraine "protagonist" because it is implicated in precipitating the migraine, whereas serotonin is termed the migraine "antagonist" because drugs that stimulate serotonin receptors in the brain can reduce or relieve symptoms of a migraine.

The typical migraine is described as unilateral, throbbing or pulsatile, having a gradual onset that progresses in intensity, having variable prodromal symptoms, associated with nausea and vomiting, and involving light and sound sensitivity. There is normally a positive past history of headache and a family history of migraines. If any of the following characteristics are found, you should consider a condition other than a migraine and search for another etiology of the headache: 1) nuchal rigidity; 2) complaint of "worst" headache; 3) change in the typical migraine presentation for that patient; 4) acute onset of headache with neurologic deficits associated with headache; 5) pain that worsens over days or weeks; 6) onset of fever, nausea, and vomiting without systemic signs of illness; or 7) first-time headache.

During the physical examination, pay attention to indications of a more serious etiology of the headache. Fever may be an indication of meningitis, sinus infection, encephalitis, or brain abscess. Severe hypertension may be the cause of the pain and can lead to an intracerebral hemorrhage or stroke. Tachypnea may be an indication of hypoxia, hypercarbia, carbon monoxide poisoning, or cyanide exposure. Pupillary changes may indicate intracranial pathology. Flexion rigidity may indicate meningitis. A thorough neurologic examination should be performed on patients complaining of headache.

During the physical examination of the suspected migraine patient, pay attention to indications of a more serious etiology of the headache.

Other migraine variants that have been discussed in the literature present with a variety of signs and symptoms that may mimic other, more serious conditions. Prehospital personnel should always treat the more serious possible condition first. Examples are hemiplegic, ophthalmic, and basilar headaches.

A hemiplegic migraine can produce hemiparesis that ranges from simple weakness to one side of the body to full hemiplegia. The neurologic deficit may persist for a period of time following resolution of the headache. When presented with a patient who complains of headache with hemiparesis or hemiplegia, you move closer to a probability of stroke, while keeping hemiplegic headache as a strong possibility or as a potential probability. You should manage this patient as a stroke patient with supportive care and rapid transport.

An ophthalmoplegic migraine is rare and seen more in young adults. The patient presents with headache, typically less intense than a classic migraine and retroorbital, with extraocular paralysis, drooping eyelid, ocular muscle weakness, and a possible pupil change. It is important in patients complaining of headache to assess the extraocular muscle movements in addition to pupillary response. This can be achieved by placing your finger in front of the patient's face and having him follow it in 90-degree direction up, down, to each side, and then in a full circle. You should note any jerky movement or lag in movement of the globe.

A basilar migraine is most common in young females, typically teenagers or those in their twenties. A basilar artery migraine, also known as a vertebrobasilar migraine, may present with severe headache and a sudden onset of neurologic deficits that include vertigo, dysarthria (difficulty in speaking due to facial muscle paralysis), ataxia (uncoordination), paresthesias (abnormal sensations), and visual disturbances. The neurologic deficits are prodromal (precede the headache) and do not persist after the headache is resolved. The headache normally lasts from 6 to 8 hours. Neurologic deficits that persist after the headache has resolved are an indication of a much more serious intracranial pathology.

Migraine equivalent is a condition in which the patient suffers autonomic system discharge during the episode. The patient may present with minimal headache and tachycardia, edema, vertigo, chest pain, and thoracic, abdominal, or pelvic pain.

Any migraine that persists for greater than 24 hours is referred to as status migrainosus. This headache is harder to control. An implication for prehospital care providers is that these patients may present as dehydrated from the long duration of the headache episodes where the patient is typically anorexic or suffering from repeated vomiting.

Patients who suffer migraines are commonly referred to as migraineurs. Migraineurs will typically suffer a migraine after being exposed to a trigger. Common triggers include smoking, foods (chocolate, cheese, nuts, MSG, alcohol), a birth control pill, missing a meal, a change in sleep pattern, stress, and tension. Also, certain conditions or diseases such as epilepsy, Tourette syndrome, depression, anxiety, ischemic stroke, and cerebral amyloid angiopathy predispose the patient to migraines.

Numerous drugs are available that will rapidly and effectively relieve migraine headache. One of the most effective groups of drugs used to stop migraines is the triptans. Triptans, also known as serotonin receptor agonists, specifically target and stimulate the serotonin receptors (5-HT1), which produces a vasconstrictive effect in the cranial arteries. This will also suppress the inflammation associated with migraine headaches. The following are triptans used to abort migraine headaches:

- Sumatriptan (Imitrex, Imigran)
- Frovatriptan (Frova)
- Eletriptan (Relpax)
- Naratriptan (Amerge, Naramig)
- Zomitriptan (Zomig, Zomig-ZMT)

Nontriptan agents may also be used to stop migraine headaches. These agents also act on serotonin receptors and may also block alpha-adrenergic receptors, resulting in cranial artery constriction. These drugs include ergotamine tartrate (Cafergot, Cafatine, Cafetrate), dihydroergotamine (D.H.E. 45, Migranal Nasal Spray), and isometheptene dichloralphenazone acetaminophen (Midrin). Other drugs that are used in management of tension-type headaches may also be used in management of migraine headaches.

Patient Assessment

As always, the primary focus of the patient assessment is to identify and manage any immediately life-threatening conditions prior to attempting to establish a differential field diagnosis of the etiology of the headache. The severity of the headache, its progress, and the accompanying signs and symptoms will be invaluable in guiding decisions on further evaluation and development of an emergency care plan.

The severity of the headache, its progress, and the accompanying signs and symptoms will be invaluable in guiding further evaluation and emergency care.

Conduct a scene size-up and initial assessment, followed by a history and physical exam. If the patient is responsive, gather the history first and use that information to guide the physical assessment, determination of the probable cause, and emergency care. In an unresponsive patient, you will proceed directly to the physical assessment, using the objective information from the physical exam findings as the basis for determining the probable etiology and for emergency medical care. An ongoing assessment is vital to identifying deterioration or improvement.

Scene Size-Up

It is first necessary to rule out a traumatic cause of the headache. Inspect the scene for evidence of a mechanism of injury consistent with head injury, such as a fall or blow to the head that may have produced an intracranial or intracerebral hemorrhage. Any patient who suffers any type of trauma to the head with subsequent onset of headache should be evaluated in the emergency department, especially the elderly.

Clinical Insight

Any patient who suffers any type of trauma to the head with subsequent onset of headache should be evaluated in the emergency department, especially the elderly.

Keep in mind that toxic inhalation can be the etiology of a headache, so be mindful of your own safety. Your suspicion of toxic inhalation should be heightened if the patient has been working with chemicals, is in a confined space or poorly ventilated area, or is in an area near a furnace or other combustion device that may be emitting carbon monoxide fumes. Patients complain of dizziness, nausea, and recurring headaches that are worst when wakening and subside once the patient leaves the structure or environment. The scene may also provide clues to the patient's associated complaints. For example, look for a bucket next to the bed or chair, which would suggest nausea and vomiting. Evidence of chronic conditions may also be noted, for example, a hospital-type bed or an oxygen tank or concentrator.

Initial Assessment

The initial assessment is designed to identify and manage immediate life threats to the airway, breathing status, and circulation. Because headache may be associated with significant illness or injury, it is imperative that the airway, breathing, and circulation be carefully assessed and closely monitored.

As you form your general impression, look for obvious trauma to the head, abnormal posturing, or vomitus. In assessing the mental status, note any decrease in cognition. An altered mental status, slurred speech, or neurologic deficit associated with headache is a significant indication of intracranial pathology, such as subarachnoid hemorrhage, stroke, subdural hematoma, encephalitis, or meningitis. (For detailed discussion of these conditions, see Chapter 7, Altered Mental Status.)

If the patient is talking with you and responding, you should expect the airway to be open. However, you should assume that any patient with an altered mental status will not be able to maintain his own airway. If necessary, establish an airway with a manual maneuver and an airway adjunct. Because vomiting is commonly associated with increased ICP and headaches in general, be prepared to suction. If no spinal injury is suspected, place the patient in a lateral recumbent position to facilitate removal of secretions and vomitus and reduce the incidence of aspiration. If profuse vomiting is present, the airway cannot be maintained, or the patient is completely unresponsive, consider tracheal intubation.

Abnormal breathing patterns associated with headache may be another indication of increased ICP associated with intracranial pathology or toxic inhalation. Respiratory patterns such as Cheyne-Stokes, Biot's, and central neurogenic hyperventilation may be found. (See the descriptions and illustrations of abnormal respiratory patterns in Chapters 5 and 7.) Carefully assess the minute ventilation, and provide positive-pressure ventilation with supplemental oxygen if an inadequate tidal volume or abnormal rate is present. Tachypnea may be an indication of hypoxia, which in turn may be causing the head pain. Significant headache can also be produced by such respiratory-related conditions as carbon monoxide poisoning, pulmonary embolus, acute exacerbation of emphysema or chronic bronchitis, cyanide poisoning, or states of decreased oxygenation found in conditions such as anemia.

Abnormal breathing patterns associated with headache may be another indication of increased intracranial pressure.

Assess the circulatory status of the patient. The pulse is typically elevated as a response to pain; therefore, tachycardia may be merely a response to the headache pain and not a symptom of an underlying condition. A slow pulse may indicate increased ICP. Warm skin may indicate fever, which is commonly accompanied by headache, and may be a sign of an infectious process as the etiology of the headache. A patient who is suffering a headache and has associated signs or symptoms of fever, rash, stiff neck or nuchal rigidity should be transported and evaluated for meningitis, encephalitis, and Lyme disease. Any patient who is older than 50 years of age and is experiencing pain in the temporal region should be evaluated for temporal arteritis. In addition, new-onset headache in patient older than 50 years of age may be an indication of a brain tumor. HIV-positive or cancer patients with new-onset headache need further evaluation to rule out meningitis, brain abscess, or brain lesion.

Clinical Insight

Be aware of possible secondary etiologies for headache in these circumstances:

- Headache with associated fever, rash, stiff neck, or nuchal rigidity—possible etiologies: meningitis, encephalitis, Lyme disease
- Temporal pain in patient older than 50—possible etiology: temporal arteritis
- New-onset headache in patient older than 50—possible etiology: brain tumor
- HIV-positive or cancer patient with new-onset headache—possible etiologies: meningitis, brain abscess, brain lesion

Any patient who presents with a headache associated with an altered mental status or with a disorder of the airway, breathing, or circulation must be considered a priority patient, and expeditious transport should be considered following your rapid medical assessment. Continuous reassessment of the mental status, airway, breathing, and circulation must be conducted to identify further deterioration or improvement trends.

Focused History and Physical Exam

If the patient is responsive and able to provide information regarding the present illness, first gather a history, and then conduct a physical exam. If the patient is unresponsive, conduct a rapid medical assessment, including a complete head-to-toe exam, prior to gathering history information from relatives or bystanders at the scene.

History Information gathered from the history is extremely important when evaluating the patient complaining of a headache. This information can assist you in determining the potential seriousness and etiology of the head pain. It is very important to determine whether the headache is typical or if it is atypical, which may indicate a more serious illness, such as intracranial bleeding. If the patient complains of a typical headache pattern, seek information about any recent change in the frequency or severity of the headaches. When evaluating a patient who has a chronic headache pattern, ask the following questions:

It is very important to determine whether the headache is typical or atypical, which may indicate a more serious illness.

1. ***Do you have a prescribed medication for your headache?***
2. ***How long have you been experiencing the headaches?***
3. ***How have the headaches changed?***
4. ***How often do the headaches occur?***
5. ***How long does each headache typically last?***
6. ***Does it hurt in one particular area?***
7. ***How would you describe the headache pain?***
8. ***How quickly does the headache reach its maximum intensity?***
9. ***Do you suffer any other complaints during the headaches?***
10. ***Is there anything that triggers the headaches?***
11. ***Do you have any warning symptoms that the headache is coming on?***
12. ***What makes the headache worse or better?***
13. ***When did the headache pattern change?***

Patients who complain of a sudden or abrupt onset of head pain are more likely to be suffering from a serious cause than those who have chronic headaches. Thus, the sudden onset and not the intensity of the pain may be the best indication that a pathological etiology other than headache is the cause of the head pain. Continuous headaches that are bilateral are typically associated with muscle tension and spasm, whereas headaches that come and go are usually migraine or cluster headaches. A throbbing headache most often has a vascular etiology. Migraine headaches are more often associated with nausea, vomiting, and visual disturbances. Patients who are experiencing headaches due to an increase in ICP may experience pain that worsens when they perform an activity that increases pressure, such as bending over, lifting, or coughing.

Clinical Insight

Sudden onset rather than intensity may be the best indication of a pathological etiology of head pain.

When gathering a history, consider the following key items, using the OPQRST format:

1. *Onset.* Determine speed of onset and its relationship to other signs and symptoms. Headaches that recur over a period of years are usually due to tension or vascular etiologies. A headache that is severe with an abrupt onset, especially when associated with altered mental status, usually indicates a significant pathology such as intracranial hemorrhage, infarction, or meningitis.
2. *Palliation/Provocation.* Headache of a vascular or inflammatory etiology is aggravated by rapid movements or movements that increase ICP or produce sudden jarring, such as coughing, sneezing, or walking. Also, foods such as

red wines, bananas, and cheese are thought to precipitate migraine headaches.

Oral contraceptives may increase migraine headaches in some patients. Also, patients who use nitrates for coronary artery disease may suffer throbbing vascular headaches. Other medical conditions such as anemia, severe hypertension, and withdrawal from certain medications may precipitate headaches. Incidentally, 80 percent of patients with migraines have a family history of migraines.

Inquire if the patient has taken any medication, such as aspirin or ibuprofen or a prescribed headache medication, and whether the medication has alleviated the pain.

3. *Quality.* Attempt to determine what the pain feels like, although this is very subjective and often difficult for patients to describe. Headaches of a vascular origin caused by vasodilation, hypertension, and fever produce a pulsating pain. Trigeminal neuralgia is usually associated with a stabbing facial pain that is transient. Brain tumors usually produce a constant, aching pain. Cluster headaches are usually very intense and recur periodically, with episodes usually lasting from 20 minutes to 2 hours.
4. *Radiation/Location.* The location of pain may be helpful in indicating the etiology. Migraine headaches are typically localized to one side of the head, but will occur on various sides during different headaches. If the headaches are recurrent and throbbing and occur on the same side during each attack, suspect the possibility of an intracranial mass, aneurysm, vascular malformation, cluster headaches, focal irritation and disease of structures of the face and neck, or trigeminal neuralgia. If the flow of the cerebrospinal fluid is interrupted, bilateral headache may occur. Tension-type headaches are typically bilateral in the frontal and occipital regions.

   The location of the pain will not be reliable in determining the site of the lesion because compression and displacement of vessels with pain-sensitive structures may occur at a distance from the actual lesion.

The location of headache pain is not a reliable indicator of the site of a lesion. The quality and intensity of headache pain is not a reliable indicator of the etiology or the severity of the patient's condition.

5. *Severity.* The severity of pain is usually measured on a scale of 1 to 10. The patient is asked to judge the intensity of the pain by assigning it a number, with 1 being little or no pain and 10 being very intense pain. However, the severity of headache pain is not a good indicator for the seriousness of the condition; a severe headache does not necessarily indicate a significant condition. The headaches that usually produce the most severe pain are trigeminal neuralgia, glossopharyngeal neuralgia, and cluster headaches.
6. *Time.* Migraine and tension headaches typically begin before the age of 40. If an elderly patient is complaining of a new onset of headache, take the complaint seriously because it usually indicates significant illness. Also, determine whether the onset was associated with an aura or prodromal (warning symptom) phase. The patient may have experienced transient autonomic, visual, motor, or sensory phenomena—symptoms such as blurred vision, light spots, or flashes. As the aura fades, the headache begins. Also, determine whether the onset was correlated with ingestion of certain foods or medications or with the menstrual cycle in women.

Headache in the elderly should always be taken very seriously.

7. *Associated Complaints.* The most significant associated sign, indicating severe illness, is an altered mental status. Nausea, vomiting, and anorexia are also common associated complaints. Other associated complaints may include flushing of the forehead, tearing, and nasal congestion. Stiff neck and altered mental status with headache strongly indicates a potential subarachnoid hemorrhage or meningeal irritation.

An altered mental status is the most significant sign that may be associated with a headache.

Physical Examination Most of the information that will differentiate a patient requiring immediate intervention from one who needs less emergent care will be determined either in the initial assessment or through the history. However, other more subtle indicators of significant pathology associated with headache may be found during the physical examination.

Inspect and palpate the head for any evidence of trauma. Inspect for contusions, abrasions, lacerations, deformity, and ecchymosis. Palpation of the head, neck, or face may actually elicit a tender response by the patient. Patients may complain of pain to the midface, teeth and gums, or temporomandibular joint. Patients with unilateral temporal pain or headache onset after age 50 may be suffering from temporal arteritis. Inspect the eyes for pupillary equality and responsiveness. Unequal, fixed, or dilated pupils may indicate head injury or severe intracranial hemorrhage. Inspect the ears, nose, and mouth for discharge of blood and, potentially, cerebrospinal fluid. Cerebrospinal fluid coming from the ears, nose, or mouth would indicate a skull fracture and possible brain injury. Ear pain may be an indication of otitis media or otitis externa.

Inspect and palpate the neck for evidence of injury. Nuchal rigidity (stiffness in the neck) is usually an indication of cervical spondylosis (arthritis), meningitis, encephalitis, or subarachnoid hemorrhage. The rigidity produced by meningeal irritation is usually found on flexion of the head and neck. You would place your hand under the head of the patient and try to flex the neck by moving it forward. Diffuse irritation of the cervical nerve roots associated with meningeal irritation will produce resistance as the neck is flexed. When flexing the neck to test for nuchal rigidity, also pay attention to the legs. If the knees flex during the nuchal flexion maneuver, it is an indication of diffuse meningeal irritation in the spinal nerve roots. This is known as Brudzinski's sign.

Also, when examining the lower extremities in the suspected meningitis patient, assess for Kernig's sign. This is done by placing the patient supine, flexing both the knee and hip on one side, and then extending the knee while the hip is still flexed. The patient will experience pain in the posterior thigh due to hamstring spasm and difficulty in extending the knee. If severe meningeal irritation exists, the opposite knee may actually flex during the test for Kernig's sign. Rarely does rotary movement produce pain. Muscular tension may produce some neck stiffness; however, it is much milder than the true nuchal rigidity associated with meningeal irritation. In a responsive patient, have him touch his chin to his chest to elicit a response of pain or stiffness.

Examine the eyes for signs of cranial nerve abnormality. Ptosis (drooping of the eyelid), dysconjugate gaze, abnormal extraocular eye movements, abnormal pupillary reactivity, or diminished visual acuity or field of vision are typical of cranial nerve deficits associated with intracranial pathology. However, migraines also are associated with visual defects. Ophthalmic ophthalmoplegia migraines may produce extraocular paralysis, eyelid droop, and pupillary changes.

Assess the extremities for pulses and motor and sensory function. Abnormal motor function is typically associated with a cerebral vascular lesion, which usually produces hemiplegic dysfunction. Hemiplegic migraines may produce muscular weakness or complete hemiplegia. The deficit may persist after the headache is resolved. Sensory deficits are not as informative as motor dysfunction in the neurologic examination. Posturing in response to noxious stimuli indicates brainstem involvement and a serious etiology of associated headache in an unresponsive patient.

Vital Signs Closely monitor the blood pressure, minute ventilation, and heart rate. Pain may normally increase the blood pressure, heart rate, and respiratory rate. Head pain with a diastolic blood pressure of greater than 120 mmHg indicates a true hypertensive headache. If associated with altered mental status or other neurologic dysfunction, a significant neurologic emergency exists.

Cushing's reflex (the body's attempt to maintain cerebral perfusion in the presence of ICP and cerebral edema) may be present. Look for increased systolic blood pressure (which results in a widened pulse pressure), decreased heart rate, and an abnormal respiratory pattern such as Cheyne-Stokes, central neurogenic hyperventilation, Biot's respirations, or apnea. In addition, respiratory changes also suggest a toxic or metabolic etiology of the head pain.

An elevated heart rate would be expected in response to severe pain; thus, tachycardia is of little significance when evaluating the headache patient. An elevated respiratory rate may suggest an etiology of headache associated with hypoxia, carbon monoxide poisoning, pulmonary embolus, cyanide poisoning, or exacerbation of a preexisting respiratory disease.

An elevated heart rate would be expected in response to severe pain.

Warm skin may be a result of fever. Meningitis, encephalitis, or abscess of the brain may present with headache and fever. These patients may also present with an altered mental status, which is a serious concern.

Laboratory Data If the patient with headache also has an altered mental status, it is necessary to gather as much information from laboratory data as possible to determine the etiology of the headache and mental status alteration. In the prehospital setting, test the blood glucose level to determine whether the patient is hypoglycemic, normoglycemic, or hyperglycemic. HHNS, also known as hyperglycemic hyperosmolar nonketotic coma, or DKA may produce alteration in mental status. Other laboratory data to collect would include arterial blood gases, hemoglobin, and white blood cell count. This information would be helpful in determining headache associated with anemia, hypoxia, and infectious processes.

Ongoing Assessment

Continually monitor the mental status, airway, and breathing and reassess vital signs. Note any trends to identify improvement or deterioration in the patient's condition.

Differential Diagnosis

Once immediate life threats have been initially managed, consider the potential cause of the headache and alteration in physiological status (Table 12-2). If the condition is life threatening and not simply a headache, further intervention and expeditious transport may be necessary.

The following indications should increase your suspicions that you are dealing with a significant etiology of the headache and warrant special consideration in assessment and management (Table 12-3):

- Headache associated with neurologic dysfunction, behavior change, seizure, or altered mental status
- Unfamiliar headache with an abrupt onset or first-time headache

TABLE 12-2 Serious Causes of Headache

Intracranial tumor	Carbon monoxide or other toxic inhalation
Subarachnoid hemorrhage	Loss of cerebrospinal fluid
Intracerebral hemorrhage	Fever
Subdural hematoma	Hypoxemia
Meningitis	Anemia
Preeclampsia	Stroke
Hypertension	Depression
Hypoglycemia	Cyanide poisoning
Brain abscess	

- "Worst headache" ever experienced
- Progressively worsening pain over days to weeks
- Fever, nausea, and vomiting without signs of systemic disease
- Worsening severity of headache when performing activities that increase ICP such as coughing, sneezing, and bending over
- Fever or stiff neck associated with headache
- Change in the quality of a chronic headache
- Headache associated with marked elevation of blood pressure

As noted earlier, headache in the elderly should always be taken very seriously. Subdural hematomas and intracranial lesions are more prevalent in the elderly. Also, keep in mind that headaches may also be due to depression and other emotional disorders.

Subarachnoid Hemorrhage

Subarachnoid hemorrhage most commonly occurs between 20 and 40 years of age. A predominant symptom is an acute onset of severe headache that is typically described as the "worst headache" the patient has ever suffered. Subarachnoid hemorrhage is usually due to an aneurysm of one of the large intracranial arteries in the circle of Willis that ruptures and leaks blood into the subarachnoid space. The onset of signs and symptoms is usually rapid. Most patients have no warning, although some patients report a sentinel headache associated with a warning leak or herald bleed days to weeks before a major bleed. Typically, the hemorrhage occurs while the patient is active.

The severe headache usually reaches its maximum intensity within a few minutes of onset. The pain is generalized and not isolated to one area of the head. The patient may lose consciousness very abruptly as a result of the increase in ICP. Some patients who are unconscious display extensor rigidity that is similar to decerebrate posturing. Also, look for bradycardia induced by vagal compression and respiratory arrest.

During the period of consciousness, the patient will complain of severe headache, stiff neck, and photophobia (sensitivity to light). You may also find

TABLE 12-3 Headache: Indications of Significant Etiology

Headache associated with . . .	
Neurologic dysfunction	Unfamiliar headache with abrupt onset
Altered mental status	Worsening with coughing, sneezing, bending over
Behavior change	Fever or stiff neck
Seizure	Change in quality of a chronic headache

diaphoresis, tachycardia, and tachypnea. A warning headache (sentinel bleed) produces a distinctive "thunderclap" headache that precedes the subarachnoid hemorrhage by days to weeks. It is caused by a small leak of blood into the arachnoid space, bleeding into the wall of the aneurysm, or thrombosis at the site of the aneurysm.

It is imperative to establish and maintain an airway. Consider tracheal intubation. Assist ventilation at a rate of 10 to 12 ventilations per minute if breathing is inadequate, at a rate of 20 ventilations per minute if evidence of brain herniation is present (follow local protocol). Maximize oxygenation by providing supplemental oxygen while ventilating or by applying a nonrebreather mask to the patient who is breathing adequately. Insert an intravenous line of normal saline running at a keep-open rate or establish a saline lock. Do not administer any glucose-containing solutions unless the patient is found to be hypoglycemic because these may worsen neurologic injury.

Consult medical direction to consider management of hypertension, especially if the systolic blood pressure is greater than 200 mmHg and the diastolic blood pressure is greater than 140 mmHg. Local protocol for antihypertensive therapy may include sublingual or intravenous nitroglycerin and sodium nitroprusside. Careful consideration must be given to antihypertensive management because, in stroke patients, this therapy may be strictly contraindicated. Rapid transport is necessary.

Consult medical direction to consider management of hypertension.

Intracerebral Hemorrhage

Rupture of a medium artery in the brain tissue will usually produce a clot that compresses and distorts the surrounding brain tissue. A sudden increase in ICP is a result of added volume within the closed cranial vault. The clinical signs and symptoms are primarily due to the cerebral edema and the mass effect of the clot because many of the bleeds will have stopped within a short period of time. The most common predisposing factor for cerebral hemorrhage is chronic hypertension.

Patients usually complain of a severe headache at the outset that continually worsens. The pain is varied, depending on the site of the bleeding. It may be generalized or a dull discomfort that is ipsilateral (on the same side as the hemorrhage). The patient will be more disturbed by the neurologic deficit associated with the hemorrhage than by the headache itself. The neurologic deficit is directly correlated to the location and size of the lesion.

Management of the patient would be the same as in the subarachnoid hemorrhage, discussed previously. Pay particular attention to the airway, breathing, and circulation. Correct any immediately life-threatening conditions while providing supportive care.

Intracranial Mass

Headaches due to mass lesions are varied. The pain is due to distortion of the meninges, innervated blood vessels or, less likely, an increase in ICP. Head pain associated with subarachnoid hemorrhage, sinusitis, and migraine are usually more severe than with an intracranial mass; however, the headache due to intracranial mass is more persistent. The pain is chronic, present on wakening, and worsens with straining activity, coughing, or any other activity that will increase ICP.

Management is limited to supportive care. Pay particular attention to reversing any life threats to the airway, breathing, and circulation.

Subdural Hematoma

Subdural hematoma is caused by bleeding beneath the dura mater. It is usually due to trauma. The event may be very minor and not memorable, especially in the elderly. Patients younger than 35 years of age usually require a much more significant blunt force to cause subdural hematoma. This age group will remember the trauma, unless suffering amnesia from a concussion or alteration in mental status from intoxication or drug influence. Focal neurologic dysfunction is a result of compression of brain tissue, whereas confusion, disorientation, and stupor are associated with increased ICP.

A chronic subdural hematoma occurs at least 2 weeks after the injury.

A chronic subdural hematoma occurs at least 2 weeks after the injury. The headache is usually transient and the neurologic deficit worsens and improves. The level of consciousness will also fluctuate, as will the associated signs and symptoms. The patient's intellectual ability may also be impaired.

Management of the patient is as previously described. Abolish any immediate life threats and provide continuous supportive care.

Meningitis

Meningitis is an infection and inflammation of the meninges, which are the fibrous coverings of the brain and spinal cord. Meningitis can be caused by bacterial, viral, or fungal infections. The patient usually presents with headache, fever, nausea, vomiting, light sensitivity, chills, and nuchal rigidity. Alteration in mental status is an ominous sign of increasing ICP. The classic triad in bacterial meningitis is fever, nuchal rigidity, and change in mental status. Mental status change may include irritability, confusion, lethargy, decreased response to pain, or coma. Seizures are more common in patients infected with *Streptococcus pneumoniae.* A rash may appear as maculopapular, petechial, or purpuric. Brudzinski's sign and Kernig's sign may be produced on examination.

Life threats to the airway, breathing, and circulation should be managed as previously noted. Be sure to take the necessary body substance isolation precautions because certain forms of meningitis are contagious, especially those of a bacterial etiology. Masks and gloves should be worn when dealing with patients with suspected meningitis. Initiate an intravenous line with normal saline and provide other supportive management. Place the patient in the recovery position to facilitate protection of the airway.

Preeclampsia

Preeclampsia, also known as toxemia in pregnancy, is typically a third-trimester complication that is associated with hypertension, proteinuria, and excessive edema. Headache and visual disturbances are common complaints of the patient. When seizures occur, the condition is known as eclampsia. Provide supportive care and expeditious transport, with gentle handling to avoid triggering seizures. Seizures are typically treated with magnesium sulfate.

Carbon Monoxide Poisoning

Patients who have inhaled carbon monoxide may present with headache, dizziness, dyspnea, visual disturbances, confusion, syncope, nausea, vomiting, altered mental status, tinnitus, chest pain, disorientation, and seizures. Headache is a very common sign. Provide supportive care, paying particular attention to the airway and ventilation status. Provide 100 percent oxygen to the patient—via positive-pressure ventilation and a reservoir device if the patient is not breathing adequately or by nonrebreather mask if adequate breathing is present. Initiate an intravenous line of normal saline, and apply a continuous ECG monitor. Provide supportive care as necessary.

Brain or Parameningeal Abscess

An abscess of the brain or parameningeal tissue can produce a variety of signs and symptoms; however, some patients may remain asymptomatic and present with no abnormal physical findings on examination. This is especially true of patients who are immunocompromised, who may look well but are very ill clinically. History and risk factors are key in differential diagnosis of brain or parameningeal abscess. Predisposing factors associated with the abscess are infectious etiologies such as otitis media, mastoiditis, sinusitis, endocarditis and congenital heart disease, and dental infection. Other predisposing factors include previous head injury, immunosuppression therapy, steroid use, and previous surgical procedure.

Some patients with brain abscess may remain asymptomatic and present with no abnormal physical findings on examination.

The patient may present with headache, focal neurologic deficit, nausea, vomiting, coma, seizure, behavioral disturbances, and personality changes. Physical examination may reveal fever, meningismus (signs of meningitis without actual meningeal inflammation), eyelid edema, and focal neurologic deficits (mild hemiparesis is the most common). The signs and symptoms have a tendency to progress rapidly in these patients. The patient is in need of high-dose intravenous antibiotics; thus, your treatment is primarily supportive.

Temporal Arteritis

Temporal arteritis, also known as giant cell arteritis, is an inflammatory disease of the external carotid arteries that most consistently affects the temporal artery. The condition is most common in patients older than 50 who present with severe headache as a common complaint. The headache can be unilateral in the temporal region or nontemporal. Other signs and symptoms include jaw pain, facial pain, decreased visual acuity or sudden loss of vision, diplopia, defects to the visual field, scalp tenderness, fever, and ptosis. Palpation over the temporal artery may reveal an abnormal cord-like, nodular, and tender temporal artery.

Temporal arteritis is very rare in African Americans and Asians. Females are affected at a rate two times greater than males. Failure to recognize and treat a patient with temporal arteritis may lead to blindness and cerebral infarction. Primary management includes steroids; thus, prehospital care is geared toward recognition and supportive care.

Management Priorities

Management priorities are focused on reversing any immediately life-threatening conditions associated with the airway, breathing, and circulation prior to attempting to establish a differential diagnosis. When considering a differential diagnosis, it is most important to identify those conditions that are life threatening, such as subarachnoid hemorrhage, intracranial mass, subdural hematoma, meningitis, hypertensive encephalopathy, preeclampsia, and carbon monoxide and other toxic poisonings.

If a head injury resulting from blunt or penetrating trauma is suspected, it is necessary to initiate manual inline spinal stabilization. If the patient has an altered mental status, open the airway using a jaw thrust maneuver. Insert an oropharyngeal or nasopharyngeal airway if the airway is difficult to maintain because of posterior displacement of the tongue. Inspect inside the mouth for evidence of vomitus, blood, or other secretions. Suction any substances from the mouth until it is clear. If no gag reflex is present, or if copious vomitus or blood is present in the airway, consider tracheal intubation. If the Glasgow coma score is less than 8, aggressive airway management with tracheal intubation should be performed. If increased ICP is suspected, consider premedication with 1 to 1.5 mg/kg of lidocaine prior to the laryngoscopy. This may reduce the sympathetic response and any associated increases in ICP.

Assess the respiratory rate and tidal volume. If either is inadequate, immediately begin positive-pressure ventilation. Supplemental oxygen must be provided when ventilating the patient. Consider controlled hyperventilation in patients with suspected increases in ICP who exhibit specific evidence of herniation (posturing, unequal size or reactivity of pupils with altered mental status, or dilated or fixed pupils). Hyperventilation must be controlled and will reduce the $PaCO_2$, vasoconstrict the cerebral vessels, reduce the cerebral blood volume, and reduce ICP. Hyperventilation should be conducted at 20 ventilations per minute with supplemental oxygenation. Extreme or uncontrolled hyperventilation may lead to excessive cerebral artery constriction and result in a reduced cerebral blood flow and cerebral perfusion pressure. If no signs of herniation are present, ventilate at 10 to 12 ventilations per minute.

Assess the respiratory rate and tidal volume. If either is inadequate, immediately begin positive-pressure ventilation with supplemental oxygen.

Clinical Insight

The following signs warrant ventilation at 20/minute:
- Unilateral or bilateral dilated pupil(s)
- Asymmetric pupil reactivity
- Nonpurposeful posturing (flexion or extension)

If the patient has an adequate respiratory status but is displaying other signs and symptoms, administer oxygen via a nonrebreather mask. If the patient is unable to tolerate the mask, coach him. If he still refuses, change to a nasal cannula.

Initiate an intravenous line of normal saline at a keep-open rate or establish a saline lock. Do not overhydrate the patient because this will worsen any cerebral edema and increase ICP. However, long-term headaches may precipitate dehydration in some patients. Draw blood for laboratory studies per local protocol. Do not use any glucose-containing solutions because research has shown worsened neurologic outcomes following administration of glucose. If the patient's blood glucose is less than 60 mg/dl with signs and symptoms of hypoglycemia, or less than 50 mg/dl with or without signs, administer 12.5 to 25 of 50 percent dextrose.

Place the patient on a continuous ECG monitor. Look for any potential dysrhythmias, and manage them accordingly.

Hypertension may be the etiology of the headache and may result in serious clinical consequences such as stroke. Nitroglycerin or sodium nitroprusside may be considered for acute antihypertensive therapy. If the diastolic blood pressure is greater than 140 mmHg, consider antihypertensive medications. Consult with medical direction and your protocol prior to managing any patient with hypertension. In occlusive stroke patients, antihypertensive therapy may not be indicated.

Place the patient in a position of comfort. If the patient has an altered mental status and no suspected spinal injury, place the patient in a recovery (lateral recumbent) position to facilitate drainage of any secretions or vomitus. Use of prehospital analgesics is not recommended. Consider oxygen therapy because high concentrations of oxygen may relieve opiate cluster headache. Toradol may be considered.

NAUSEA AND VOMITING

In the prehospital environment, you will encounter various complaints that are sometimes associated with serious illness and that other times are annoying but medically insignificant. Nausea and vomiting are in this category: complaints that may or may not be indicative of a serious underlying etiology. Nausea and vomiting are included in this chapter because, as discussed earlier, they so frequently occur with headache. Other etiologies of nausea and vomiting are addressed here.

Nausea is the unpleasant "queasy" sensation that often, but not always, precedes vomiting. (Vomiting can occur without being preceded by nausea; nausea can occur without leading to vomiting.) Vomiting occurs as a reflex caused by stimulation of the vomiting center in the medulla of the brain, which is responsible for motor control of vomiting. Stimulation of the vomiting center can arise from several different sources, including:

Nausea is the unpleasant "queasy" sensation that often, but not always, precedes vomiting.

- Stimulation of nerve fibers resulting from irritation or infection in the gastrointestinal viscera
- Stimulation of the vestibular system of the inner ear by motion or infection
- Disorders of the higher CNS or certain sights, smells, or emotional experiences
- Stimulation of chemoreceptors located outside the blood–brain barrier in the area postrema of the medulla by agents or conditions such as drugs, chemotherapeutic agents, radiation therapy, toxins, uremia, hypoxia, or acidosis

The process generally proceeds from nausea to retching to vomiting. Reverse peristalsis of the small bowel and positive intraabdominal and intrathoracic pressures result in expulsion of the gastric and intestinal contents from the mouth.

Remember that vomiting is a sign, not an illness in itself. It can be an indicator of very serious illness or injury, or it can be a simple condition with no further significance.

Although vomiting is a sign of another condition, vomiting itself can lead to serious complications. Some of these are life threatening. Conditions that may result from vomiting are severe dehydration, metabolic alkalosis, severe electrolyte disturbances (potassium, sodium, chloride), esophageal hemorrhage, gastric bleeding, and tear near the esophageal and gastric junction (Mallory-Weiss tear). There are numerous causes of vomiting that are not associated with the gastrointestinal tract (Table 12-4).

Cyclic Vomiting Syndrome

Cyclic vomiting syndrome (CVS) is a condition in which the patient experiences episodes of severe nausea and vomiting, which can last for hours or up to days, that alternate with periods when the patient has absolutely no symptoms. The condition

TABLE 12-4 Common Causes of Vomiting Not Associated with a GI Disorder

Common Causes of Vomiting Not Associated with a GI Disorder
Pneumonia
Meningitis
Sepsis
Diabetic ketoacidosis
Uremia
Toxicologic ingestion (digoxin, theophylline, aspirin, iron)
Hydrocephalus
Cerebral edema
Renal calculi
Ovarian or testicular torsion
Pregnancy
Rupture ectopic pregnancy
Myocardial ischemia
Stroke (posterior circulation)

was first identified in 1882 and has received much more attention since the mid-1990s. The pathophysiology of CVS is not well understood; however, there is some support for a brain-gut mechanism in which, some believe, the mechanisms are similar to those of migraine or involve neuronal hyperexcitability. Supporting this hypothesis is the fact that approximately 82 percent of patients with CVS also have a family history of migraines. Children with CVS who don't have a family history of migraines will typically develop migraines as they grow older. Many of the migraine triggers also trigger CVS. Migraines and CVS both have an abrupt onset, terminate quickly, and are followed by longer periods in which the patient is symptom free.

CVS occurs in all races. It is slightly more prevalent in females than males. The median age of onset is 5.2 years; however, it has been reported in neonates as young as 6 days and in elderly as old as 73 years. Because there is no test that leads to a diagnosis, CVS must be diagnosed based on a pattern of recurrence of the episodes. As already noted, the patients are symptom free between bouts of CVS.

Each episode of CVS is similar to the previous episode and creates a typical pattern of signs and symptoms. Most episodes begin around the same time of day and will have approximately the same duration and severity. The episodes occur more frequently in children and less often in adults; however, individual episodes have a tendency to last longer in the adult patient. Like migraines, CVS has triggers that are more easily identified in children than in adults. The triggers include stress, infection, excitement, colds, allergies, certain foods (chocolate, MSG, cheese), eating too much, eating just prior to bedtime, hot weather, motion sickness, menstruation, and physical exhaustion. The most common trigger is infection, usually associated with a sinus infection.

The pattern of CVS usually includes the following:

- Severe episodes of vomiting that recur
- Symptom-free periods that vary in length
- Vomiting episodes that span hours to days
- No diagnosis of the etiology of the vomiting
- Each episode is similar in time of onset, duration, intensity, frequency, and associated signs and symptoms
- Onset and cessation of the episode is abrupt
- Episodes are self-limited and resolve without any intervention

Associated signs and symptoms that patients may experience while suffering a CVS episode include

- Severe nausea
- Abdominal pain
- Motion sickness
- Headache
- Photophobia
- Lethargy
- Fever
- Pallor
- Diarrhea
- Dehydration
- Excessive salivation

The primary signs and symptom of CVS are severe vomiting, retching, and nausea. The vomiting episodes often begin early in the morning (2:00 A.M. to

4:00 A.M.) or on awakening. Patients may vomit up to 12 times per hour with a median of 6 times per hour. The duration of the episodes is anywhere from 1 to 5 days; however, cases have reported some episodes lasting up to 10 days.

The vomiting is often projectile with no retching. The vomit may contain bile, mucus, and blood. In addition to the vomiting, the patient may complain of abdominal pain. In some cases, the abdominal pain is severe enough to present as an acute abdomen. Retching and nausea also frequently accompany the vomiting. The nausea has been described by patients as being the worst symptom in the episodes. The patient typically gets no relief from the nausea, even after vomiting, and it doesn't resolve until the episode is completely over. Other signs to look for include fetal positioning, as well as turned-off lights, television, and radio as an attempt to lessen the nausea. About 30 percent of CVS patients will also experience fever and diarrhea. The patient may exhibit lethargy, which can be profound, and he will often look pale. Excessive salivation and drooling may be noted.

Patients who have been diagnosed with CVS are typically treated prophylactically with antiemetic agents or agents to reduce the triggers of the condition. Drugs commonly used to reduce the specific trigger mechanism, prevent the episode, or abort the episode include

- Benzodiazepines (Lorazepam, Diazepam) to reduce stress triggers
- Propranolol (Inderal)
- Cyproheptadine (Periactin)
- Amitriptyline (Elavil)
- Phenobarbital (Luminal)
- Erthromycin (E.E.S, Eryc, E-Mycin, Erythrocin)
- Ondansetron (Zofran)
- Sumatriptan (Imitrex)
- Diphenhydramine (Benadryl)

Prehospital management of CVS is mostly supportive. However, it is most important for prehospital personnel to recognize that the condition exists, especially when being called to the scene at 3:00 A.M. for a patient with severe sustained vomiting. In severe cases, the patient may suffer from dehydration and electrolyte imbalance, which may precipitate syncopal episodes and cardiac dysrhythmias. Severe vomiting in CVS has also been associated with peptic esophagitis from frequent gastric reflux, hemataemesis from esophageal irritation, and Mallory-Weiss tear at the gastroesophageal junction from retching and forceful vomiting. In your physical assessment, inspect the teeth for excessive tooth decay associated with gastric acid corroding of the tooth enamel. It is important to note that the average time it takes to diagnose the condition is about 2.5 years from the onset because the patients often don't seek medical attention immediately and because a pattern of the condition must be established.

Patient Assessment

The focus of patient assessment is to identify and manage any life-threatening problems before attempting to identify the underlying etiology of the condition. With vomiting, the life threat is the potential for airway obstruction.

Scene Size-Up

During the scene size-up, note clues that the patient has been vomiting, such as a bucket or large pan placed next to the patient's bed or chair or vomitus on bed clothes, furniture, or floor. Also observe any evidence of a meal, drugs, or other substances the patient may have ingested that might trigger vomiting.

Initial Assessment

During the initial assessment, your major concern is control of the airway. A patient with an altered mental status who is vomiting is a prime candidate for aspiration of gastric contents. Position the patient to assist with drainage of vomitus and secretions, and be prepared to suction the oral cavity aggressively. In the presence of severe and continuous vomiting in a patient with an altered mental status, place the patient in a lateral recumbent position and consider tracheal intubation. Evaluate the patient's perfusion status and pulse for indicators of shock. Profuse vomiting may lead to dehydration. Also, electrolyte disturbances and alkalosis may result from prolonged vomiting.

Focused History and Physical Exam

History When taking a history where vomiting is the complaint, use the relevant parts of the OPQRST format, as follows:

1. *Onset.* Determine whether the patient vomits prior to or after eating. Determine the time of day and the length of time after a meal when the patient has begun to vomit. Vomiting associated with pregnancy, uremia, alcoholic gastritis, and increased ICP is usually seen in the early morning and before eating. Vomiting after eating is usually present in peptic ulcer disease. Vomiting after eating fatty foods is common in cholecystitis. Projectile vomiting occurs without nausea or retching. It is most often associated with increased ICP. Ask about onset with headache or chest pain.
2. *Palliation/Provocation.* Determine what makes the vomiting better or worse. Vomiting in peptic ulcer disease is made worse by eating. Vomiting due to gastritis is often relieved after eating. Inner ear infections will result in vomiting with movement of the head. Activity that increases ICP, such as straining or bending over, may induce projectile vomiting.
3. *Quality.* Determine the characteristics of the vomit. Various colors and consistencies of vomit may indicate the presence of blood or suggest various disease processes and levels of potential obstruction. Acute gastritis will produce vomitus that consists of stomach contents mixed with a small amount of bile. A patient suffering from a torsion of an abdominal or pelvic organ will retch but vomit very little. Intestinal obstruction will progress from gastric contents to bilious material to brown feculent material. This is characteristic of a small bowel obstruction. Vomiting blood indicates gastrointestinal bleeding.
4. *Radiation/Location.* Does not apply to vomiting.
5. *Severity.* Find out if the vomiting has been mild or forceful. Encourage the patient to describe the severity in his own words.
6. *Time.* Determine how long the patient has been vomiting. A patient who has been vomiting every half-hour or so all night is likely to be dehydrated.
7. *Associated Complaints.* Look for evidence of other signs and symptoms, including pain, fever, headache, stiff neck, blurred vision, vertigo, double vision, or weakness. Also, obtain a history regarding menstruation in females in their childbearing years.

During the history, ask about recurrent episodes of vomiting. If a pattern of recurrent episodes exists, especially if it is associated with a trigger mechanism, the patient may be suffering from cyclic vomiting syndrome.

Physical Examination Conduct a focused medical assessment on the patient who is responsive and a rapid medical assessment (head-to-toe exam) on the unresponsive patient. Observe the patient's general appearance. What is the posture? For example, a patient lying completely still may have a central organic etiology to the vomiting. A restless patient may be suffering from a kidney stone. Assess for evidence of dehydration. Abdominal tenderness may be present or not in a variety of conditions associated with vomiting. However, a rigid abdomen indicates peritonitis, a serious condition.

Assess the breath sounds and place the patient on the cardiac monitor. Assess the abdomen. Inspect and palpate for distention, which may indicate a bowel obstruction. Palpate for tenderness and rigidity. Check the pulses and motor and sensory function in all four extremities. Determine if any neurologic deficits exist. Inspect for skin rashes that may indicate meningitis.

Vital Signs When assessing vital signs, it is important to check for orthostatic (postural) hypotension. This should provide an indication of the degree of dehydration associated with the vomiting. Tachypnea may be indicative of metabolic acidosis. Kussmaul's respirations may occur from diabetic ketoacidosis, (DKA), alcoholic acidosis, and uremia; also consider drug overdose or intoxication from aspirin, methanol, or ethylene glycol. Assess the blood glucose level to rule out DKA. Warm skin may indicate fever and an infectious etiology to the episode.

Ongoing Assessment

Continue to monitor the patient's airway, breathing, circulation, and vital signs. Note any trends in the patient's condition.

Differential Diagnosis

In the presence of vomiting, consider both gastrointestinal causes and etiologies from other organs and organ systems. It is important to assess all body systems to detect signs or elicit symptoms that may be unrelated to the GI system. See Table 12-5 for possible etiologies.

Management Priorities

Because vomiting is a sign of illness and not a true condition, it is most important to concentrate on managing the airway and preventing aspiration. In severe cases, intubation may be necessary to ensure a patent airway. Apply a continuous ECG monitor and initiate an intravenous line of normal saline. Run the intravenous infusion based on the patient's signs and symptoms. Consider the use of an antiemetic agent such as ondansetron (Zofran), Compazine, or Phenergan, based on local protocol.

Vomiting is a sign, not an illness in itself. It is most important to concentrate on managing the airway and preventing aspiration.

SUMMARY

Headache, nausea, and vomiting are complaints that often present together but also exist independently. All may be chronic or episodic, subtle or severe, not associated with any serious underlying condition, or an indication of a life-threatening injury or illness.

TABLE 12-5 Serious Causes of Nausea and Vomiting

Increased intracranial pressure
Intracranial hemorrhage (stroke)
Intracranial mass lesion
Hypertensive crisis
Acute myocardial infarction (especially a posterior wall infarct)
Pericarditis
Drugs, including nonsteroidal antiinflammatory drugs, aspirin, codeine, erythromycin, other antibiotics, chemotherapy agents, and other narcotics
Increased ocular pressure
Gastrointestinal disorders
Diabetic ketoacidosis
Ovarian cyst or torsion
Pelvic inflammatory disease
Pregnancy
Endometriosis
Testicular torsion; testicular disorders
Pneumonia
Spinal fracture
Electrolyte imbalances

Headache is one of the most common complaints. The three main types are tension-type headaches, vascular headaches (including migraines), and cluster headaches. Tension-type headaches are likely caused by neurochemical imbalances leading to an increased sensitivity to pain. Migraines are caused by vascular dilation and/or contraction triggered by pathological mechanisms of the brainstem, vasomotor centers, or trigeminal nerve, also associated with neurochemical imbalances. Other etiologies of headache include fever, hypoxemia, anemia, intracranial tumor or hemorrhage, loss of cerebrospinal fluid, toxic inhalation, depression, and hypertension.

Nausea is the queasy feeling that may precede vomiting. Vomiting is a reflex caused by stimulation of the vomiting center in the medulla of the brain from factors as diverse as gastrointestinal irritation, inner ear infection, certain sights, smells or emotional experiences, chemotherapy or radiation therapy, toxins, uremia, hypoxia, and acidosis.

Remember that headache, nausea, and vomiting are not illnesses in themselves. In fact, they may be distressing but not serious events. However, they may be signs of a serious underlying etiology. The patient with headache, nausea, or vomiting must always receive a complete assessment to detect and manage any immediate life threats and to form an impression of the probable underlying etiology.

Management priorities for headache, nausea, and vomiting (Figure 12-1) include support of the airway, breathing, and circulation. Be especially vigilant about the airway in the presence of vomiting. If the patient has an altered mental status, consider performing tracheal intubation to guard the airway. Apply an ECG monitor for continuous cardiac monitoring. With vomiting leading to dehydration, establish an IV line for fluid replacement therapy.

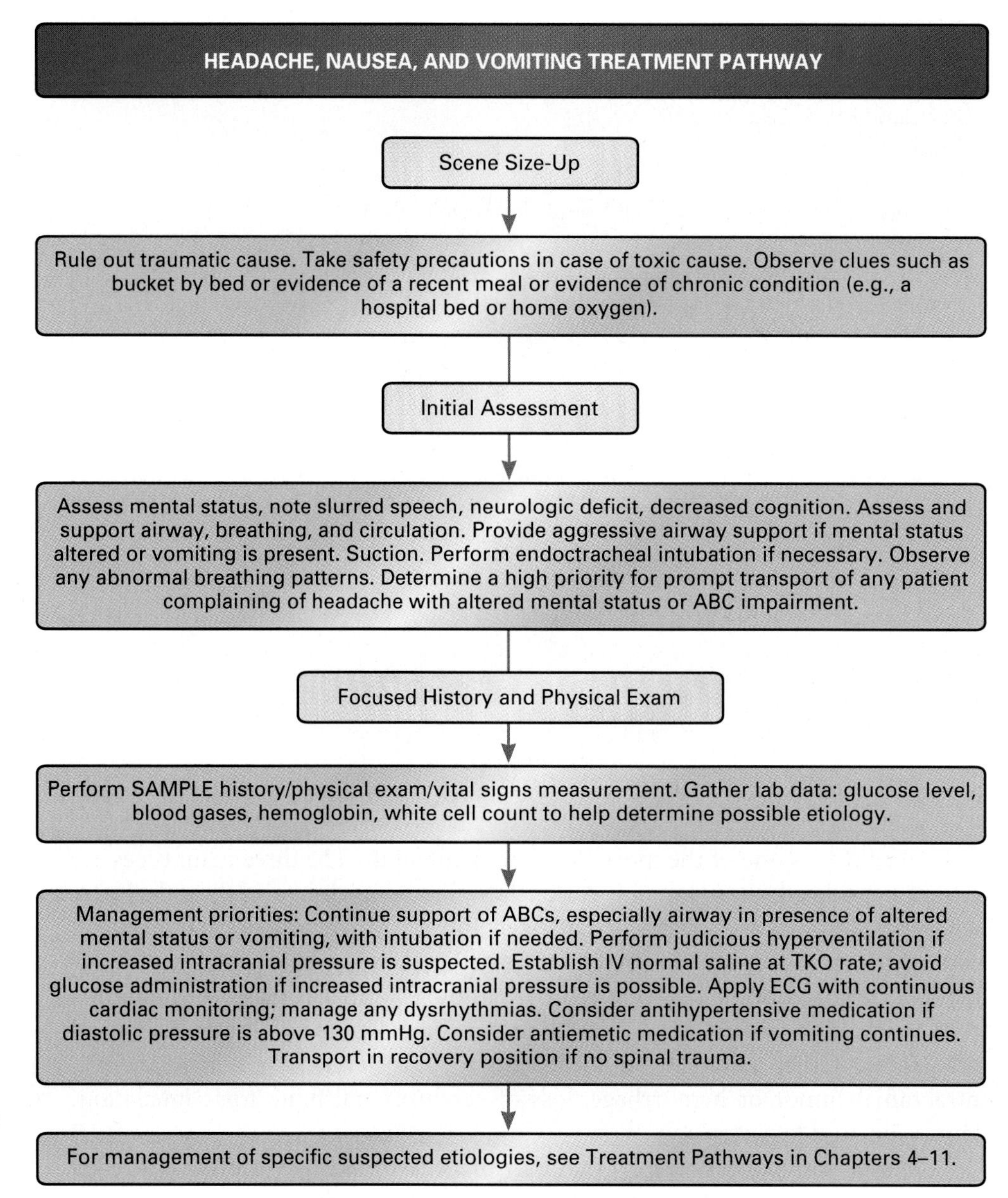

FIGURE 12-1 Headache, nausea, and vomiting treatment pathway.

SCENARIO FOLLOW-UP

You are called to a gymnasium for a patient who "passed out." Upon arrival, you find a 39-year-old male patient who was playing basketball lying supine on the floor in a pool of vomitus. He is postured with extensor rigidity. He is not responding to verbal stimuli. Prior to losing consciousness, the patient complained of a very severe headache, stiff neck, and nausea. He had two episodes of projectile vomiting before your arrival.

As you approach the patient, you note gurgling sounds on inspiration and exhalation. Your partner immediately suctions the airway clear of the vomitus and secretions and maintains an airway by using a head tilt, chin lift maneuver. The patient's rigid posture with extension of the extremities is similar to decerebrate posturing. The patient does not respond to a pinch to the web between his thumb and finger. The respiratory rate is very irregular at a rate of 30 breaths per minute with a shallow tidal volume. You immediately begin bag-valve-mask ventilation with supplemental oxygen attached to the reservoir. The radial pulse is present and full with a rate of approximately 50 beats per minute. The skin is clammy to the touch.

As you continue with the rapid medical assessment, the patient begins to projectile vomit again. Because of your concern with protecting his airway, you elect to intubate the patient with a tracheal tube. You perform orotracheal intubation and confirm proper tube placement. Your partner resumes ventilating the patient, with the bag-valve device now attached to the tracheal tube.

You inspect and palpate the patient's head, looking for any evidence of trauma, as you ask the bystanders if the patient was struck in the head or struck his head. Everyone at the scene denies having seen the patient strike his head. The pupils are equal but dilated and very sluggish to respond to light. The ears, nose, and mouth are clear of any discharge. Nuchal rigidity is present on palpation and manipulation of the neck.

The extremities remain extended and rigid. Pulses are present in all extremities. No response to pain is noted in any extremity. You run your thumb up the lateral edges of the soles of the feet and note that the Babinski reflex is abnormal on both the right and the left.

The blood pressure is 178/84. The cardiac monitor shows a sinus bradycardia at a rate of 52 beats per minute. The pulse oximeter shows an SpO_2 reading of 98 percent. The skin is a normal temperature and slightly diaphoretic.

You initiate an intravenous line of normal saline at a keep-open rate. You draw blood and test the glucose level, which is 95 mg/dl.

While performing the assessment, you question the bystanders about the events prior to the patient becoming unresponsive. The bystanders state that they were playing basketball when the patient suddenly stopped and began to complain of a severe headache, stiff neck, and nausea. He sat down in the middle of the court, lay back on the floor, and slowly began to lose consciousness. After about 10 minutes, he began to throw up profusely and got "real stiff." No one at the scene knows anything about the patient's medical history.

You prepare the patient for expeditious transport. En route, you continue to ventilate him and monitor his mental status for any change, of which there is none. You reassess breath sounds for tube placement and ensure the intravenous line is still patent and running. You assess the vital signs several times while en route. The presentation of the patient is consistent with an intracranial hemorrhage, and you suspect a subarachnoid hemorrhage based on your findings. You notify the hospital about the patient's condition.

Your emergency care has been primarily supportive with expeditious transport. Upon arrival at the hospital, you quickly transfer the patient and give your report to the emergency department staff. They continue to manage the patient as you gather your equipment and prepare to write your written report.

During a later stop at the hospital, you ask about your patient. You learn that he has, as you surmised, suffered a subarachnoid hemorrhage. The prognosis for recovery is uncertain.

FURTHER READING

1. Bickley, L.S., and P.G. Szilagyi. *Bates' Guide to Physical Examination and History Taking.* 8th ed. Philadelphia: Lippincott Williams & Wilkins, 2003.
2. Sargeant, L., and M. Blanda. "Headache, cluster," *eMedicine Journal,* March 10, 2005.
3. Blanda, M., and J. Wright. "Headache, migraine," *eMedicine Journal,* November 16, 2004.
4. Blanda, M. "Headache, tension," *eMedicine Journal,* June 3, 2004.
5. Bledsoe, B.E., R.S. Porter, and R.A. Cherry. *Paramedic Care: Principles and Practice—Volume 3.* 2nd ed. Upper Saddle River, NJ: Pearson/Prentice Hall, 2006.
6. Davis, M., S. Votey, and G. Greenough. *Signs and Symptoms in Emergency Medicine.* St. Louis: Mosby, 1999.
7. Ferri, F. *Clinical Advisor: Instant Diagnosis and Treatment.* St. Louis: Mosby, 2002.
8. Guyton, A.C., and J.E. Hall. *Textbook of Medical Physiology.* 10th ed. Philadelphia: Saunders, 2001.
9. Huether, S.E., and K.L. McCane. *Understanding Pathophysiology.* 4th ed. St. Louis: Mosby, 2004.
10. Ignatoff, W.B. "Migraine headache: evidence-based treatment guidelines for emergency management," *Emergency Medicine Reports,* 1999;20(23): 238-247.
11. Kaspor, D.L., E. Braunwald, A.S. Fauci, S.L. Hauser, and D.L. Longo. *Harrison's Principles of Internal Medicine.* 16th ed. New York: McGraw-Hill, 2004.
12. Markovchick, V., and P. Pons. *Emergency Medicine Secrets.* 2nd ed. Philadelphia: Hanley & Belfus, 1999.
13. Marx, J., and R. Hockberger. *Rosen's Emergency Medicine.* 5th ed. St. Louis: Mosby, 2002.

14. MAY, H.L., ed. *Emergency Medicine.* 2nd ed. Boston: Little Brown and Company, 1992.
15. PONS, P., and D. CASON. *Paramedic Field Care: A Complaint-Based Approach.* St. Louis: American College of Emergency Physicians, Mosby–Year Book, 1997.
16. PORTH, C.M. *Pathophysiology: Concepts of Altered Health States.* 5th ed. Philadelphia: Lippincott-Raven, 1998.
17. RUND, D., R. BARKIN, P. ROSEN, and G. STERNBACH. *Essentials of Emergency Medicine.* 2nd ed. St. Louis: Mosby–Year Book, 1997.
18. SEIDEL, H., J. BALL, J. DAINS, and G. BENEDICT. *Mosby's Guide to Physical Examination.* 4th ed. St. Louis: Mosby, 1999.
19. SUNDARAM, S., and B. UK LI. "Cyclic vomiting syndrome," *eMedicine Journal,* August 10, 2002.
20. SWARTZ, M. *Textbook of Physical Diagnosis: History and Examination.* 4th ed. Philadelphia: Saunders, 2002.
21. TIERNEY, L.M., S.J. MCPETH, and M.A. PAPADAKIS, eds. *Current Medical Diagnosis and Treatment 1997.* 36th ed. Stamford, CT: Appleton & Lange, 1997.
22. ZOLLO, A. *Medical Secrets.* 2nd ed. Philadelphia: Hanley & Belfus, 1997.

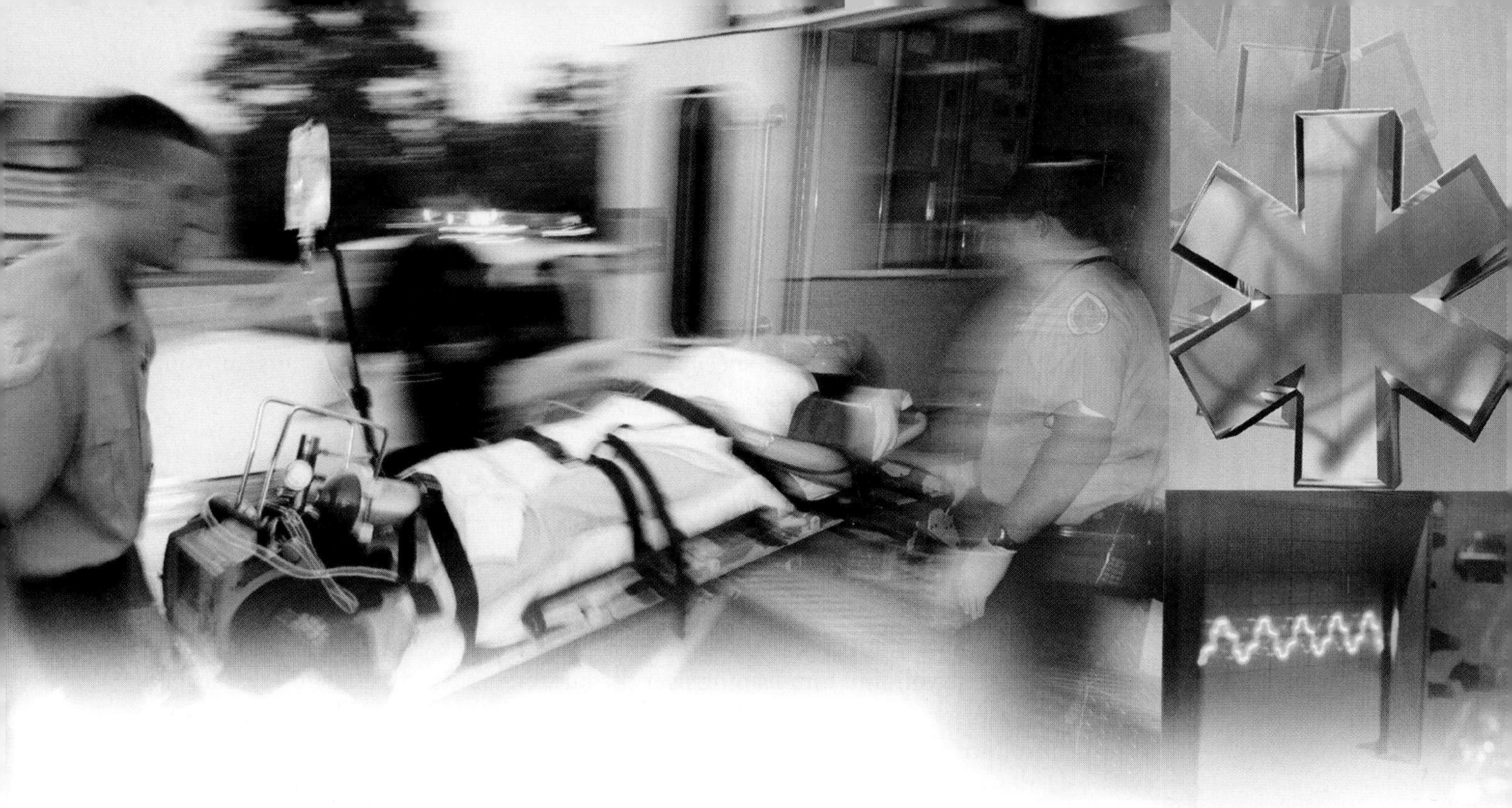

PUTTING IT ALL TOGETHER: SCENARIOS

13

The scenarios in this final chapter invite you to use your critical thinking skills to "put it all together." Each case features a patient with a chief complaint or presenting condition that will be familiar to you from your study of the prior chapters. But, like all patients, the patient at hand is an individual with specific signs, symptoms, history, and physical findings. As in the cases you actually encounter in EMS practice, you will be challenged to put together knowledge from more than one source—the prior chapters of this book, knowledge you bring from your own background and experiences in EMS, and the facts of the particular patient—to help you analyze and "solve" each case.

This chapter includes the following scenarios:

- Scenario 1: Difficulty Breathing
- Scenario 2: Difficulty Breathing
- Scenario 3: Shock
- Scenario 4: Shock
- Scenario 5: Abdominal Pain
- Scenario 6: Altered Mental Status
- Scenario 7: Altered Mental Status
- Scenario 8: Chest Pain
- Scenario 9: Sudden-Onset Paraplegia
- Scenario 10: Unconscious Woman

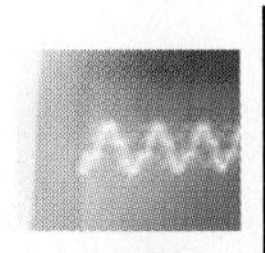

INTRODUCTION

The scenarios that follow include two kinds of material: a running narrative of the case and, in *italics,* a commentary on the case. Each segment ends with a question or two in purple type to encourage you to think about what you have just read—to ponder, analyze, speculate, or discuss with fellow students or your instructor—before you read the commentary or the next section.

THE SCENARIOS

SCENARIO 1: DIFFICULTY BREATHING

At 18:00 hours, you are dispatched to a 56-year-old male with difficulty breathing. On arrival, you find him leaning over the kitchen table, struggling to breathe. He is awake and appears very pale. He is clutching an inhaler in his left hand. As you introduce yourself and begin an assessment, you note that his skin is cool and clammy. He has a radial pulse of 100, respirations of 24 with intercostal retractions, and a blood pressure of 156/90. He talks in two- to three-word sentences. He tells you he started having trouble breathing this afternoon and has been getting steadily worse. He has had no relief from his inhaler. He denies chest pain but does admit to feeling a "weight" on his chest. He is on Ventolin (albuterol) and Vasotec (enalapril). Pulse oximetry reads 86 percent. When asked to rank the "weight" on a 1 to 10 scale, he states, "It's a 6." What is this patient's problem? Have you noted any clues, so far, to the underlying cause? What is your immediate task?

This patient has several signs of acute dyspnea. The inability to talk in complete sentences indicates inadequate minute volume, which, at rest, is abnormal. His respiratory rate is 24 with intercostal retractions, which indicates labored breathing, and his pulse oximetry is 86 percent, well below normal. His tachycardia may be due to his hypoxia. The feeling of "weight" on his chest suggests cardiac involvement. This man is in acute respiratory distress. The task here is first to support vital functions, and then to figure out the most likely cause so appropriate treatment can be implemented. How should you proceed with assessment? with care?

You have the patient rinse his mouth with water before you administer sublingual nitroglycerin. Then, you place the nonrebreather mask with reservoir on the patient at 15 lpm. Your partner is attaching the cardiac monitor while you get more history.

The patient reports a history of asbestosis, hypertension, and insulin-dependent diabetes. Last year, he underwent a triple coronary artery bypass. He has bilateral wheezes, most pronounced in the bases. You also note mild pitting edema in his ankles, which is normal for him but, he reports, has been getting worse over the last month. The ECG rhythm is a sinus tachycardia. You decide to do a 12 lead (Figure 13-1).

The 12 lead is suggestive of left ventricular hypertrophy (V1 S 22 mm + V5 R 17 mm = 39 mm) with left ventricular strain pattern (asymmetric ST depression and T-wave inversion that looks almost biphasic in V5, V6), but there are no acute injury patterns. Why did you have the patient rinse his mouth? Why did you give nitroglycerin? Why did you decide to do a 12 lead? What additional clues to the etiology of his problem have you gathered?

The concern here is the cardiac implication of the patient feeling a "weight" on his chest. It is prudent to interpret this as a description of cardiac involvement, although patients with COPD or asthma will also report chest "tightness" with bronchospasm. This patient's choice of words and cardiac history are more typical of cardiac ischemia, which is a logical result of poor oxygenation of heart muscle (pulse oximetry value of 86 percent). However, you don't know if the

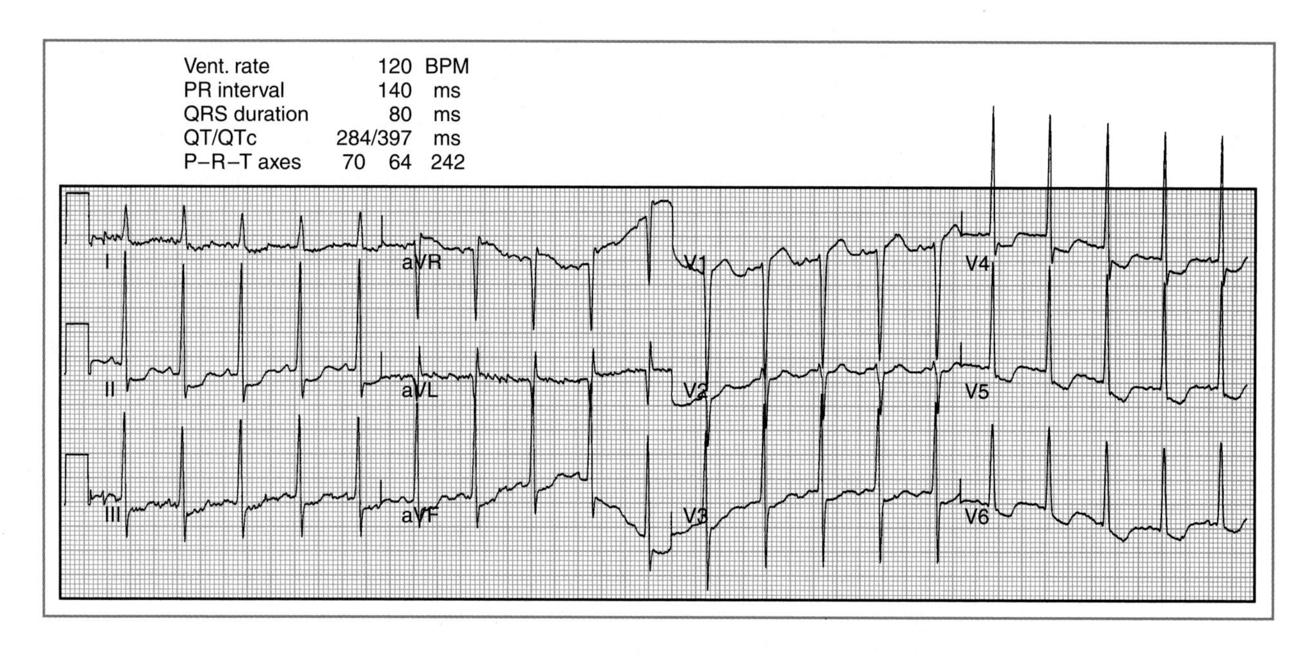

FIGURE 13-1
12-Lead ECG tracing suggestive of left ventricular hypertrophy with left ventricular strain pattern. (From Bob Page. *12-Lead ECG for Acute and Critical Care Providers*. Upper Saddle River, NJ: Pearson/Prentice Hall, 2005.)

poor oxygenation of heart muscle is the result of his respiratory distress or the cause of his respiratory distress (poor oxygenation of heart muscle leads to impaired cardiac function, which can precipitate pulmonary edema).

Additional contributing factors include his cardiac history (bypass last year) and being an insulin-dependent diabetic. Diabetics are very prone to peripheral neuropathies, which frequently interfere with normal pain sensation. The absence of a clear description of chest pain is not reliable and heightens the suspicion for a "silent" AMI; thus the need for a 12 lead.

Assessment factors of importance include the presence of mild pitting edema. Fluid retention in a patient with a cardiac history suggests the presence of a decreased efficiency in the pumping action of the heart and pulmonary edema. Patients with COPD are prone to developing right-sided heart failure or cor pulmonale. This results in decreased cardiac output as well as backup of venous pressure. Distended neck veins and, eventually, pitting edema will result. The body's own compensatory mechanisms, intended to increase cardiac output, also increase the cardiac workload. Eventually, the backup of venous pressure extends to the arterial system and the left heart. Left heart involvement results in pulmonary edema, which can cause bronchospasm ("cardiac wheezing"). Pulmonary edema can cause, or can be the result of, bronchospasm. Thus, the presence of bilateral wheezing, particularly in the bases, could be due to this patient's chronic asbestosis, pulmonary edema, or both.

The fact that his inhaler was ineffectual could be due to an expired medication, to the medication adhering to the mucous membranes of the mouth (from improper and frequent use), or to the fact that his bronchospasm was caused by something other than asbestosis. Rinsing the mouth with water will prevent side effects of inhaled medications and improve the effectiveness of additional nebulized medications.

Because this patient has wheezing, a history of asbestosis, and a cardiac history supported by evidence of left ventricular hypertrophy with left ventricular strain pattern, nitroglycerin can be a useful diagnostic agent in the field. Sublingual nitroglycerin works as a vasodilator, especially within the pulmonary capillary beds and the coronary arteries. The combined effect will improve oxygenation of the pulmonary blood supply, thus improving oxygenation of cardiac muscle, in turn leading to improved cardiac function; it will also result in lower preload, which will reduce oxygen demand and the workload of the heart. In cases of pulmonary edema, the work of breathing should improve. In cases of bronchospasm due to hyperreactivity of bronchioles, nitroglycerin should have no effect. After administering nitroglycerin, what are the next steps?

After administration of nitroglycerin, you take another set of vital signs. The patient's pulse remains at 100, but he states that his breathing is easier despite his continued wheezing. His blood pressure is 148/88 and, when questioned, he states his chest pressure is better. Pulse oximetry shows saturation at 92 percent. Based on these results, you administer a second nitroglycerin, along with 40 mg of Lasix and a nebulized albuterol treatment. Reassessment shows a pulse of 90, respirations 18, and a blood pressure of 140/76. Was the nitroglycerin effective for this patient? How do you know? Why did you administer more nitroglycerin, Lasix, and albuterol?

Because there was improvement noted in both the chest discomfort and his breathing, the cause is more clearly suggested, and further treatment for pulmonary edema is continued.

Nitroglycerin is the mainstay of treatment for pulmonary edema. Because of its effect on both the pulmonary vasculature and coronary arteries, nitroglycerin remains the drug of choice. Lasix (furosemide) is a good second choice. Lasix is best known for its diuretic effect, but it also has a localized vasodilating effect on the pulmonary vasculature that takes place within minutes. Both agents reduce preload, which reduces oxygen demand on the heart. The net effect in this patient is improved cardiac output. Together with the diuretic effect, furosemide is a potent and valuable pharmacologic aid in treating pulmonary edema, especially when used in conjunction with nitroglycerin.

Albuterol was also considered for treatment of bronchospasm because of the patient's history of asbestosis. Bronchospasm can be a result or cause of pulmonary edema. In this case, when a preexisting chronic disease causing bronchospasm is present, and wheezing persists despite treatment for pulmonary edema, use of a bronchodilator may be advisable.

Administration of further nitroglycerin, furosemide (Lasix), and albuterol should help boost the patient's oxygen saturation to or above the desired minimum of 95 percent. Pulse oximetry can be a helpful tool to guide treatment choices. Morphine is also preferred as a treatment for pulmonary edema of cardiac origin. In this case, the patient experiences substantial improvement using nitroglycerin, furosemide, and albuterol. What do you think the ultimate diagnosis of this patient's condition will be?

On arrival at the hospital, your patient's color is much better. He is talking in complete sentences, denies any chest discomfort, and his skin is warm and dry. Admitting vital signs are pulse 88, respirations 18, blood pressure 142/86, and pulse oximetry 96 percent. He is eventually admitted for congestive heart failure and medication adjustment.

SCENARIO 2: DIFFICULTY BREATHING

At 13:30 hours, you are dispatched to a 32-year-old female who is complaining of difficulty breathing. On arrival, you find her sitting at her desk on the second floor of an office building. She appears pale but is awake and alert and does not appear to be in acute distress. Coworkers are standing around her, and a cup of water is on her desk.

She tells you that she was working at her computer when she had a sudden, sharp chest pain that came and went. Then, she states, "I just couldn't catch my breath." She had gotten up to go to the bathroom when she felt very weak and sank to the floor. She denies fainting or passing out. Now she feels much better and thinks she can wait for her husband to take her home. Coworkers tell you she looks much better now than she did. The office manager tells you your patient appeared "the color of putty" and "broke out in a sweat." Your patient clearly feels and looks pretty well just now, but is she? What should your next assessment steps include?

Although, when you arrive, the patient is in no apparent distress, her history is worrisome. She had a sudden onset of sharp chest pain followed by dyspnea, weakness, pallor, and diaphoresis. This combination of signs and symptoms is suspicious for an event that triggered an epinephrine/norepinephrine release (pallor with diaphoresis). Such an event has a high probability for either a respiratory or a cardiovascular cause, both of which have the potential for serious problems and bear further investigation. Vital signs will be important.

An additional tool to help evaluate the respiratory system in the normotensive patient is pulse oximetry. To help evaluate the cardiovascular system, a cardiac monitor, along with vital signs, is also a useful assessment tool. (Remember that angina in women does not always have the same clinical presentation as in men, and sudden cardiac dysrhythmias can precipitate similar epinephrine/norepinephrine releases.)

Furthermore, the patient's episode of weakness indicates that a central nervous system event, such as a stroke, hypoglycemia, or a hypoperfusion event to the brain, might also be present. So, although the presence of chest pain and spontaneous improvement makes that a low probability, her blood sugar, as well as her vital signs, should also be checked. What further findings do you anticipate? How will you continue with the assessment?

Initial assessment findings revealed an alert, oriented female who was somewhat pale but warm and dry. Her vital signs are pulse 86, respirations 24, and blood pressure 142/88. Lung sounds are clear to auscultation bilaterally with no discomfort on inspiration or expiration.

Pulse oximetry is 98 percent. It is a normal value, but that does not rule out a pulmonary problem. (However, abnormal values would confirm the presence of a problem.) The cardiac monitor shows a sinus rhythm consistent with her radial pulse, right axis deviation, and a P wave that is tall and peaked. You check her blood sugar, and it is 110 mg/dl, which is normal.

She has no complaints of pain, no edema, and is on no medications but does take birth control pills. She has no allergies and has no medical problems. She recently tried to quit smoking, using patches, but has been unsuccessful. The patient's heart rate, respirations, and blood pressure are on the high side, but not alarmingly so. Pulse oximetry and blood glucose are normal. No dysrhythmias were detected. Would you conclude, at this point, that her condition is probably not serious?

This patient's assessment findings contribute to a subtle picture of a potentially major problem. Although she has a normal pulse rate at rest, she has a slightly elevated respiratory rate. Her ECG shows a right axis deviation, which is unusual, and she has a tall peaked P wave, elevated over 2 mm in height, suggestive of P pulmonale. She has a history of taking birth control pills and smoking, both of which are implicated in blood clot formation and cardiac dysfunction. It is important to pursue the nature and character of her chest pain to try to discriminate between the probability of pleuritic pain versus cardiac pain. How would you continue your assessment to form an impression of the etiology of her chest pain?

When you ask the patient to describe the sudden chest pain, she states it was in the right side of her chest, points to the midclavicular line, midchest, and denies radiation. She is very clear that the pain disappeared as fast as it came, she has no pain now, and she feels much better. This has never happened to her before. When asked if anything made the pain worse, she states that it happened so fast and disappeared so fast that she does not know. You are trying to differentiate between a possible cardiac or a possible pulmonary origin to her pain. Which seems more likely at this point—and why?

Her description of the chest pain is more suggestive of a pulmonary problem than of a cardiac event. Cardiac pain is usually not so sudden in onset and disappearance, whereas a pulmonary condition can present this way. Because of her associated signs and symptoms (weakness, pallor, sweating, tachycardia, elevated respirations) and her history (smoking, birth control pills), the probability is of a serious underlying problem. She needs to be transported to be evaluated by a physician. Because of the body systems involved (cardiac and respiratory) and life-threatening nature of the suspected condition, waiting another day would be risky. You need to persuade her to let you take her to the hospital. Will this patient agree to transport? How do you think this case will turn out?

After some conversation, you persuade your patient to let you take her to the hospital. You start her on a nasal cannula at 4 lpm and start a saline lock. You recheck a set of vital signs, check the monitor, and decide to do a 12 lead before you leave (Figure 13-2). The 12 lead reveals a sinus rhythm with right atrial enlargement (P wave greater then 2 mm in height), right axis deviation, right ventricular hypertrophy (positive R in V1), and left heart strain pattern (decreased T wave amplitude in Lead I, aVL, V3-6). This pattern is highly suggestive of a patient with long-standing pulmonary disease, pulmonary hypertension, or right-sided valvular heart disease, although the patient has no known history of any of these. When her history is taken into consideration with her 12 lead, the probability of pulmonary emboli becomes more clear.

At the completion of the 12 lead, you load her for transport. There is no change in her condition en route. On arrival at the hospital, you give your report, point out the abnormalities on the 12 lead, help get her settled, and complete your paper work.

Suddenly, you note a flurry of increased activity at your patient's door. You discover that she has developed pleuritic chest pain and is considerably paler than when you saw her last. Her blood gases are PaO_2 58 torr, pH 7.47, $PaCO_2$ 29 torr, and HCO_3^- 21 mEq/l on a nasal cannula at 4 lpm. The suspicion is acute pulmonary emboli. A CT pulmonary angiogram is done and interpreted as "high probability" for PE. She is admitted to the ICU for acute pulmonary emboli. What is the meaning of the blood gas values?

Most paramedics learn about blood gases in the classroom and have some exposure to them in their clinical training. Paramedics who work in other areas, such as in the emergency department or on critical care transport programs, often have further exposure. However, many paramedics do not pay attention to blood gases of patients once they are out of school. If blood gases are done prior to leaving for the hospital, the information they reveal can give valuable feedback on your decision making prior to arrival.

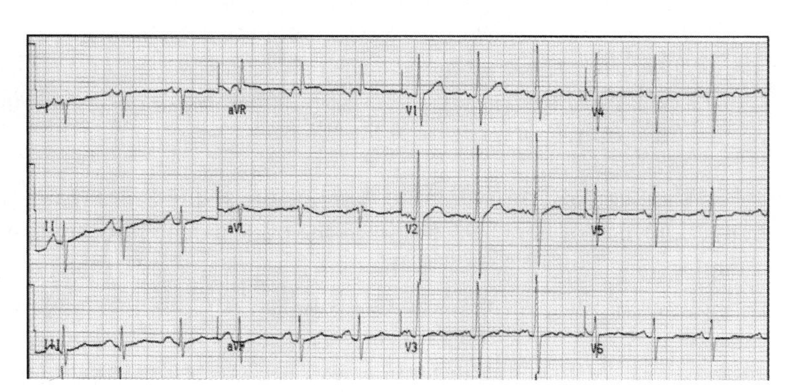

FIGURE 13-2
12-Lead ECG tracing revealing a sinus rhythm with right atrial enlargement and right heart strain. (Courtesy of Bob Page.)

In this case, the pH (7.47) shows the patient is alkylotic, and this is supported by her $PaCO_2$ (29), which is low. This is consistent with a patient who is hyperventilating. Normally, you would expect that a hyperventilating patient with normal alveolar exchange on 4 lpm of oxygen would have a PaO_2 around 100 torr. Your patient does not. Instead, she has a PaO_2 of 58, well below what would be expected.

Pulse oximetry will not detect early changes with pulmonary emboli because the initial problem is not with exchange across the alveolar membrane (ventilation); rather, the problem is blocked blood vessels (perfusion of lung tissue). A pulse oximetry reading of 98 percent reflects detected saturation of available hemoglobin. The decision to oxygenate and transport this patient was a wise one.

SCENARIO 3: SHOCK

At 22:30 hours, you are dispatched to a 42-year-old woman with "flu." On arrival, her husband greets you at the door and tells you his wife is really sick. As he leads you down the hallway to their bedroom, he explains that she has had a bad cold for the last several days. Tonight, she took several aspirin along with an over-the-counter cold and flu medication and went to bed after dinner. When the husband went to bed, he thought she looked "funny, kind of swollen in the face." When he tried to wake her, she could "barely open her eyes, they were so swollen," and when she tried to talk, her breathing was "noisy." He tells you she has no previous medical problems and is not allergic to any medication but does have hay fever every fall. From the dispatch information and what the husband has told you—before you even see the patient—what do you suspect may be this patient's problem?

This history is particularly suspicious for an allergic reaction. Although there is no history of an allergy to a medication, this woman does have an allergy history (hay fever). The husband's description of her appearance and "noisy" breathing is particularly worrisome. You have enough information to suspect that airway control will be an immediate concern and cardiovascular support may be needed. What do you anticipate finding as you make contact with the patient?

As you enter the bedroom, you see your patient lying under the covers. Her face is extremely puffy with her eyes swollen shut. Her color is flushed with mottling, and her lips are gray. As you make contact, she moves her head toward you and tries to talk, but the sound is harsh with crowing on inspiration. She tells you in halting speech that she cannot breathe. Faint wheezes are audible, with a respiratory rate of about 30 with neck muscle use. You cannot find a radial pulse, but she has a weak, thready carotid. Her hands are so swollen that the skin is taut. What are this patient's immediate needs? How will you proceed?

At this point, you do not need any other information to know that this patient is in acute respiratory distress and is in danger of respiratory arrest. You noticed the harsh "crowing" sound when she inhaled to try to talk. Her crowing is a result of swelling of the subglottic and glottic soft tissues, which creates turbulent flow in the inhaled air, causing the distinctive sound. Faint wheezes are also audible, which is an indication of the amount of bronchoconstriction that is occurring. Her halting speech confirms the presence of inadequate minute volume, another indicator of the amount of airway obstruction present.

Her skin characteristics are typical of the massive fluid shifts that occur with acute allergic reactions. The absence of a radial pulse indicates diminished cardiac output. Her tachycardia is expected as a result of the hypoxia and lack of perfusion. Because there is more than one body system involved, as indicated by the presence of crowing and low cardiac output, anaphylactic shock is a very strong possibility. She needs immediate treatment to prevent respiratory arrest. What interventions will you and your partner perform?

While you were doing your assessment, your partner was preparing and administering a nebulized albuterol/Atrovent combination by mask. You start looking for a vein to start an IV, and your partner is trying to get a blood pressure. Your partner tells you that he hears a faint pressure at 50 systolic and asks if you have the IV yet. Fortunately, you hit a vein and start delivering a fluid bolus of 500 ml of normal saline.

Your partner has the epinephrine ready and delivers 0.1 mg of 1:10,000 IV push, then continues with the fluid bolus and looks for a second IV site. By this time, you have her hooked up to the cardiac monitor, where a supraventricular tachycardia at 160 is apparent. Why have you and your partner chosen to administer epinephrine—and to administer it in this manner? Why the albuterol/Atrovent combination treatment?

Administration of epinephrine by IV bolus is seldom done outside an arrest situation. This case is extreme and is the exception. The patient has little perfusion as evidenced by her skin and hypotension, and she is in immediate danger of respiratory arrest from swelling of the airway. Nebulized albuterol/Atrovent is an option because it is readily available and quickly administered. Albuterol is a bronchodilator and, when combined with cool oxygen from the tank, can help reduce swelling of the respiratory mucosa. Atrovent (ipratropium) works on the parasympathetic system to inhibit mucus production and enhance bronchodilation. This will buy you time by treating the symptoms but will not stop the allergic reaction.

Albuterol and Atrovent are selective for the respiratory system. Because multiple body systems are involved (respiratory, cardiovascular, and cutaneous), the patient needs epinephrine. Epinephrine has several important actions in allergic reactions. It stabilizes the cell walls of basophils and mast cells, thus limiting release of histamine. Alpha receptor stimulation causes needed vasoconstriction, while beta 1 receptor stimulation increases cardiac contractility, automaticity, and other functions. Beta 2 receptor stimulation further promotes bronchodilation. All these properties of epinephrine make it the drug of choice in acute allergic reactions. However, epinephrine is short acting and should be followed by long-acting medications.

Sometimes, there is concern regarding administration of epinephrine, especially IV, to a person who is already tachycardic. In the case of allergic reactions, however, the tachycardia is not because of a sick heart but because of reaction to the allergen, hypoxia, and hypoperfusion.

Age is an important consideration, due to the prevalence of underlying cardiac problems in older patients. In this case, your patient is relatively young and has no previous history of cardiac problems. In any patient who receives a cardiac stimulant, cardiac status must be monitored. In the case of severe allergic reactions, the rate usually comes down after epinephrine administration, even when it is given IV push, due to relief of hypoxia—as in this acute situation. What trends do you expect to note when you reassess your patient?

The second IV line has been established, and your partner administers 50 mg of Benadryl (diphenhydramine). You maneuver the cot next to the bed, and you and your partner carefully transfer your patient to the cot. The albuterol treatment has finished, and your partner replaces the nonrebreather mask. You rapidly reassess. The patient's color seems to be improving, but the light in the bedroom is not very good and you are not sure whether that is just wishful thinking. Her breathing seems to be getting easier with a rate of 24, down from 30, and the monitor shows her SVT of 160 slowing to 148. She now has a blood pressure of 66, up from 50, and you prepare to transport.

In the back of the ambulance, you reassess once more. The patient's vital signs seem to have improved to a pulse of 140 and systolic pressure of 70. Her breathing is easier, but lung sounds are not yet clear. It has been at least 10 minutes since your last administration of epinephrine. You administer another fluid bolus, continue with another nebulized albuterol treatment, hang an IV drip of 300 mg of cimetidine in a 100-ml bag to run in over 15 to 20 minutes, and then administer 125 mg of methylprednisolone (Solu-Medrol) in your second IV line. While en route to the hospital, you notice that the patient's color seems to be improving and her breathing continues to become easier. Her radial pulse returns, and you palpate a systolic pressure of 72. Your patient seems to be doing better. So why have you administered more fluid, albuterol, diphenhydramine, cimetidine, and Solu-Medrol?

Your patient is slowly improving. Because of the massive fluid shifts that occur in an anaphylactic reaction, repeated boluses of fluid are often necessary to help restore circulating volume. Repeated nebulizer treatments are appropriate and will help augment the bronchodilating effects of epinephrine. Diphenhydramine is an H1 (histamine) blocker and is long acting. H1 receptor sites are known to exist in the skin, mucous membranes, and vascular walls. By administering an H1 blocker, you hope to enhance the vascular stabilization begun by epinephrine and control the angioedema. Diphenhydramine is also helpful in preventing delayed reactions. It can be given any time after epinephrine. Cimetidine is an H2 blocker that is also helpful in minimizing the effects of histamine. Solu-Medrol is an antiinflammatory agent that will stabilize the mast cell walls, preventing restimulation of the degranulation by leukotrienes. Recent research suggests that the onset of action of Solu-Medrol is actually about 20 minutes, with its full effect occurring in about 45 minutes to an hour. What measures are needed to further stabilize your patient en route to the hospital?

Reassessment after the second dose of epinephrine shows a pulse of 134, respirations of 28, and a systolic pressure of 74. The patient's color looks better, and she is able to speak without crowing. She has received a total of 1,500 milliliters of normal saline and has completed her second nebulized albuterol treatment. Because her blood pressure continues to be hypotensive, you consider your options of epinephrine drip or dopamine. After delivering another fluid bolus, her blood pressure seems to stabilize at 78 systolic. Because this blood pressure is still very low, you opt for dopamine. You grab a premix of 400 mg of dopamine in 250 ml of D_5W. Your patient continues to slowly improve and, on arrival at the ED, her vital signs are pulse 112, respirations 20, and systolic blood pressure 84, with the dopamine at a drip rate of 10 μg/kg/min. Why is dopamine the drug of choice at this point?

Anaphylactic shock is a serious threat to life. Although your patient is improving, she is not out of danger. Both an epinephrine drip and dopamine are additional options after bolus epinephrine for management of a severe anaphylactic reaction.

Diphenhydramine is an antihistamine that, although it does not act as rapidly as epinephrine, has longer effects. Diphenhydramine also inhibits histamine by blocking H1 receptors. In this manner, it helps stabilize vessel walls. It is also effective in prevention of delayed reactions to allergens in the body. Diphenhydramine could be given any time after the first epinephrine. Many protocols also call for the administration of an H2 blocker, such as cimetidine or ranitidine. By blocking H2 receptor sites, these medications provide an additional benefit, particular in severe reactions.

When hypotension persists after epinephrine, several options are available. Fluid administration should be ongoing, due to the massive fluid shifts that occur during anaphylaxis. Additional options include an epinephrine drip and/or dopamine, due to the inotropic and vasoconstrictive actions (increasing cardiac contractile force and constricting blood vessels) these medications have. Both options are acceptable. The choice is up to medical direction, local protocols, and the condition of the patient. Regardless of the drug chosen, the effect is dose related, so titration is often necessary. How do you expect your patient to be doing by the time you reach the hospital?

On arrival at the hospital, your patient is able to talk in four- to five-word sentences and looks much better. Admission vital signs are pulse 110, respirations 20, and blood pressure 90/74. After another fluid bolus, chest X-rays, and blood work, the IV of cimetidine (H2 blocker) is continued. She is admitted for persistent wheezing and observation overnight.

SCENARIO 4: SHOCK

At 09:22 hours, you are dispatched to a 78-year-old female complaining of abdominal pain. On arrival, you find the woman lying on her side on the couch in her living room. She is very pale. She is awake and alert but seems disoriented to time and place. Her daughter tells you that her mother has not been feeling well for the last 2 weeks. She has had a "cold" that she "just couldn't shake." Today, her mother complained of abdominal pain and dizziness when she got up. When her daughter came over to check on her, she believed her mother's color was bad, so she called EMS. Based on what you have heard and seen so far, do you think this patient's condition is serious or not? Why?

The importance of history in this case cannot be overestimated. This patient has a 2-week history of a "cold" with no improvement. Her pallor and disorientation create the impression of a woman who is very ill, with more than a simple upper respiratory infection.

If she has had a fever, an infection is likely, and with a productive cough, pneumonia might be suspected. However, the history of abdominal pain is unusual, and dizziness when getting up is suspicious for orthostatic hypotension. Although the abdomen can be the site for referred pain from pneumonia, orthostatic hypotension is not a usual result of pneumonia. There is more to this patient than meets the eye. Additional information is needed. What more do you want to find out about this patient? How should you proceed with assessment and care?

While your partner prepares to administer oxygen by nonrebreather mask, you begin your assessment. You note that your patient has a frequent cough and seems out of breath when she talks. Her skin remains extremely pale and is warm and dry with poor turgor. Her lung sounds have basilar wheezes and crackles bilaterally, and pulse oximetry is 87 percent on room air. Your partner starts an IV of normal saline and places a cardiac monitor while you get vital signs. The vital signs are pulse 110 and irregular, respirations 24, and blood pressure 102/56. There is no pedal edema. A rapid blood glucose check shows 90 mg/dl.

Her daughter tells you that her mother is on an over-the-counter medication (Robitussin) for her cough and has been taking Tylenol (acetaminophen) when she felt feverish. She is also on Lanoxin (digoxin [Digitek]), Lasix (furosemide), and Aldactone (spironolactone). By comparing the date her prescriptions were filled with the number of pills present, you conclude that she takes her medication regularly. The cardiac monitor shows atrial fibrillation at a rate consistent with her pulse. Here is her 12 lead (Figure 13-3). What do the patient's medications suggest about her history? Are her present vital signs and other findings consistent with this history? What factors can be responsible for her lung sounds? breathlessness? confusion? tachycardia? hypotension? What does the 12 lead suggest?

Her medication and cardiac rhythm are consistent with congestive heart failure and hypertension. Although no pedal edema is noted, crackles and wheezes are present in her lungs. This suggests a primary cardiac problem. The pulmonary edema may be something more serious than would normally occur with congestive failure. Because the number of medications remaining in the bottles is reasonable, an overdose is not likely.

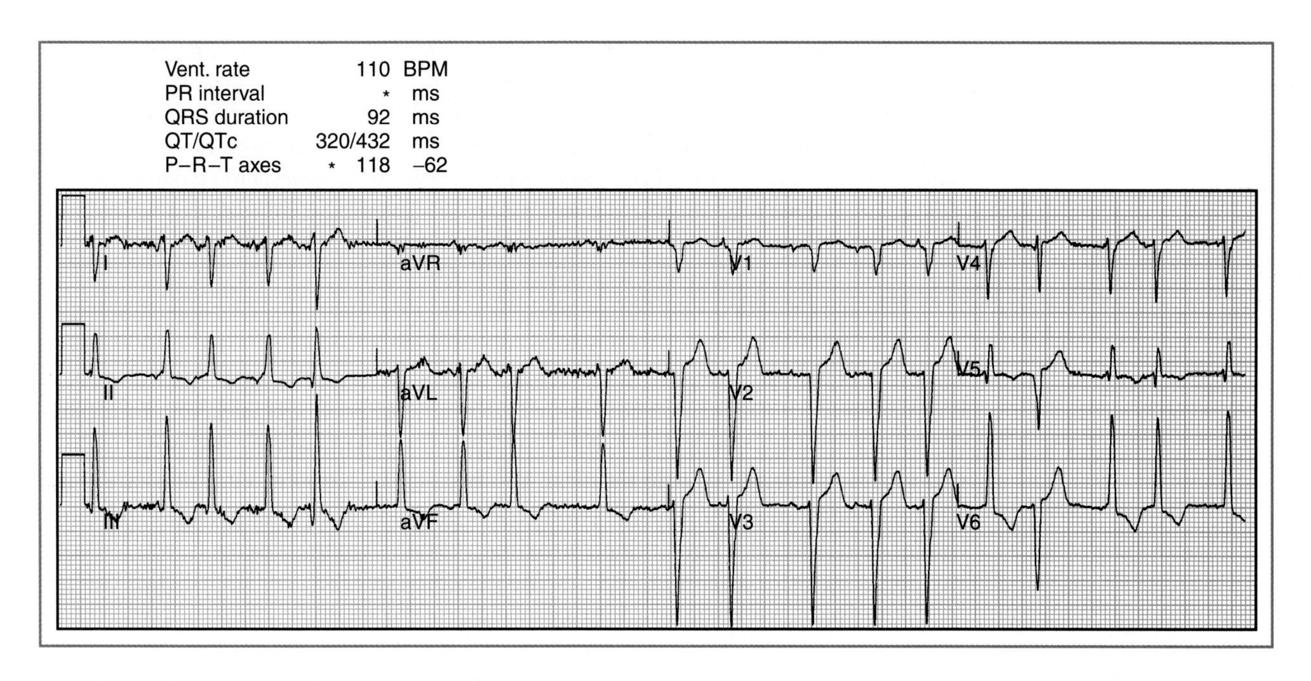

FIGURE 13-3
12-Lead ECG tracing showing atrial fibrillation with paroxysmal ventricular contraction, posterior hemiblock, and left ventricular hypertrophy with strain. (From Bob Page. *12-Lead ECG for Acute and Critical Care Providers*. Upper Saddle River, NJ: Pearson/Prentice Hall, 2005.)

The 12 lead shows atrial fibrillation with PVC, posterior hemiblock, and left ventricular hypertrophy with strain. There is no AMI injury pattern. These findings are consistent with the suspicion of congestive heart failure.

Your assessment findings suggest that the fluid in her lungs is enough to interfere with minute volume (she is out of breath when she talks). This suspicion is supported by a respiratory rate of 24 and a pulse oximetry value of 87 percent.

Her confusion may also be a result of hypoxia, as well as dehydration and infection. The presence of confusion in this patient underscores the seriousness of her situation.

Her vital signs suggest that some cardiovascular compensation is also occurring. A pulse of 110 may be due in part to hypoxia (and anaerobic metabolism) and/or may be a direct effect of catecholamine release. However, a tachycardia in the presence of a systolic of 102 in a patient who, previously, was hypertensive also suggests that there is another problem. You wonder: Could this patient be in early shock? What test could you perform to confirm your suspicion?

After the oxygen is applied and the IV started, you and your partner explain to your patient that you are going to sit her up to see how she feels. Supporting her on either side, with one hand on her radial pulse, you gently bring her to a sitting position. She immediately turns ashen in color and tells you she is going to "pass out." You also lose her radial pulse. After you lay her back down, a quick set of vital signs shows an irregular carotid pulse of 142 and a systolic pressure of 80/54. What do the results of this tilt test indicate?

Her tachycardia, relatively low systolic pressure (in the presence of a history of hypertension), and history of dizziness when she gets up suggest the presence of shock. The positive tilt test confirms your suspicions. The question now becomes: What type of shock?

The presence of a productive cough and fever is highly suspicious for an infection. An infection severe enough to produce orthostatic hypotension is particularly troubling and points in the direction of septic shock. However, because of her cardiac history, this patient is also at risk for cardiogenic shock. While the 12 lead does not overtly reveal AMI injury pattern, she still has a sick heart, and left ventricular failure is possible. Atrial fibrillation deprives the heart of the "atrial kick," further contributing to lower cardiac output. Elements of hypovolemia are also present with her poor skin turgor. The issue of her abdominal pain, reported in the dispatch, is also of concern, although she has not complained of it since your arrival. Given the confirmation of early shock and the possible etiologies, what interventions would you perform for this patient?

You have decided that this patient needs to be immediately transported to the nearest hospital. You direct your partner to prepare a dopamine drip of 400 mg in 250 ml of D_5W, while you prepare a nebulized treatment of albuterol. As your patient is receiving the albuterol, you administer a 200-ml bolus of normal saline. Your partner has determined the drip rate for a 5 μg/kg/min dopamine dose and programmed that into the portable IV drip monitor. You begin reassessment. Vital signs are pulse 126 and irregular, respirations 26, and blood pressure 92/60. Lung sounds have not changed since the albuterol, but pulse oximetry is now up to 91 percent. You tell your partner to start the dopamine and prepare to transport. The fluid bolus administered is a small one—why? Why your choices of dopamine and albuterol?

A small bolus of fluid is appropriate in this case because of the patient's signs of dehydration and history of being on a diuretic (furosemide). The presence of pulmonary edema does not absolutely contraindicate a fluid bolus; however, it does highlight the need for extreme caution if fluid is necessary and is administered.

This patient is in shock. Both cardiogenic and septic shock are major possibilities. Furthermore, elements of both can occur together, especially in the elderly, with sepsis triggering cardiac insufficiency.

Determining the amount of fluid to administer can be tricky. Fluid is restricted in cardiogenic shock but is given more liberally (however, with close monitoring) in the septic shock patient. Closely monitor lung sounds and degree of respiratory distress as your guide. Consult medical direction when in doubt.

After assuring adequate oxygenation and fluid volume, dopamine is the drug of choice. Starting doses can range from 2 to 10 μg/kg/min for more of the beta 1 effect of increased cardiac contractility. In this case, 5 μg/kg/min is a starting dose set by your physician medical director. Close monitoring of the blood pressure and heart rate is also required whenever this medication is used.

Albuterol was administered to help with bronchospasm (as revealed by the wheezing) that result from her pulmonary edema. Although albuterol will not cure the problem, its bronchodilatory action will counter the bronchospasm, offering temporary relief. Based on your prehospital findings, this patient's shock could be caused by a cardiac etiology, a pulmonary etiology, or both. What is your instinct about the ultimate diagnosis?

En route to the hospital, you administer a second fluid bolus of 200 ml and reassess. Your patient's mental status seems to improve, and her blood pressure stabilizes at 106 to 110 systolic. On arrival at the hospital, a chest X-ray and blood work seem to indicate pneumonia with sepsis. The patient is directly admitted to the ICU. After several other blood tests and radiologic tests (including a CT scan), her abdominal pain is determined to be referred pain from her pneumonia. It diminishes on day two and is gone by day three.

SCENARIO 5: ABDOMINAL PAIN

It is 16:12 hours when you are dispatched to a 56-year-old male who is complaining of abdominal, low back, and leg pain. On arrival, you find your patient lying in bed in a crowded bedroom. He is a very large, overweight man, who appears older than his stated age. He is pale, and from the expression on his face, he appears to be in pain. He greets you with, "Its about time you're here! A person could die waiting for help!" What is your general impression of the patient so far?

A patient who is talking in complete sentences has an adequate minute volume at rest. He is irritable, but the fact that he is coherent and making sense indicates that he is most likely perfusing his brain. After completing the initial assessment and finding no immediate life threats, what is your next step?

As your partner calls for backup, you begin getting a history. The patient tells you he got up this morning not feeling well but with no real complaint of pain. The back pain began as an ache around noon and now, 4 hours later, it is so bad he cannot stand it. He describes the pain as steady, "a terrible tearing pain," and ranks it as a 10 (the worst) on a scale of 1 to 10. It is located in his lower back and radiates to his abdomen and down both legs. Relying on your knowledge of abdominal organs and abdominal pain, what can you infer from the patient's description of his pain? Why has your partner called for backup?

His description of the pain is typical of a hollow organ stretching (tearing pain). If contractions were present, it is likely he would complain of pain that comes and goes, but this pain is constant. Because of the location (lower back) and the radiation (to the abdomen and legs), the organ system most likely affected is the aorta. As the aorta dilates, pressure is exerted on surrounding structures—in this case, nerve roots supplying the abdominal wall—thus causing radiation of pain to the abdomen. As the aorta continues to dilate downward, the iliac arteries supplying the legs are also affected, producing pain in the groin.

Your partner has called for backup because this patient is just too heavy for the two of you to move by yourselves, especially with the gentle handling his condition will require. What facts might you obtain during the remainder of the history?

The patient interrupts your history by yelling at you to "do something," he hurts so bad "I'm dying!" Because of the patient's skin color and description of pain, your partner has already applied oxygen with a nonrebreather mask with a reservoir at 15 lpm. As you continue with a history from his wife, your partner begins a physical assessment.

His wife tells you, "Don't pay him any mind. He's always like that." You find out that the patient has a history of hypertension and is on Tenormin (atenolol). According to his wife, he is noncompliant, taking the medication only when he thinks he needs to. She also states that his doctor recently told him he had a "sugar problem," but her husband did not believe him, and he was not going back. What does this additional history suggest regarding etiology of the patient's condition?

A history of hypertension, especially with the question of diabetes, is very suggestive of atherosclerosis. Vascular disease is a strong possibility and a risk factor for aneurysms. What do you expect the physical exam may reveal?

While you were gathering this information, your partner has discovered that your patient has a distended, tender abdomen with mottling that extends from his chest to his feet. His skin is cool and dry. There were no masses felt, but he is extremely tender to palpation. His vital signs are radial pulse 110 and regular, respirations 22 and shallow, and blood pressure 90/56. Lung sounds are equal and clear bilaterally. Pulses in his legs are diminished, and capillary refill is delayed. Your partner is preparing an IV. You attach a cardiac monitor and find a regular sinus rhythm with no ectopy. How would you interpret these physical findings?

Palpating masses in a patient with a large abdomen is difficult. What is more important is to key in on the presence of mottling, with an abdomen tender to palpation and a history of steady pain. Mottling is more suggestive of the type and degree of shock that an abdominal aneurysm might produce, probably because of the diminished circulation to the tissues caused by the aneurysm. Although the aneurysm has not yet ruptured, it is leaking and is at risk for rupture. Even though he is on a beta-blocker (atenolol), the body may override the beta-blocking effect if there is enough sympathetic stimulus. That seems to be the case here.

The patient's vital signs are indicative of compensated shock moving toward progressive shock. You know that the shock is still compensated because the patient remains alert and oriented. However, the patient's elevated heart rate, rapid, shallow respirations, and falling blood pressure—hypotension in a patient with a history of hypertension—indicate that progressive shock is developing. How would you continue the care of this patient?

You adjust the IV to flow rate to maintain perfusion and, as backup arrives, prepare to move to your vehicle and transport the patient to the hospital. You and the backup team move him as gently as possible. En route, you are careful to keep him as comfortable as you can and to keep him warm. A blood sugar check reads "HIGH." You monitor his blood pressure and pulse every 5 minutes. There is no appreciable change in vital signs. On arrival at the ED, vital signs continue to be stable and the patient continues to complain loudly of his pain and that no one is doing anything. Blood work is rapidly done, and a quick CT is obtained. An abdominal aneurysm is confirmed, and he is taken directly to surgery.

The next day you are picking up equipment at the same ED. The physician on duty was the same one who took care of your patient yesterday. You ask how the patient turned out. He survived surgery, the physician tells you, but the aneurysm was 10 cm, almost too big for the graft, and was leaking so much they evacuated 2 liters of blood from his retroperitoneal space. He congratulates you on recognizing the problem and getting him to the hospital so quickly. The patient is in the ICU now. The doctors expect him to survive, but he has been a definite challenge to the staff!

SCENARIO 6: ALTERED MENTAL STATUS

At 17:30 hours, you are dispatched to an unconscious 54-year-old female. On arrival, her husband tells you that earlier today his wife had complained of a headache. Later this afternoon, she returned from a meeting early because she did not feel well and vomited. She told him her headache was worse, so she went to the bedroom to lie down. That was at about 1:30 P.M. When her husband went in to wake her for dinner, at about 5:30 P.M., he could not arouse her. You find your patient supine in bed. She is softly snoring, has normal color, and appears to be sleeping. As you make contact, she does not arouse. This patient presents with a number of troubling signs and symptoms. What is the most important intervention to perform right now?

A snoring person has an obstructed airway. Turning the head to one side or doing a head-tilt, chin-lift will often clear the airway. The obstruction is often caused by either the tongue or the soft tissues at the back of the throat. How should the assessment proceed from this point?

While you concern yourself with the patient's airway and initial assessment, your partner obtains more history. The husband reports that your patient has suffered no trauma and is on Glucophage (metformin hydrochloride) for her diabetes but is no longer taking any other medication. When questioned further, he states that his wife used to have a blood pressure problem, but she does not any longer so has not taken her pills recently. When asked what made her think she no longer had a problem, he states that she has not had high blood pressure for "months" so she is "cured."

The husband produces two empty bottles, one of Capoten (captopril) and Cardizem (diltiazem). The last refill was 3 months ago with pills enough for 2 months. When questioned about her health during the last few weeks, he says that his wife thought she was coming down with something because she has had a headache "off and on" for about 2 or 3 days, but today it was worse. He said she came home complaining that she had "the worst headache of my life." Then she started vomiting, so she believed she had a bad case of the flu and went to bed. When questioned about the presence of any trauma, he stated he had no knowledge of any. What clues have you gathered to the etiology and severity of this patient's problem?

In this case, as with most medical emergencies, the history gives the clues to the most likely cause of the problem. She is a hypertensive patient who is not taking her medication. She is also a type II diabetic, a condition that predisposes to hypertension and cardiovascular problems.

With an altered mental status, you know that the central nervous system is affected. The pattern of complaint, with headache and vomiting preceding unresponsiveness, suggests increasing intracranial pressure. The description her husband relayed of this being "the worst headache of her life" helps confirm the suspicion of an intracranial process.

Her pattern of complaints indicates a high potential for a threat to life. How would you proceed with assessment and care?

While your partner is obtaining this information, you have been managing the airway and beginning a physical exam and vital signs measurements.

The patient did not respond to verbal stimuli and continued to snore, so you performed a head-tilt, chin-lift. The snoring stopped, and now her breathing seems easier at a rate of 24. She accepts an oral airway with no gag reflex. Lung sounds are clear with a good tidal volume. Pulse oximetry shows 98 percent, so you apply a nonrebreather mask with a reservoir at 15 lpm. Her radial pulse is strong at 54, and her blood pressure is 180/130. A quick check of her pupils shows them to be equal but sluggish. Her blood glucose level is 210 mg/dl. What do these findings tell you?

The assessment findings confirm the suspicion you already formed from the history. The pattern of slower heart rate with high blood pressure (two parts of Cushing's triad), altered mental status, and sluggish pupils points to a CNS problem that has a high probability for increasing intracranial pressure. Together with the history of hypertension and lack of medication compliance, you conclude that this patient may well be suffering a hemorrhagic stroke. Note: This patient was also an untreated type II diabetic. It was this fact, as well as the presence of a body stressor (the release of epinephrine/norepinephrine will also stimulate gluconeogenesis), that resulted in her high blood glucose level. What interventions are required now?

Your patient showed no gag reflex when the oral airway was inserted, so she cannot protect her airway. With a history of vomiting, securing an airway is a priority. At this moment her airway is intact, so you need to make a decision about whether to secure her airway now or wait until you obtain the remaining baseline assessment findings.

Based on your experience, you decide to intubate the patient immediately—but at that moment she begins to vomit thin, watery stomach fluid. You turn her on her side as she begins to display seizure-like activity. Your partner hands you the suction while he reaches for the diazepam. Maintaining her in position, you attempt to open her mouth and suction. Her seizure activity ends prior to the diazepam; however, trismus is present and you cannot open her mouth. You quickly assess her breathing and determine that, at a rate of 6, it is inadequate. You change the nonrebreather mask to a bag-valve mask and start carefully ventilating at a rate of 14 to 16. You note that it is difficult to get good chest rise and fall despite repositioning of the airway. You realize that managing her airway is a priority. The presence of trismus eliminates that option of oral intubation. Now that the patient has clamped her jaws shut, how can intubation be accomplished?

This patient needs to have her airway secured as soon as possible. In this situation, with her jaws clamped shut, there are two choices: a nasotracheal intubation or a rapid sequence induction (RSI). Your partner quickly ascertains that the patient has had surgery on her nose and nasal passages. Due to her slow respiratory rate and history of nasal surgery, you decide that nasally intubating is not appropriate. Because the distance between the prominence of the mandible and the hyoid bone is four fingers, and the horizontal distance between the angles of the jaw appears wide, you decide that RSI is a good option for managing her airway.

Several of the sedating, amnesic, and paralytic drugs that may be used with RSI are known to produce hypertension or an increase in intracranial pressure. Some of these drugs also produce cardiac depression. This patient has a history of hypertension and a high probability of increased intracranial pressure, with a slowing of the heart rate already noticed. These factors guide you when you consider RSI and the medications you carry. In this case, you are authorized to administer etomidate as a sedative and vecuronium as a nondepolarizing, paralytic agent. What are the next steps?

An IV is started, pulse oximetry is attached, a monitor is applied, and your partner ventilates the patient. Pulse oximetry is 92 percent with clear lung sounds, and the monitor shows a sinus rhythm with no ectopy. After preparing your medications and your tracheal tube, you administer lidocaine and the sedative/hypnotic etomidate followed by succinylcholine. The patient's jaws visibly relax. You insert your laryngoscope, visualize the vocal cords, and insert your tracheal tube. After assuring correct placement, you secure the tube, attach capnography, and place a c-collar to ensure the patient's head does not move and inadvertently dislodge the tube. You are able to maintain a capnography reading of 40 at a ventilatory rate of 12/min with no sign of bronchospasm. What is the reasoning behind maintaining a capnography reading of 40?

Even though the patient's pulse oximetry is 98 percent, increasing intracranial pressure creates hypoxia in the brain through local tissue ischemia. (It's a vicious cycle: The initial insult triggers local edema, compressing blood vessels and leading to local ischemia, creating tissue hypoxia, which builds up metabolic acids, causing local vessel dilation, triggering more edema, further compressing blood vessels, and so on.) So, ensuring good tidal volume and exhalation of carbon dioxide is a priority. Capnometry measures exhaled carbon dioxide accurately in real time. Because there is a helpful correlation between capnometry values and blood gas values of CO_2*, 35 to 45 is the desired range for capnometry values. Not only does capnometry guide ventilatory rate, but, by measuring* CO_2 *exhalation, capnometry is also the gold standard for recognizing a misplaced tracheal tube.* What are the chances, do you think, of an uneventful transport to the hospital?

You load your patient and proceed to the hospital. En route, she suddenly has a generalized tonic-clonic (grand mal) seizure. You quickly grab a preloaded syringe of diazepam 10 mg. By the time you are ready to administer the medication, her seizure activity has stopped. So, you hold the diazepam, quickly check capnometry for tube placement, and then check her pupils. A capnometry value of

64 quickly reveals that the tube is still in place, but the left pupil is fixed and dilated while the right is sluggish. A recheck of her vital signs shows a radial pulse of 50 and a blood pressure of 200/100. You adjust your ventilations to lower the CO_2 level to 40 and keep the diazepam ready. You know that, although the numbers are significant, it is the trend in the numerical values that is most helpful and important. Why were you planning to administer diazepam—and why didn't you administer it? What is the significance of the pupil exam? the rechecked vitals?

Her bradycardia and wide pulse pressure are of two of the three typical signs of Cushing's reflex for increased intracranial pressure. The seizure-like activity is typical of irritation of the brain, either due to the pressure or due to free blood in contact with brain tissue. When a seizure occurs, intracranial pressure increases, creating further damage. Consequently, stopping the seizure activity is critical.

In the field, diazepam (Valium) is the drug of choice to stop a seizure. However, diazepam does not prevent seizures, so diazepam is usually administered during a seizure but not once the seizure has stopped.

Her fixed pupil indicates increased pressure from the left side, which has caused the dilated and unreactive pupil. Because a "blown pupil" is strongly suggestive of increased intracranial pressure, hyperventilation may be authorized as a last resort to buy time by helping perfuse the brain. The ventilation effort is aimed at reducing CO_2 levels, thus reducing vasodilation that may be occurring and, in turn, limiting swelling. With the advent of capnography and the ability to take frequent or continuous measures of exhaled CO_2, trending of the numerical values can be observed and used as a basis for adjusting ventilatory rates to maintain desired CO_2 levels.

Posturing would also be common at this point, but your patient does not display the typical extremity rigidity during transport. What might be the outcome for this patient?

The patient has no further seizure activity and, on arrival at the hospital, the ED staff takes over the ventilations. Blood gases are done and then, during initial baseline assessments, the patient begins posturing. She is taken immediately to the CT scan where an intracranial bleed is discovered. Her prognosis is poor.

As you are leaving, you see your patient's husband, looking bewildered and confused, in the hallway. You stop to see how he is doing and ask if he has any questions regarding your care of his wife. He tells you that he is grateful for everything you have done and asks if they have told you that his wife might not make it. You tell him yes, you were told that, and you express how sorry you were to hear it. After a few more minutes of conversation you leave, feeling unsettled and a bit angry, wondering if this would have happened had this patient taken her medication as she should have.

SCENARIO 7: ALTERED MENTAL STATUS

It is 13:00 hours, and you are dispatched to a 70-year-old male who has fallen. On arrival, you find your patient lying on the floor of the entryway to a church. He had been attending a meeting and was on his way out to lunch when he paused, turned to the man next to him, and said he felt faint. The other man helped him to the floor and sought help. From the few facts you have gathered so far, do you have any clues to the etiology of this episode?

The patient's description of feeling "faint," versus feeling "dizzy," can be a clue to the origin of the episode. Feeling "dizzy," as if the room were spinning, is more indicative of the balance organ being affected. Feeling "faint," or light-headed, is more indicative of another type of problem. This description needs to be verified. What would you look for as you begin to assess the patient?

Your 70-year-old patient is awake and focuses on you as you approach. He appears pale and is moving all extremities. You kneel beside him, taking his hand and feeling for a pulse in his wrist as you begin talking. He is alert and oriented and states he feels fine now. He is talking in complete sentences, and his arm feels cool and dry with an irregular radial pulse of about 90. His skin turgor is good. What are your first impressions of this patient's condition?

The patient's ability to focus on you, his orientation, and the movement of all extremities seems to lessen the probability of a stroke. A full assessment of extremity function is necessary, however, and may reveal more information. His talking in complete sentences indicates adequate minute volume at rest. For the moment, his mental status implies adequate perfusion to the brain. His irregular pulse needs to be checked. However, as long as he is lying down, he looks pretty stable. What's next in assessing this patient?

While your partner brings over the cardiac monitor, you proceed to get a full set of vital signs. The monitor shows atrial fibrillation at a rate of 86 to 90. Vital signs are pulse 88 and irregular, respirations 18, and blood pressure 146/82. The patient tells you that he is on Lanoxin (digoxin [Digitek]) for his heart. Lasix (furosemide) is his water pill, Diazide (hydrochlorothiazide) is for his blood pressure, and Isordil (isosorbide) is for his heart. He says he is allergic to "some blood pressure medication, I can't remember which one." He assures you that he takes his medications regularly. Have you formed any further ideas about the etiology of the episode of faintness?

So far, the patient's assessment is pretty normal. From his medications, you know he has chronic heart problems, including angina. His atrial fibrillation is also confirmed by his medications. However, atrial fibrillation can predispose to the development of clots and subsequent embolic stroke, so a thorough check of neurologic function, including movement and sensation of his extremities, is warranted. Cardiac dysrhythmias can cause faintness, but faintness in the elderly, especially, has myriad possibilities. To help sort it out, more of an assessment should be completed. What more would you try to find out?

The patient states he felt fine this morning and does not know why he suddenly felt faint. When he describes the incident, he says he was feeling fine when he got up from his meeting but then, as he was walking out, he felt "light-headed." He denies any sensation of spinning. He denies any pain or discomfort prior to the incident; denies losing consciousness, which his friends confirm; and denies previous episodes.

Further questioning reveals that he has been on his medications for about a year, with isosorbide added about 6 or 8 months ago. He did eat breakfast this morning, but not too much, because his stomach has been "bothering" due to a hiatal hernia. He last saw his doctor about 2 months ago, and everything was okay. In fact, he has been feeling pretty good lately. He also denies melena (blood in the stool) and denies hematuria (blood in the urine). You perform a gross cranial nerve exam along with the Cincinnati Prehospital Stroke Scale. Everything looks normal.

You ask those with him if his color is normal for him. They tell you his normal coloring is pale, but maybe he is just a little more pale than usual. So far, this patient seems pretty normal. Have you identified any further clues to the etiology of his problem?

A loss of brain perfusion can be a factor of age, medication, or pathology. Even though we may not be able to tell which is likely, testing for it can determine whether there is a problem. So far, you have checked his mental status and cognitive function. His gross motor movement seems fine, and his cardiovascular system seems adequate with no sign of dysrhythmia or chest pain. A problem with his medication is unlikely because he has not had any recent changes. His paler-than-usual color is the only thing that seems to be out of character for him.

By the way, although your patient felt faint, the fact that he did not actually lose consciousness means that, by definition, he did not suffer from true syncope. So just what is the underlying problem? Two more things still need to be checked as you try to determine the probable etiology. What would you check next?

Your partner gets the blood glucose monitor and tests the patient's blood sugar. His blood sugar reading is 50. You ask your patient what time he ate breakfast this morning, and he tells you "About 6 A.M." It is now a little over 7 hours later. When you ask whether he has had anything to eat since breakfast, he tells you no, he passed over the refreshments at the meeting and just had some water because he was going out to lunch with his friends and did not want to spoil his appetite. You explain that his blood sugar is a little low and ask his friends if there is something left over from the meeting refreshments that he might eat. While they are going to get a piece of cake, your patient sheepishly looks at you and says, "You know, my doctor told me my blood sugar was a little low and I needed to eat regularly, but he didn't tell me this might happen if I didn't!" He chuckles and tells you that sometimes his doctor is right. You laugh with him and agree.

You also explain that you need to check one more thing, and you proceed with a tilt test. After explaining what you are going to do, you sit the patient up and take his pulse and blood pressure. His pulse is 96 and irregular, and his blood pressure is 138/78. You ask how he feels, and he says he feels a little weak but otherwise feels fine. By that time the cake arrives, along with a cup of punch, and you have him eat the cake and drink the punch, watching him carefully to be sure that he does not get faint again while he is eating. Within 5 minutes his pallor is much improved, and he is laughing with his friends and embarrassed that you were called. You try to persuade him to go to the hospital to be checked, but he refuses—with a smile, but quite firmly. What do you conclude from the results of the blood sugar test and the tilt test?

A low blood glucose level usually presents with symptoms that are more gradual than the symptoms you seem to be seeing in this patient; in the elderly, however, changes are sometimes seen only when body need arises. Therefore, blood glucose levels should be checked if there is the suspicion of hypoglycemia, even in the nondiabetic elderly. A tilt test should be conducted to rule out orthostatic hypotension as a cause of the faintness. Orthostatic hypotension may result from a variety of causes, including blood loss or other hypovolemic states; medications such as vasodilators, diuretics, and beta-blockers; or autonomic neuropathy, which is common in diabetics and the elderly. In elderly men, orthostatic hypotension may be a chronic condition and with no apparent cause.

Your patient passed the tilt test—his results were negative for orthostatic hypotension. This leaves low blood sugar as the culprit in the case, and his quick improvement after eating pins this down as the likely etiology. Because the patient has refused transport to the hospital, how should you conclude the call?

Having determined that your patient's refusal of transport is final, you check his blood sugar once more and make sure that he can get up and walk around without any problem. You encourage him to see his doctor once more about his diet, complete your instructions, and have him sign the refusal form.

Several months later, you run into this patient again. He remembers you and thanks you for your help that day. He tells you he is now eating more regularly and more often and feels "great." In fact, he tells you that you changed his life for the better. It seems he is dating one of the ladies at the church, and he credits you with making her notice him that day. According to him, she is a great cook, and he's taking advantage of it—by his doctor's order, of course!

SCENARIO 8: CHEST PAIN

It is 10:00 hours. You are dispatched to a 38-year-old male with chest pain. On your arrival, his wife greets you at the door and tells you her husband has been up for several hours with chest pain. He woke from sleep at 5 A.M. with an ache in his chest that has steadily gotten worse. She also tells you he is a cancer patient with a relapse of leukemia and is undergoing chemotherapy for the second time. The description of chest pain is suspicious for cardiac involvement. However, this is a fairly young man, and he is suffering from a chronic disease. What possibilities immediately enter your mind?

The presence of a chronic disease implies that his problem may not be isolated to a single body system and/or may be a result of the chronic disease process. Another implication is that normal compensatory mechanisms are already being taxed, leading to decompensation more quickly than in someone without a chronic disease. You have not yet made contact with the patient—but what steps are you already planning?

As the patient's wife leads you into the bedroom, you find your patient sitting upright in bed. He is awake, but his color is ashen and he is diaphoretic. As you approach, you pull out a nonrebreather mask while your partner is getting the cardiac monitor ready. What is your general impression as you approach the patient?

His ashen color implies poor perfusion, and his diaphoresis implies that a sympathetic response has occurred. These signs, in the presence of chest pain, are consistent with cardiac involvement and imply a serious problem is present. You have all the information you need to justify high-flow, high-concentration oxygen and the need to evaluate the cardiac rhythm. But more of an assessment is needed to determine the exact nature of the problem and whether pharmacologic intervention is necessary. Simultaneous assessment and care are clearly required. How will you proceed?

You apply the nonrebreather mask at 15 lpm while your partner applies the monitor, and you start asking the patient about his pain. He describes it as substernal but denies radiation. He explains that he felt a heaviness in his chest last night when he went to bed but did not think much of it because he had not felt good all day. He was awakened about 5 A.M. by an "ache" in his chest that got steadily worse. He put off calling EMS because he really did not want to go to the hospital again. He describes his pain as "terrible pressure" and ranks it as a 10 on a scale of 1 to 10.

He seems out of breath when he talks, and his skin is cold and clammy. Your partner is getting an IV ready, and you check the monitor. His ECG shows a regular sinus tachycardia of 128. You quickly obtain a set of vital signs. He has respirations of 22, blood pressure 88/72, and, in spite of the regular sinus tachycardia, the palpated radial pulse seems to be irregular at a rate of 116. What clues have you obtained so far to the possible etiology of the chest pain?

The patient's description of pain is highly suggestive of cardiac involvement. His cold, clammy skin and rapid pulse support the suspicion of an epinephrine/norepinephrine response. His vital signs confirm that he is in shock. From the assessment so far, cardiogenic shock is implied.

However, because of his history of chronic disease, the cause of his cardiogenic shock should be explored further. The palpated irregular intensity of his pulse in the presence of a regular heart rate by cardiac monitor is suspicious for a paradoxical pulse. This is not typical of cardiogenic shock from ventricular muscle failure due to an AMI. Although his breathlessness bears further assessment, determining the most likely cause of his irregular pulse is of primary importance. How will you continue to assess this patient's respiratory and cardiac status?

While you listen to lung sounds, you also note the patient's heart sounds. Lung sounds are equal and clear, but his heart sounds are hard to hear. You also note that his neck veins are distended. A rapid check of his hands also reveals peripherally distended veins. A careful check of the radial pulse reveals that the pulse disappears on inspiration. On expiration, the pulse returns. The ECG continues to show a regular QRS tracing. What do these findings indicate?

Distended jugular and peripheral veins are strongly suggestive of a backup of venous pressure. When peripheral veins are distended in both extremities, the problem is somewhere in the chest. The disappearance of the radial pulse on inspiration is indicative of increased intrathoracic pressure interfering with cardiac output. Such an increase in intrathoracic pressure occurs when there is either enough air trapping to cause that amount of pressure (tension pneumothorax) or there is something interfering with the filling of the ventricles (cardiac tamponade) so that normal breathing causes enough pressure for a paradoxical pulse to occur.

Listening to lung sounds will help determine whether air trapping is present. His are equal and clear, implying that air trapping is not the case. The heart sounds, however, are hard to hear, which implies that something is interfering with either the transmission of sound or the amount of blood filling the heart. This is strongly suggestive of a cardiac tamponade. Cardiac tamponade in a medical patient? This seems highly unusual. Is your suspicion accurate? Have you done the right thing for this patient?

Your partner adjusts the IV to deliver a fluid bolus of 500 ml. A rapid recheck of the patient's blood pressure shows 90/78, with no change in his cardiac rate. The ECG monitor shows low voltage on the monitored lead.

You load him up and prepare for rapid transport. En route, his color remains the same, but he seems less alert. Vital signs remain at pulse 118 and irregular with a monitored heart rate of 130, respirations 22, and blood pressure 82/70. Fortunately, the transport time is relatively short. Your radio report of your assessment findings has alerted the hospital to your suspicion. On arrival at the ED, the patient's color remains ashen and he is very restless.

After quickly assessing heart sounds and lung sounds and completing a rapid chest X-ray, the physician does a pericardiocentesis and begins withdrawing blood-tinged, serous fluid. The patient begins to look better right away. After observing for a few more minutes, you leave the room to complete your paper work. The doctor finds you at the desk and commends you on your radio report. "Good job, guys. You told me exactly what I needed to be able to identify the problem."

"Gee, doc," your partner replies, "this is the first patient I've seen with a cardiac tamponade and no trauma. I didn't know that could happen."

"It doesn't happen often, but sometimes cancer patients, or even people with pericarditis, develop a pericardial effusion that is bad enough to create a cardiac tamponade. But usually it occurs more slowly and symptoms are more gradual. Didn't this fellow start having symptoms earlier?"

"Yeah, he did," you reply, "and I'm sure he thought he was having a heart attack. So did I, at first."

"Well, you guys did a good job. I think he's going to be okay, at least for now. See you around," he says.

"Thanks doc, see ya," you both say as you turn to leave.

SCENARIO 9: SUDDEN-ONSET PARAPLEGIA

It is 21:00 hours. You are dispatched to an assisted-living apartment building for a 78-year-old female who suddenly became unable to move her legs. On arrival, you are greeted by an attendant who leads you to the patient. Rose is lying on the couch, with her head elevated on several cushions. She appears pale but is awake, alert, and oriented. She tells you that she was watching TV and decided to get up but could not move her legs. So she called the attendant, who called you. Rose tells you that she normally walks with her walker but has not had any trouble and is very distressed to discover that now she cannot move her legs. This is a very unusual case. Usually, trauma is a factor with paraplegia. What is significant about her history that might help you focus your assessment?

Significant history includes her sudden onset. The description of her problem suggests that the central nervous system, specifically the spinal cord, is involved. Usually, medical problems involving the central nervous system that result in difficulty walking are either more gradual in onset, such as Guillain-Barré syndrome, or result in unilateral deficits, such as a stroke. The fact that Rose uses a walker suggests a predisposing factor that will need to be explored. Can gathering further history from the attendant and Rose shed some light?

The attendant tells you that Rose normally uses her walker because of bilateral hip fractures that required replacement surgery. Rose is normally healthy but has not had much energy the last several days. She was at dinner and did not seem to have any problem walking then. Dinner was at 5 P.M., and Rose did not eat anything but her JELL-O because she was not that hungry. After dinner, Rose states, her gastric reflux was "acting up," so she returned to her room, took her "purple pill" (Nexium), and propped herself up on the couch to watch the news. She fell asleep, and when she woke up she was unable to walk. She denies any trauma. Rose's lack of hunger and gastric reflux after eating JELL-O (typically, JELL-O does not aggravate gastric reflux) are puzzling. To discover what might be causing these symptoms, as well as what might cause paraplegia without trauma, you need to gather some past medical history.

Further conversation with Rose reveals that she has a history of coronary artery disease, hypertension, type II diabetes, gastric reflux disease, glaucoma, and osteoporosis, with bilateral hip replacement about a year ago. She is on Isordil (isosorbide), Blocadren (timolol), Vasotec (enalapril), Tricor (fenofibrate), Ticlid (ticlopidine), Skelaxin (metaxalone), and Nexium (esomeprazole). She takes her medicine regularly and is allergic to aspirin. Rose denies pain or discomfort, although she does admit to "not feeling well." When asked to define "not feeling well," she tells you she has no energy, does not feel like eating and, for the last several days, gets light-headed if she gets up too fast. What is significant about Rose's past medical history that influences your assessment?

The fact that Rose is a diabetic, is on a chronic muscle relaxant (Skelaxin), and does not feel well is suggestive of peripheral neuropathy with medication masking her pain. Her description of getting light-headed if she gets up too fast, gastric reflux "acting up," and a previous history of lack of energy is suggestive of a more serious problem. You just do not exactly know what underlying problem may be present. Now that you have gathered the history, how should you proceed with the physical exam?

You continue your assessment while your partner applies oxygen by nonrebreather mask at 15 lpm and gets a set of vital signs. Rose is alert, oriented, and anxious over her inability to move her legs. Her skin is pale with poor turgor. She has a radial pulse of 72, respirations of 20 with clear lung sounds, and a BP of 106/78. Her abdomen is soft and nondistended. She does complain of feeling "uncomfortable" on palpation in the upper quadrants. When asked to describe the "uncomfortable" feeling, she tells you it makes her feel "nauseated" and "just uncomfortable." On a scale of 1 to 10, 10 being the worst discomfort, she tells you that it is an 8. Her pelvis is intact, as are her legs. You note that her legs are very pale, and you cannot find pedal pulses. Your partner starts 2 IVs, one a large-bore IV and the other a blood pump, while you attach the monitor. Your partner tells you her blood glucose is 150 mg/dl. What is significant about Rose's physical assessment?

Rose's pale skin, poor turgor, and lack of pedal pulses is significant for a volume problem. This seems to be confirmed by her description of light-headedness when she gets up too fast. Her systolic pressure is low for someone with a history of hypertension. Her pulse should be faster if hypotension is present, but she is on a beta-blocker (Blocadren) and an ACE inhibitor (Vasotec), which could be preventing an increase in pulse rate. In geriatric patients especially (due to inefficient sympathetic response), a gradual decrease in body volume together with a beta-blocker could result in a normal pulse rate in the presence of hypovolemia.

If her report of taking her medication and just eating JELL-O are accurate, a blood glucose level of 150 suggests that a sympathetic response, enough to release glycogen stores, is occurring.

Lack of pedal pulses in the presence of abdominal pain is suggestive of an aneurysm. An aneurysm resulting in an inability to walk would mean that the aneurysm is at the level of the vertebral artery. That would suggest the presence of further deficit in her abdomen and extremities. It also suggests presence of a threat to life and the need for rapid transport. How should you now continue with assessment and care?

You note a regular sinus rhythm on the monitor, administer a 500-ml bolus of fluid, and load your patient for transport. You decide to take Rose to the closest trauma center for their vascular surgical capability. Repeat assessment shows no change in heart rate, lung sounds remaining clear, and an increased BP of 112/82. En route to the hospital, you administer another 500-ml bolus, rechecking lung sounds and blood pressure. On arrival to the emergency department, Rose has a pulse of 78, no change in respirations, and a systolic blood pressure of 118/84.

You give your report and are finishing your paperwork when you see Rose being taken to the CT scan. Later, after delivering another patient, you ask the ED physician what happened. He tells you Rose was the most interesting case he has seen in a long time. She had a thoracic aneurysm that occluded the vertebral artery, resulting in paraplegia. She was taken to surgery straight from CT; he did not know the outcome, but the prognosis was poor.

SCENARIO 10: UNCONSCIOUS WOMAN

It is 14:35 hours. It is a hot, humid summer day when you are dispatched to a private residence in an older part of town. You arrive to find a man in his fifties waving you into a small, well-kept home. He is busy throwing all the windows open and tells you his mother is in the kitchen. When you enter the home, you note how hot it is. Before you even reach the patient, your shirt is sticking to you. Betty is lying on the floor. She appears to be in her eighties. Her face is very red, and her lips are cyanotic. You note weak, rapid movement of her chest wall. She is not responding to your voice or touch. Her skin is dry and very hot to the touch. What is significant about the immediate surroundings?

It is a very hot environment, and a heat-related illness is your first thought. How will you continue your assessment?

You immediately check Betty's respirations and pulse. Respirations are 50/min, and she has no radial pulse with a weak, thready carotid at around 160. You quickly ask the son what happened. He tells you his mother called and said the air conditioner was not working. He states she must have gotten confused and turned on the heat instead of the air conditioner. She takes some pill for hypertension and has been healthy until this. While you were talking to the son, your partner has immediately applied oxygen by nonrebreather mask at 15 lpm. Both of you move Betty to the stretcher and to your ambulance. You ask for a driver from the engine crew and get on the way to the hospital immediately. Why do you apply oxygen and then move her to the ambulance prior to starting further treatment?

Betty is critically ill. She must be removed from the hot environment as soon as possible. Even though her respirations are not adequate, applying oxygen by mask will start cooling her through her respiratory system while you are moving her. What care should you provide en route?

Once in the ambulance, you turn on the air conditioner to cool the environment and start one IV while your partner applies the monitor and starts another IV, checking her blood glucose level. The monitor shows a left axis, left bundle branch block and tachycardia. Her blood glucose level is 138. You move to ventilate her with a bag-valve mask, while your partner checks her blood pressure and gets ready to intubate. Her BP is 60/38. Betty has no gag reflex and is readily intubated with a 7.5 tracheal tube. While your partner takes over ventilations, you check lung sounds. You confirm placement and note pulmonary edema in all lobes. You secure the tube, apply capnography, and note a blunted alpha angle, suggesting bronchoconstriction, and a capnometry value of 60. Your partner adjusts ventilations to achieve a value closer to 40. What is the significance of the ECG changes? What is the connection between pulmonary edema and hyperthermia? What is the significance of a capnometry value of 60?

Severe hyperthermia results in an increased oxygen demand, metabolic acidosis, and multisystem failure. The ECG changes are reflective of the severe demand on her heart. Betty's entire body is in an extreme state of stress. Her heart is failing, unable to keep up with the increased metabolic demand, most likely producing ischemia, extreme tachycardia, and breakdown of muscle enzymes due to hyperthemia, resulting in pulmonary edema. She is also in respiratory failure with a carbon dioxide level of 60. What should you do to help stabilize Betty's condition?

Your partner administers positive-pressure ventilation to help blow off the carbon dioxide and to help cool Betty through her respiratory system. Bronchoconstriction is a protective mechanism of the lungs. Positive-pressure ventilation with 100 percent oxygen is the initial treatment of choice followed by reassessment to determine further treatment.

You strip off Betty's clothing, cover her with a sheet, and break out the sterile water, soaking the sheet. You also make sure to wet Betty's hair and fan her. You then turn up the air conditioner. While your partner continues to monitor capnography and adjust ventilations, you check the flow rate of the IVs. You now have 300 ml of fluid on board. You recheck vital signs. Her pulse rate is 150, respirations are being assisted, and her BP has not changed. You now consider more fluid and an inline nebulized treatment of albuterol. Why would you wet Betty's hair? Why more fluid if she has pulmonary edema? Why nebulized albuterol if she has pulmonary edema?

The head is a primary route *of releasing body heat, and evaporation of water has a cooling effect. By wetting her hair, you are helping Betty's body cool off. She is severely dehydrated due to her extreme body heat and insensible loss of body water (usually through respirations). Even though she has pulmonary edema, she still needs replacement fluid for her dehydration and to dilute her metabolic acidosis. Administering controlled fluid replacement along with positive pressure will help dilute her acidosis, improve preload, oxygenate the heart muscle, and bring her heart rate under control, thus controlling pulmonary edema. Bronchoconstriction is a protective mechanism, in this case protecting against edema and possibly her extreme body heat. Unfortunately, bronchoconstriction will also prevent exchange of oxygen and carbon dioxide. As long as positive pressure is being administered and cooling methods begun, nebulized albuterol may help oxygen/carbon dioxide exchange and thus help provide the heart with needed oxygen.* What care should you now provide before arrival at the hospital?

After an additional 400-ml bolus, Betty's BP has increased to 70/48, and her pulse has decreased to 142 bpm. You assemble an inline nebulized treatment and attach it to the tracheal tube. Your partner continues to adjust ventilations, and now has a capnometer reading of 45. You rewet the sheet, rewet her hair, and reassess her lung sounds. You no longer hear crackles but are hearing wheezes bilaterally.

On arrival at the emergency department, you have administered a total of 1 liter of fluid. Betty's skin is still flushed and hot. Her lung sounds are now bilateral wheezes in all lobes with pulse of 136 and BP of 78/56. Her core temperature is 106.5 degrees Fahrenheit. The staff immediately places her in a cooling blanket, establishes a central line, draws blood chemistries, and begins further treatment. The ED physician tells you that brain protein begins to break down at 106 degrees Fahrenheit. He is not sure she will make it, and if she does, he is not sure she will be neurologically intact. In general, hyperthermia in the elderly has a poor prognosis. However, he compliments you on your aggressive treatment, without which Betty would probably have no chance at all.

Two months later, you are ready to sit down to lunch when the door bell rings. An elderly woman comes in, bringing a batch of chocolate chip cookies. She is with a man you vaguely recognize. Betty introduces herself, and you recognize the name but cannot place it. She reminds you that you were the ones to "save her life" when she nearly "cooked to death." You remember now and cannot believe this is the same woman. She tells you she is doing fine and is now living with her son and his wife. She made the cookies as a thank you. After chatting for a while, Betty and her son leave. To this day, you still marvel at her recovery.

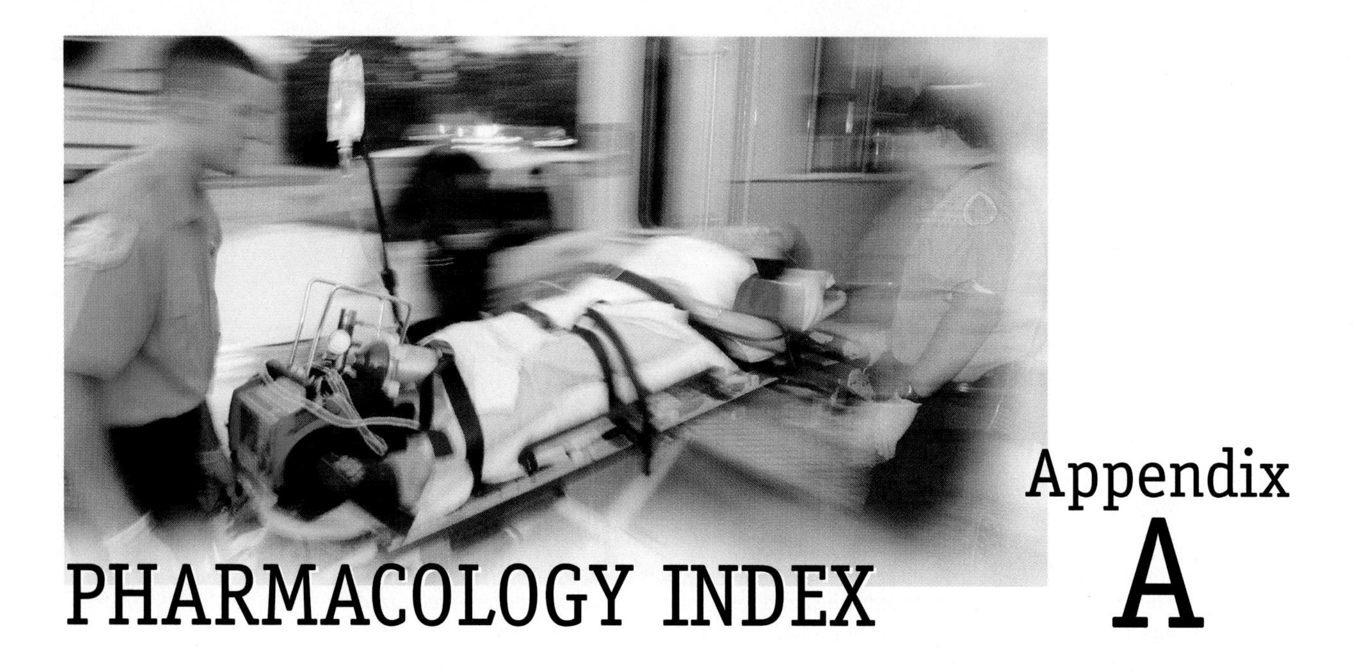

Appendix A
PHARMACOLOGY INDEX

The following is an index of drugs that are referred to in the chapters of this text and that are commonly administered in adult medical emergencies. This index can be used as a quick-reference guide. The drugs are listed alphabetically by generic name with brand names in parentheses. Several sources were consulted in compiling this index. Keep in mind that sources vary with regard to indications and dosages. Always consult your medical protocol or medical director for appropriate indications and dosages.

Acetylcysteine (Airbron, Mucomyst, Mucosol)

Class
- Mucolytic; antidote

Action
- Reduces hepatotoxicity in acetaminophen poisoning
- Reduces viscosity of purulent and nonpurulent pulmonary secretions
- Permits expectoration or removal by suction

Indications
- Antidote in acetaminophen poisoning
- Adjunct in treatment of acute and chronic bronchitis, emphysema, tuberculosis, pneumonia, bronchiectasis, and atelectasis

Contraindications
- Sensitivity to drug

Side Effects/Precautions
- Increased incidence of bronchospasm in patients with asthma
- Use with caution in the elderly
- Bronchial and tracheal irritation

- Tightness in chest
- Bronchoconstriction
- Nausea and vomiting
- Rash
- Fever
- Drowsiness
- Rhinorrhea
- Dizziness

Dosage

- Acetaminophen overdose: 140 mg/kg initially followed by 70 mg/kg every 4 hours for a total of 17 doses
- 1 to 10 ml of a 20% solution or 2 to 10 ml of a 10% solution three to four times daily by nebulizer for management of pulmonary secretions

Activated Charcoal (Aqua, Actidose, Liqui-Char)

Class

- Powerful pharmaceutical adsorbent and general-purpose antidote

Action

- Adsorbs ingested toxic substances that are still within the gastrointestinal tract and prevents gastrointestinal absorption

Indications

- Ingested poisoning and overdose by ingestion of medications or drugs

Contraindications

- Oral administration to an unresponsive patient
- Corrosives and caustic agents
- Petroleum distillates
- GI bleeding

Side Effects/Precautions

- Nausea and vomiting
- Abdominal cramping
- Constipation
- Syrup of ipecac and n-acetylcysteine may be inactivated by activated charcoal

Dosage

- 1 to 2 g/kg mixed with water to form a slurry
- May be given by nasogastric tube or orogastric tube
- Use larger dose if food is present in stomach

Adenosine (Adenocard)

Class

- Endogenous nucleoside, antidysrhythmic

Action

- Natural nucleoside that slows conduction through the AV node without negative inotropic effects
- Decreases chronotropic effect from direct activity on sinus pacemaker cells and vagal nerve terminals

Indications

- Supraventricular tachycardia, except for atrial fibrillation and flutter

Contraindications

- Adenosine hypersensitivity
- Bradycardia
- Second- or third-degree block
- Sick sinus syndrome

Side Effects/Precautions

- Transient dysrhythmias including second- or third-degree AV blocks, asystole, sinus bradycardia, premature atrial contractions, or premature ventricular contractions
- Facial flushing
- Headache
- Shortness of breath
- Dizziness
- Nausea
- Chest discomfort
- Bronchoconstriction
- Methylxanthines may decrease effectiveness, may require larger dose
- Dipyridamole may potentiate effect, may need to reduce dose

Dosage

- 6-mg rapid IV push followed by a 20-ml saline flush, repeated in 1 to 2 minutes at 12 mg to a total cumulative dose of 30 mg

Albuterol (Proventil, Ventolin, Salbutamol)

Class

- Beta 2-specific agonist, sympathomimetic, bronchodilator

Action

- Primarily a beta 2 agonist that dilates bronchial smooth muscle
- Relaxes vascular smooth muscle

Indications

- Reverse bronchoconstriction associated with asthma, emphysema, chronic bronchitis, and other conditions that cause bronchospasm

Contraindications

- Hypersensitivity to drug
- Symptomatic tachycardia
- Hypertension

- Tachycardia greater than 150 bpm
- Acute myocardial infarction

Side Effects/Precautions
- Tachycardia
- Hypertension
- Chest pain
- Anxiety
- Headache
- Dizziness
- Sweating
- Nausea and vomiting
- Tremors
- Dysrhythmia
- Antidepressants may potentiate vasodilation

Dosage
- 2.5 to 5.0 mg in 2.5 to 3 ml of normal saline via nebulizer over 5 to 15 minutes
- Repeat if severe bronchospasm persists

Aminophylline (Amoline, Somophyllin, Theophylline)

Class
- Methylxanthine

Action
- Smooth muscle relaxant
- Bronchodilation
- Mild diuretic
- Cardiac stimulant
- CNS stimulant

Indications
- Reversal of bronchospasm associated with asthma, chronic bronchitis, and emphysema
- Congestive heart failure
- Pulmonary edema
- Rarely used in the acute setting

Contraindications
- Hypersensitivity
- Tachydysrhythmias
- Peptic ulcer disease and acute gastritis
- Dysrhythmia

Side Effects/Precautions
- May cause atrial and ventricular dysrhythmias
- Use with caution for a patient who has liver disease or congestive heart failure or a patient on theophylline

- Draw blood for a theophylline level
- Palpitations
- Chest pain
- Headache
- Nervousness
- Seizures
- Tremors
- Anxiety
- Dizziness
- Nausea and vomiting

Dosage
- 5 to 6 mg/kg IV infusion over a 20- to 30-minute period
- If the patient is on a theophylline or aminophylline drug, reduce the loading dose to 2.5 to 3 mg/kg

Aspirin (A.S.A, Bayer, Ecotrin, St. Joseph, Others)

Class
- Platelet aggregation inhibitor
- Antiinflammatory agent
- Analgesic
- Antipyretic

Action
- Inhibits platelet aggregation and reduces clot formation
- Decreases inflammation
- Blocks pain impulses in the central nervous system

Indications
- Acute myocardial infarction
- Acute ischemic stroke

Contraindications
- Hypersensitivity
- Hemorrhagic stroke
- Bleeding disorder
- GI bleeding

Side Effects/Precautions
- GI bleeding
- Nausea and vomiting
- May cause wheezing
- Heartburn

Dosage
- 81- to 325-mg tablet chewed or swallowed

Atropine Sulfate

Class
- Parasympatholytic (anticholinergic, vagolytic)

Action
- Anticholinergic agent that blocks acetylcholine receptors blocking the parasympathetic nervous system influence on the heart, smooth muscle, and glands
- Increases heart rate by reducing parasympathetic tone on sinoatrial node
- Increases atrioventricular conduction
- Decreases gastrointestinal secretions

Indications
- Hemodynamically significant bradycardia
- Asystole
- Organophosphate poisoning or nerve gas exposure
- PEA with slow complex rate

Contraindications
- Asymptomatic bradycardia
- Tachycardia
- Hypersensitivity
- Thyrotoxicosis

Side Effects/Precautions
- Tachycardia
- Palpitations
- Seizures
- Hypertension
- Respiratory failure
- Dizziness
- Anxiety
- Dry mouth
- Pupillary dilation
- Blurred vision
- Urinary retention

Dosage
- Symptomatic bradycardia: 0.5 to 1.0 mg IV repeated in 3 to 5 minutes at dose of 0.5 to 1.0 mg to a total maximum cumulative dose of 0.04 mg/kg
- Asystole: 1 mg repeated every 3 to 5 minutes to a total maximum cumulative dose of 0.04 mg/kg
- Organophosphate poisoning: 2 mg repeated until blood pressure and heart rate are stable
- Tracheal dose is 2 to 2.5 times the intravenous dose

Calcium Chloride

Class
- Calcium salt (electrolyte)

Action

- Increases calcium levels (calcium is necessary for normal function of nerves, muscles, skeletal system, and for cell membrane and capillary permeability)
- Has a role in the release of neurotransmitters and hormones
- Increases cardiac contractile state
- May increase ventricular automaticity

Indications

- Acute hypocalcemia
- Acute hyperkalemia
- Calcium channel blocker overdose
- Hypermagnesemia

Contraindications

- Hypercalcemia
- Digitalis toxicity
- Renal or cardiac disease

Side Effects/Precautions

- Extravasation may cause tissue damage and necrosis
- Will precipitate if mixed with sodium bicarbonate
- Rapid injection may cause vasodilation, hypotension, bradycardia, cardiac dysrhythmia, syncope, and cardiac arrest

Dosage

- 2 to 4 mg/kg of a 10% solution repeated at 10-minute intervals

Calcium Gluconate (Kalcinate)

Class

- Calcium salt

Action

- Increases calcium levels (calcium is necessary for normal function of nerves, muscles, skeletal system, and for cell membrane and capillary permeability)
- Has a role in the release of neurotransmitters and hormones
- Increases cardiac contractile state
- May increase ventricular automaticity

Indications

- Acute hypocalcemia
- Acute hyperkalemia
- Calcium channel blocker overdose

Contraindications

- Hypercalcemia
- Patient on digitalis
- Renal or cardiac disease

Side Effects/Precautions

- Extravasation may cause tissue damage and necrosis
- Will precipitate when mixed with sodium bicarbonate

- Rapid injection may cause vasodilation, hypotension, bradycardia, cardiac dysrhythmia, syncope, and cardiac arrest

Dosage
- 2.25 to 14 mEq intravenously repeated in 1 to 2 minutes

Cimetidine Hydrochloride (Tagamet)

Class
- Histamine H2 receptor antagonist

Action
- Inhibits the action of histamine at the H2 receptors

Indications
- Anaphylactic or anaphylactoid reaction

Contraindications
- Hypersensitivity

Side Effects/Precautions
- Dysrhythmias
- Hypotension from rapid administration
- Diarrhea
- Headache

Dosage
- 300 mg IV diluted with 50 to 100 ml of normal saline and administered over 15 to 20 minutes

Dextrose 50% (D_{50})

Class
- Carbohydrate

Action
- Increases blood glucose level

Indications
- Hypoglycemia

Contraindications
- Do not use for altered mental status due to stroke, head injury, or other intracranial pathology unless hypoglycemia is documented

Side Effects/Precautions
- Local venous irritation
- Infiltration may cause tissue necrosis
- Collect a blood sample before administration
- Consider thiamine administration in suspected thiamine-deficient patients

Dosage
- 25 g (50 ml) intravenous injection

Diazepam (Valium)

Class
- Benzodiazepine

Action
- CNS depressant
- Anticonvulsant
- Anxiolytic
- Sedative
- Skeletal muscle relaxant

Indications
- Status epilepticus or actively seizing patient
- Skeletal muscle relaxant
- Sedation prior to cardioversion
- Reduction of extreme anxiety

Contraindications
- Hypersensitivity

Side Effects/Precautions
- Local venous irritation and burning at the intravenous injection site that often produces pain on injection
- CNS depression
- Respiratory depression
- Hypotension when injected too rapidly
- Use with caution in patients with narrow-angle glaucoma and those with increased intraocular pressure

Dosage
- Seizures: 5 to 10 mg over a 3-minute period repeated every 5 minutes to a total of 20 mg
- Acute anxiety: 2 to 5 mg IV or IM
- Premedication prior to cardioversion: 5 to 15 mg IV
- For induction, 0.2 mg/kg can be used

Diltiazem (Cardizem) Injectable

Class
- Slow calcium channel blocker

Action
- Slows conducton through the atrioventricular node
- Increases refractoriness in the atrioventricular node
- Causes coronary and peripheral vasodilation
- Decreases myocardial oxygen demand
- Decreases the ventricular response

Indications
- Control ventricular response rates in atrial fibrillation, atrial flutter, multifocal atrial tachycardia, and paroxysmal supraventricular tachycardia

Contraindications
- Hypotension
- Wolff-Parkinson-White syndrome
- Wide complex tachycardia
- Conduction system defects
- Should not be used in patients receiving intravenous beta-blockers

Side Effects/Precautions
- Hypotension
- Nausea and vomiting
- Dizziness
- Incompatible with concurrent furosemide injection
- Bradycardia
- Sweating
- Syncope
- Dry mouth
- Headache
- Chest pain
- Ventricular dysrhythmias

Dosage
- 0.25 mg/kg (typically 15 to 20 mg) IV over 2 minutes; may be repeated in 15 minutes at 0.35 mg/kg (typically 20 to 25 mg) IV over 2 minutes; maintenance infusion of 125 mg (25 ml) in 100 ml infused at 5 to 15 mg/hour and titrated to heart rate

Diphenhydramine (Benadryl)

Class
- Antihistamine (H1 histamine blocker)

Action
- Blocks histamine H1 receptor sites
- Anticholinergic effects
- Reduces vasodilation, hypotension, tachycardia associated with histamine release in anaphylaxis

Indications
- Severe allergic reaction
- Anaphylaxis
- Dystonic (extrapyramidal) reaction as a result of phenothiazines and antipsychotic drugs

Contraindications
- Hypersensitivity
- Asthma
- Narrow-angle glaucoma

Side Effects/Precautions

- Hypotension
- Drowsiness
- Disturbed coordination
- Epigastric distress
- Dry mouth
- Dry nose
- Tachycardia
- Urinary retention
- Thickened bronchial secretions
- Wheezing
- Nausea and vomiting

Dosage

- 25 to 50 mg IV or deep IM

Dobutamine (Dobutrex)

Class

- Synthetic catecholamine (sympathomimetic) with primary beta-adrenergic reception stimulation

Action

- Positive inotrope (increases myocardial contractility)
- Increases stroke volume and cardiac output
- Minimal chronotrope (increased heart rate)

Indications

- Cardiogenic shock from left ventricular dysfunction
- Acute congestive heart failure

Contraindications

- Atrial fibrillation, atrial flutter
- Bradycardia-induced hypotension

Side Effects/Precautions

- May increase myocardial infarction size
- May cause ventricular irritability
- May be deactivated by alkaline solutions
- Headache
- Hypertension
- Palpitations

Dosage

- 2 to 20 μg/kg/min intravenous infusion

Dopamine (Intropin)

Class

- Sympathomimetic

Action
- Precursor to norepinephrine
- Dose-dependent action may include increased renal and mesentery blood flow, beta-adrenergic effects such as increased heart rate and myocardial contractility, and increased systemic vascular resistance from vasoconstriction
- Acts on alpha-, beta-, and dopaminergic-adrenergic receptors

Indications
- Cardiogenic shock with hemodynamically significant hypotension (systolic BP of 70 to 100 mmHg)

Contraindications
- Hypotension due to hypovolemia prior to fluid resuscitation efforts
- Pheochromocytoma (tumor of adrenal gland)

Side Effects/Precautions
- Tachydysrhythmias
- Hypertension
- Palpitations
- Nausea and vomiting
- Chest pain
- Nervousness
- Headache
- Dyspnea
- May be deactivated by alkaline solution
- Reduce the dose if patient is taking MAO inhibitor (antidepressant)
- May cause hypotension if administered concomitantly with phenytoin (Dilantin)

Dosage
- 2 to 5 μg/kg/min will increase renal and mesentery blood flow
- 2 to 10 μg/kg/min for predominant beta-adrenergic effects for increasing heart rate and myocardial contractility
- 10 to 20 μg/kg/min for predominant alpha-adrenergic effects for vasoconstriction and an increase in systemic vascular resistance

Epinephrine (Adrenalin)

Class
- Sympathomimetic

Action
- Alpha and beta agonist
- Alpha effects are vasoconstriction and an increase in peripheral vascular resistance (PVR)
- Beta 1 is a positive inotrope that increases myocardial contractility and a positive chronotrope that increases heart rate
- Beta 2 dilates bronchial smooth muscle and skeletal vasculature
- Increases myocardial automaticity
- Increases myocardial electrical activity
- Vasoconstriction of arterioles in the skin, muscle, and splanchic (visceral) areas
- Stabilize mast cell and basophil membranes in anaphylactic and anaphylactoid reactions

Indications

- Cardiac arrest
- Anaphylaxis
- Status asthmaticus
- Reactive airway disease

Contraindications

- None in cardiac arrest
- Hypertension
- Pregnant patient
- Cardiovascular or hyperthyroid disease

Side Effects/Precautions

- Protect drug from light
- Tachycardia
- Palpitations
- Hypertension
- Dysrhythmia due to myocardial irritability
- Increased myocardial oxygen demand
- Headache
- Tremors
- Anxiety
- Nausea and vomiting
- Use with caution in males > 40 years of age or females > 50 years of age

Dosage

- Cardiac arrest: 1 mg of 1:10,000 IV every 3 to 5 minutes
- Anaphylaxis: 0.3 to 0.5 mg 1:1,000 dilution IM or SQ or 0.3 to 0.5 mg IV 1:10,000 dilution if hypotension and poor perfusion
- Asthma with severe bronchoconstriction: 0.3 to 0.5 mg 1:1,000 SQ
- Infusion: 1 mg in 500 ml D_5W—infuse at 1 to 2 μg/min and titrate to desired response to 10 μg/min
- Tracheal dose: 2.0 to 2.5 mg

Etomidate (Amidate)

Class

- Nonnarcotic, nonbarbiturate sedative/hypnotic

Indications

- Sedation prior to paralyzing a patient for tracheal intubation or premedication for cardioversion

Contraindications

- Hypersensitivity

Side Effects/Precautions

- Pain at injection site
- Involuntary muscle movement
- Nausea and vomiting
- Tachycardia
- Apnea

- Dyspnea
- Hypotension
- Hypertension

Dosage

- 0.3 to 0.6 mg/kg IV over 30 to 60 seconds

Famotidine (Pepcid I.V.)

Class

- Competitive inhibitor of histamine H2 receptors

Action

- Inhibits histamine H2 receptors and blocks the secretion of histamine

Indications

- Anaphylaxis

Contraindications

- Hypersensitivity to the drug or other H2 blockers

Side Effects/Precautions

- Nausea and vomiting
- Dry mouth
- Anorexia
- Anxiety
- Paresthesia
- Fatigue
- Palpitations
- AV block, bradycardia, and other dysrhythmias

Dosage

- 20 mg (2 ml) mixed in 100 ml of normal saline administered over 15 to 30 minutes

Fentanyl Citrate (Sublimaze)

Class

- Opioid narcotic

Action

- Central nervous system depressant
- Potent analgesic

Indications

- Sedation prior to paralyzing a patient for tracheal intubation
- Severe pain

Contraindications

- Shock
- Severe hemorrhage

- Hypersensitivity
- Undiagnosed abdominal pain

Side Effects/Precautions

- Hypotension (typically caused by parasympathetic-induced bradycardia)
- Respiratory depression (reversible with naloxone)
- Nausea
- Dizziness
- Altered mental status
- Bradycardia
- Muscular rigidity (particularly, the chest wall muscles)

Dosage

- 3 to 5 μg/kg IV

Flumazenil (Romazicon)

Class

- Benzodiazepine receptor antagonist

Action

- Reverses the effects of benzodiazepines in the central nervous system by blocking the benzodiazepine receptor sites

Indications

- Reversal of sedation, impairment of recall, psychomotor impairment, and respiratory depression associated with administration of benzodiazepines; it is not as effective in reversing the hypoventilation of the benzodiazepines

Contraindications

- Hypersensitivity to drug
- Cocaine or other stimulant intoxication
- Tricyclic antidepressant overdose
- Should not be used to rule out benzodiazepine overdose in the same manner as naloxone

Side Effects/Precautions

- Headache
- Nervousness and agitation
- Dizziness
- Fatigue
- Cutaneous vasodilation
- Careful administration in patients with known benzodiazepine dependency

Dosage

- 0.2 mg IV over 15 to 30 seconds with additional doses of 0.3 to 0.5 mg to a maximum dose of 3.0 mg

Furosemide (Lasix)

Class

- Loop diuretic

Action

- Inhibits reabsorption of sodium and chloride in loop of Henle, promoting diuresis
- Intravenous administration causes vasodilation that results in an increase in venous capacitance and decreases cardiac preload

Indications

- Congestive heart failure
- Pulmonary edema associated with left ventricular failure

Contraindications

- Anuria (relative)
- Hypovolemia
- Dehydration
- Pregnancy
- Hypersensitivity

Side Effects/Precautions

- Protect drug from light
- Dehydration
- Hypokalemia
- Hyperglycemia
- Hypercalcemia
- Hyponatremia
- Hypochloremia

Dosage

- 20 to 40 mg (0.5 to 1.0 mg/kg) slow IV push over 1 to 2 minutes not to exceed 20 mg/min

Glucagon

Class

- Antihypoglycemic counterregulatory hormone
- Beta-blocker and calcium channel blocker toxicity antidote

Action

- Causes glycogenolysis (conversion of glycogen to glucose)
- Increases blood glucose level (only if liver glycogen is available)
- Positive inotrope (increased myocardial contractility) and positive chronotrope (increased heart rate)
- Increases AV conduction
- Decreases renal vascular resistance
- Inhibits glycogenesis (synthesis of glycogen from glucose)

Indications

- Hypoglycemia
- Beta-blocker and calcium channel blocker toxicity
- Can be used in patients suffering from an anaphylactic or anaphylactoid reaction who are taking beta-blockers following the administration of epinephrine

Contraindications
- Hypersensitivity
- Hyperglycemia

Side Effects/Precautions
- Nausea
- Vomiting
- Headache
- Tachycardia
- Hypotension
- Use with caution in patients with cardiovascular or renal disease

Dosage
- Hypoglycemia: 0.5 to 1 mg IM or IV
- Beta-blocker or calcium channel toxicity: 1 to 5 mg IV bolus

Hydrocortisone Sodium Succinate (Solu-Cortef)

Class
- Corticosteroid

Action
- Antiinflammatory
- Immunosuppression

Indications
- Status asthmaticus and chronic obstructive pulmonary disease
- Anaphylaxis and angioedema

Contraindications
- None in emergency setting

Side Effects/Precautions
- None from single-dose use

Dosage
- 50 to 250 mg IV

Ipratropium Bromide (Atrovent)

Class
- Anticholinergic, bronchodilator

Action
- Inhibits acetylcholine action at the receptor sites on the bronchial smooth muscle resulting in bronchodilation
- Dries respiratory secretions

Indications
- Asthma
- Chronic obstructive pulmonary disease with reversible bronchospasm

Contraindications
- Hypersensitivity to drug
- Not a primary acute treatment of bronchospasm

Side Effects/Precautions
- Dry mouth
- GI distress
- Nausea and vomiting
- Cough
- Nervousness
- Dizziness
- Headache
- Palpitations
- Blurred vision

Dosage
- 0.5 mg or 500 μg by nebulizer
- Usually used in conjunction with beta agonists

Ketamine (Ketalar)

Class
- Sedative
- Analgesic
- Amnestic

Action
- Dissociative anesthesia
- Functional and electrophysiological dissociation between the cortical and limbic system by blocking afferent transmission of impulses associated with pain perception

Indications
- Sedation prior to paralyzing a patient for tracheal intubation

Contraindications
- Hypersensitivity to drug
- Stroke
- Increases intracranial pressure
- Severe hypertension

Side Effects/Precautions
- Increased heart rate and myocardial oxygen demand
- Use with caution in patients with severe coronary artery disease
- Hallucinations
- Hypotension and respiratory depression
- Increased bronchial secretions
- Bronchodilation

Dosage
- 1 to 2 mg/kg IV over 1 minute

Levalbuterol (Xopenex)

Class
- Beta 2 sympathetic agonist

Action
- Bronchodilation by relaxing the smooth muscles of all airways from the trachea to the terminal bronchiole

Indications
- Acute asthma
- Treatment of bronchospasm in adults, adolescents, and children 6 years of age and older with reversible obstructive airway disease

Contraindications
- Contraindicated in patients with a history of hypersensitivity to the drug or to racemic albuterol

Side Effects/Precautions
- Palpitations
- Headache
- Dizziness
- Anxiety
- Tachycardia
- Hypertension
- Use with caution in patients with cardiovascular disorders, especially coronary insufficiency, cardiac dysrhythmias, and hypertension
- May produce ECG changes, such as flattening of the T wave, prolongation of the QT interval, and ST segment depression

Dosage
- For adult patients (12 years of age and older), 0.63 mg diluted in 3.0 ml of normal saline administered every 6 to 8 hours by nebulization
- A dose of 1.25 mg diluted in 3.0 ml of normal saline administered via nebulization may be used

Lidocaine (Xylocaine)

Class
- Antidysrhythmic

Action
- Decreases automaticity by slowing rate of phase four depolarization
- Reduces reentry by converting unidirectional block to bidirectional block in ischemic tissue
- Increases the ventricular fibrillation threshold

Indications
- Prevents a rise in intracranial pressure associated with administration of succinylcholine and the intubation procedure
- Suppression of ventricular dysrhythmia

Contraindications
- Hypersensitivity
- Second- or third-degree block
- PVCs with a heart rate less than 60 bpm

Side Effects/Precautions
- Hypotension
- Drowsiness
- Confusion
- Anxiety
- Seizures at high doses
- Muscle twitching
- Agitation
- Blurred vision
- Lightheadedness
- Reduced conduction velocity at large doses

Dosage
- 1 to 1.5 mg/kg IV repeated at 0.5 to 0.75 mg/kg every 3 to 5 minutes to a total cumulative dose of 3 mg/kg
- 2 to 2.5 mg/kg tracheally
- After suppression of ectopy or dysrhythmia, initiate an infusion at 2 to 4 mg/min

Lorazepam (Ativan)

Class
- Benzodiazepine
- Antianxiety

Action
- Anticonvulsant
- Stimulates GABA neurotransmitters that decrease presynaptic neuron stimulation and suppresses propagation of seizure activity originating in the cortex, thalamus, and limbic areas

Indications
- Status epilepticus
- Motor seizure of a nonepileptic origin
- Acute anxiety
- Premedication prior to cardioversion

Contraindications
- Hypersensitivity to drug
- Severe hypotension

Side Effects/Precautions
- Use with caution in renal and hepatic disease
- May precipitate when mixed with other drugs
- Drowsiness
- Confusion
- Hypotension
- Ataxia
- Respiratory depression or apnea

Dosage
- 1 to 4 mg slow IV push over 2 to 5 minutes; prior to IV administration, dilute lorazepam with an equal volume of sterile water or normal saline
- May be repeated in 15 to 20 minutes to a maximum dose of 0.1 mg/kg
- May be given IM (do not dilute when administered IM) and rectally

Magnesium Sulfate

Class
- Anticonvulsant
- Electrolyte
- Antidysrhythmic

Action
- Magnesium depresses central nervous system and blocks neuromuscular transmission

Indications
- Seizures associated with eclampsia
- Hypomagnesemia
- Torsades de pointes
- Severe asthma
- Refractory ventricular fibrillation
- Refractory pulseless ventricular tachycardia

Contraindications
- Heart block
- Shock

Side Effects/Precautions
- CNS depression
- Flushing
- Hypotension
- Myocardial depression
- Diaphoresis
- Respiratory depression
- Hypothermia
- Decreased heart rate
- Use with caution in patient with renal failure or in patient taking digitalis

Dosage
- Anticonvulsant: 1 to 4 g IV 10%-20% solution or 1 to 5 g IM 25%-50% solution

- Antidysrhythmia: 1 to 2 g (2 to 4 ml of 50% solution) mixed in 100 ml or 10 ml of D_5W administered IV over 1 to 2 minutes

Mannitol (Osmotrol)

Class
- Osmotic diuretic

Action
- Increases osmolarity of the glomerular filtrate, which increases the reabsorption of water, increasing sodium and chloride excretion; promotes the movement of intracellular fluid into the extracellular space

Indications
- Acute cerebral edema
- Reduction of intracranial pressure

Contraindications
- Anuria (severe renal disease)
- Pulmonary edema
- Dehydration
- Congestive heart failure
- Hypovolemia
- Hypotension
- Hypersensitivity

Side Effects/Precautions
- Sodium depletion
- Transient volume overload
- Pulmonary edema
- Hypotension (excessive diuresis)
- Angina-like chest pain
- Dizziness
- Headache
- Nausea and vomiting
- Chills
- Drug may crystallize at temperatures of 45°F or lower
- Use an inline filter

Dosage
- 0.5 to 1.5 g/kg of a 20% solution IV infusion over 20 minutes

Metaproterenol (Alupent, Metaprel)

Class
- Sympathomimetic, beta 2-specific agonist, bronchodilator

Action
- Beta 2 agonist causing bronchodilation by smooth muscle relaxation

Indications
- Asthma
- Chronic obstructive pulmonary disease with reversible bronchospasm

Contraindications
- Patient experiencing cardiac dysrhythmia
- Hypersensitivity
- Significant tachycardia (usually heart rate greater than 150 bpm)

Side Effects/Precautions
- Dose-related tachycardia
- Palpitations
- Nervousness and anxiety
- Headache
- Nausea and vomiting
- Peripheral vasodilation
- Dizziness
- Tremor
- Constantly monitor the ECG rhythm, blood pressure, and heart rate

Dosage
- 0.2 to 0.3 ml diluted in 2 to 3 ml of normal saline administered by nebulizer over 5 to 15 minutes

Methohexital (Brevital)

Class
- Rapid-acting barbiturate

Action
- Sedation

Indications
- Sedation prior to paralyzing patient for tracheal intubation

Contraindications
- Hypersensitivity to drug
- Seizure disorder

Side Effects/Precautions
- Moderate fall in systolic blood pressure
- Significant increase in heart rate
- Decreased respiratory drive
- Respiratory depression
- Apnea
- Pain at injection site

Dosage
- 0.75 to 1.5 mg/kg IV

Methylprednisolone (Solu-Medrol)

Class
- Glucocorticoid

Action
- Synthetic steroid that suppresses the inflammatory response
- Used for reduction of edema associated with spinal cord injury; however, this practice is controversial
- Immunosuppression

Indications
- Anaphylaxis
- Asthma
- Chronic obstructive pulmonary disease
- Spinal cord injury

Contraindications
- None in the emergency setting

Side Effects/Precautions
- Headache
- Hypertension
- Hyperglycemia
- Hypocalcemia
- Sodium retention
- Nausea and vomiting
- Use with caution in patients with renal disease, CHF, and diabetes mellitus

Dosage
- 125 to 250 mg IV bolus or IM
- Spinal cord injury: 30 mg/kg IV bolus over 15 minutes followed by an infusion of 5.4 mg/kg/hr

Midazolam (Versed)

Class
- Benzodiazepine

Action
- Sedation
- Amnesia
- Hypnotic
- Anticonvulsant

Indications
- Sedation prior to paralyzing a patient for tracheal intubation
- Sedation before cardioversion

Contraindications
- Hypersensitivity
- Hypotension
- Shock
- Narrow angle glaucoma

Side Effects/Precautions
- Drowsiness
- Hypotension

- Headache
- Amnesia
- Respiratory depression (more common than with other benzodiazepines)
- Pain at injection site
- Cough or hiccup
- Blurred vision
- Nausea and vomiting

Dosage

- 0.05 to 0.1 mg/kg IV with a typical adult dose of 2.5 to 5.0 mg IV; an induction dose is typically 0.1 mg/kg

Morphine Sulfate (Astramorph, Duramorph, Infumorph, Kadian, Morphine, Roxanol, Statex)

Class

- Opioid (narcotic) analgesic

Action

- Binds to opiate receptors in the central nervous system
- CNS depressant
- Peripheral vasodilation
- Analgesia
- Reduces myocardial preload
- Anxiolytic

Indications

- Management of pain
- Chest pain associated with myocardial infarction
- Acute cardiogenic pulmonary edema (controversial—morphine sulfate has been shown to increase incidence of respiratory depression and arrest with resultant need to intubate and ventilate the patient; the venodilatory and increased venous capacitance theory is limited in effect and does not outweigh the consequence of respiratory depression)

Contraindications

- Hypersensitivity to the drug
- Respiratory depression
- Volume-depleted patient
- Head injury
- Undiagnosed abdominal pain
- Severe hypotension

Side Effects/Precautions

- Decreased mental status
- Respiratory depression
- Hypotension
- May decrease the seizure threshold
- Nausea and vomiting
- Dizziness
- Tachycardia

- Bradycardia
- Palpitations
- Dry mouth

Dosage

- 2 to 5 mg slow IV push over 1 to 5 minutes followed by 2-mg increments until pain is resolved or until respiratory depression occurs

Naloxone (Narcan)

Class

- Narcotic antagonist, opioid antagonist

Action

- Competes for and displaces narcotic molecules at the opiate receptor sites in the brain
- Inhibits the action of the narcotic
- Reverses respiratory depression secondary to narcotic use

Indications

- Known or suspected narcotic overdose
- Used to stabilize vital signs and reverse respiratory depression in narcotic overdose

Contraindications

- Hypersensitivity to the drug

Side Effects/Precautions

- Hypertension if pushed rapidly
- Nausea and vomiting if pushed too rapidly
- Dysrhythmias
- Use with caution in patients who are dependent on narcotics because it may cause withdrawal

Dosage

- 0.4 to 2.0 mg IV, IM, or SQ
- Tracheal dose: 2 to 2.5 times IV dose

Nitroglycerin (Nitrostat)

Class

- Vasodilator
- Antianginal analgesic

Action

- Vascular smooth muscle dilation
- Reduction in myocardial workload
- Coronary artery dilation
- Reduction of systemic vascular resistance

Indications

- Angina pectoris
- Chest pain associated with myocardial infarction

- Hypertensive emergency
- Congestive heart failure

Contraindications
- Hypersensitivity
- Hypotension
- Increased intracranial pressure
- Head injury
- Volume depletion
- Patient recently used tadalafil (Cialis), vardenafil (Levitra), or sildenafil (Viagra)

Side Effects/Precautions
- Hypotension
- Reflex tachycardia
- Headache
- Syncope
- Burning sensation in mouth
- Dizziness
- Nausea and vomiting

Dosage
- 1/150 grain (0.4 mg) sublingual repeated every 3 to 5 minutes up to three doses
- 1 to 2 metered-dose sprays (0.4 mg/spray) repeated every 3 to 5 minutes up to three doses
- 10 to 100 μg/min for IV infusion

Norepinephrine (Levophed)

Class
- Sympathomimetic

Action
- Alpha- and beta 1-adrenergic agonist
- Intense peripheral vasoconstriction
- Positive inotrope (increases myocardial contractility)

Indications
- Hypotension due to vasodilation (systolic BP < 70 mmHg refractory to other sympathomimetic agents)
- Neurogenic shock

Contraindications
- Hypotension secondary to hypovolemia

Side Effects/Precautions
- Increases myocardial demand and oxygen consumption
- Potential cardiac dysrhythmia
- Palpitations
- Headache
- Hypertension
- Severe tissue necrosis may occur in infiltration
- Tachycardia
- Angina pectoris

Dosage
- ▶ 0.5 to 1.0 µg/min up to 30 µg/min IV infusion titrated to desired effect

Pancuronium Bromide (Pavulon)

Class
- ▶ Nondepolarizing neuromuscular blockade paralyzing agent

Action
- ▶ Paralyzes skeletal muscle by binding to the acetylcholine receptor site at the neuromuscular junction without causing depolarization of the muscle

Indications
- ▶ Paralyzing agent for long-term paralysis for induction to facilitate tracheal intubation or to maintain paralysis after tracheal intubation

Contraindications
- ▶ Hypersensitivity to drug

Side Effects/Precautions
- ▶ Hypertension
- ▶ Increased heart rate
- ▶ Excessive salivation
- ▶ Transient hypotension
- ▶ Prolonged paralysis
- ▶ Dysrhythmias
- ▶ Pain and burning at injection site

Dosage
- ▶ 0.04 to 0.1 mg/kg slow IV produces paralysis in 2 to 3 minutes; repeat at 0.01 to 0.02 mg/kg every 20 to 40 minutes

Phenobarbital Sodium (Luminal Sodium)

Class
- ▶ Barbiturate
- ▶ Anticonvulsant

Action
- ▶ Depresses central nervous system
- ▶ Interferes with neural transmission in the cerebral cortex that stops the propagation of seizure impulse transmission
- ▶ Interferes with the reticular activating system

Indications
- ▶ Major motor seizures
- ▶ Status epilepticus

Contraindications
- ▶ Hypersensitivity to the drug

Side Effects/Precautions
- ▶ Drowsiness
- ▶ Respiratory depression

- Hypotension
- Tissue necrosis may occur if infiltrated

Dosage

- 100 to 250 mg slow IV push

Phenytoin (Dilantin)

Class

- Anticonvulsant
- Antidysrhythmic

Action

- Inhibits seizure activity in the cerebral cortex by promoting sodium efflux from neurons stabilizing the neuron and making it less susceptible to excitability and excessive stimulation
- Negative inotrope
- Improves AV conduction and decreases ventricular automaticity by stabilizing the sodium influx in the Purkinje fibers of the conduction system

Indications

- Major motor seizures (generalized tonic-clonic)
- Digitalis toxicity with dysrhythmias
- Status epilepticus

Contraindications

- AV blocks
- Hypersensitivity to the drug
- Dysrhythmia, especially bradycardia (except those associated with digitalis toxicity)

Side Effects/Precautions

- Hypotension (associated with rapid IV push)
- CNS depression
- Nausea and vomiting
- Incoordination
- Diplopia
- Nystagmus
- Do not mix with glucose-containing solution
- Bradycardia
- Ataxia
- Respiratory depression

Dosage

- Major motor seizures or status epilepticus: 10 to 18 mg/kg slow IV push not to exceed 50 mg/min
- Digitalis toxicity: 100 mg over 5 minutes until dysrhythmia is suppressed or until a maximum of 1,000 mg has been administered or CNS depression occurs

Promethazine (Phenergan)

Class

- Antihistamine (H1 antagonist)

Action

- Histamine 1 receptor antagonist
- Blocks action of histamine
- Sedative
- Antimotion effects
- Antiemetic
- Anticholinergic activity

Indications

- Reduce the incidence of nausea and vomiting associated with narcotic administration
- Motion sickness
- Potentiate the effects of analgesics
- Sedation

Contraindications

- Hypersensitivity to drug
- Unresponsive patients
- CNS depression from alcohol, narcotics, barbiturates, or other CNS depressants

Side Effects/Precautions

- Decreased mental status
- Impaired physical ability
- Dizziness
- Dysrhythmia
- Nausea and vomiting
- Hyperexcitability
- Dystonic reactions (muscle contractions)

Dosage

- 12.5 to 25 mg IV or deep IM

Propofol

Class

- Phenol

Action

- Rapid anesthesia

Indications

- Sedation prior to paralyzing a patient for tracheal intubation

Side Effects/Precautions

- Pain on rapid injection
- Profound cardiac depression, especially in elderly

Dosage

- Total dose of 2.0 to 2.5 mg/kg IV in adults, typically at 40 mg every 10 seconds to effect; reduce the dose by one-half in the elderly

Ranitidine Hydrochloric (Zantac Injection)

Class

- Histamine H2 receptor antagonist

Action

- Inhibits the action of histamine at the histamine H2 receptor sites

Indications

- Anaphylaxis

Contraindications

- Known hypersensitivity to the drug

Side Effects/Precautions

- Bradycardia in rapid administration
- Pain at the IM or IV injection site
- Headache, malaise, dizziness, vertigo
- Tachycardia, asystole, AV blocks, PVCs
- Abdominal discomfort or pain

Dosage

- 50 mg (2 ml) mixed in normal saline to a dilution concentration of no greater than 2.5 mg/ml (20 ml); inject no faster than 4 ml/min (over 5 minutes)

Reteplase (Retevase)

Class

- Fibrinolytic

Action

- Recombinant plasminogen activator that creates plasmin for plasminogen, which is responsible for destroying the fibrin matrix associated with thrombus formation

Indications

- Acute myocardial infarction in adults after confirmation with 12-lead ECG

Contraindications

- Active internal bleeding
- History of stroke
- Recent cranial or spinal surgery
- Intracranial tumor, arteriovenous malformation, or aneurysm
- Bleeding disorder
- Severe hypertension

Side Effects/Precautions

- Bleeding
- Anaphylactoid reaction
- Dysrhythmias
- Nausea and vomiting
- Hypotension
- Fever

Dosage

- 10 + 10 unit double bolus injection; each bolus is administered IV over a 2-minute period; the second bolus is given 30 minutes after the initial bolus

Rocuronium Bromide (Zemuron)

Class
- Nondepolarizing neuromuscular blocker

Action
- Blocks acetylcholine
- Prevents neuromuscular transmission
- Paralyzes skeletal muscle

Indications
- Facilitate intubation
- Paralyze skeletal muscle

Contraindications
- Hypersensitivity

Side Effects/Precautions
- Dysrhythmia
- Tachycardia
- Nausea and vomiting
- Laryngospasm
- Bronchospasm
- Wheezing
- Rhonchi
- Hiccups
- Rash
- Injection site edema
- Itching
- Use with caution in liver disease and obese patients

Dosage
- 0.6 to 1.2 mg/kg IV

Sodium Bicarbonate

Class
- Alkalinizing agent, electrolyte

Action
- Sodium bicarbonate combines with hydrogen ions to form water and carbon dioxide
- Buffers metabolic acidosis
- Forces an intracellular shift of excess potassium in hyperkalemia
- Increases pH

Indications
- Severe metabolic acidosis in cardiac arrest refractory to ventilation
- Tricyclic antidepressant overdose
- Hyperkalemia
- Alkalinization agent for specific toxins

Contraindications

- Metabolic or respiratory alkalosis
- Hypocalcemia
- Hypokalemia
- Hypernatremia

Side Effects/Precautions

- Metabolic alkalosis may occur
- Precipitates when mixed with calcium chloride
- May increase intracellular acidosis
- May cause electrolyte imbalance
- May deactivate catecholamine
- Large solute load may lead to fluid overload

Dosage

- 1 mEq/kg IV repeated at 0.5 mEq/kg every 10 minutes

Succinylcholine (Anectine)

Class

- Depolarizing neuromuscular blocker

Action

- Binds with receptor sites and paralyzes skeletal muscle to include respiratory muscles

Indications

- Paralyzing agent to facilitate tracheal intubation
- Terminate laryngospasm
- Muscle relaxation

Contraindications

- Hypersensitivity to drug
- Penetrating eye injury
- Inability to control airway or ventilate patient
- Acute renal failure
- Burns or crush injury more than 8 hours old

Side Effects/Precautions

- Elevation in serum potassium level
- Rise in intracranial, intragastric, and intraocular pressure
- Bradycardia
- Hypotension
- Dysrhythmia
- Muscle fasciculation
- Prolonged paralysis

Dosage

- 1.0 to 1.5 mg/kg (40 to 100 mg) rapid IV over 10 to 30 seconds

Syrup of Ipecac

Class

- Emetic agent

Action
- Stimulates the emetic center of brain and irritates the gastric mucosa
- Gastric mucosal irritant

Indications
- Induction of vomiting in toxic ingestion

Contraindications
- Hypersensitivity
- Known caustic or corrosive ingestion
- Decreased level of consciousness
- Patient with no gag reflex
- Petroleum product ingestion
- Ingestion of rapidly acting CNS depressant
- Tricyclic antidepressant overdose
- Camphor ingestion

Side Effects/Precautions
- CNS depression
- Prolonged vomiting
- Dysrhythmia
- Hypotension
- Diarrhea

Dosage
- 15 to 30 ml by mouth followed by 16 ounces of water
- Repeat once at 15 ml if not effective within 20 to 30 minutes

Tenectaplase (TNKase)

Class
- Fibrinolytic agent

Action
- Tissue plasminogen activator

Indications
- Acute myocardial infarction in an adult patient following confirmation by 12-lead ECG

Contraindications
- Active internal bleeding
- History of stroke
- Recent cranial or spinal surgery
- Intracranial tumor, arteriovenous malformation, or aneurysm
- Bleeding disorder
- Severe hypertension

Side Effects/Precautions
- Bleeding
- Allergic reaction (rare)
- Dysrhythmias
- Nausea and vomiting
- Fever

Dosage
- The dose is based on weight in kilograms; the total dose should not exceed 50 mg; a single bolus is administered over 5 seconds

<60 kg	30 mg
60 to <70 kg	35 mg
70 to <80 kg	40 mg
80 to <90 kg	45 mg
>90 kg	50 mg

Terbutaline (Brethine)

Class
- Sympathomimetic

Action
- Beta 2-specific bronchodilator
- Dilates peripheral vascular smooth muscle
- Relaxes uterine smooth muscle

Indications
- Bronchospasm associated with asthma, chronic bronchitis, and emphysema
- Prevent uterine contractions

Contraindications
- Hypersensitivity
- Tachydysrhythmias
- Tachycardia due to digitalis administration

Side Effects/Precautions
- Nausea
- Tachycardia
- Palpitations
- Restlessness
- Anxiety
- Tremors
- Headache
- Chest pain
- Coughing
- Facial flushing

Dosage
- 0.25 mg SQ may be repeated in 15 to 30 minutes to a maximum dose of 0.5 mg/4 hr
- 400 µg (two inhalations, with each ventilation 1 minute apart) every 4 to 6 hours
- 0.15 to 1.0 mg/dose in 2 ml of normal saline by nebulizer

Thiamine (Bedizen, Betaxin)

Class
- Vitamin B_1

Action
- Combines with ATP to form a coenzyme in glucose metabolism

Indications
- Known or suspected thiamine deficiency
- Alcoholism
- Coma of unknown origin
- Wernicke's encephalopathy
- Korsakoff's syndrome

Contraindications
- None in emergency setting

Side Effects/Precautions
- May cause allergic reaction
- Hypotension in rapid push
- Nausea and vomiting
- Anxiety
- Diaphoresis

Dosage
- 100 mg slow IV or IM
- Ideally, 50 mg IV and 50 mg IM

Thiopental

Class
- Barbiturate

Action
- Produces sedation

Indications
- Sedative prior to paralyzing a patient for tracheal intubation

Contraindications
- Hypersensitivity to drug

Side Effects/Precautions
- Respiratory depression
- Hypotension
- Use with extreme caution in hypertensive patients and those with decreased circulating volume
- May cause laryngospasm
- Profound vagal response with increased mucous secretions
- Use with caution in severe cardiac disease, airway obstruction, and asthma

Dosage
- 3 to 5 mg/kg IV

Vecuronium (Norcuron)

Class
- Intermediate-acting nondepolarizing agent

Action

- Combines with acetylcholine receptors on muscle cells, causing an inability to generate muscle contraction

Indications

- Paralytic used to facilitate tracheal intubation and for prolonged paralysis

Contraindications

- Hypersensitivity to drug

Side Effects/Precautions

- Hypotension
- Laryngospasm
- Prolonged paralysis
- Bradycardia
- Paralysis lasts for approximately 30 minutes

Dosage

- .08 to 0.1 mg/kg IV

Further Reading

Valuable sources of information about drugs include the following:

1. *AMA Drug Evaluation,* a manual published by the American Medical Association, addresses all drug groups with dosage, prescribing, and usage information.
2. Drug inserts that are provided in the packaging of most drugs provide excellent information and may be kept in a notebook for ready reference.
3. *Hospital Formulary,* a loose-leaf book published by the American Society of Hospital Pharmacists. It is best consulted at a location, such as a hospital pharmacy, where pages are promptly replaced as updates become available.
4. *Physicians' Desk Reference (PDR),* published by the Medical Economics Company, lists most drugs currently on the market with comprehensive information provided by the drug manufacturers.
5. BLEDSOE, B. and D. CLAYDEN. *Prehospital Emergency Pharmacology*. 6th ed. Upper Saddle River, NJ: Pearson/Prentice Hall, 2005.

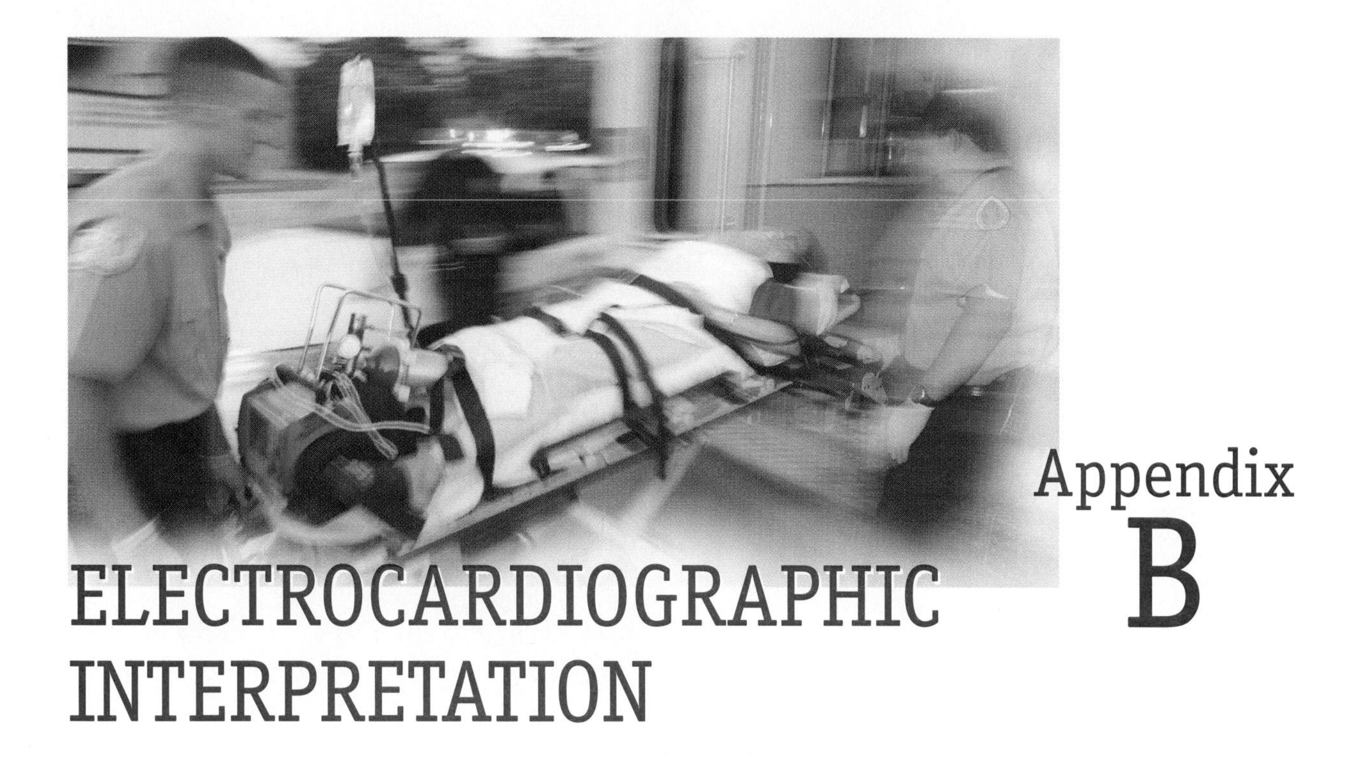

Appendix

B

ELECTROCARDIOGRAPHIC INTERPRETATION

Rationale

This appendix is a primer—not a comprehensive text—on ECG interpretation. It is intended to familiarize the reader with the basic tenets of ECG interpretation. We briefly discuss use of the ECG in recognizing several medical conditions that we have addressed in the chapters of this text. The major focus is recognition of the characteristic changes associated with an acute myocardial infarction (AMI), with particular emphasis on recognition of ST segment elevation in the presence of AMI, because this condition merits rapid identification and treatment.

Introduction

The treatment of acute coronary syndromes has changed dramatically since the early 1990s. Although prehospital care providers have teamed with emergency physicians and surgeons to rapidly deliver the patient with traumatic injuries to the operating suite, only recently have patients with AMI been treated using a similar approach. Because of the progressive destruction of myocardial muscle during infarction, the expression that should guide the emergency provider is "Time is Muscle."

In addition to the important element of obtaining a careful clinical history, the ability to obtain and rapidly interpret a 12-lead ECG is essential to activating the emergency care system to respond to the cardiac patient. The first step in reestablishing blood flow in patients with AMI is obtaining a diagnostic ECG. By recognizing the characteristic changes on the ECG, the emergency care provider can set in motion a series of steps designed to restore blood flow to the affected myocardium.

The ECG and rhythm strip can also be useful adjuncts in the care of many other patients in the out-of-hospital setting. A variety of conditions, including heart rhythm disturbances, pericarditis, pulmonary disease, and other disorders (e.g., hyperkalemia, hypocalcemia, hypothermia), can be detected by the provider who has a good working knowledge of ECG interpretation. In addition, the ECG can be used as a guide to determining the patient's response to certain therapies.

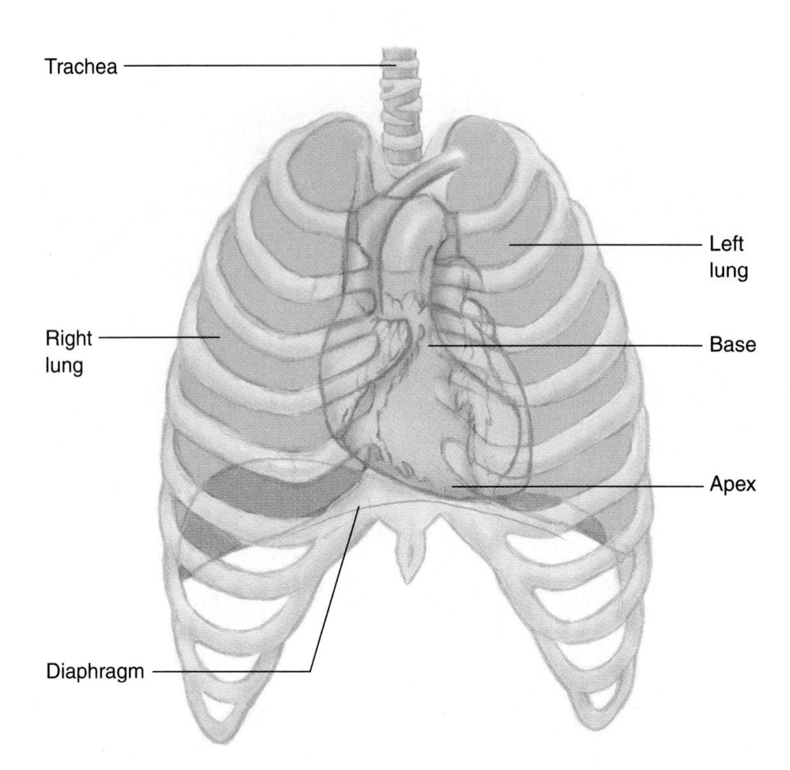

FIGURE B-1
The location of the heart within the chest.

There are several excellent texts on ECG rhythm interpretation to which the reader is referred (see "Further Reading" at the end of this appendix).

For these reasons, a basic understanding of ECG and rhythm strip interpretation is an important skill for the out-of-hospital health care provider.

Cardiac Anatomy and Physiology

Remember that the heart is a fist-shaped organ that sits posterior to the sternum and anterior to the thoracic spine (Figure B-1). The apex of the heart protrudes slightly into the left chest cavity.

The heart is divided into the left heart and the right heart. The right side of the heart receives deoxygenated blood from the rest of the body and delivers this blood to the lungs for reoxygenation. Oxygenated blood then returns from the lungs into the left side of the heart, which pumps blood into the aorta. Blood is then distributed to the entire body via the arterial system.

Each side of the heart, both left and right, contains a single atrium and a ventricle. The atria are the smaller upper chambers that are responsible for delivering the last 30 percent of blood volume into the lower chambers, the ventricles, prior to ventricular contraction. (The ventricles fill to 70 percent capacity by passive filling during diastole, the period when the heart relaxes between contractions.) The interatrial septum separates the right and left atria, while the interventricular septum divides the two ventricles.

Coronary Arteries

The heart is served by two major arteries: the right and left coronary arteries (Figure B-2). Each artery originates from the aorta just above the aortic root. The unique feature of coronary artery perfusion is that it occurs during *diastole* in contrast to other arteries in the body that fill during systole.

The left coronary artery (LCA) is typically the larger of the two major arteries serving the heart. The LCA provides blood supply to the anterior wall of the left

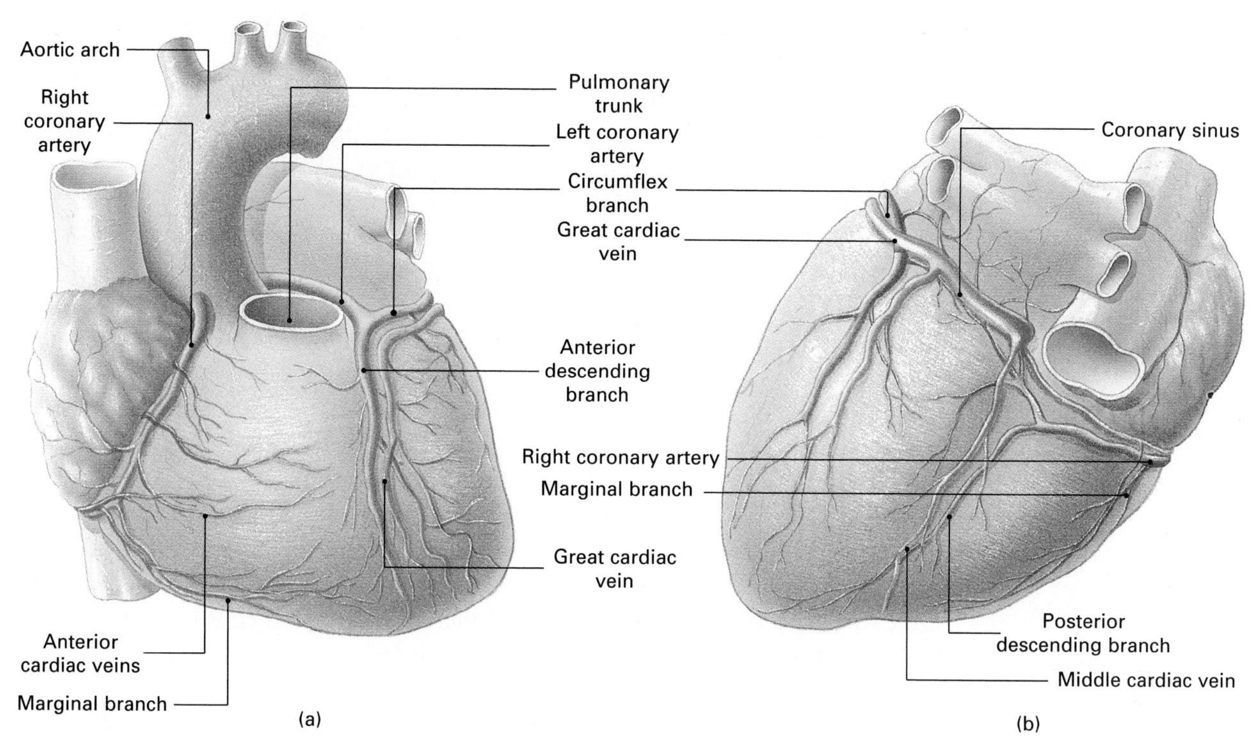

FIGURE B-2
The coronary circulation: (a) anterior view (b) posterior view.

ventricle, the lateral wall of the left ventricle, the posterior wall of the left ventricle, and the left interventricular septal wall. Almost immediately after leaving the aorta, the LCA divides into the left anterior descending (LAD) artery and the left circumflex artery. The LAD supplies the anterior ventricular wall, whereas the circumflex artery provides circulation to the posterior wall. A marginal branch of the LCA provides circulation to the lateral ventricular wall.

Understanding this portion of the coronary anatomy can help explain why patients who suffer an occlusion of the LCA or its major branches develop an infarction of the anterior wall of the left ventricle (anterior AMI). It also explains why patients with anterior AMIs may have associated infarctions of the posterior or septal wall.

The right coronary artery (RCA) is typically smaller than the LCA. The RCA supplies blood to the right ventricle, as well as to the lateral and inferior portions of the left ventricle. It also supplies the upper portions of the conduction system (SA node, AV node, and His bundle). Occlusion of the RCA is often associated with an infarction of the inferior wall of the left ventricle (inferior AMI). A patient with an inferior AMI can also have an associated right ventricular infarction. In addition, because the RCA supplies the conducting system, cardiac dysrhythmias such as bradycardia and heart blocks can occur in patients with inferior AMIs.

Fundamentals of Electrical Cardiac Activity

Remember that the ECG is a representation of electrical events that are occurring within the heart as viewed by a variety of "cameras" (limb leads and precordial leads) placed on the surface of the body. These cameras provide different views of the same electrical events that occur during the cardiac cycle.

The heart is composed of at least two types of cells. The first type of heart cells are the *myocardial cells,* which contain contractile elements that require an electrical impulse to produce myocardial contraction. Such cells form the muscular chambers of the heart. Once the electrical stimulus reaches a certain threshold, the process of contraction proceeds to completion. To produce an orderly contraction of the heart muscle, a specific series of electrical events (which can be seen on the ECG) must occur.

The second group of cells are the specialized *pacemaker cells* located throughout the heart. Pacemaker cells form the conduction system of the heart. These cells contain little contractile material, but rather are primarily responsible for generating and conducting the electrical impulses throughout the heart.

Cardiac cells possess four characteristics: automaticity, excitability, conductivity, and contractility. *Automaticity* is the ability of cardiac cells to generate their own electrical impulses and is a function of the pacemaker cells. The sinoatrial (SA) node is the dominant pacemaker for the heart. It has a spontaneous rate of between 60 and 100 bpm. Other cells, including cells in the atria, the atrioventricular (AV) junction, and portions of the ventricular conduction system, can drive cardiac contraction at their own inherent rate. Atrial cells pace at between 60 and 80 bpm, the AV junction spontaneously fires at a rate between 40 and 60 bpm, while the spontaneous rate of the ventricles is between 20 and 40 bpm.

Excitability is the ability of cardiac cells to respond to an electrical stimulus. The related term *irritability* implies that a cell or group of cells may generate an impulse with only a slight amount of stimulation. The more irritable a group of cardiac cells is, the less the stimulus that is required to produce an impulse. Stimuli such as hypoxia, ion shifts, and inflammation can increase cardiac irritability. Any area (also referred to as a "focus") in the conduction system can become irritable and can depolarize at a rate faster than the inherent pacing rates listed previously. An example is ventricular tachycardia in which an irritable focus in the ventricle becomes the dominant pacemaker for the heart.

Conductivity is the ability of cardiac cells to transmit an impulse. Cardiac cells do this effectively, resulting in the organized activity seen during the cardiac cycle. *Contractility,* the ability of cells to contract, was discussed previously in relation to myocardial cells.

Cardiac Conduction

In a normal heart contraction, there is a systematic flow of an electrical impulse down the heart's conduction system (Figure B-3). The normal impulse begins in the SA node located in the upper portion of the right atrium, near the junction with the superior vena cava. As stated previously, the normal spontaneous impulse rate generated by the SA node (automaticity) is 60 to 100 beats per minute. This rate can be modified by actions of the autonomic nervous system. Sympathetic stimulation increases the resting heart rate, while parasympathetic stimulation slows the normal heart rate.

From the SA node, the impulses are conducted down three internodal pathways, as well as Bachman's bundle, to the left atrium, resulting in contraction of the atria and stimulation of the AV node. The AV node is located at the base of the right atrium just above the tricuspid valve. In most patients, the AV node is the portal for impulse transmission to the ventricles. At this point in impulse transmission, there is a delay of 0.5 seconds to allow for effective cardiac output during ventricular contraction. The electrical impulse then passes through the AV junction to the bundle of His. As noted earlier, the AV junction is capable of spontaneous depolarization, but at a rate slower than the SA node.

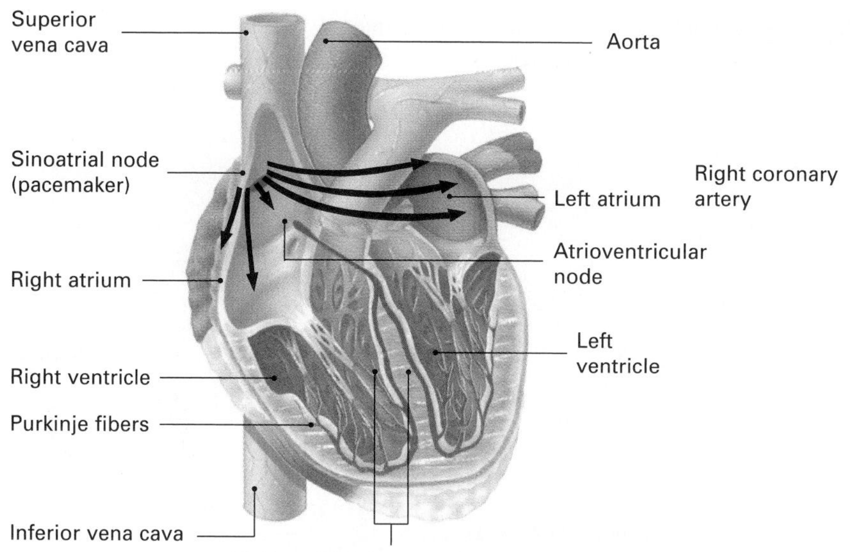

FIGURE B-3
The cardiac conduction system.

The bundle of His divides into two main branches at the upper portion of the interventricular septum: the left bundle branch and the right bundle branch. While the right bundle branch transmits impulses to specialized Purkinje fibers, which depolarize the right ventricle, the left bundle branch divides into an anterior and posterior fascicle before terminating in the Purkinje fibers of the left ventricle. The Purkinje fibers are also capable of spontaneous depolarization at between 20 and 40 beats per minute.

All electrical impulses within the heart are the result of movements of ions across the myocardial cell membrane. Potassium, sodium, and calcium are the major ions that effect cardiac impulses; magnesium is involved in the cardiac cycle to a lesser degree. Potassium and sodium are involved in impulse generation, while calcium is involved in both impulse generation and cellular contraction. Calcium is the major ion propagating the signal through the AV node. In the resting state of the myocardial cell, sodium is actively concentrated outside the cell, whereas potassium is concentrated inside the cell. The inside of the myocardial cell maintains a negative charge relative to fluid outside the cell in the resting state. The concentration of ions on both sides of the cell membrane and the resting negative charge are established by energy-requiring ion transport pumps located within the myocardial cell membrane.

During *cardiac depolarization,* an impulse is conducted throughout the myocardium that is generated by the free flow of ions across the cell membrane. This leads to a reversal of the normal negative charge inside the cell. This change in polarity is called an *action potential.* Cardiac depolarization is coordinated by the conduction system so myocardial contraction proceeds in an organized fashion. During the process of *cardiac repolarization,* the normal resting ionic relationships are reestablished and the cell interior resumes a negative charge. When this occurs, the cardiac cells are *refractory* (resistant) to any additional electrical impulses that would otherwise initiate the process of depolarization.

Basics of the Electrocardiogram

As suggested earlier, the ECG represents a picture of the electrical activity of the heart as viewed from the body surface with a variety of cameras. These electrical pictures are projected on a screen or recorded on paper after being amplified by the

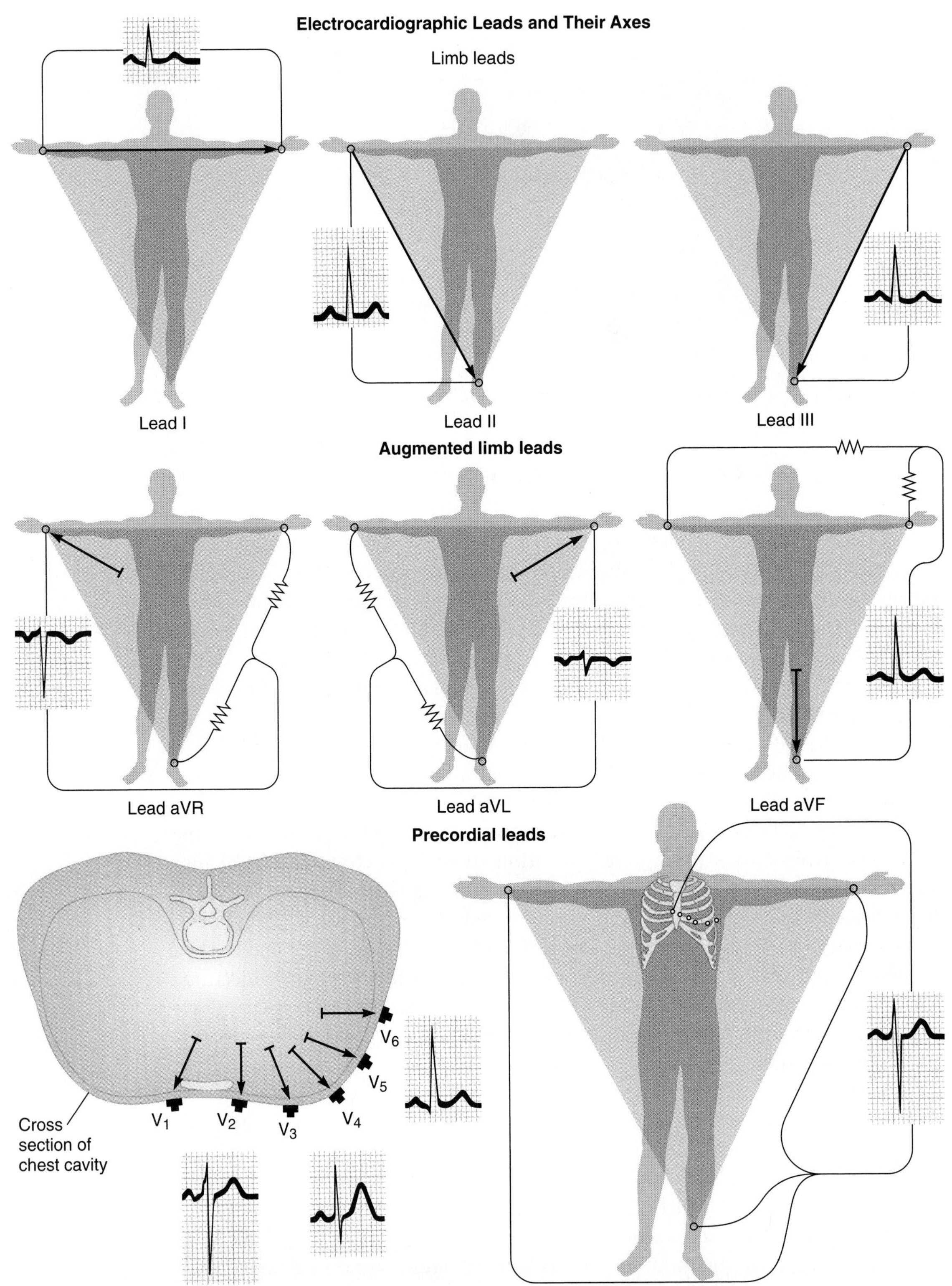

FIGURE B-4
ECG leads and their axes.

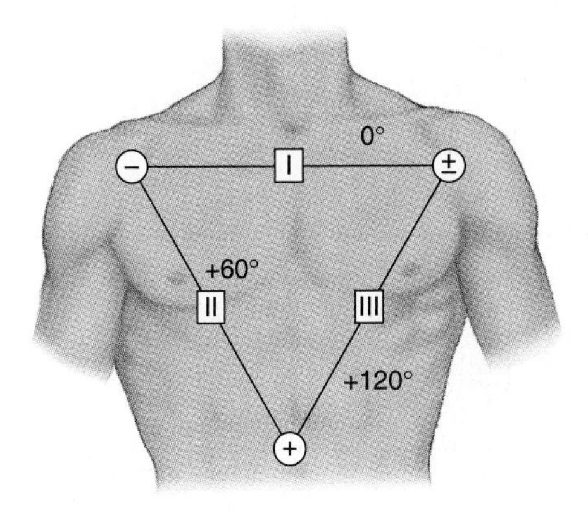

FIGURE B-5
Einthoven's triangle as formed by the bipolar leads.

ECG machine. The ECG is captured using a series of gel electrodes that are attached to the patient in a standard fashion. The wires that connect to these electrodes are typically labeled so the tracing is properly recorded.

In general, each standard camera view (called a lead) consists of a positive and a negative electrode. Leads I, II, and III are called *limb leads* (Figure B-4). The electrodes are classically placed on the left arm, right arm, and left leg. However, prehospital providers typically place three electrode pads on the trunk, rather than on the arms and legs (some manufacturers require placement of a fourth electrode on the right lower trunk), to record the limb leads. These leads form an imaginary triangle on the surface of the body referred to as *Einthoven's triangle* (Figure B-5). These leads capture the ECG from the perspective of the frontal plane. By convention, lead II is typically used when continuously monitoring the patient's cardiac rhythm. This is done because electrical evidence of atrial contraction (P waves) are best seen in lead II.

Three additional *augmented leads* (review Figure B-4) that view the electrical currents traveling from the center of the heart to the right arm (AVR), left arm (AVL), and left foot (AVF) are also obtained in a standard 12-lead ECG (Figure B-6). As you can see from the figure, leads II, III, and AVF provide information about the inferior portions of the heart. Lead I and AVL are considered the lateral leads.

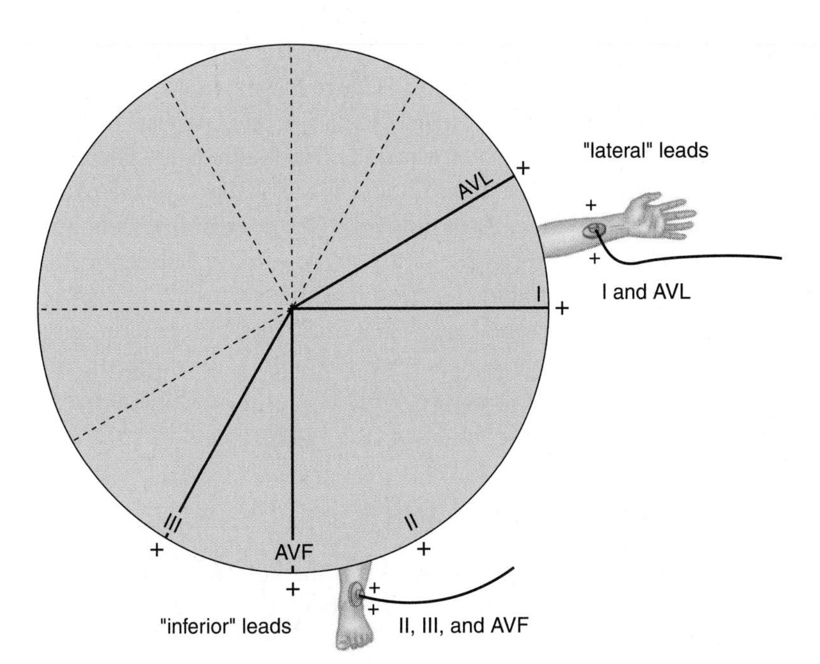

FIGURE B-6
The conventional placement of limb lead electrodes. A positive left arm electrode records lateral leads I and AVL. A positive left foot electrode records inferior leads II, III, and AVF.

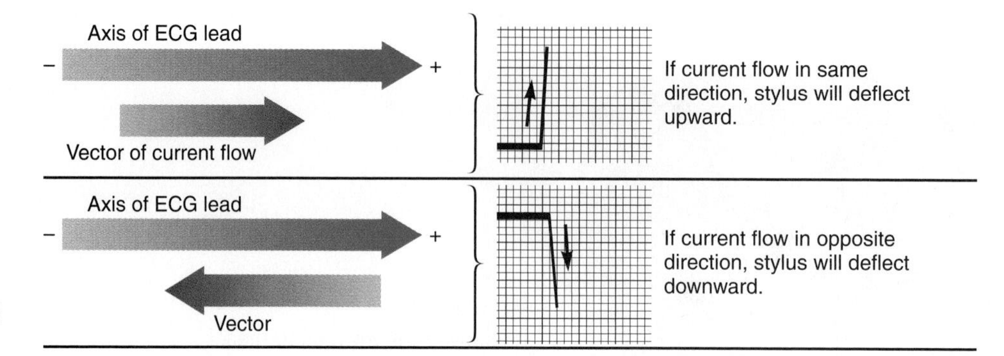

FIGURE B-7
Relationships between current flow direction and ECG lead axis.

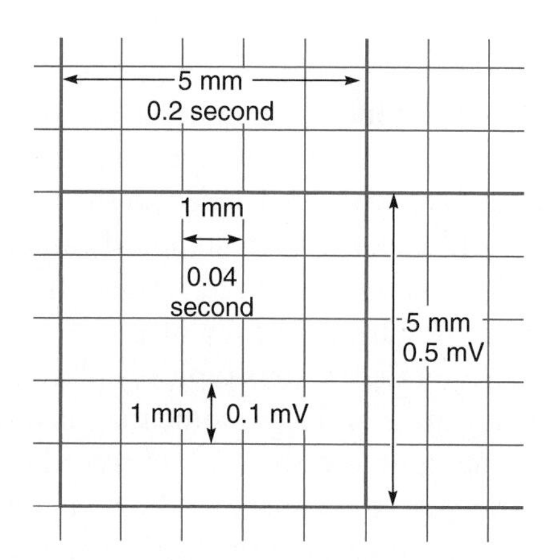

FIGURE B-8
ECG grid: Relationships between horizontal axis and time and between vertical axis and amplitude.

Six additional views are obtained by examining the heart along the horizontal plane. These leads are referred to as the *precordial leads,* and the positive electrode for each lead proceeds from the right side of the chest (V1) to the left chest (V6) (review Figure B-4). V1 and V2 provide information about the interventricular septum, V3 and V4 view primarily the anterior wall of the left ventricle, and V5 and V6 demonstrate the lateral wall of the left ventricle.

The ECG records the electrical activity of the heart from the perspective of each of the 12 electrodes defined previously. Electrical activity of the heart that travels in the direction of a lead's positive electrode results in a positive deflection above the baseline, or *isoelectric line,* whereas a current moving away from the positive electrode is recorded as a negative deflection (Figure B-7).

The ECG tracing is recorded using a standard format on lined paper. The ECG paper is scored to make interpretation of the tracings easier (Figure B-8). There are thick lines that are further divided by five light lines. The vertical axis of the paper records the amplitude of the ECG deflection in millivolts (mV). Typically, each light horizontal line represents 0.1 mV, although the common convention is to report the elevation in millimeters (mm). Each 1-mm elevation is actually 0.1 mV.

Time is measured along the horizontal axis. Each thick vertical line represents 0.2 seconds, so each light vertical line equals 0.04 seconds. Knowing both the amplitude measurements and the time measurements is important for interpreting the ECG tracing.

Elements of the Cardiac Cycle

Each cycle of atrial contraction, impulse conduction to the ventricles, ventricular contraction, and repolarization of both cardiac chambers is represented by a series of electrical waveforms on the ECG tracing.

P Wave

Completion of atrial excitation

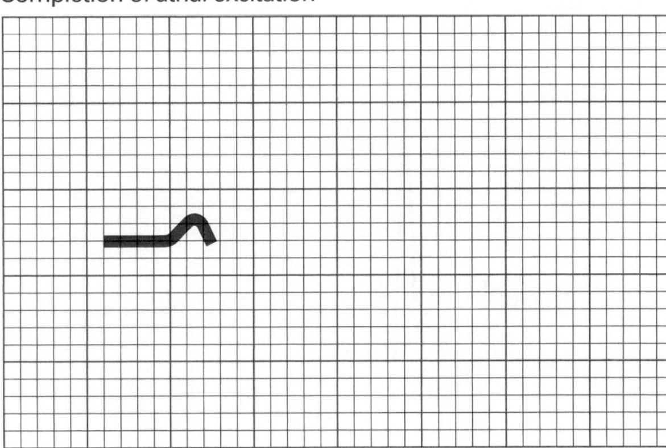

FIGURE B-9
The P wave.

The *P wave* is the first upward rounded deflection of the electrical waveform and represents atrial contraction (Figure B-9). This is best seen in leads II and V2.

The electrical impulse is then conducted through to the ventricles. The *PR interval* represents the time from the beginning of atrial contraction to ventricular contraction and is calculated from the beginning of the P wave to the beginning of the QRS complex (Figure B-10). The normal PR interval measures between 0.12 and 0.20 seconds (three to five small squares on the ECG tracing).

The *QRS complex* is the electrical representation of the beginning of ventricular contraction (Figure B-11). Any downward deflection from the isoelectric line before the positive deflection is called a *Q wave.* The presence of Q waves is particularly important in diagnosing AMI. Q waves are best seen in leads I and II. The first upward deflection of the QRS complex is known as the *R wave,* and any subsequent negative deflection is an *S wave.* Note that if the first component of the QRS complex is a positive deflection, this is by convention an R wave and the subsequent negative deflection is the S wave.

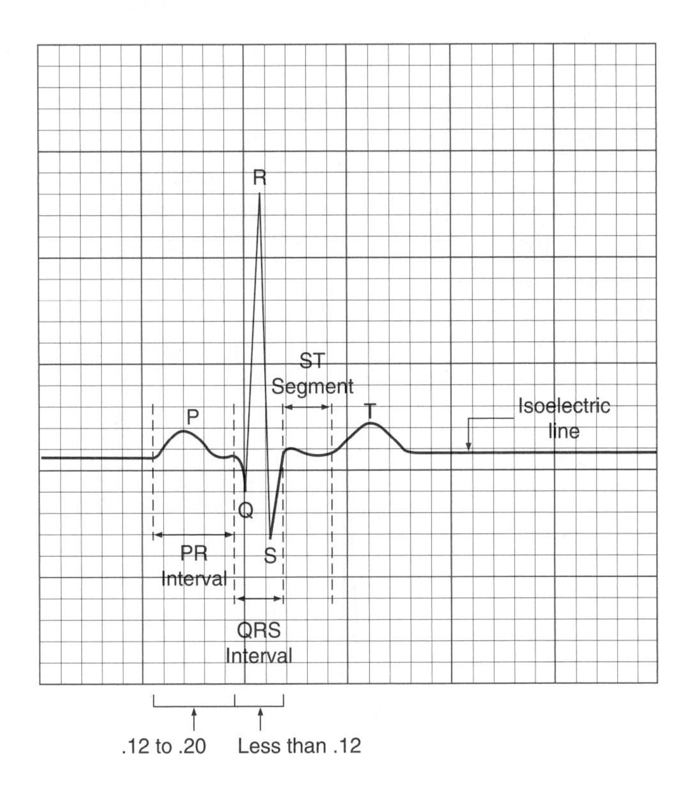

FIGURE B-10
ECG waveforms.

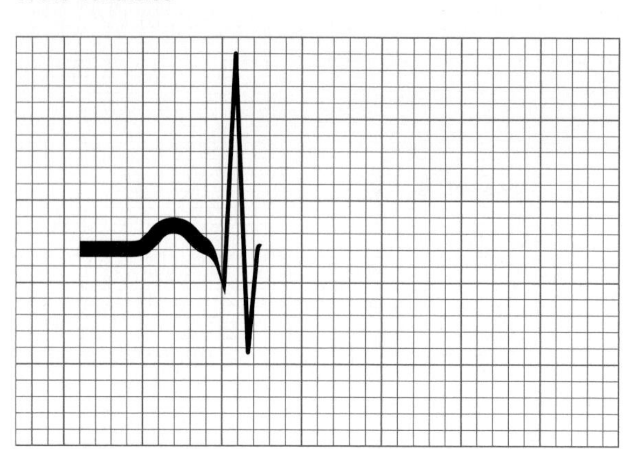

FIGURE B-11
The QRS complex.

The appearance of the QRS complex varies by patient and appears different in each ECG lead. The normal QRS complex should be less than 0.12 seconds. It should also be mentioned that the electrical events that represent atrial repolarization occur during this time, but remain hidden by the appearance of the QRS complex.

An important point along the ECG tracing is the *J point*, which represents the point where the QRS complex ends and the ST segment begins (Figure B-12). The tracing from the J point to the beginning of the T wave is called the *ST segment* (review Figure B-10). The ST segment represents the initial phases of ventricular repolarization. Normally, the ST segment lies along the isoelectric line. In patients with cardiac disease, the ST segment may be either elevated or depressed. Other conditions, such as hypothermia, pericarditis, and certain normal variants, may also alter the ST segment.

When interpreting an ECG in a patient with suspected coronary disease, it will be important to know whether the J point is elevated above the isoelectric line (ST segment elevation) or depressed below this line (ST segment depression).

Finally, the *T wave* is a rounded electrical waveform at the end of the cardiac cycle. This represents the final stages of ventricular repolarization (Figure B-13). The T wave is typically represented by a positive deflection. However, if the QRS complex has a large S wave, then it may be normal to have the T wave appear as a negative deflection. With a normal QRS complex, T-wave inversion may be a sign of underlying cardiac disease. Note that ventricular systole lasts from the beginning of the QRS complex to the end of the T wave.

During the ST segment and early portions of the T wave, the heart is in its *absolute* refractory period (Figure B-14). This means that it cannot be stimulated to contract by any electrical impulses. During the last half of the T wave, the heart

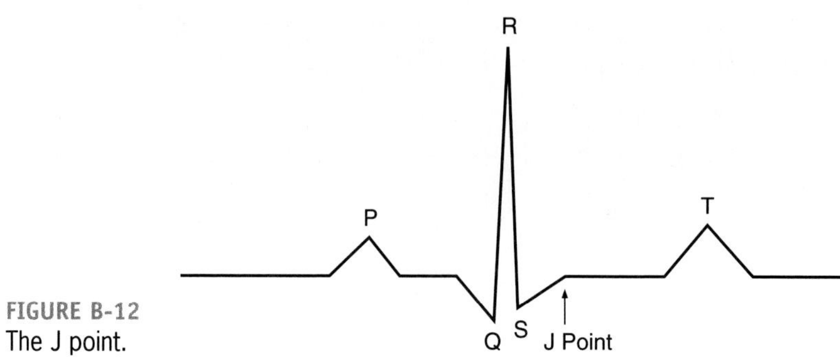

FIGURE B-12
The J point.

T Wave
Ventricular repolarization

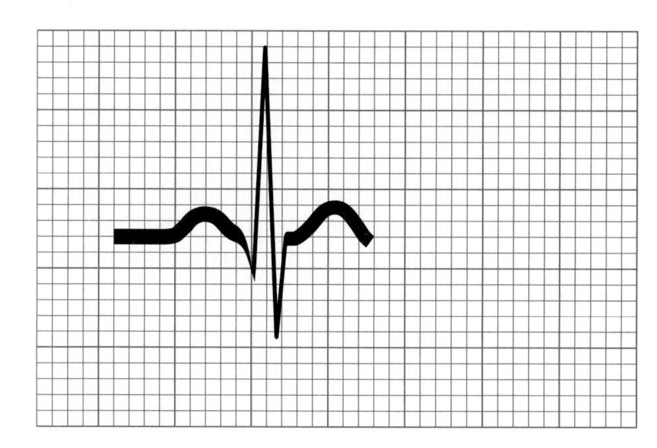

FIGURE B-13
The T wave.

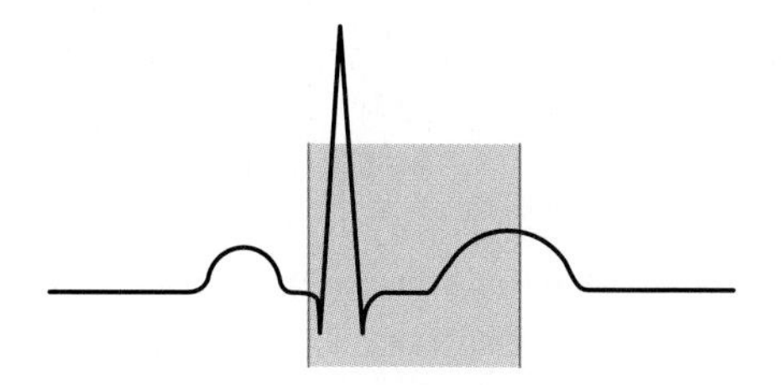

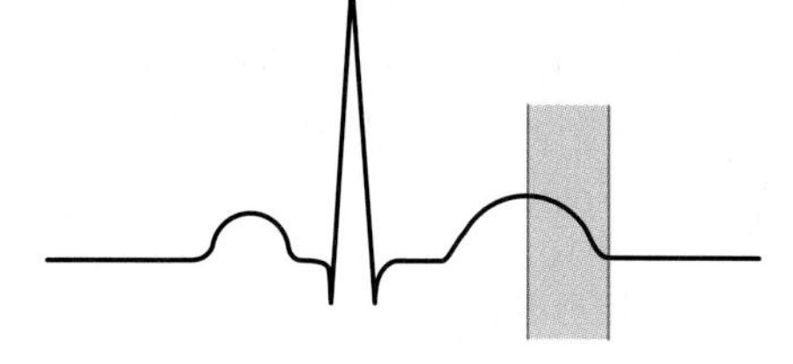

FIGURE B-14
Refractory periods.

enters its *relative* refractory period. The heart cannot be stimulated at this time unless a large electrical stimulus is applied.

Two other terms must be recognized. The *QT interval* is represented by the time from the beginning of the QRS complex to the beginning of the T wave (review Figure B-10). The QT interval is a reflection of ventricular repolarization. Because the QT interval varies with the heart rate, you may see a more accurate measurement (QT_c) used; this is the QT interval that is mathematically corrected for the heart rate. In general, the duration of the QT interval should be less than half of the R-to-R measurement. Patients with prolonged QT intervals may be prone to fatal ventricular dysrhythmias. In addition, ions such as calcium and magnesium can alter the duration of the QT interval.

Finally, it should also be noted that there may occasionally appear a rounded waveform after the T wave that appears before the next P wave. By convention, such a wave is called a *U wave.* The U wave represents repolarization of the Purkinje fibers, which are the last portion of the ventricles to undergo repolarization. Usually, this phase of the cardiac cycle is not evident on the tracing. However, U waves may be seen in patients with alterations in ion concentration, such as hyperkalemia.

Basics of ECG Interpretation

When viewing ECGs, you should always approach the tracings in a systematic manner. There are at least six areas that you should view as you analyze the ECG:

Rate
Rhythm
Axis
PR interval

QRS complex

ST segment

With each ECG that you obtain, you should review each of these areas in a systematic fashion to determine whether there are any abnormalities.

Rate

The normal resting heart rate of an adult is between 60 and 100 bpm. A resting heart rate less than 60 bpm is referred to as *bradycardia.* A rate greater than 100 bpm is called *tachycardia.* There are basically two methods of determining the rate as you review the ECG.

The first method is to count the number of beats that occur over a known length of time, similar to the method used in obtaining a pulse rate. Most ECG printouts have a marking on the top of the tracing denoting 3-second intervals (15 large boxes). Two of these markings would mark 6 seconds of elapsed time.

Remember that, in most patients, each ventricular contraction (QRS complex) is preceded by an atrial contraction (P wave). Thus, by counting the number of QRS complexes that occur over the 6-second interval and multiplying by 10, we arrive at the heart rate over 1 minute (60 seconds). This is known as the 6-second method (Figure B-15). The result represents the number of cardiac cycles per minute.

It should be noted that some patients with abnormal cardiac rhythms may have different atrial rates and ventricular rates. This could occur if the atrial and ventricular rates are independent of each other, as in a patient with third-degree heart block. In this instance, one could calculate both the number of P waves in 6 seconds and the number of QRS complexes to determine both rates. This method is particularly useful for calculating ventricular rates in patients that may have an irregular ventricular rhythm, such as patients with atrial fibrillation.

In patients with a regular rhythm, this calculation can be simplified by remembering that each large box represents 0.2 seconds. If two QRS complexes are separated by a single large box (called R-R interval), this suggests that each beat occurs every 0.2 seconds or that 300 beats will occur over a period of 60 seconds. Similarly, if the next QRS complex occurs after two large boxes (0.4 seconds), then the heart rate is 150 beats per 60 seconds. Thus, by counting the number of large boxes between each R-R interval, we can estimate the underlying heart rate.

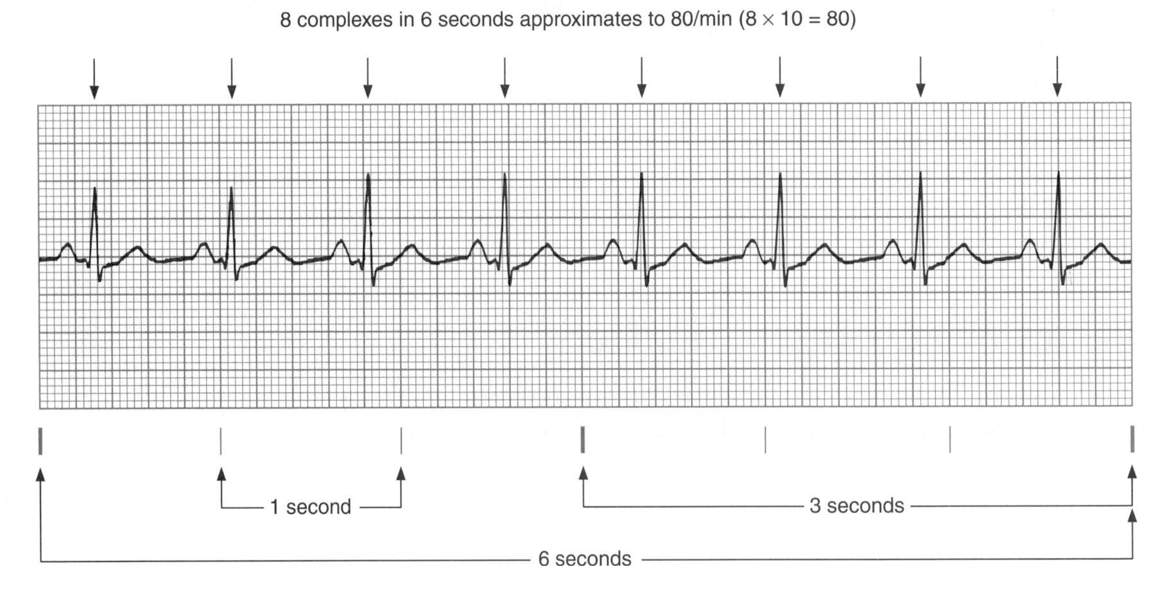

FIGURE B-15
The 6-second method.

Number of Boxes	Heart Rate
1	300
2	150
3	100
4	75
5	60
6	50

Alternatively, use the formula

300/(the number of large boxes between each R-R interval) = heart rate (bpm)

Rhythm

In a normal ECG, each cardiac cycle begins with a P wave. Each P wave is followed by a QRS complex and, subsequently, a T wave. When this PQRST pattern is found during each beat, the ECG is described as a normal sinus rhythm (Figure B-16).

Although a detailed discussion of the various dysrhythmias is beyond the intent of this appendix, heart rhythms can be described as either *regular* or *irregular* based on the pattern of R waves. If the R-R interval is constant, the rhythm is regular. If the R-R interval varies, then the rhythm is irregular.

Irregular rhythms can be further subdivided into regularly irregular, occasionally irregular, and irregularly irregular. The most common form of a *regularly irregular* pattern is sinus dysrhythmia in which the patient's heart rate fluctuates in a pattern that follows the respiratory cycle.

Occasionally irregular rhythms describe cardiac rhythm disturbances in which early atrial or ventricular beats cause a disruption of the normal R-R interval. Patients with premature atrial or ventricular contraction will have an ECG tracing that is occasionally irregular (Figure B-17).

When there appears to be no underlying pattern to the R-R interval, the patient is said to have an *irregularly irregular rhythm.* This is most commonly due to atrial fibrillation/flutter in which disorganized atrial electrical activity is conducted through to the ventricles in a random fashion (Figure B-18).

Also, remember that when each complex is preceded by a P wave, the rhythm is described as a *sinus* rhythm. Rates greater than 100 bpm are sinus tachycardia and less than 60 bpm are sinus bradycardia. If no P wave precedes each normal QRS, then the rhythm is *junctional.* Wide complex rhythms (greater than 0.12 seconds) are usually ventricular in origin, although this may occasionally represent an abnormal conduction pathway into the ventricles from the atria ("supraventricular rhythm with aberrant conduction").

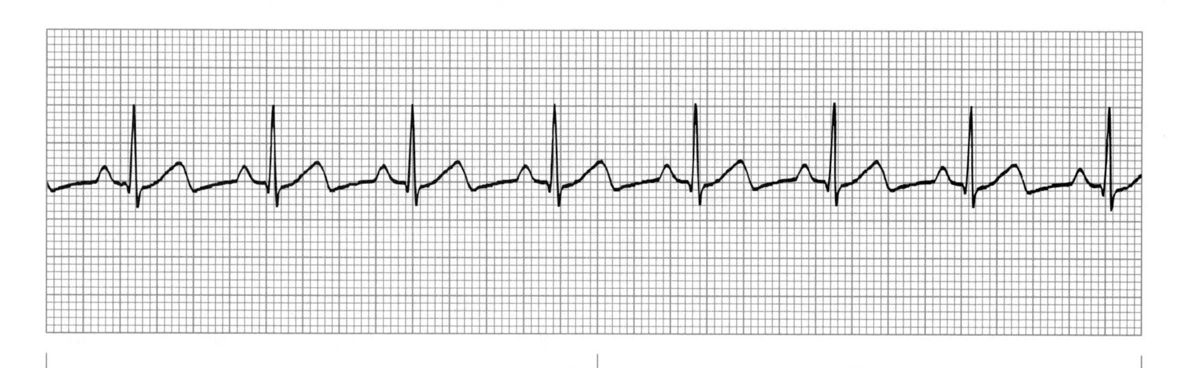

FIGURE B-16
Normal sinus rhythm.

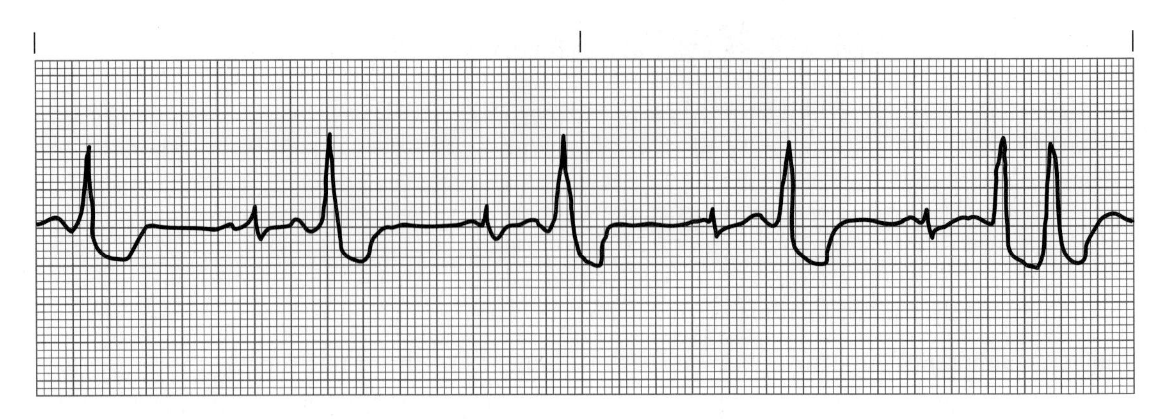

FIGURE B-17
Premature ventricular contractions.

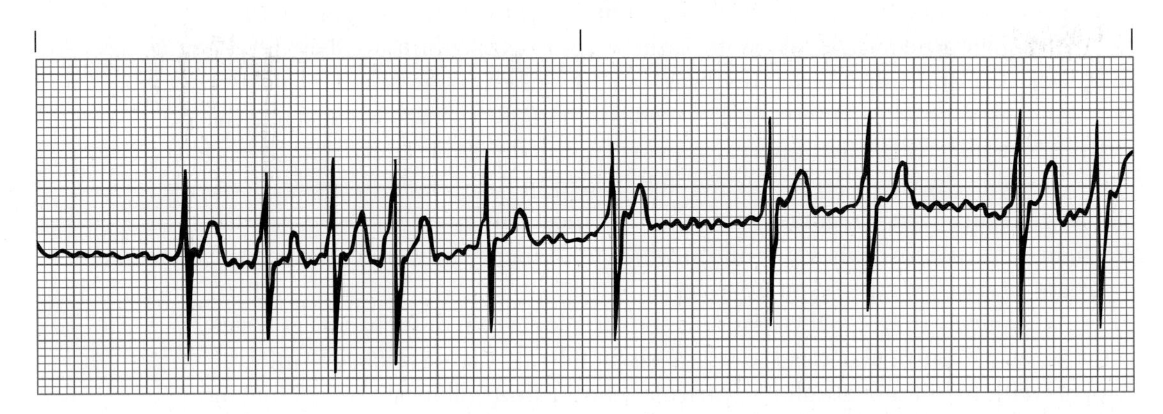

FIGURE B-18
Atrial fibrillation.

Axis

The cardiac axis describes the overall direction of ventricular depolarization. It can be thought of as an arrow pointing in the direction of the QRS complex (Figure B-19). Because the larger left ventricle is oriented downward and to the left, in most normal patients the QRS axis points in that direction.

The body can be visualized as a 360-degree circle present along the frontal plane (Figure B-20). Pointing due left on the patient is 0 degrees. The circle proceeds down to +90 degrees through +180 degrees toward the right arm. Similarly, proceeding upward is −90 degrees. The normal QRS axis is between 0 degrees and +90 degrees.

The easiest method of estimating the axis is by reviewing lead I and AVF on the ECG (see the following chart). Remember that a positive deflection of the ECG tracing for a given lead indicates current flow in the direction of the lead. Therefore, a positive deflection of the QRS complex (large R wave) in both lead I and AVF indicates that the major electrical depolarization is in the direction between 0 degrees and +90 degrees.

If there is a positive deflection in lead I (large R wave) and a large S wave in AVF, then the axis lies between 0 degrees and −90 degrees. This is called *left axis deviation.* Similarly, if the axis falls between +90 degrees and +180 degrees, then the patient has *right axis deviation.* A patient with a calculated axis of between −90 degrees and −180 degrees is described as *extreme right axis deviation.*

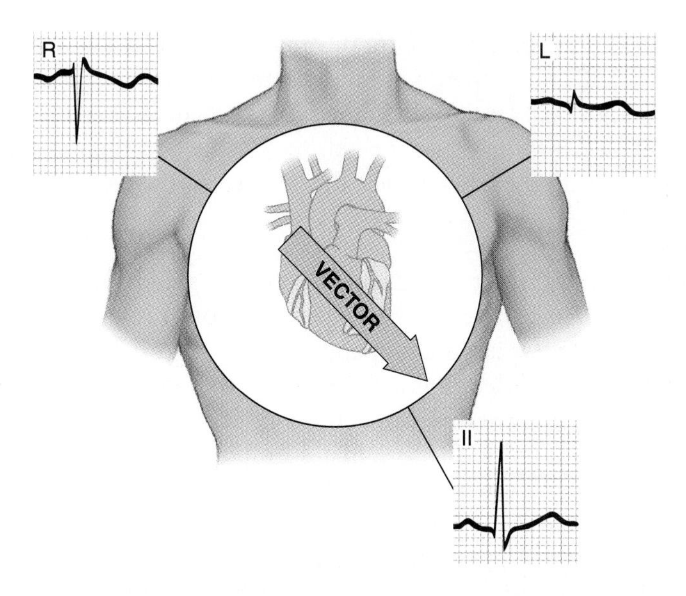

FIGURE B-19
Cardiac vector (QRS axis).

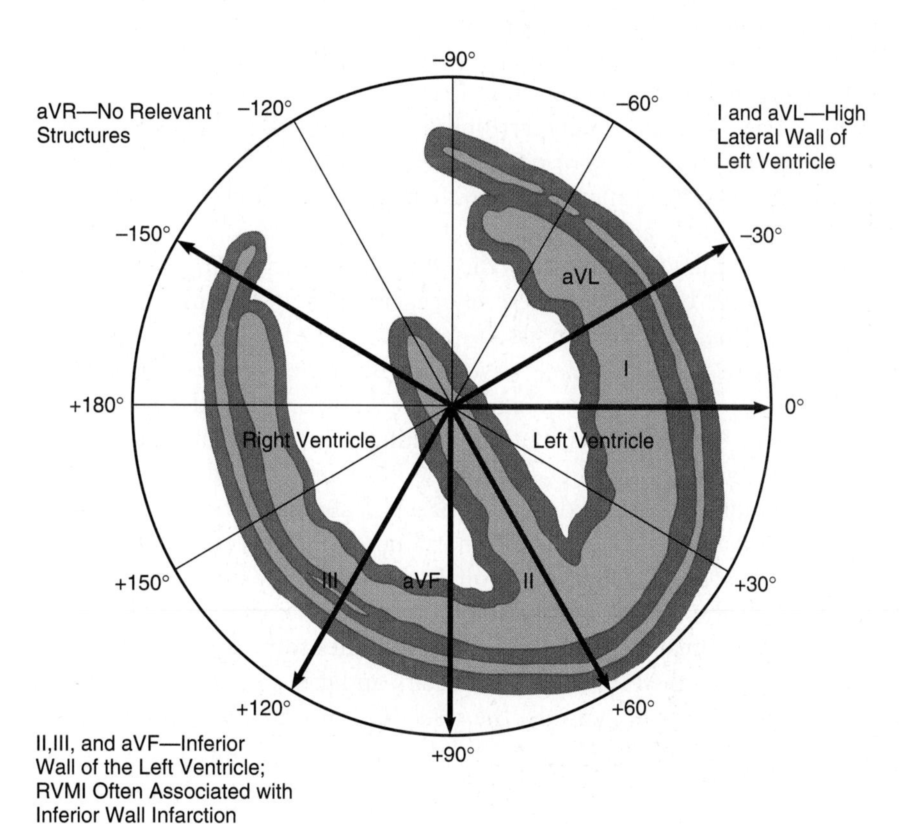

FIGURE B-20
Detailed hexaxial reference system. (Illustration courtesy of Ricaurte Solis, NREMT-P.)

Axis	Lead 1	Lead AVF	Description
0° and +90°	+	+	Normal axis
0° and −90°	+	−	Left axis deviation
+90° and +180°	−	+	Right axis deviation
−90° and −180°	−	−	Extreme right axis deviation

Left axis deviation is produced by those conditions that result in an abnormal enlargement of the left side of the heart. Such conditions as ischemic heart disease, hypertension, and aortic valve disease can lead to left axis deviation.

Right axis deviation may occur in those conditions that strain the right side of the heart. Patients with COPD, pulmonary emboli, pulmonary hypertension, and cor pulmonale may have right axis deviation on their ECG. In addition, damage to the left ventricle from an AMI will cause the axis to shift toward the right because there is a loss of forces from the left ventricle due to myocardial damage.

P Wave and PR Interval

The normal P wave is smooth symmetric rounded wave that is best seen in leads II and V2 (review Figure B-9). When reviewing the ECG, you should review the P waves in each lead to make sure they are similar in appearance. Any difference in appearance suggests that there may be electrical activity originating in other portions of the atria (not the SA node) that are stimulating the conduction system. This is typical of a premature atrial contraction that originates from an ectopic (other than the normal SA location) focus in the atria. The appearance of the P wave in this beat would be different from its appearance in the other PQRST complexes.

Also review the P wave to ensure it is not biphasic (with two peaks) in appearance (Figure B-21), which suggests that one of the atria may have thickened (hypertrophied) from stress on the muscular wall. When this occurs, conduction through the hypertrophied atria is delayed, resulting in asynchronous atrial contraction. If the major positive deflection of the P wave is seen in the early V leads (V1-V2), this suggests right atrial hypertrophy. This might occur in patients with tricuspid valve stenosis. If the major positive deflection is seen in the later V leads (V5-V6), this suggests left atrial hypertrophy. In addition, you may see a large negative deflection in leads V1 and V2 with left atrial enlargement.

Quickly review the PR intervals on the entire ECG tracing. You should consider a diagnosis of AV block when there is an increase in any PR interval or you find a P wave that does not have an associated QRS complex. The PR interval is measured from the beginning of the P wave to the beginning of the QRS complex (review Figure B-10). The PR interval is normally 0.12 to 0.2 seconds. Because the PR interval represents the time that impulse conduction is occurring between the atria and the ventricles, any prolongation of the PR interval is called AV block. A PR interval of less than 0.12 seconds may indicate an abnormal conduction pathway between the atria and the ventricles. An example is a delta wave that is characteristically seen in some patients with Wolf-Parkinson-White (WPW) syndrome (Figure B-22). Here, the P wave slopes gently into the QRS complex.

Any PR interval greater than 0.20 seconds indicates some form of AV block. In first-degree AV block, the PR interval is constant and measures greater than 0.20 seconds (Figure B-23). This is typically the result of abnormal functioning of the AV node.

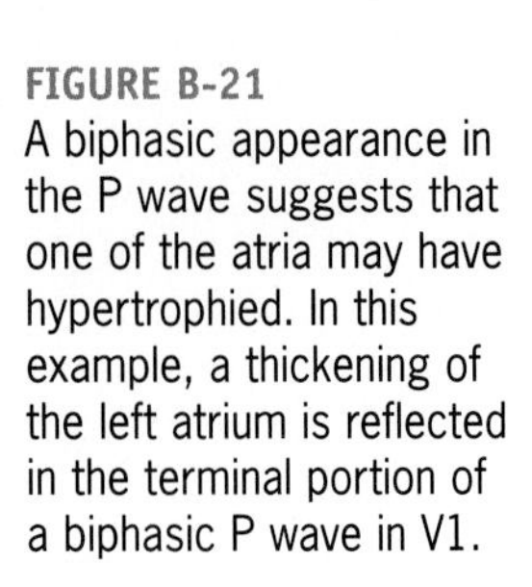

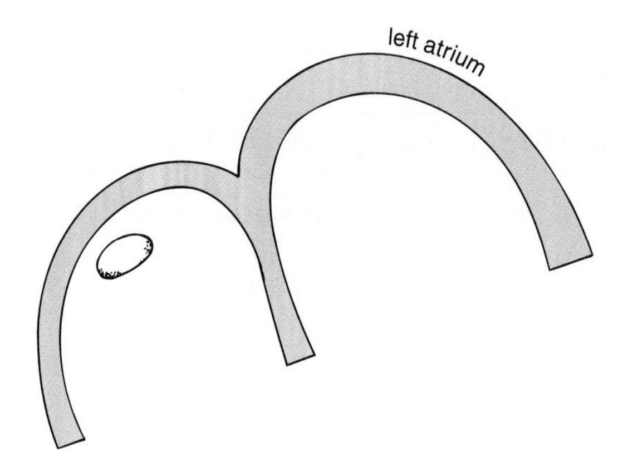

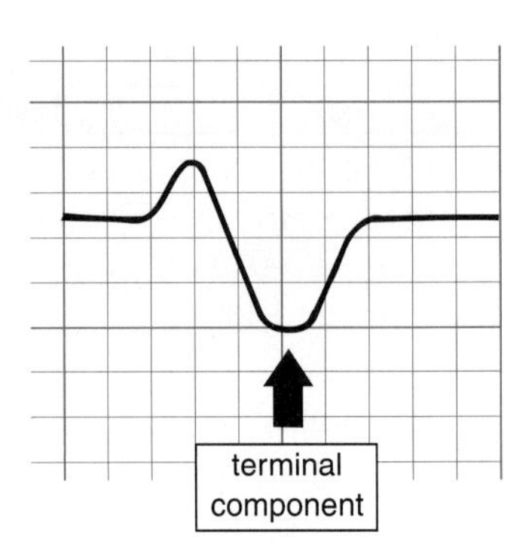

FIGURE B-21
A biphasic appearance in the P wave suggests that one of the atria may have hypertrophied. In this example, a thickening of the left atrium is reflected in the terminal portion of a biphasic P wave in V1.

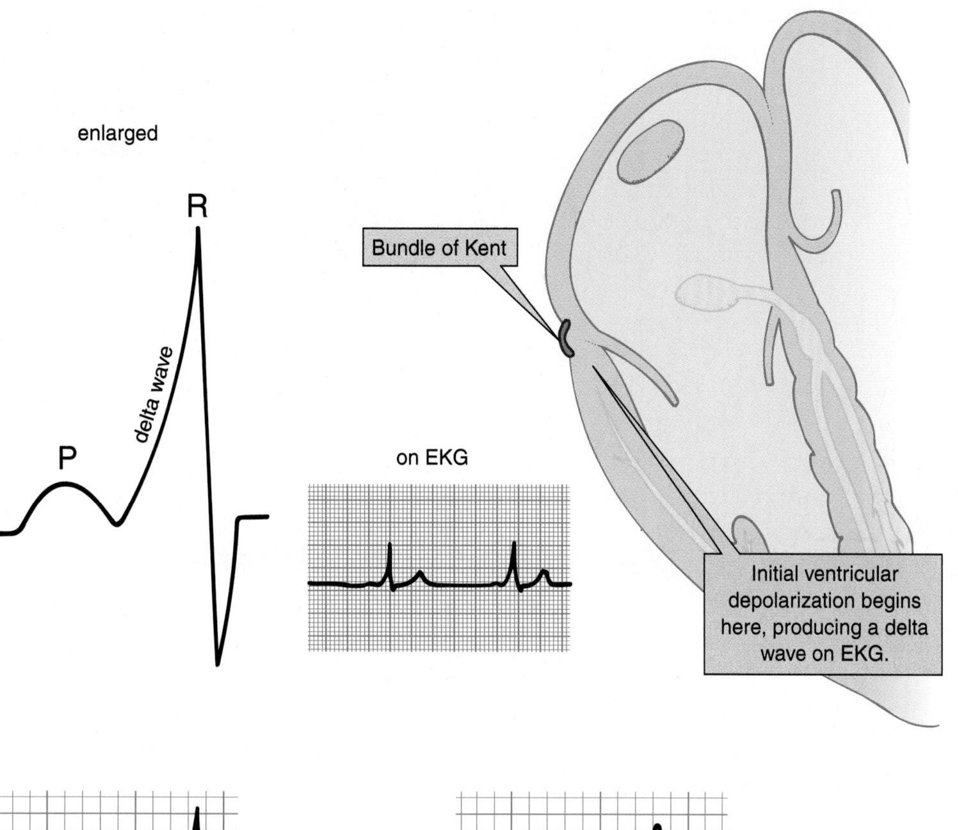

FIGURE-B22
A PR interval less than 0.12 seconds may indicate an abnormal conduction pathway between atria and ventricles. Shown here: The delta wave characteristic of some Wolf-Parkinson-White (WPW) patients where the P wave slopes gently into the QRS complex.

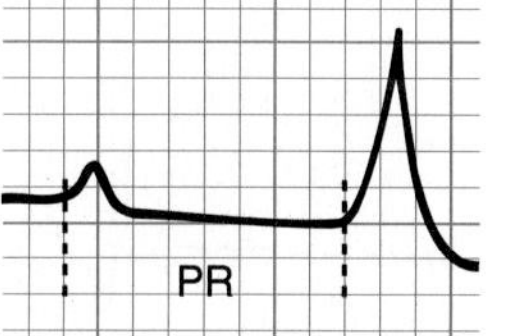

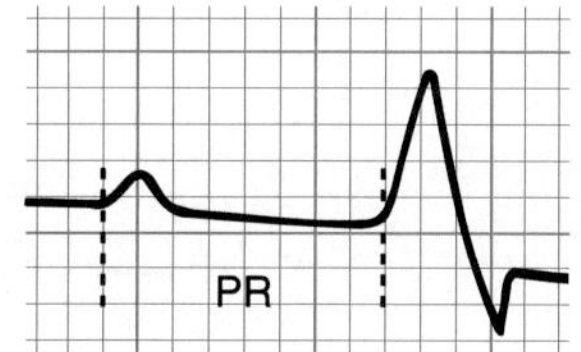

"Measure" PR by observation (one large square).

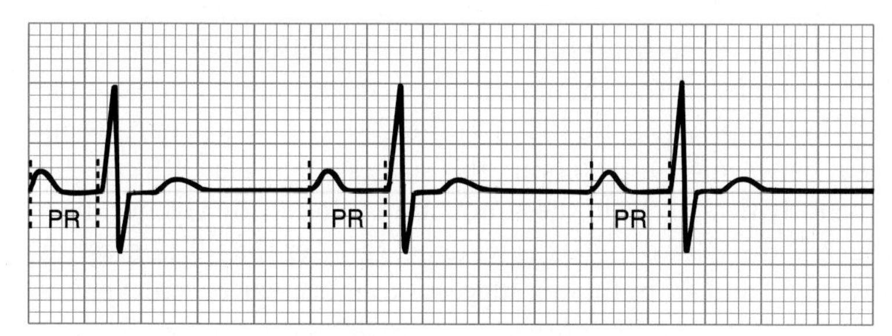

PR remains consistently lengthened cycle to cycle.

FIGURE B-23
A PR interval greater than 0.20 seconds indicates some form of AV block. Shown here: Prolonged PR intervals typical of first-degree AV block.

In second-degree AV block, there is intermittent malfunction of conduction through the conduction system to the ventricle. Two types of second-degree blocks are commonly identified: Wenkebach blocks and Mobitz blocks. In Wenkebach blocks, there is a malfunction of the AV node, and on the ECG, there is progressive lengthening of the PR interval until a QRS complex is dropped (Figure B-24). Wenkebach blocks are characterized as 2:1, 3:2, 4:3, and so forth, depending on the number of P waves in relation to the QRS complexes. Mobitz blocks involve the conduction segments below the AV node, including the His bundle and the left and right bundle branches. In Mobitz blocks, the AV node depolarizes several times until one beat is completely conducted (Figure B-25). Mobitz blocks are characterized as 2:1, 3:1, 4:1, and so forth.

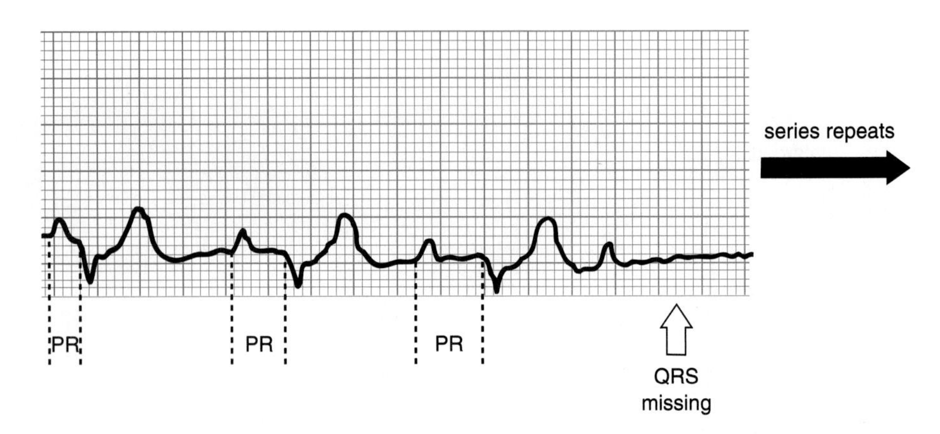

FIGURE B-24
In Wenkebach blocks, the ECG records a progressive lengthening of the PR interval until a QRS complex is dropped.

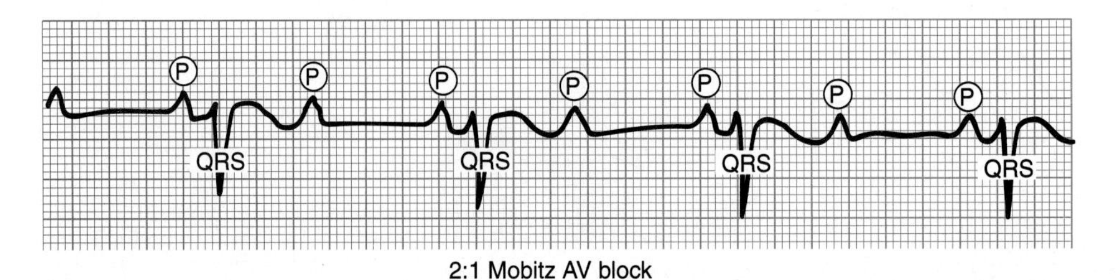

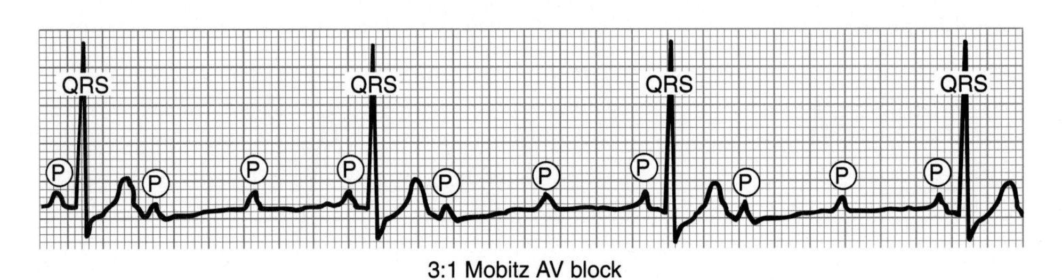

FIGURE B-25
In Mobitz blocks, the AV node depolarizes several times until one beat is completely conducted. There may be two P waves to one QRS (2:1 Mobitz block), three P waves to one QRS (3:1 Mobitz block), or more.

In complete, or third-degree, heart block, there is no relationship between the P waves and the QRS complexes. You should be able to map out the P waves independently of each QRS complex (Figure B-26). If the QRS complex is narrow and the underlying rate is between 40 and 60 bpm, this suggests that the QRS complex is paced by spontaneously firing cells in the conduction system (the His bundle or the bundle branches). If the QRS complex is widened (greater than 0.12 seconds) and the rate is between 20 and 40 bpm, this suggests a ventricular pacemaker.

In addition to measuring one PR interval, you should inspect successive complexes to make sure the PR interval is uniform for each cardiac cycle. Variations occur in various types of AV blocks.

QRS Complex

The QRS complex represents the electrical events surrounding ventricular contraction. We have already stated that, because the heart possesses a coordinated conduction system, contraction of the left and right ventricles occurs almost simultaneously under normal conditions. On the ECG tracing, the normal duration of the QRS complex is 0.12 seconds (three small squares) or less.

In addition, because of the relatively larger size of the left ventricle, the average electrical forces during ventricular contraction appear to be oriented toward the left side of the heart. As a result, cardiac leads that are directed toward the left side of the heart (e.g., lead I, AVL, and precordial leads V5 and V6) will demonstrate a primarily positive QRS complex (large R wave). If you examine

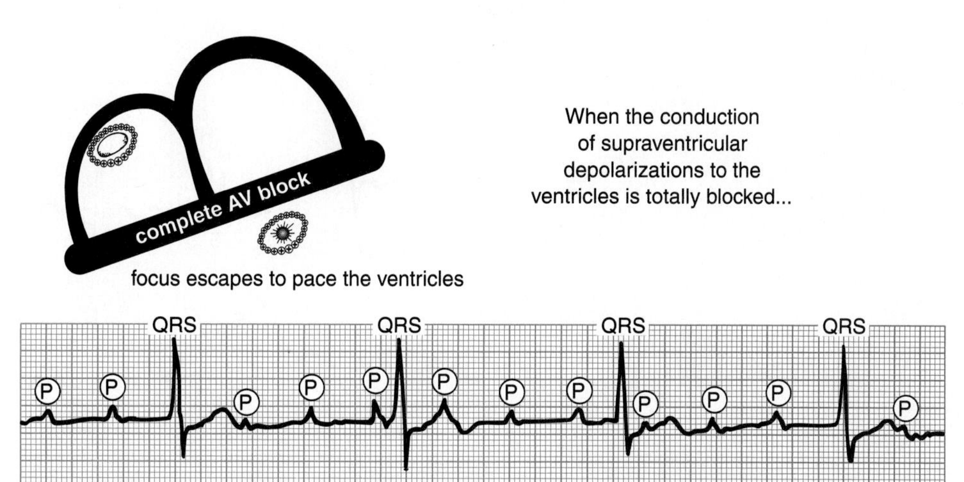

FIGURE B-26
In complete, or third-degree, heart block, there is no relationship between the P waves and the QRS complexes. You should be able to map out the P waves independently of each QRS complex.

the precordial leads, you will notice that there is a tendency of the R wave to become more prominent as the tracing is viewed from V1 through V6 (called "R-wave progression") (Figure B-27).

When the QRS complex is greater than 0.12 seconds, the conduction system may not be functioning appropriately. A condition known as a bundle branch block may have occurred. Under these circumstances, the electrical impulse is carried down the AV node through the bundle of His. From this point, there may be a blockage either in the left bundle branch or in the right bundle branch.

A right bundle branch block (Figure B-28) is a fairly common finding on an ECG. It is often seen in patients who have suffered an AMI involving the anterolateral portion of the left ventricle. It is recognized by a widened QRS complex and a second positive deflection in the QRS complex (called an RSR′ [RSR prime] pattern) in the early precordial leads (V1 and V2).

In the case of a left bundle branch block (Figure B-29), conduction proceeds into the right bundle and the right ventricle contracts. Conduction then proceeds through the cardiac muscle more slowly to the left ventricle, which then contracts. Thus, the QRS complex is widened and reflects the nonsimultaneous contraction of each ventricle.

A left bundle branch block is a more concerning problem than a right bundle branch block because it is usually associated with significant cardiac damage. This pattern is recognized by a QRS duration of greater than 0.12 seconds and a broad, sometimes notched R wave in the lateral precordial leads. In addition to

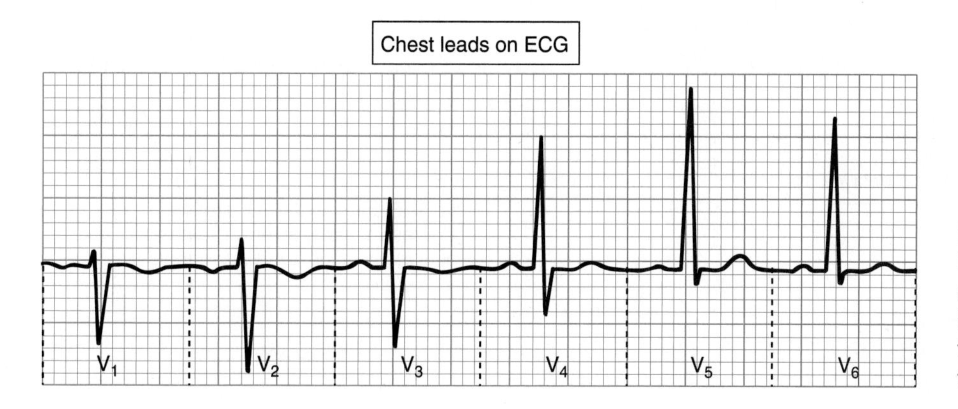

FIGURE B-27
In the precordial leads, there is a tendency for the R wave to become more prominent as the tracing is viewed from V1 through V6.

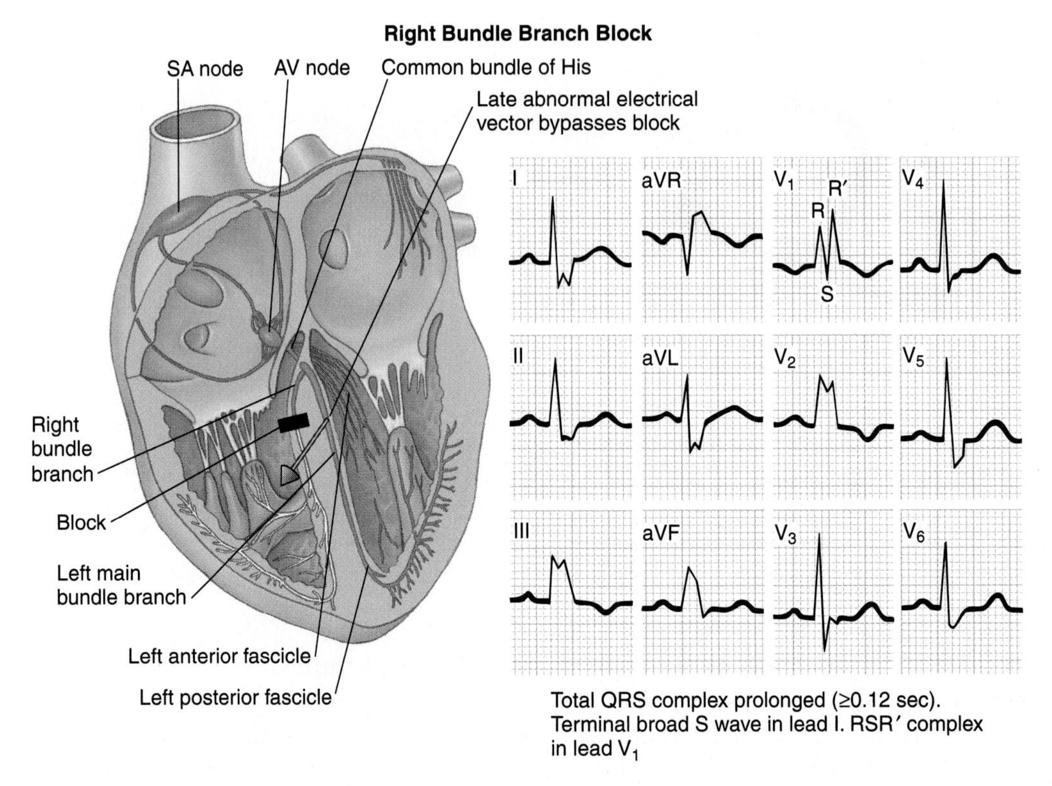

FIGURE B-28
Right bundle branch block.

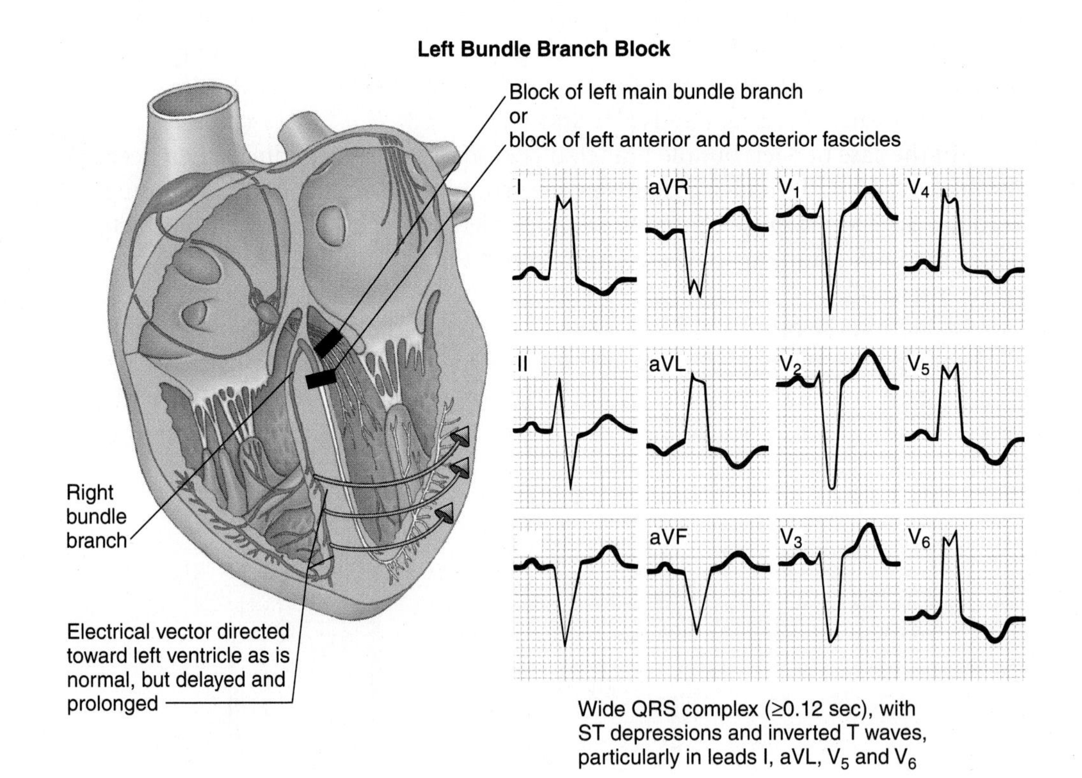

FIGURE B-29
Left bundle branch block.

suggesting significant underlying cardiac disease, the presence of a left bundle branch pattern can make interpretation of the ECG difficult, especially in the setting of an AMI. In fact, the presence of a new left bundle branch block in a patient with signs and symptoms consistent with cardiac chest pain is an indication to consider fibrinolytic therapy or immediate angioplasty. These patients are also at high risk of developing complete heart block and cardiogenic shock.

You should also be aware that the main two branches of the left bundle branch, the left anterior fascicle and left posterior fascicle, can also become disrupted. A discussion of the ECG findings associated with these lesions is beyond the intent of this appendix.

ST Segment and T Wave

Reviewing the ST segment and the T wave is one of the most important aspects of interpreting the ECG in a patient with suspected cardiac disease. Remember that the ST segment begins at the J point and ends at the beginning of the T wave (review Figure B-12). In a normal ECG, the ST segment should rest along the isoelectric line. Changes in the ST segment can result from myocardial ischemia, but other conditions such as ventricular hypertrophy, conduction defects, and drugs may also produce ST changes.

The T wave is a smooth, rounded deflection that occurs after the QRS complex (review Figure B-10). This represents the end of ventricular repolarization. You should review the shape of the T wave and specifically look for "peaking" of the T wave. Also remember that the T wave tends to move in the same direction as the QRS complex. That is, if the QRS complex has a large positive component (R wave), then the T wave tends to be represented by a positive deflection. However, if the QRS complex has a significant negative component (large S wave), then the T wave may be primarily negative in orientation.

Ischemia, Injury, and Infarction

Acute coronary syndromes occur when there is a difference between the oxygen requirements of the heart and the oxygen supplied to the heart by the coronary arteries. Findings can vary from transient symptoms, primarily angina (chest pain) caused by a temporary rise in the work of the heart, to permanent heart damage caused by a complete blockage of the blood supply to the heart from a thrombus (clot). The inciting event in these cases is most commonly atherosclerotic narrowing of the coronary arteries, which leads to a cascade of events that may ultimately cause complete obstruction of the blood supply to the heart. Commonly, the final obstructing event is the development of a clot (thrombus) within the coronary arteries. Early recognition of this process can minimize the damage to the heart muscle and a better functional recovery.

Even in the setting of complete coronary occlusion, there are different areas of the heart that can be defined by their ultimate prognosis (Figure B-30). Although some areas are clearly permanently damaged by the lack of blood supply, other areas are potentially salvageable if there is prompt recognition and initiation of appropriate therapy.

AMI produces a characteristic progression of changes in the ECG, particularly during the period of ventricular repolarization. As a result, initial changes are found in the ST segment and T wave. Early recognition of these changes by emergency personnel can set in motion a series of steps designed to produce the best outcome in the patient suffering an AMI.

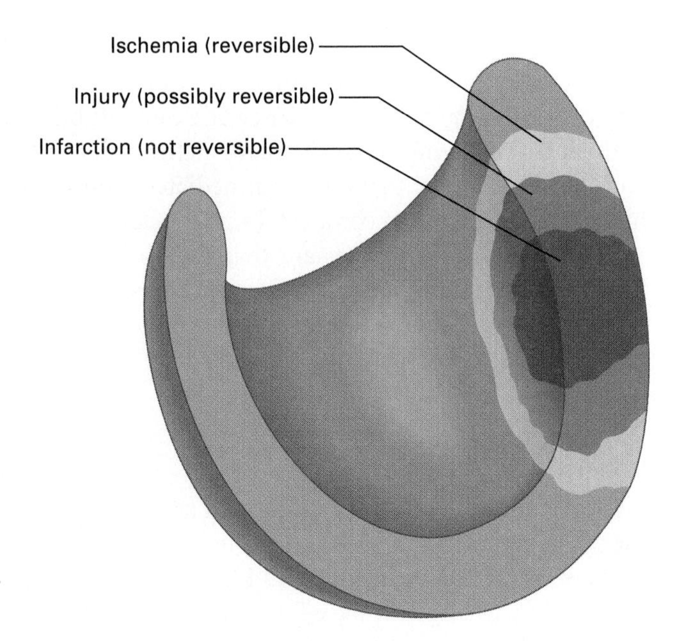

FIGURE B-30
Sectors of myocardial damage resulting from coronary occlusion: ischemia, injury, and infarction (necrosis).

The earliest findings in patients with cardiac disease include *myocardial ischemia* in the area of involved blood supply (Figure B-31). This is characterized by depression of the ST segment, T-wave inversion (opposite to the major direction of the QRS complex), and peaked T waves. ST segment depression is considered significant when the ST segment (measured from the J point) is depressed at least 1 mm below the isoelectric line.

As the hypoxic insult progresses, evidence of *myocardial injury* is present (Figure B-32). Myocardial injury is characterized by ST segment elevation and T-wave inversion. Again, ST segment elevation is considered significant when it is greater than 1 mm above the isoelectric line. You should also note that when the ST segment is viewed in leads that are opposite in orientation to an ECG lead

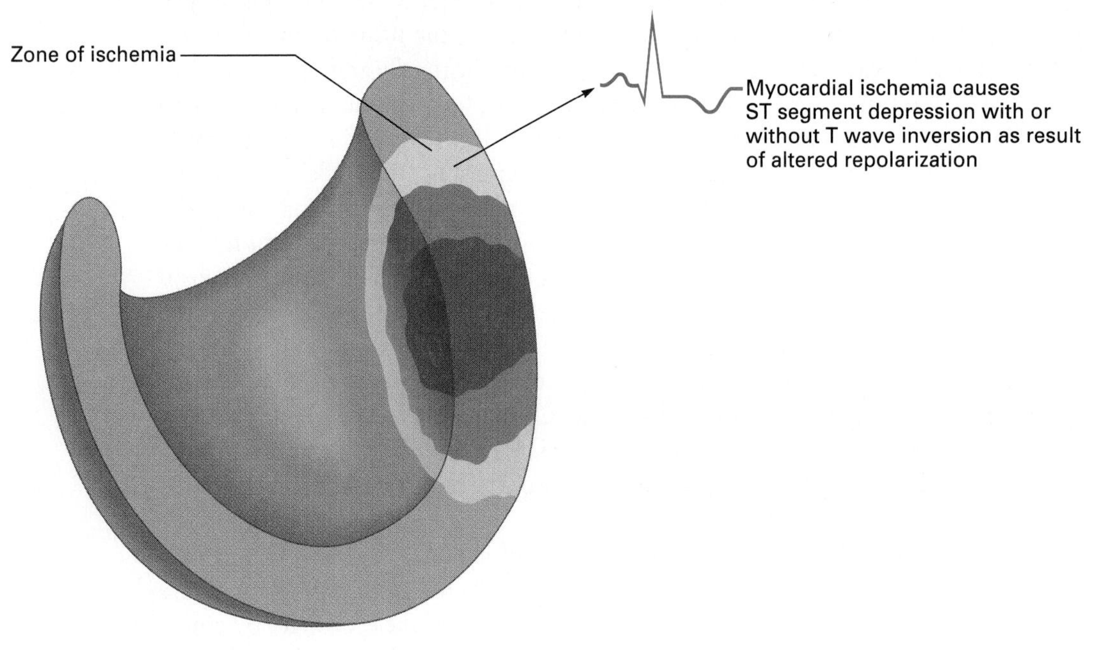

FIGURE B-31
ECG changes reflecting myocardial ischemia.

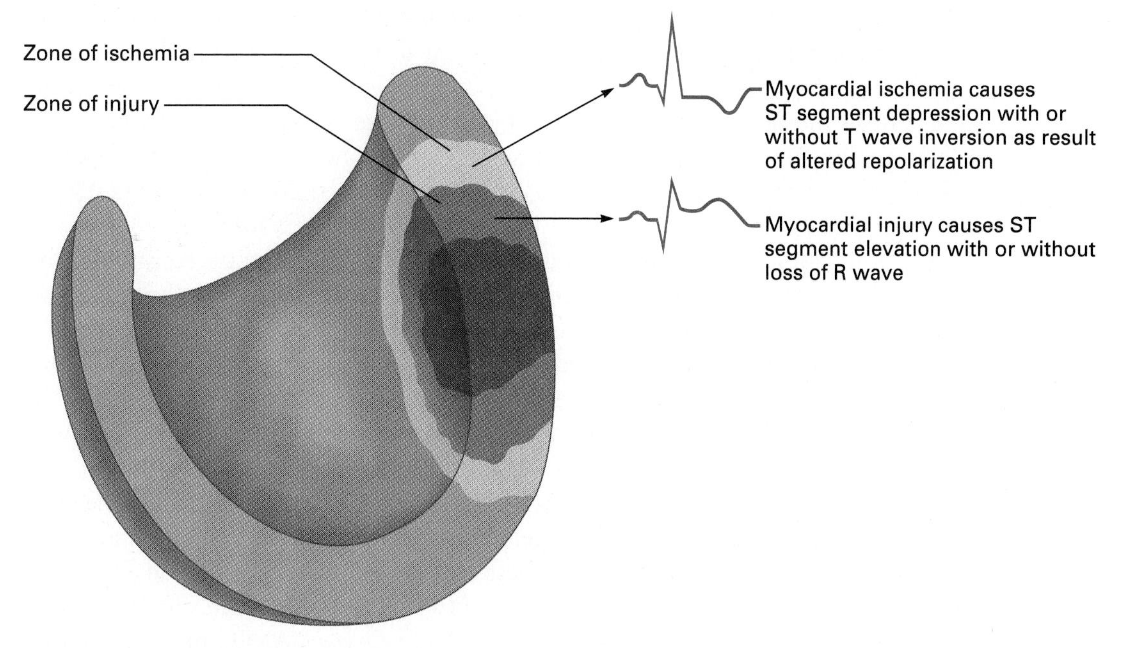

FIGURE B-32
ECG changes reflecting myocardial injury.

demonstrating ST elevation (e.g., ST changes in AVR when there is ST elevation in lead II), the ST segments may appear depressed. This is referred to as *reciprocal change.*

Finally, as cellular death occurs following complete occlusion, ECG changes of *myocardial necrosis,* or tissue death, are seen (Figure B-33). This is heralded by the presence of significant, or pathological, Q waves. We have already defined Q waves as the first negative deflection of the QRS complex, signifying the initial unopposed depolarization away from the direction of the involved lead. A

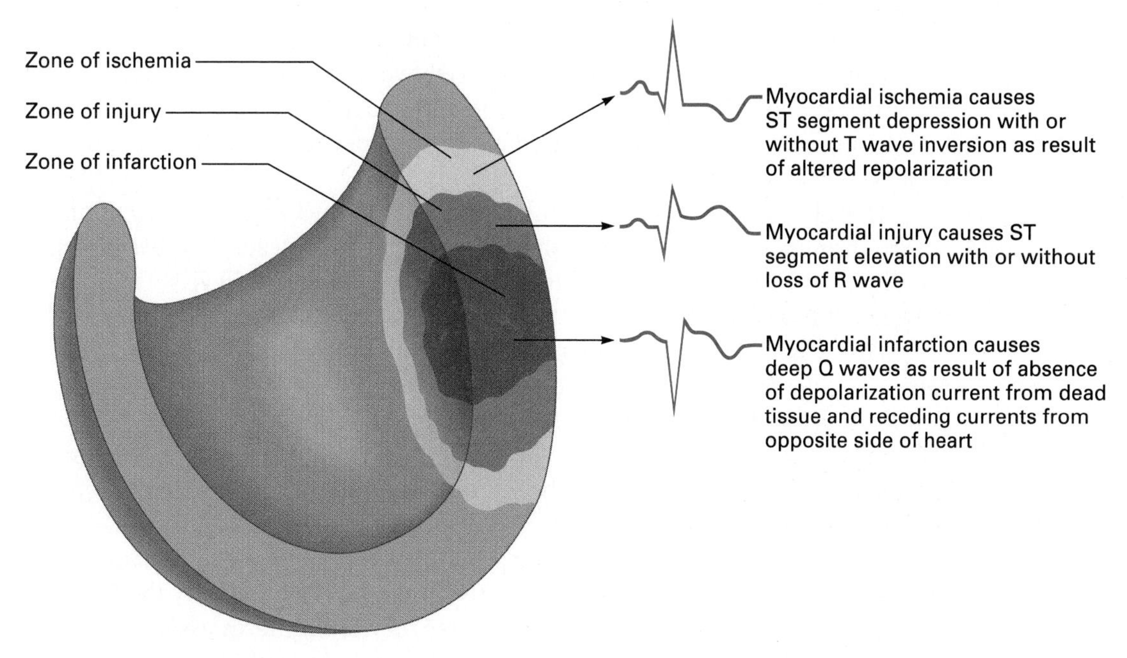

FIGURE B-33
ECG changes reflecting myocardial infarction (necrosis, or tissue death).

Q wave is defined as significant or pathological if it is 1) greater than 0.04 seconds (one small box) and 2) more than 25 percent of the height of the R wave. Such pathological changes in the Q wave result from the absence of a depolarization current from the necrotic tissue. These Q wave changes develop over the course of hours following an AMI and persist on subsequent ECGs. As a result, it may be impossible to determine the age of myocardial necrosis based solely on the presence of significant Q waves unless there is some historical context for these findings.

You should also be aware that the classic ECG findings are consistent with those patients who experience a coronary artery occlusion affecting the entire wall of the heart. This is referred to as a *transmural AMI* (*transmural* means "through the wall") because the damage occurs across all three layers of the heart: the epicardium, the myocardium, and the endocardium. These cases tend to develop the full progression of changes described previously and are thus called "Q-wave AMIs" or "transmural AMIs."

Often, the entire heart wall is not affected by an occlusion, with only the most susceptible portions suffering damage. Because the endocardium (innermost portion of the myocardium) has the highest oxygen demand, it is most likely to sustain injury. In these cases, the spectrum of ECG changes described previously does not necessarily occur; such cases are called "non-Q-wave AMIs" or "subendocardial AMIs." Patients with subendocardial AMI tend to demonstrate ST depression rather than the classic ST elevation. In addition, these patients do not ultimately develop significant Q waves.

Findings in Inferior AMI

As we have stated earlier, "Time is Muscle." Therefore, the emergency care provider must not only be efficient in obtaining a focused history that suggests an acute coronary syndrome, but also be able to set in motion the series of steps that will lead to opening an occluded coronary artery in the shortest possible time. Perhaps the most important element of this process is the recognition of characteristic ECG findings of AMI. A familiarity with the coronary anatomy is essential and guides the clinician in understanding the two dominant patterns of AMI: *inferior myocardial infarction* and *anterior myocardial infarction.*

Remember that the RCA supplies the right ventricle, the posterior wall of the left ventricle, and the inferior wall of the left ventricle. The RCA also provides blood supply to portions of the conduction system, including the SA node, AV node, and His bundle.

The ECG simply represents the electrical activities of the cardiac cycle as viewed through several "cameras": the limb and precordial leads. Our basic understanding of the cardiogram reminds us that leads II, III, and AVF view the inferior portions of the heart.

This tells us that if the patient has a history that is consistent with an acute coronary syndrome, we should also see evidence of ischemia, injury, or infarction in leads II, III or AVF (Figure B-34). By convention, ST elevation is considered significant if it occurs in two or more of these leads and measures at least 1 mm in height. T-wave inversion may also be seen in conjunction with ST changes in the setting of an inferior AMI.

Also be aware of other ECG changes that may be found in association with an inferior AMI. We have already noted the other areas supplied by the RCA. As stated in Chapter 6, right ventricular infarcts may be found in association with an acute inferior MI. These patients tend to present with hypotension that responds to fluid therapy, which increases right ventricular filling pressure. Preload-reducing agents such as morphine or nitrates can produce disastrous

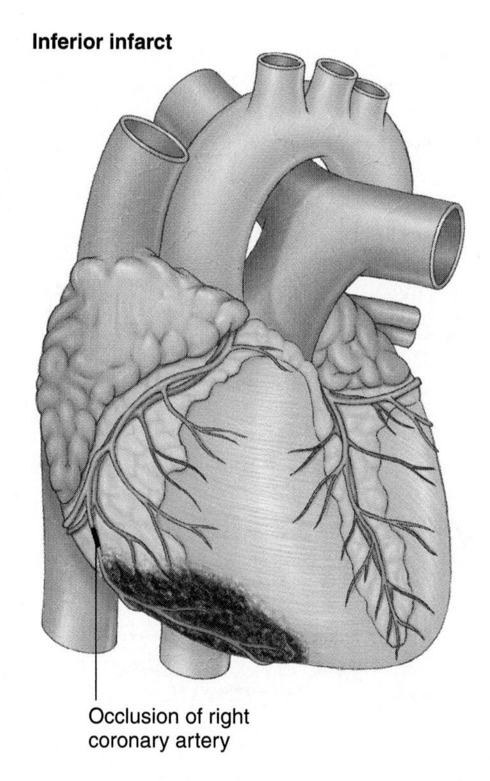

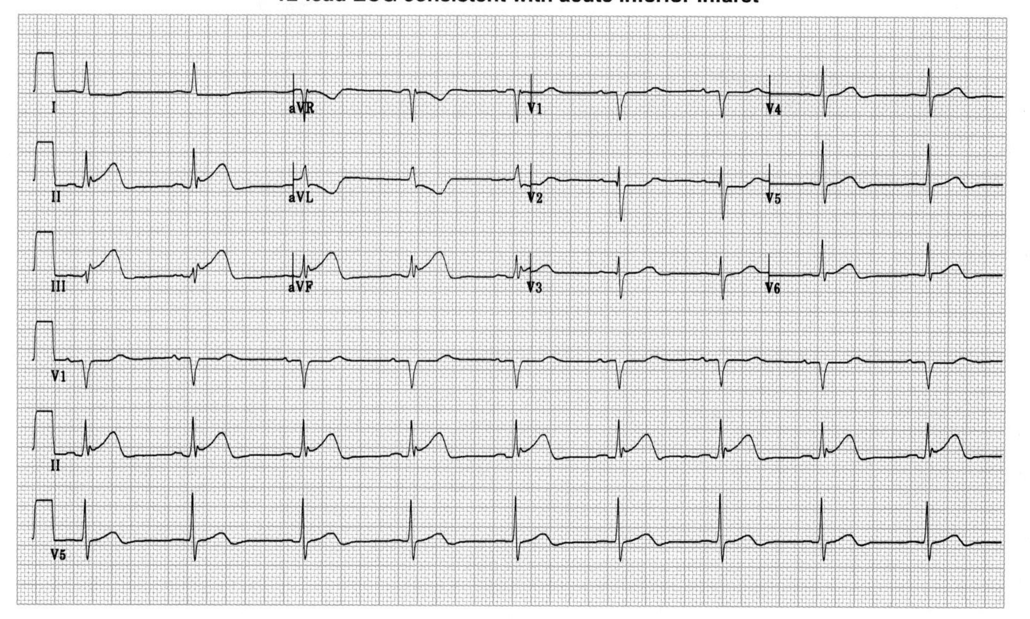

FIGURE B-34 Inferior myocardial infarction with typical ECG findings.

results when given to a patient with a right ventricular infarct. The classic ECG findings of RV infarct may be difficult to demonstrate. You must use special ECG leads placed on the right side of the heart in a position analogous to V4 and V5 (Figure B-35).

Remember that the RCA also supplies the posterior wall of the left ventricle. The difficulty in recognizing posterior AMIs is that none of the ECG leads is directed posteriorly; therefore, none of our "cameras" will directly demonstrate the classic ECG findings of a posterior AMI. This leaves us with evaluating the leads that face in the *exact opposite* direction of the posterior wall: V1

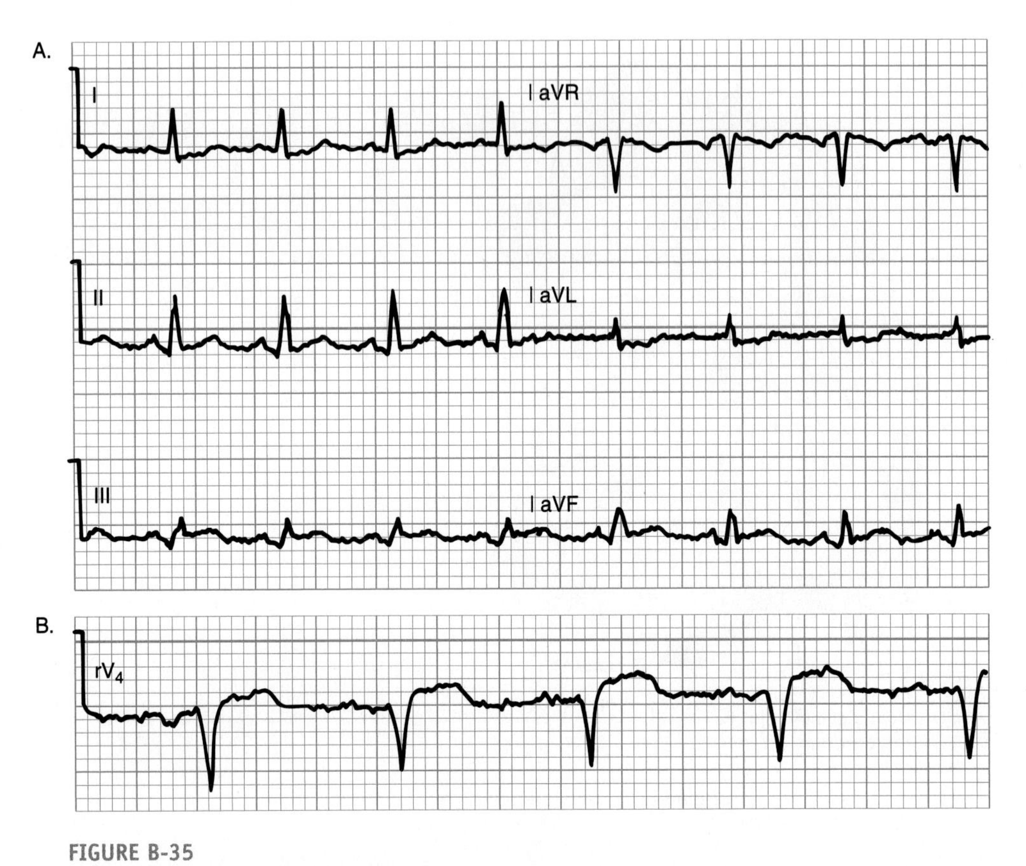

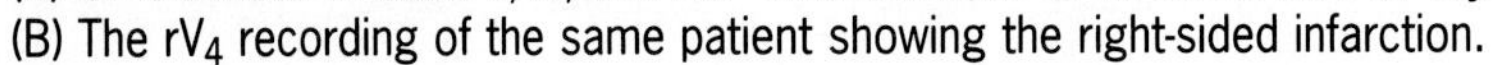

FIGURE B-35
(A) ST elevation in leads II, III, and AVF characteristic of an acute inferior myocardial infarction. (B) The rV_4 recording of the same patient showing the right-sided infarction.

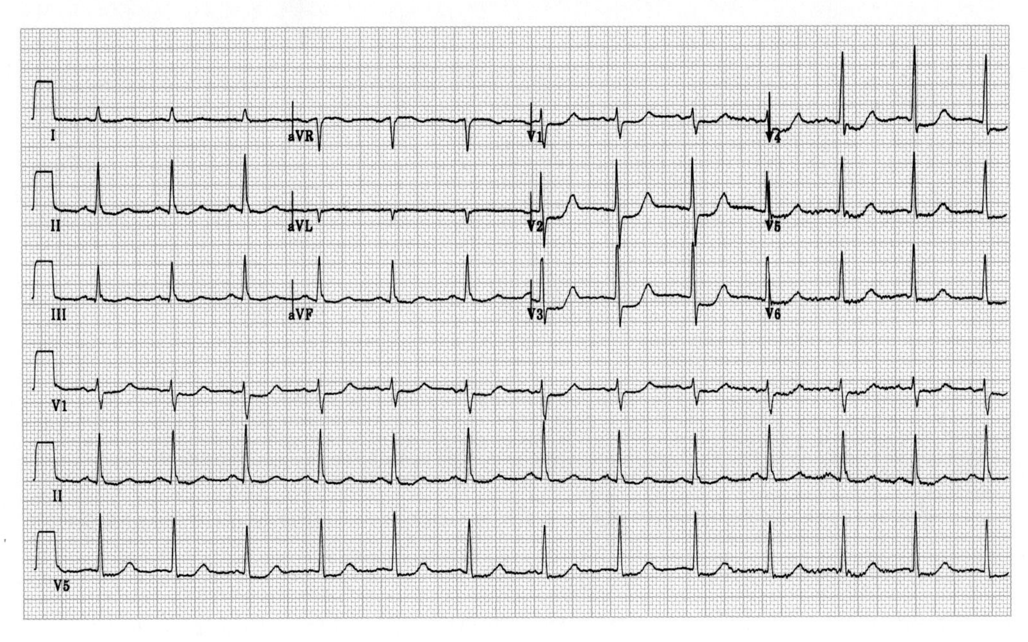

FIGURE B-36
ECG findings consistent with posterior myocardial infarction.

through V4. Because these leads face in the opposite direction, the findings of a true posterior AMI would be "reciprocal" to the classic anterior AMI pattern (Figure B-36). As such, we will see ST *depression* in the involved leads. In the later stages, large R waves (the equivalent of deep Q waves) develop in the early precordial leads.

It has been suggested that a mirror can be used to determine posterior ST elevation by viewing the tracing with the ECG inverted. Alternatively, one could hold the ECG upside down and backward toward bright light to visualize the classic ST pattern of AMI.

Posterior V leads (also labeled V7 through V9) obtained with the patient in the right lateral decubitus position (right side down) have been suggested (Figure B-37). Patients with a posterior AMI in conjunction with an inferior AMI tend to have more significant ventricular dysrhythmias in association with their disease.

In some patients with "right dominant" cardiac circulation, the RCA also supplies the lateral wall of the left ventricle. In such cases, ST elevation may be seen in leads V5 and V6 in conjunction with an inferior AMI.

Because the RCA provides blood supply to some portions of the conduction system, there are dysrhythmias that are seen in patients with acute inferior MI. Classically, first-degree AV block and Wenkebach AV blocks are seen. These are believed to be relatively benign dysrhythmias.

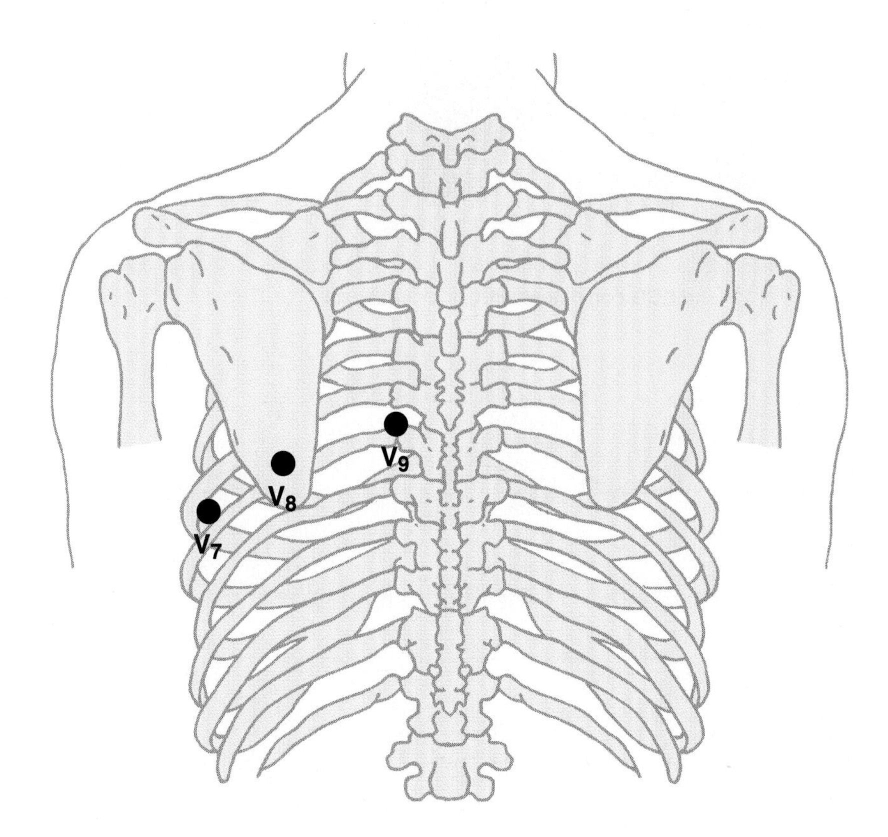

V_7—5th intercostal space, posterior axillary line
V_8—5th intercostal space, midscapular line
V_9—5th intercostal space, 2 cm left of spinal column

FIGURE B-37
Posterior V lead placement. (Illustration courtesy of Ricaurte Solis, NREMT-P.)

Findings in Anterior AMI

The LCA divides into the descending branch, which supplies the anterior wall of the left ventricle, and the circumflex branch, which supplies the lateral wall of the left ventricle (except in right-dominant circulation, as noted), portions of the posterior wall of the left ventricle, and the interventricular septum.

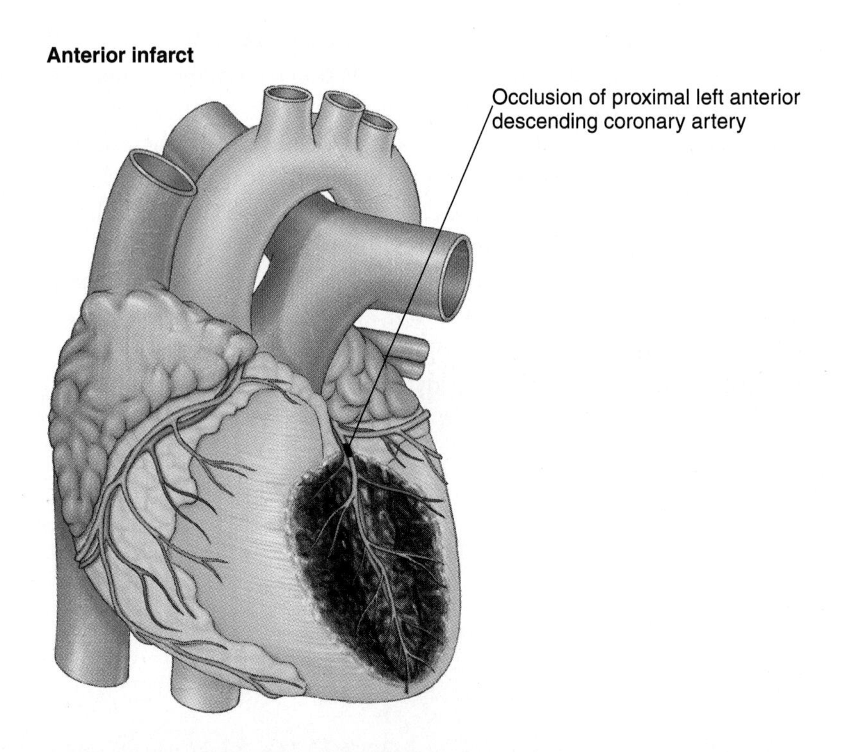

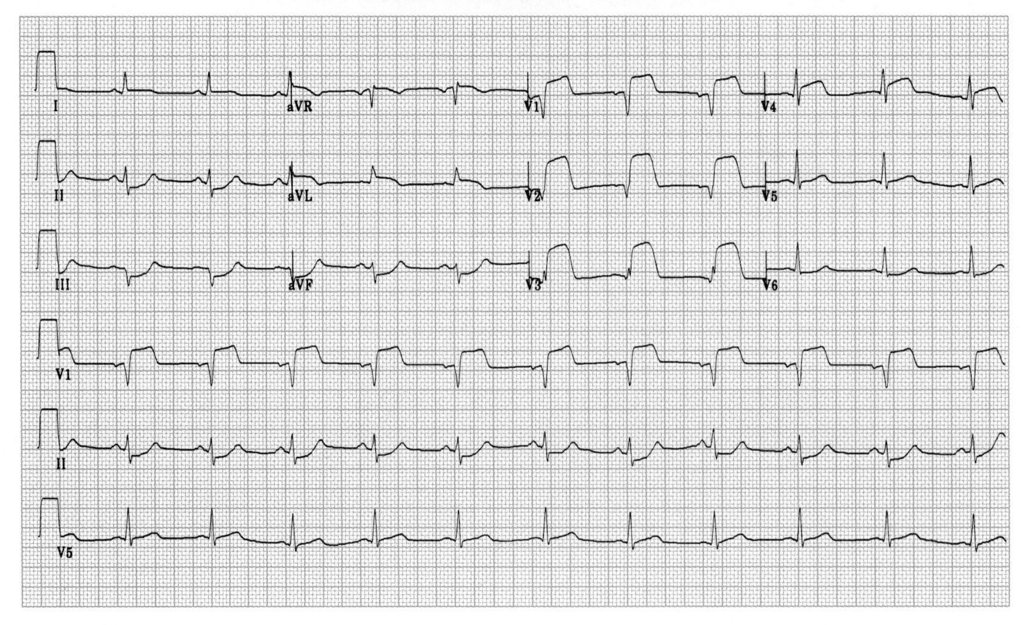

FIGURE B-38
Anterior myocardial infarction with typical ECG findings.

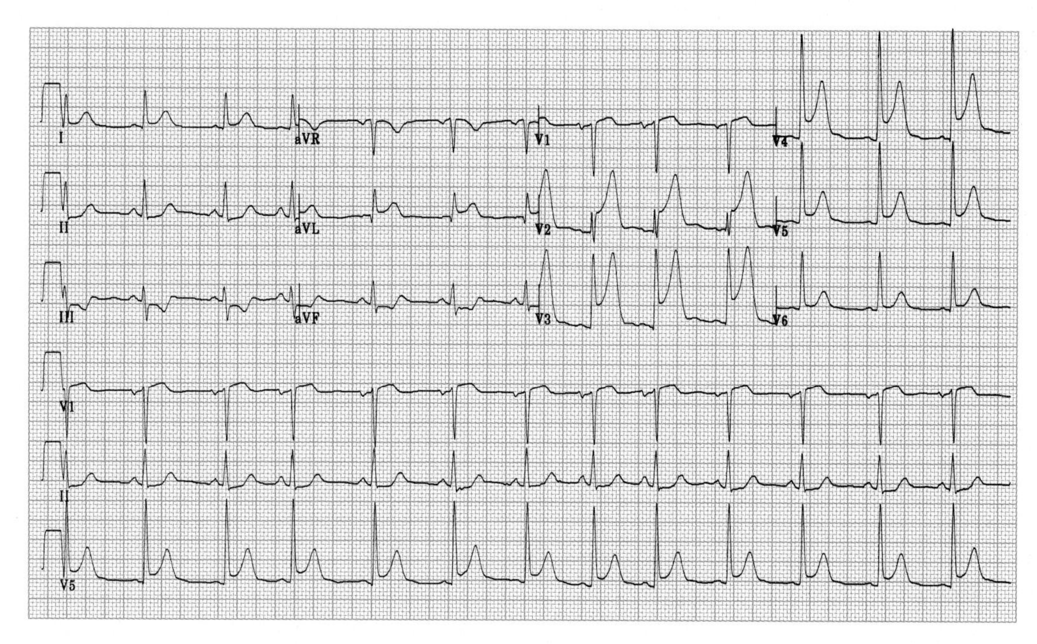

FIGURE B-39
Anterolateral myocardial infarction.

Occlusions of the LCA can effect the septal (V1 and V2), anterior (V3 and V4), and lateral (V5 and V6) precordial leads. By convention, ST elevation of 2 mm or more in three contiguous precordial leads is diagnostic of an anterior AMI (Figure B-38). If the elevation is found in V1 through V4, the term *anteroseptal AMI* is used. For leads V3 through V6, the term *anterolateral AMI* is applied (Figure B-39). Here again, T-wave inversion may be associated with ST changes in the presence of an AMI.

Anterior AMIs tend to involve a significant amount of cardiac damage. As a result, significant ventricular rhythm disturbances (ventricular tachycardia and ventricular fibrillation), cardiogenic shock, and severe conduction system blocks are associated with anterior AMIs. In particular, Mobitz AV block and complete heart block may be seen.

ECG Findings in Other Medical Conditions

There are characteristic patterns on the ECG that can suggest other significant diagnoses. However, these ECG patterns must be considered in the context of the patient's history and physical examination.

Pericarditis

Pericarditis is an inflammatory condition involving the fluid surrounding the heart. This condition may be caused by a variety of bacterial or viral pathogens and other inflammatory mediators. Patients with acute pericarditis may present with diffuse ST elevation in most of the cardiac leads except AVR and V1. Several features distinguish the ECG findings of pericarditis from findings of AMI. The T waves are generally upright. ST segment elevation is not limited to the a few isolated leads as with acute inferior or anterior myocardial injury. Also, the ST segments are classically described as having an initial flattened or concave appearance (Figure B-40). The T wave may also appear to be elevated off the isoelectric line.

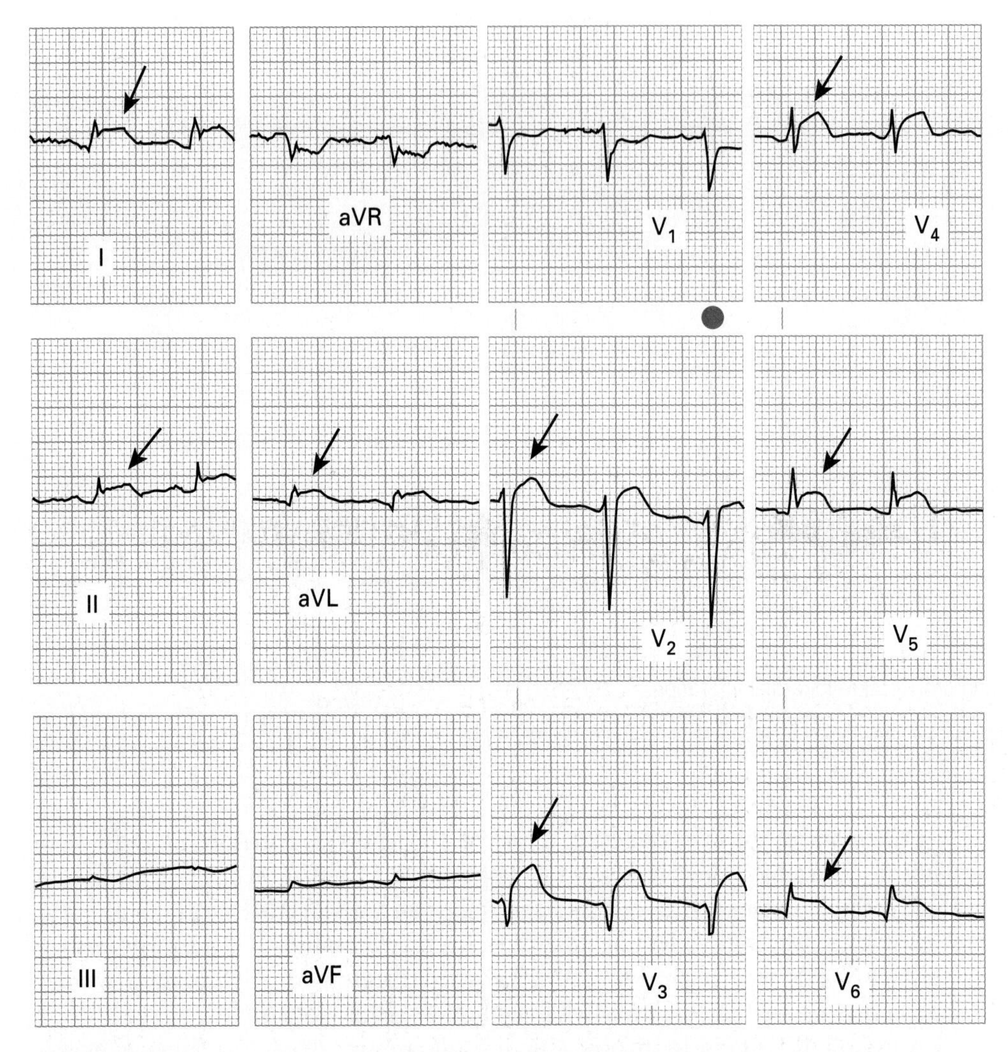

FIGURE B-40
ECG of patient with acute pericarditis. Note the diffuse ST elevation in most of the cardiac leads except AVR and V1.

As the disease process continues, the ST segments return to baseline with the T waves becoming flattened or even inverted. In the final stages, the ECG demonstrates a pattern of diffuse ST depression. With resolution of the disease, the ECG returns to normal.

Pulmonary Embolism

The most consistent finding in patients with a pulmonary embolism is an ECG demonstrating sinus tachycardia. However, there is a classic ECG pattern in patients with pulmonary embolism referred to as the "S1Q3T3" pattern (Figure B-41). These patients will have a large S wave in lead I, a Q wave in lead III, and an inverted T wave in lead III. Patients with pulmonary embolism may also demonstrate ST depression in lead II. Additionally, there may be evidence of right atrial enlargement in lead II or V2. Finally, patients with this condition may

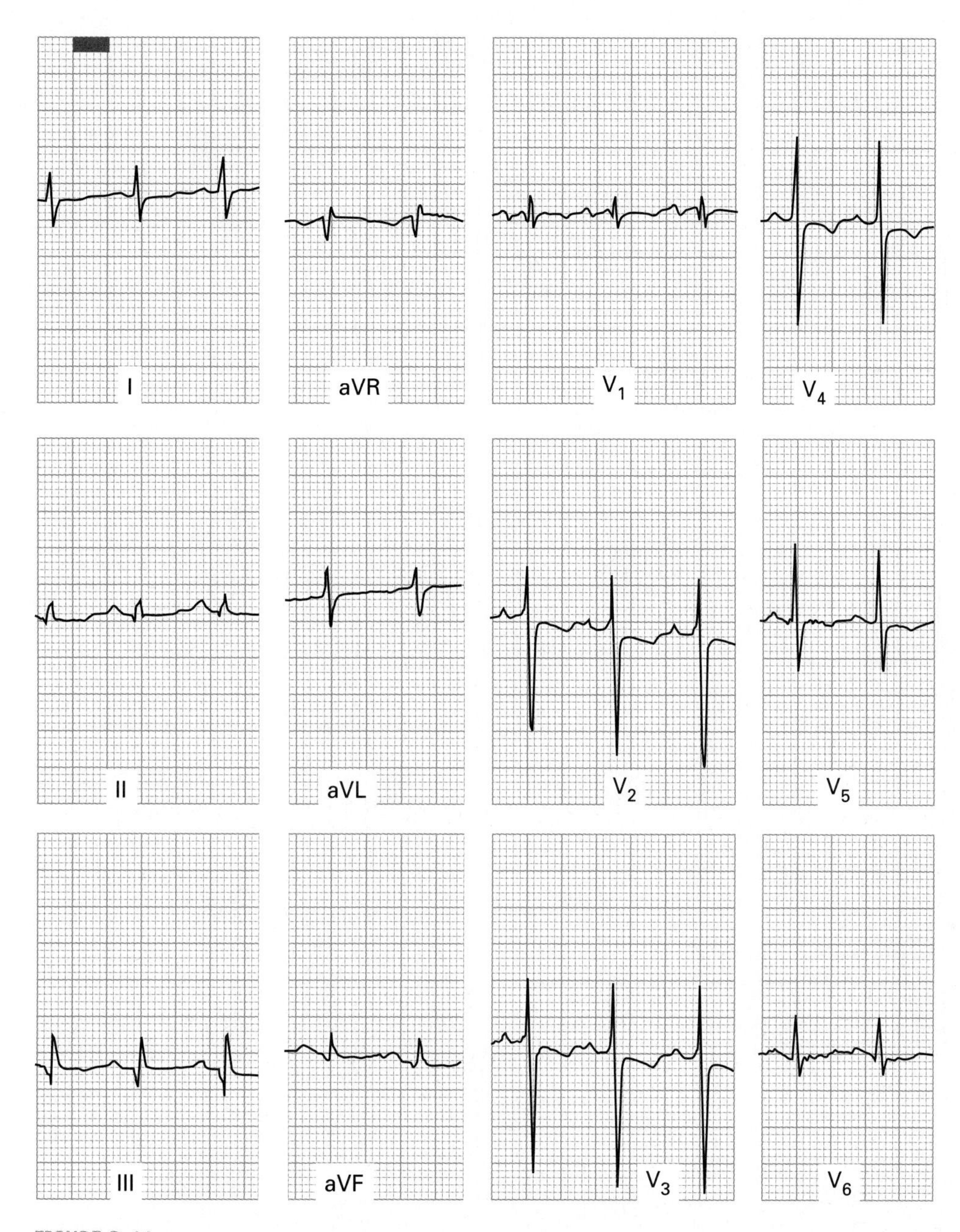

FIGURE B-41
ECG of patient with pulmonary embolism. Note the characteristic S1Q3T3 pattern (large S wave in lead I, Q wave in lead III, and inverted T wave in lead III).

also demonstrate T-wave inversion in leads V1 through V4 with a right bundle branch pattern.

Hyperkalemia

Potassium is one of the most important ions in regulating the electrical activity of the heart. As such, changes in potassium ion concentration will produce significant

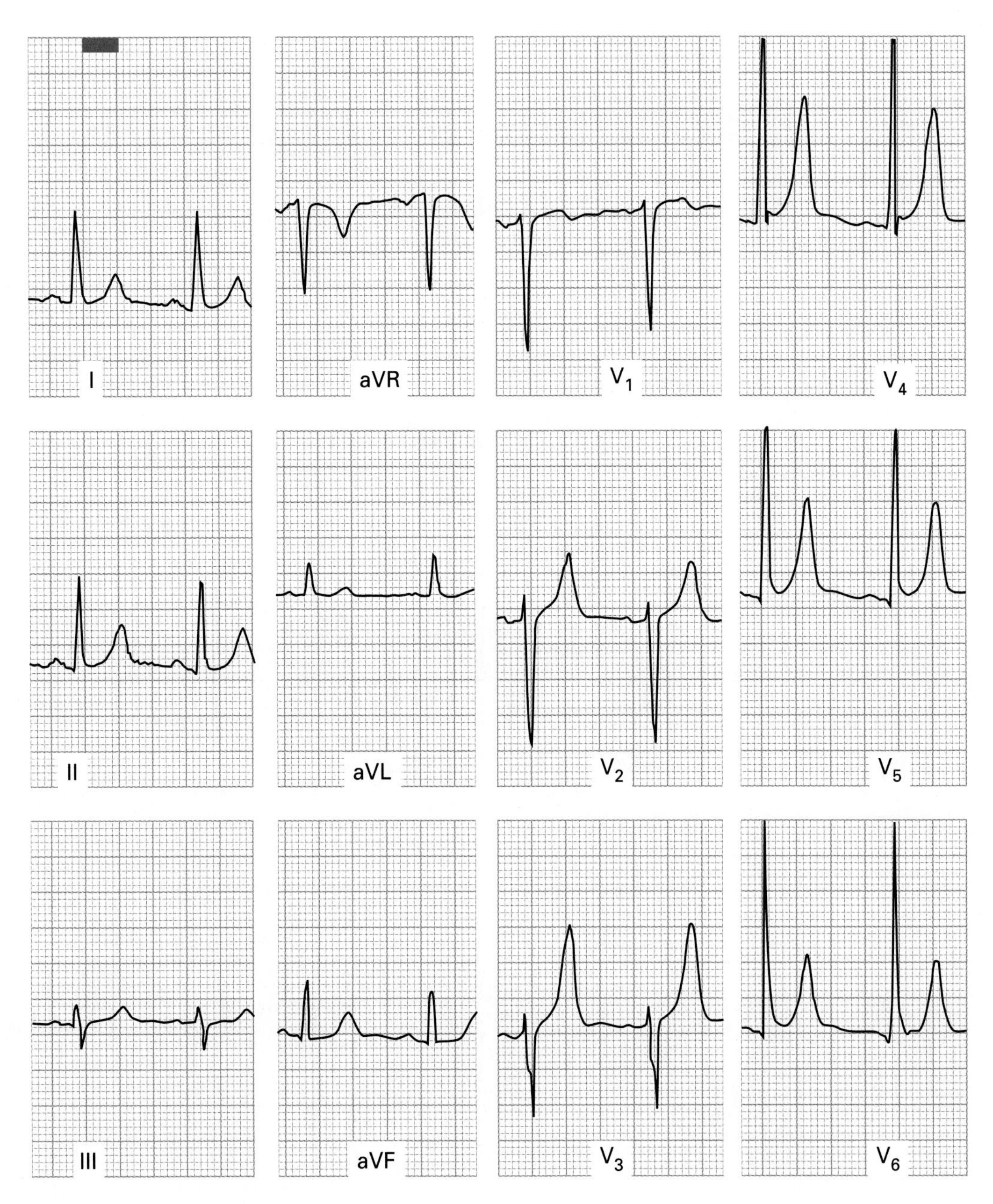

FIGURE B-42
ECG of patient with hyperkalemia, showing characteristic tall, peaked T waves.

ECG findings. The most striking feature in patients with hyperkalemia (elevated serum potassium) is the appearance of tall, peaked T waves (Figure B-42). These are best seen in leads II, III, and V2. As the level of potassium increases, the P waves begin to disappear and ventricular conduction slows. This results in a widening of the QRS complex into what are called "sine waves" (Figure B-43). Eventually, with increasing serum potassium levels, marked bradycardia and cardiac arrest ensue.

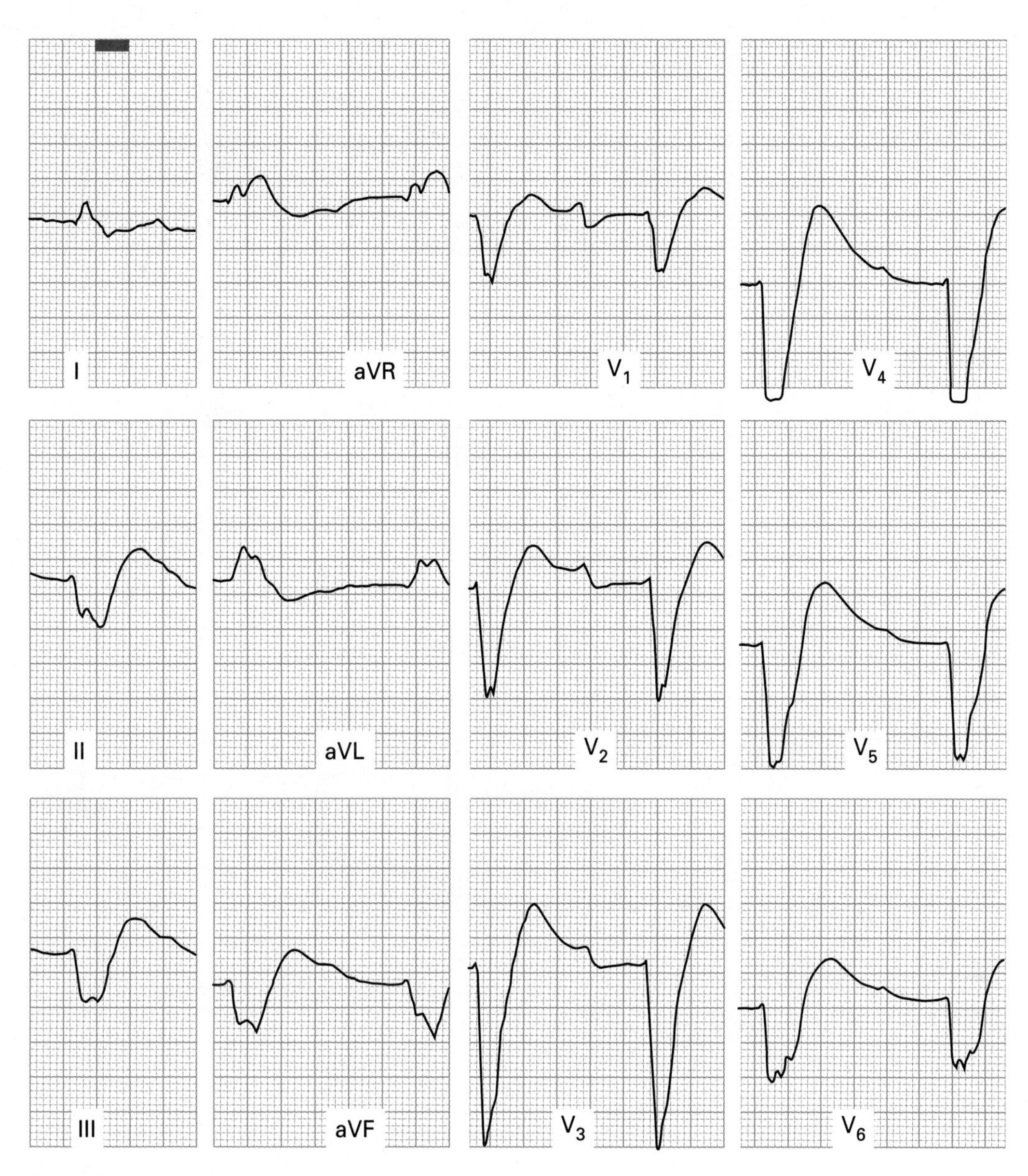

FIGURE B-43
ECG of patient with hyperkalemia that has progressed to show widened QRS complexes blending into inverted T waves in a sine-shaped configuration.

Hypokalemia

Patients with low serum potassium demonstrate the opposite findings as those described for hyperkalemic patients. These patients will develop flattening of the T wave and may also develop prominence of the U wave (Figure B-44). Finally, because hypokalemia increases ventricular irritability, ventricular dysrhythmias such as PVCs, ventricular tachycardia, ventricular fibrillation, and Torsades de Pointes can develop.

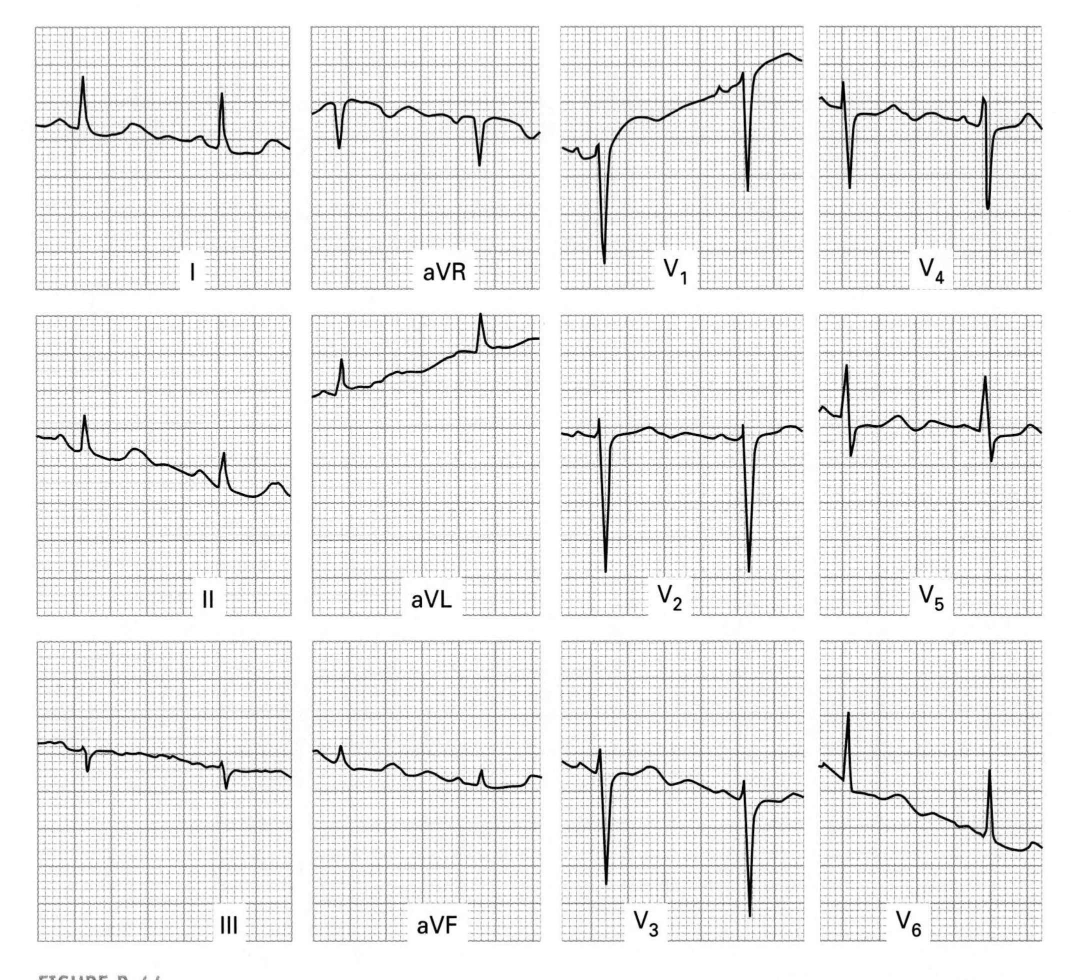

FIGURE B-44
ECG of patient with hypokalemia with opposite findings as those for a hyperkalemic patient. Note the fattening of T waves and appearance of U waves.

Hypocalcemia

Calcium is the major ion that contributes to cardiac repolarization. This is primarily reflected in the length of the QT interval, measured from the beginning of the QRS complex to the beginning of the T wave. Patients with hypocalcemia will demonstrate a prolonged QT interval, primarily due to a long ST segment (Figure B-45). By definition, the QT interval is greater than 50 percent of the entire cardiac cycle. Conversely, patients with hypercalcemia will demonstrate a shortened QT interval.

Hypothermia

Patients with hypothermia will demonstrate several different ECG findings, which often depend on the severity of the exposure. Initially, patients develop

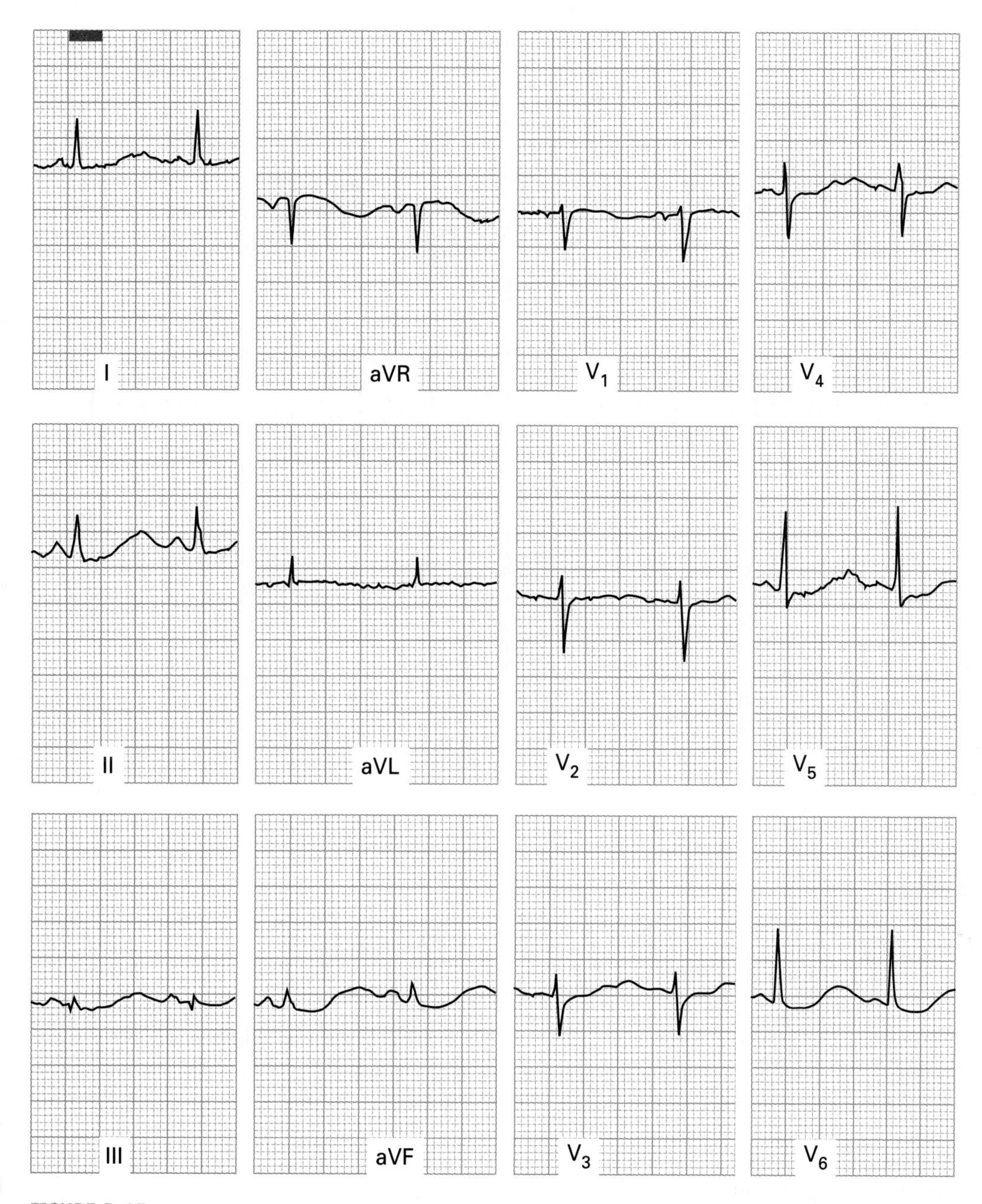

FIGURE B-45
ECG of a patient with hypocalcemia showing a typical prolonged QT interval, primarily due to a long ST segment.

sinus tachycardia, which can progress to a profound bradycardia as the patient's core temperature drops. All types of atrial or ventricular dysrhythmias may be seen. The ECG pattern in hypothermia may be characterized by elevation of the J point, called a J wave or an Osborn wave (Figure B-46). The J wave appears as a hump that occurs just after the QRS complex. It is most characteristically seen in lead II or V6 but can be seen in virtually all leads. The J wave may be confused with ST changes in AMI.

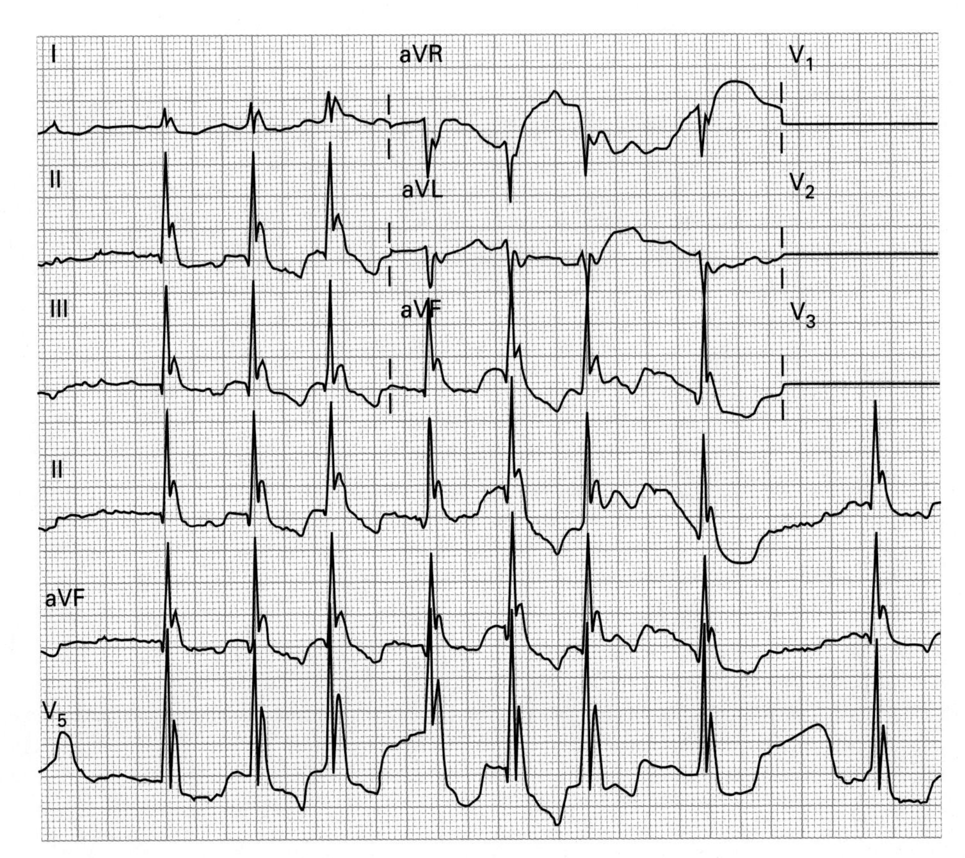

FIGURE B-46
ECG of patient with hypothermia. Note the appearance of J waves just after the QRS complexes.

Further Reading

1. BEASLEY, B.M., and M.C. WEST. *Understanding 12-Lead EKGs.* 2nd ed. Upper Saddle River, NJ: Pearson/Prentice Hall, 2005.
2. BLEDSOE, B.E., R.S. PORTER, and R.A. CHERRY. *Paramedic Care: Principles & Practices, Volume 3: Medical Emergencies.* 2nd ed. Upper Saddle River, NJ: Pearson/Prentice Hall, 2006.
3. DUBIN, D. *Rapid Interpretation of EKG's.* 6th ed. Tampa, FL: Cover Publishing Company, 2000.
4. PAGE, B. *12-Lead ECG for Acute and Critical Care Providers.* Upper Saddle River, NJ: Pearson/Prentice Hall, 2005.
5. SPRINGHOUSE. Patricia Schull, ed. *ECG Interpretation Made Incredibly Easy!* 3rd ed. Philadelphia: Lippincott Williams & Wilkins, 2004.

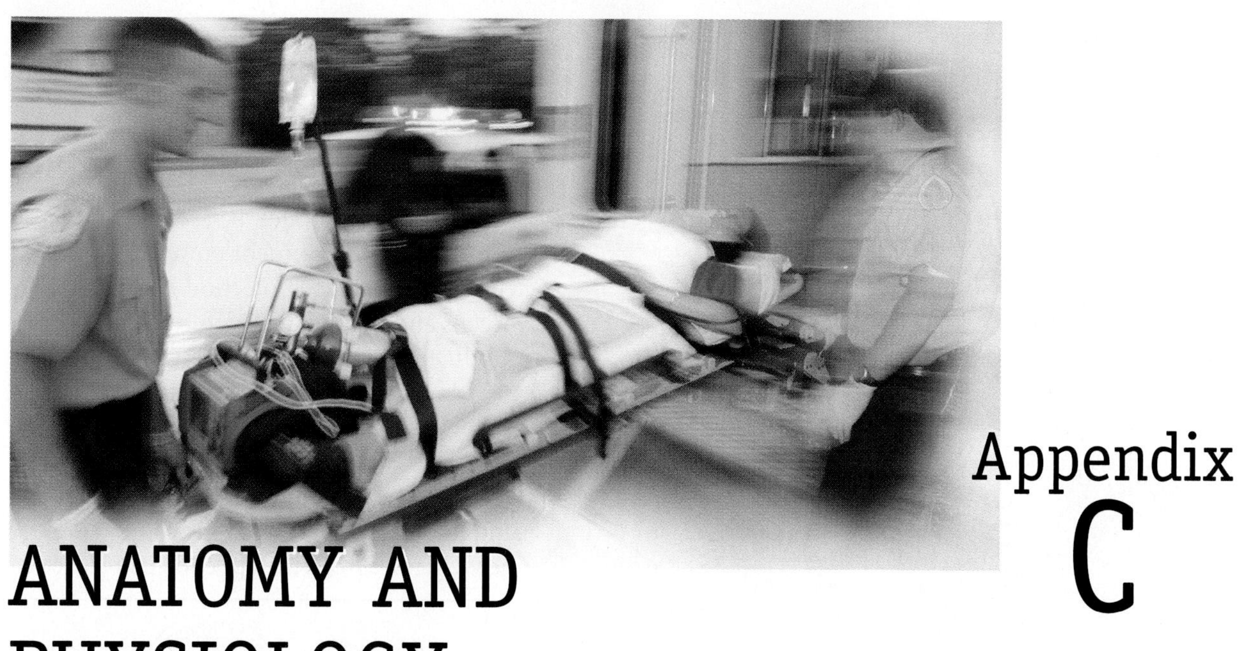

Appendix C

ANATOMY AND PHYSIOLOGY ILLUSTRATIONS

Musculoskeletal System

Skeleton

The skeleton is a living framework made by the joining of bones. It serves to provide support, body movement powered by muscular contractions, protection for the vital organs and other soft structures, blood cell production, and storage for essential minerals. There are 206 bones in the adult body, forming the two divisions of the skeletal system. The axial skeleton is comprised of skull, vertebrae, rib cage, and sternum. The upper and lower extremities and the shoulder and pelvic girdles from the appendicular skeleton.

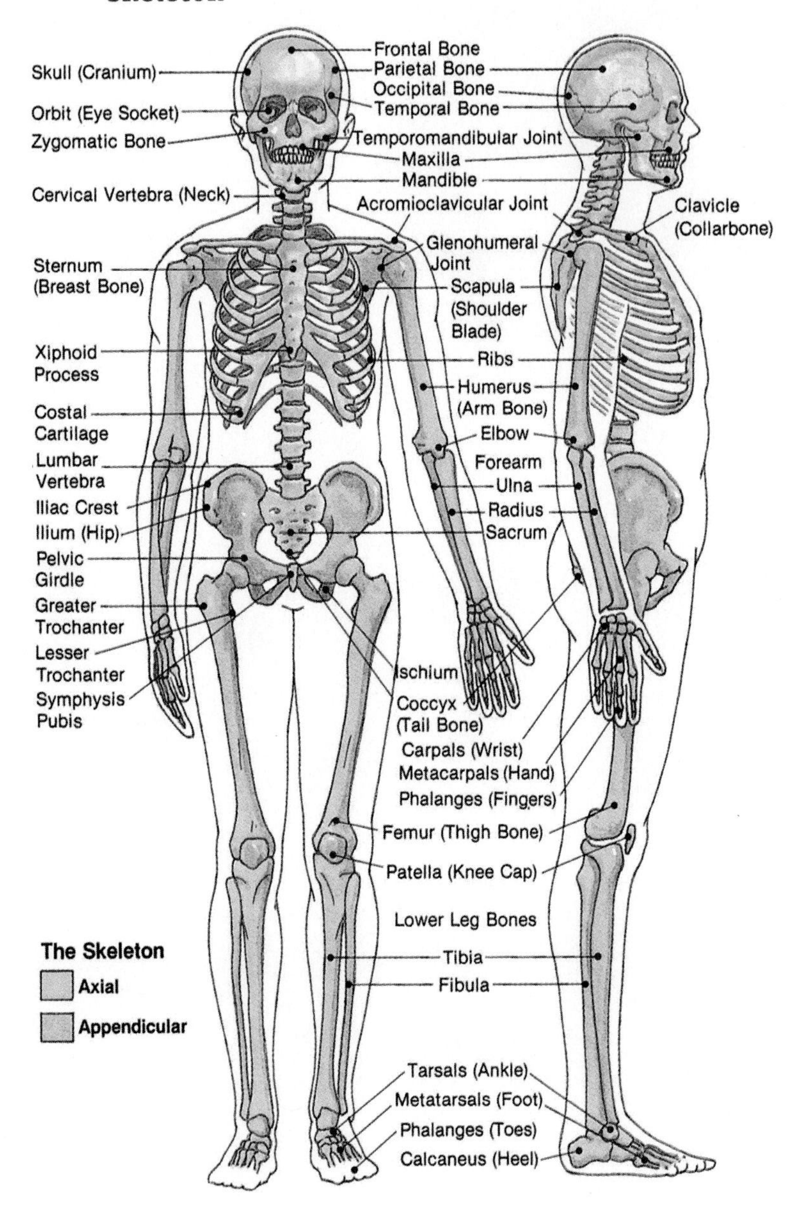

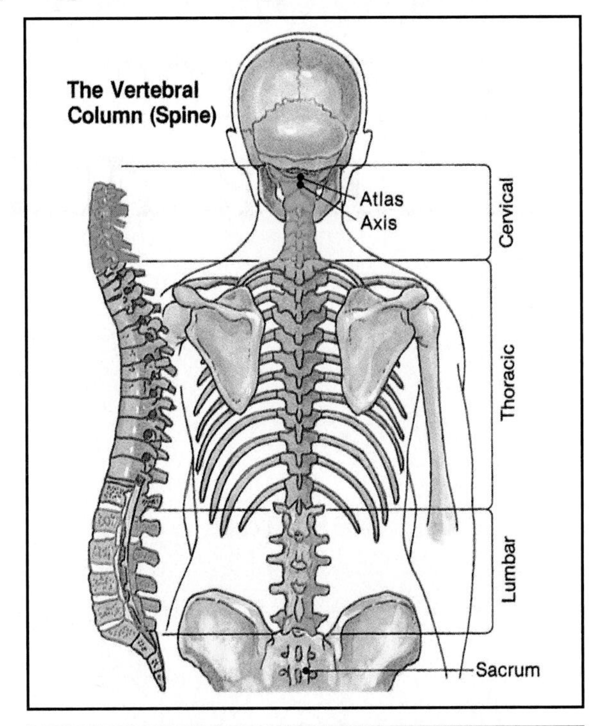

Talus
Metatarsals (Foot Bones)
Calcaneus (Heel)
Tarsals (Ankle Bones)
Phalanges (Toes)
Carpals (Wrist)
Metacarpals (Hand Bones)
Phalanges (Fingers)
The Hand

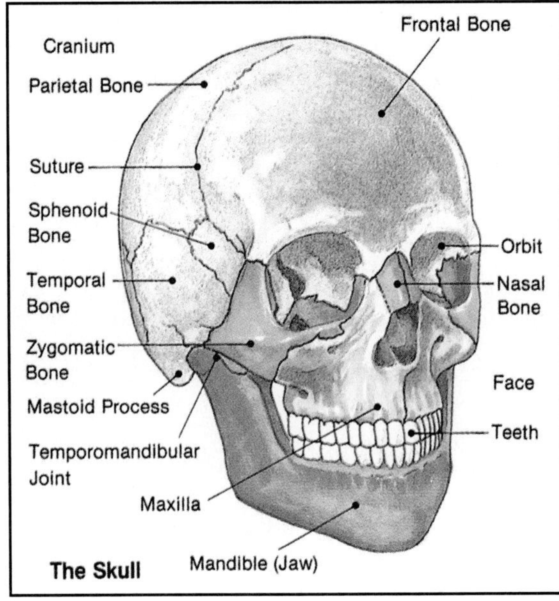

Musculoskeletal System

Muscles

The tissues of the muscular system comprise 40 to 50% of the body's weight. The skeletal muscles of the body are voluntary muscles, subject to conscious control. They exhibit the properties of excitability; that is, they will react to nerve stimulus. Once stimulated, skeleton muscles are quick to contract and can relax and very quickly be ready for another contraction. There are 501 separate skeletal muscles that provide contractions for movement, coordinated support for posture, and heat production. Muscles connect to bones by way of tendons.

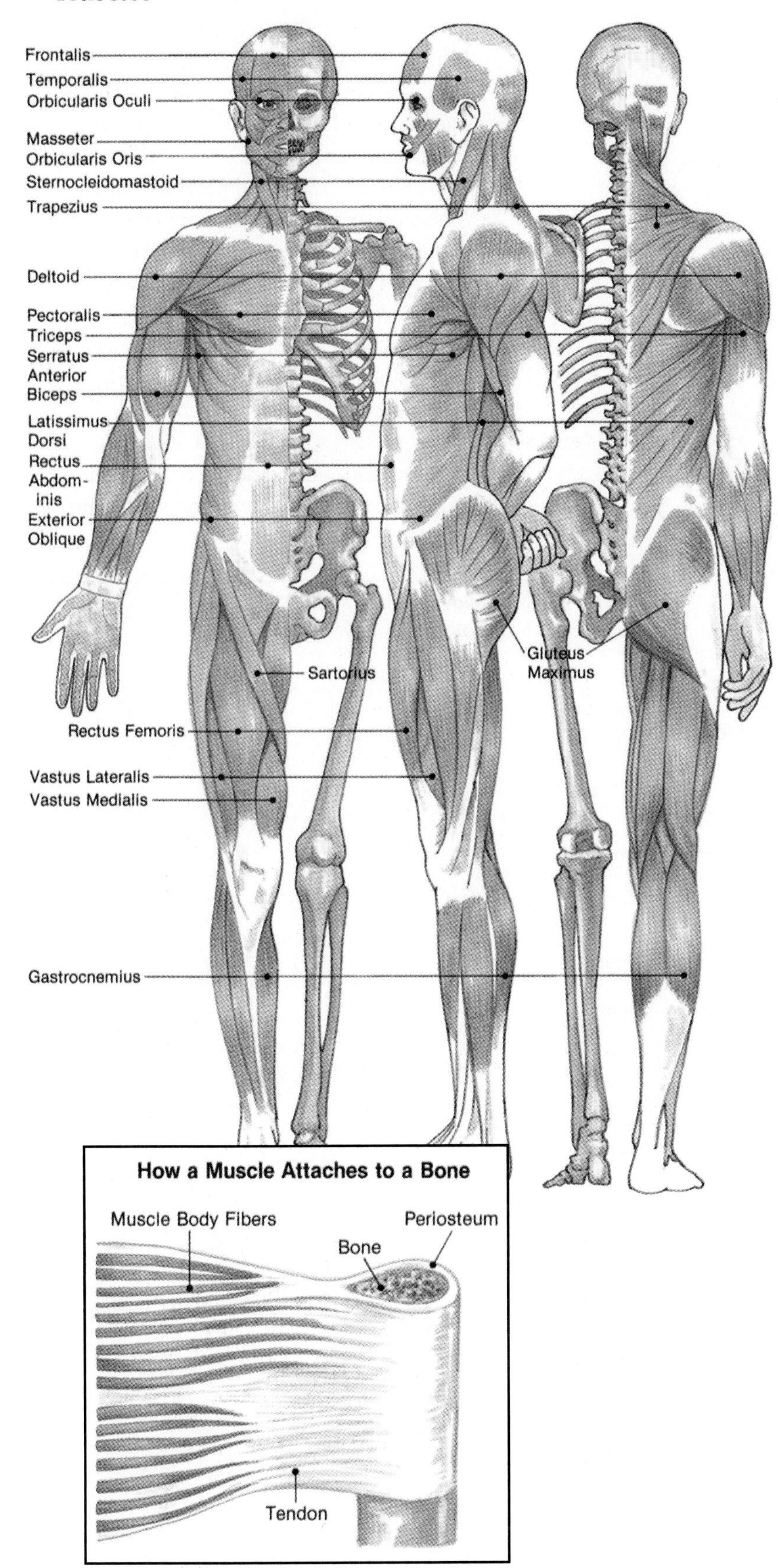

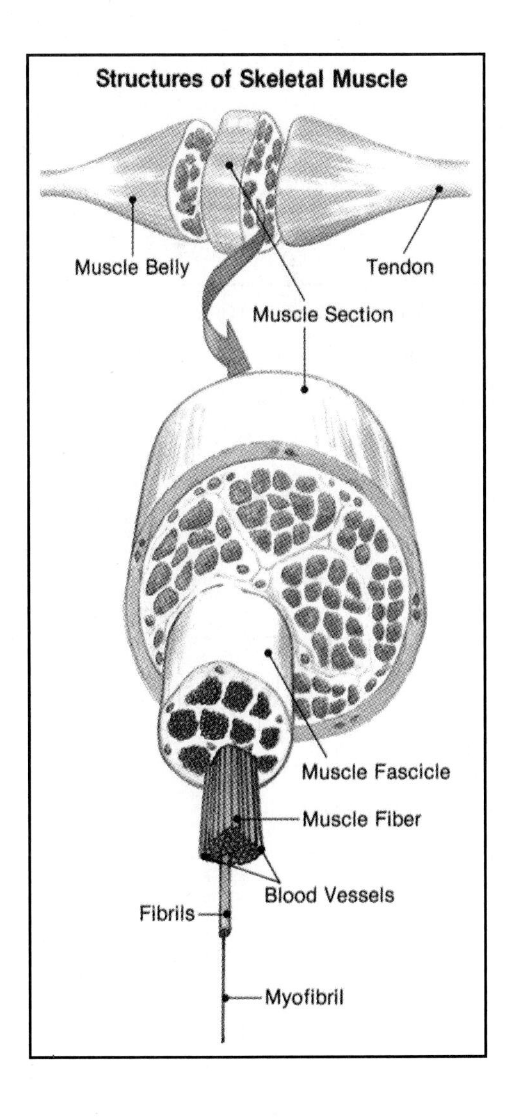

Nervous System

Brain and Spine

The nervous system includes the brain, spinal cord, and nerves. Structures within the system may be classified according to divisions: central, peripheral, and autonomic divisions of the nervous system. The central nervous system includes the brain and spinal cord. The sensory (incoming) and motor (outgoing) nerves make up the peripheral nervous system. The autonomic nervous system has structures that parallel the spinal cord and then share the same pathways as the peripheral nerves. This division is involved with motor impulses (outgoing commands) that travel from the central nervous system to the heart muscle, blood vessels, secreting cells of glands, and the smooth muscles of organs. The impulses will stimulate or inhibit certain activities.

The Brain

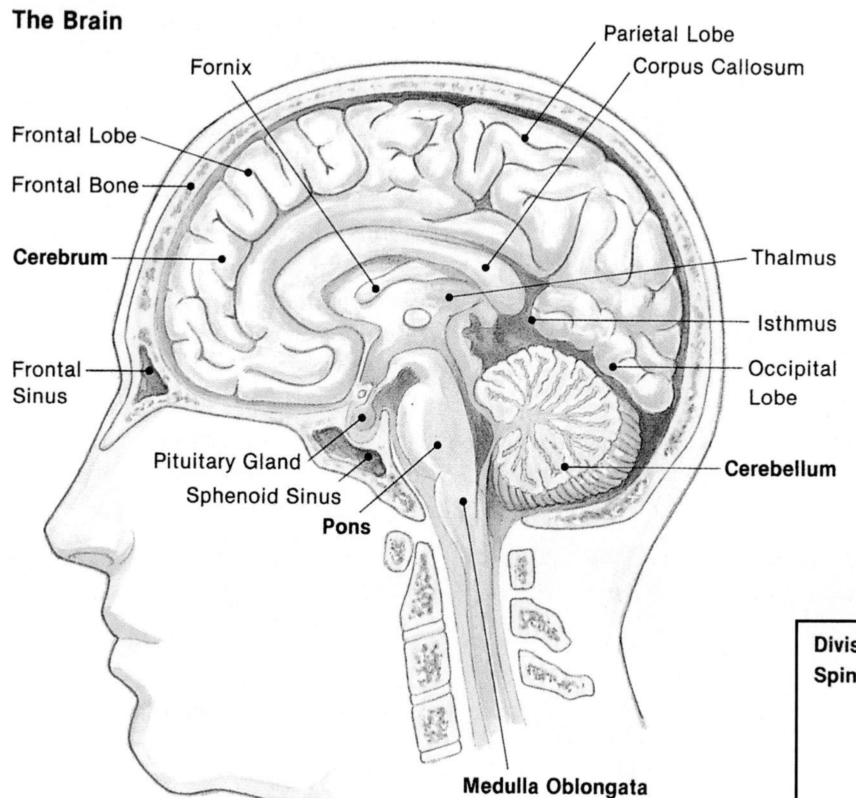

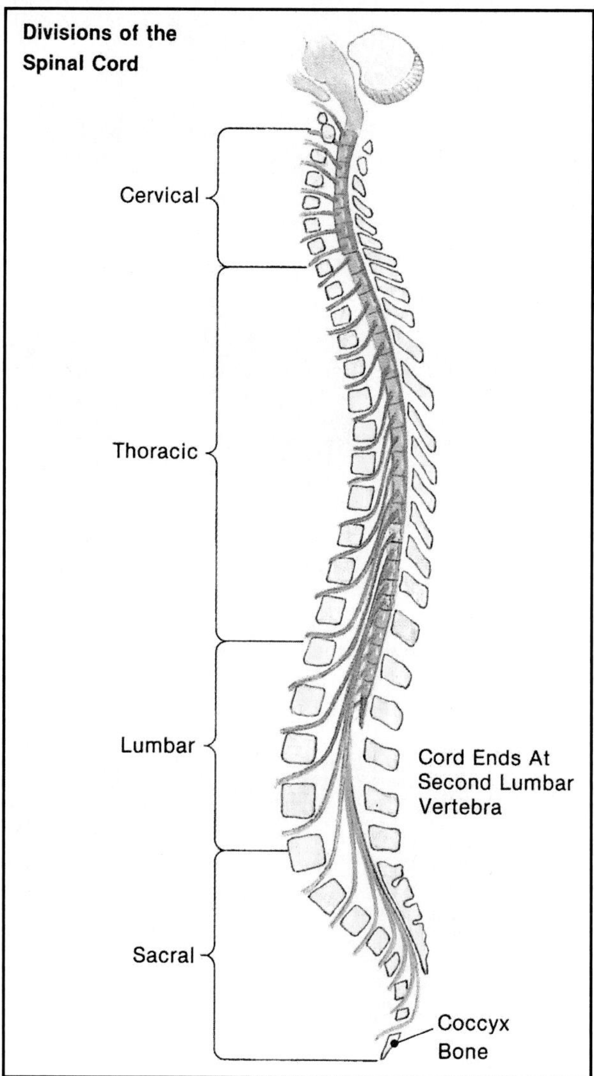

The Spinal Cord

Sympathetic Trunk
Spinal Cord
Spinal Ganglion
Posterior Root
Anterior Root
Pia Mater
Arachnoid
Spinous Process of Vertebra
Dura Mater
Spinal Nerves
Body of Vertebra
Intervertebral Disk
Sympathetic Ganglion
Transverse Process of Vertebra

Nervous System

Nerves

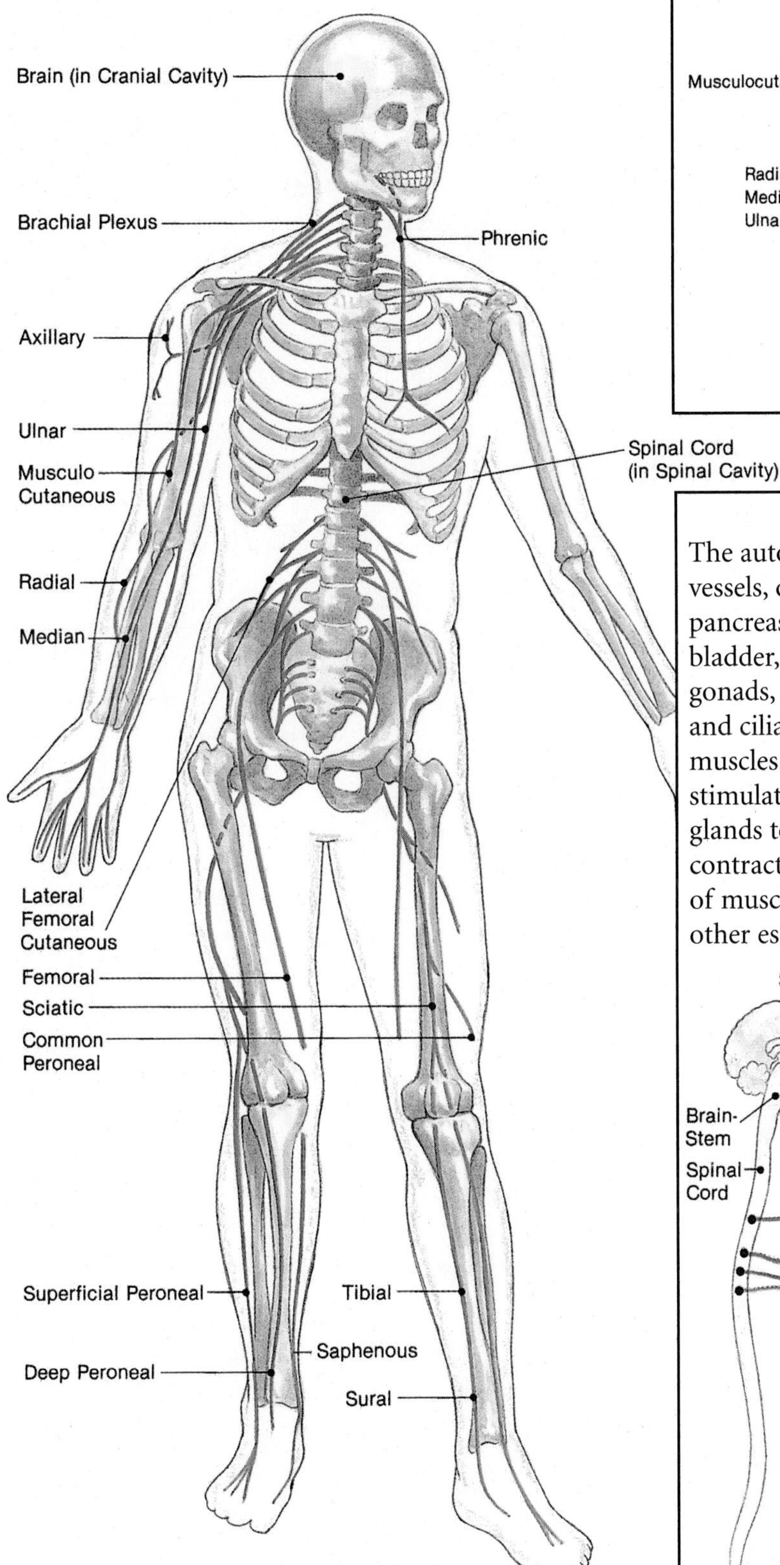

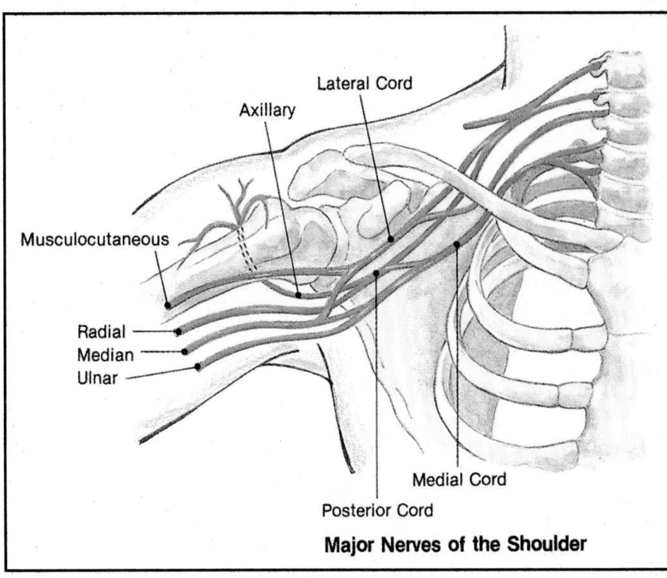

Major Nerves of the Shoulder

Autonomic Nervous System

The autonomic nervous system affects the heart, blood vessels, digestive tract, salivary and digestive glands, pancreas, liver, spleen, anal sphincter, kidneys, urinary bladder, urinary sphincter, adrenal glands, thyroid gland, gonads, genitalia, nasal lining, larynx, bronchi, lungs, iris and ciliary muscles of the eyes, tear glands, and hair muscles. Impulses can increase or slow heart rate, stimulate dilation or constriction of blood vessels, cause glands to secrete or decrease secretion, initiate or inhibit contractions in the bladder, stimulate or decrease a wave of muscle contraction along the digestive tract, and many other essential body activities.

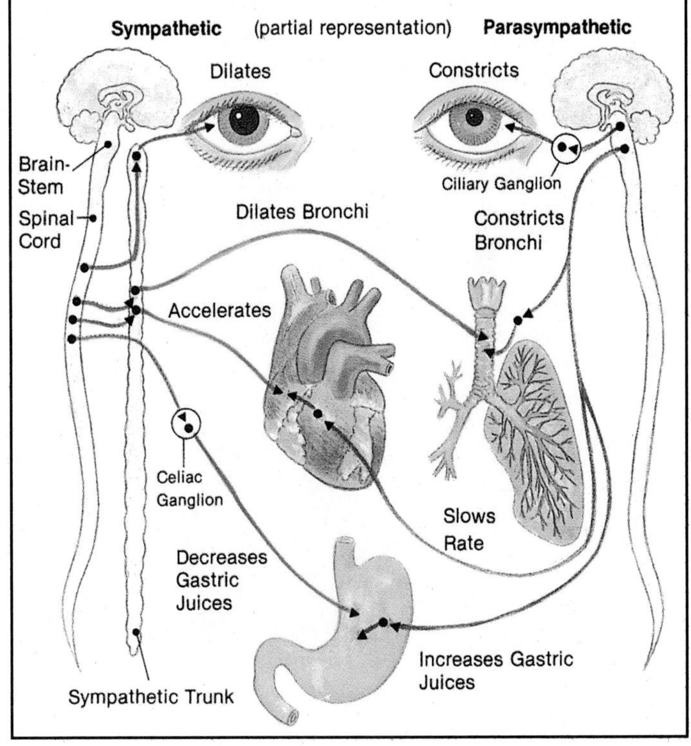

Cardiovascular System

Heart

The heart is a hollow, muscular organ that pumps 450 million pints of blood in the average lifetime. Its superior chambers, the atria, receive blood. Both atria fill and then contract at the same time. The inferior chambers are the ventricles. They pump blood out of the heart. Both ventricles fill and then contract at the same time. When the atria are relaxing, the ventricles are contracting.

The right side of the heart receives blood from the body and sends it to the lungs (pulmonic circulation). The heart's left side receives oxygenated blood from the lungs and sends it out to the body (systemic circulation).

The heartbeat originates at the sinoatrial node (pacemaker) and spreads across the atria to stimulate contraction. After a slight delay, the impulse is sent from the atrioventricular node, down the bundles of His, and out across the ventricles. This stimulates the ventricles to contract while the atria are relaxing.

The heart muscle (myocardium) receives its blood supply by way of the right and left coronary arteries. These vessels are the first branches of the aorta.

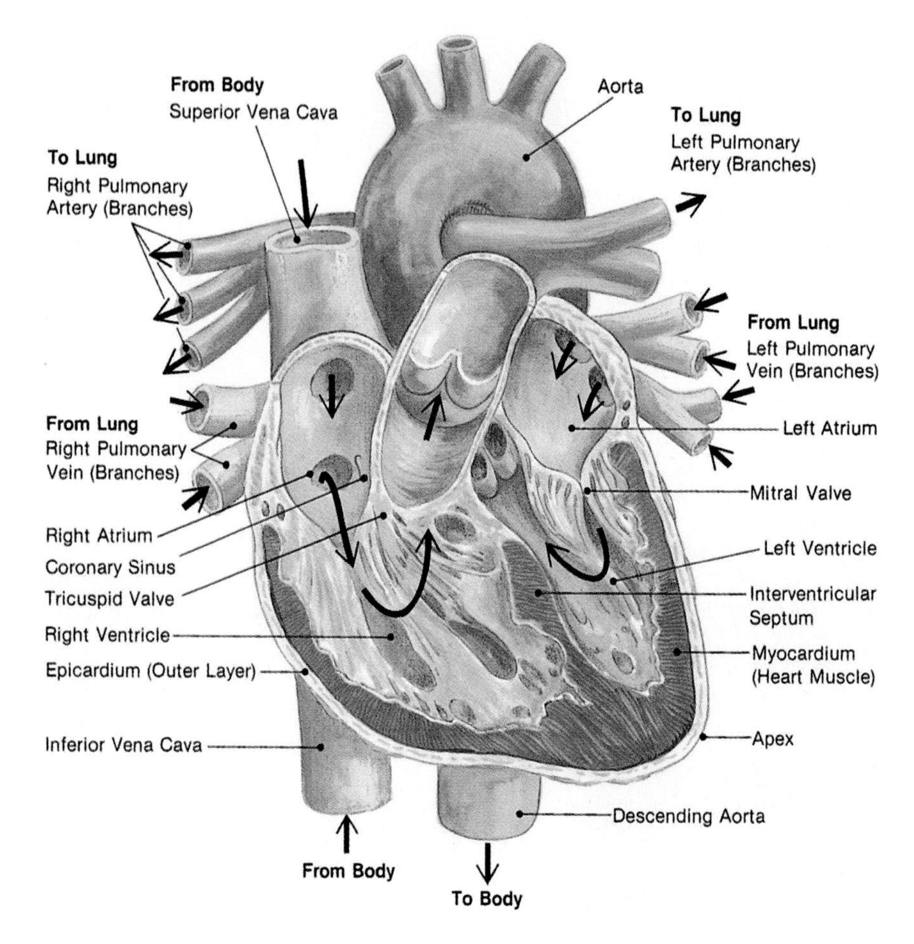

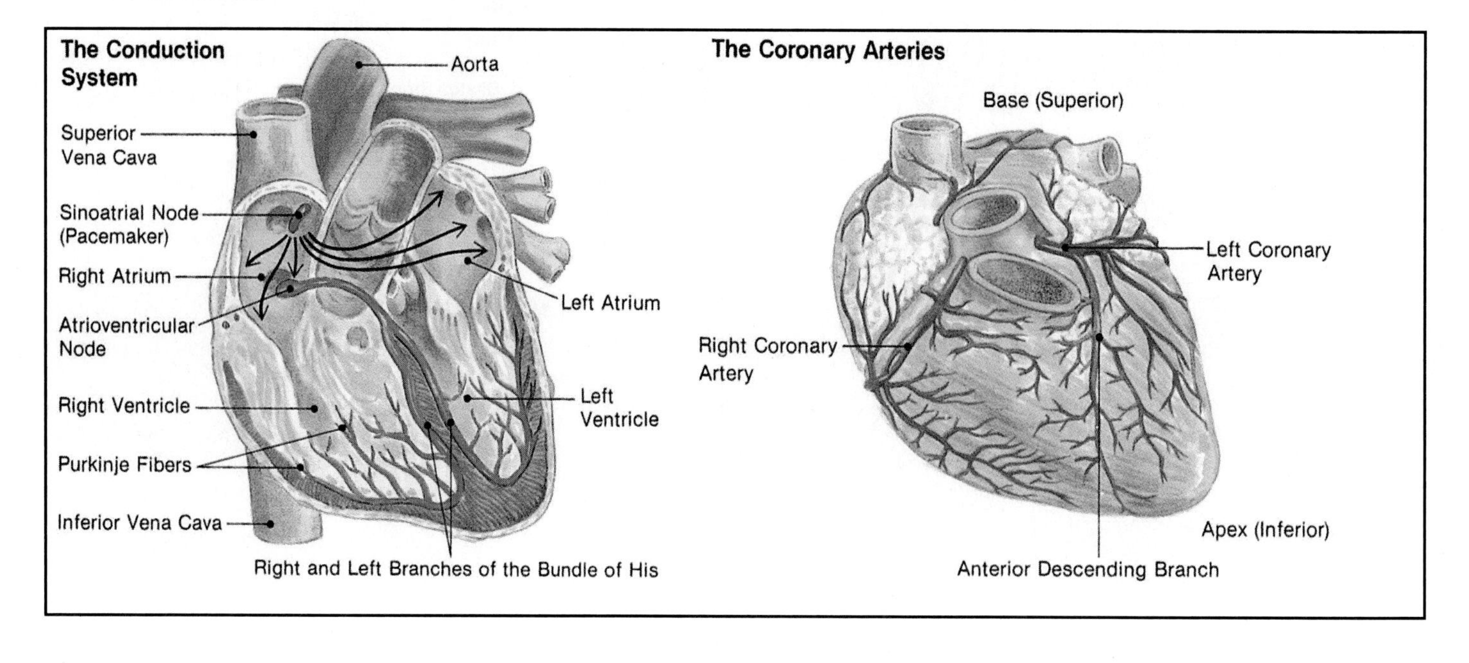

Circulatory System

Blood Vessels

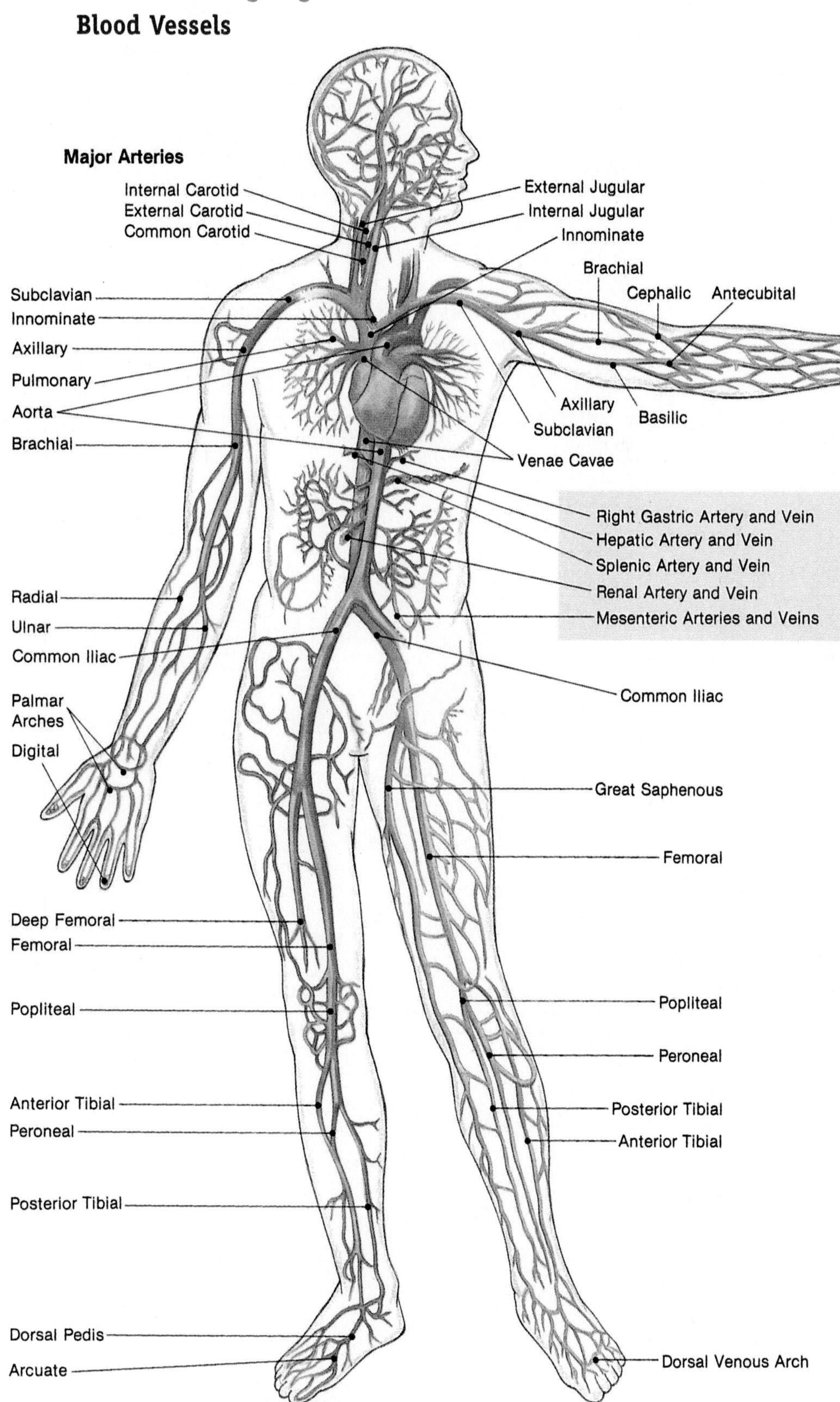

Any blood vessel that carries blood away from the heart is an artery. Arteries have strong muscular walls and are very elastic, changing their diameter as the heart contracts to force blood into circulation. They decrease in diameter to become arterioles. These structures join with capillary beds. A capillary is thin-walled, being no thicker than the lining of an arteriole. Blood moves through the capillaries in a constant flow known as **perfusion.** During perfusion, oxygen and nutrients are given up to the body's tissues and cellular carbon dioxide and wastes are picked up.

Any blood vessel that carries blood back to the heart is a vein. The small-diameter veins that leave capillary beds are called venules. These join with larger veins. The walls of the veins are not as thick or elastic as those of the arteries. Some veins have valves to prevent the backward flow of blood.

Respiratory System

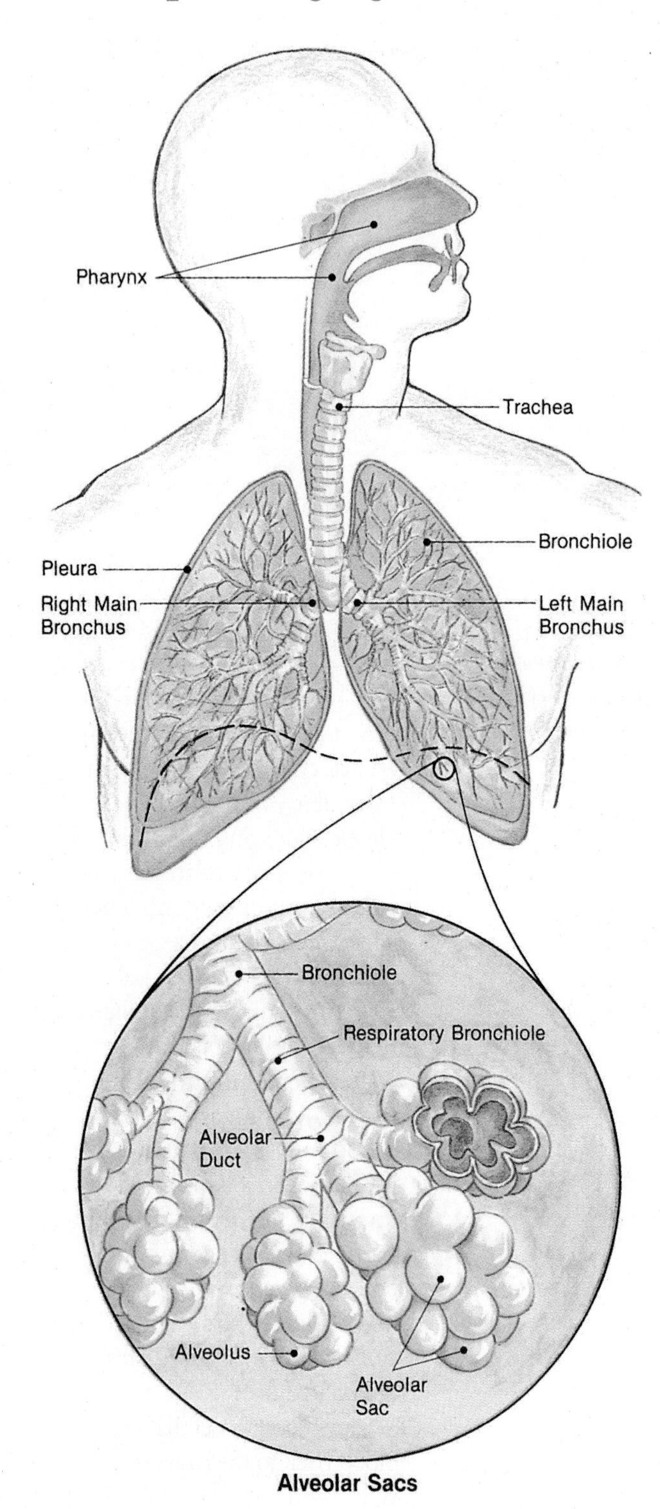

Alveolar Sacs

The airway consists of structures involved with the conduction and exchange of air. Conduction is the movement of air to and from the exchange levels of the lungs. Air enters through the nose (primary) and mouth (secondary) and travels down the pharynx to enter the larynx. After passing through the larynx, air enters the trachea. At its distal end, the trachea branches into the left and right primary bronchi. These bronchi branch into secondary bronchi, which then branch into the bronchioles. Some of the bronchioles end as closed tubes. Air movement in them helps the lungs expand. The rest of the bronchioles carry the air to the exchange levels of the lungs.

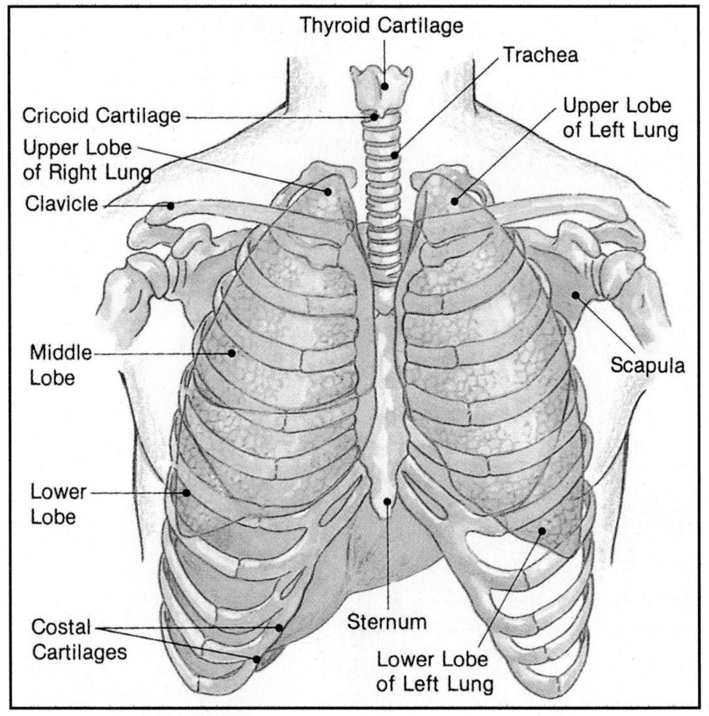

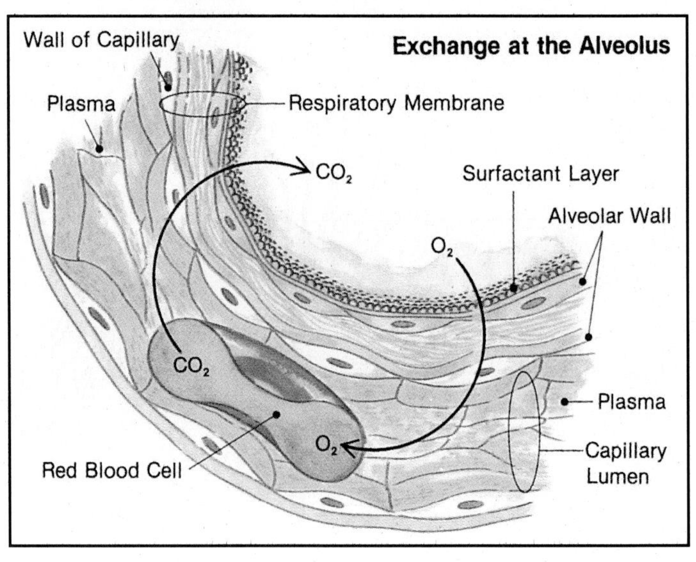

The respiratory bronchioles turn into alveolar ducts. These form alveolar sacs that are made up of the alveoli. Gas exchange takes place between the alveoli and the capillaries in the lungs.

Digestive System

The digestive system includes the digestive tract and various supportive structures and accessory glands. The tract begins at the oral cavity with the teeth and tongue. The salivary glands release saliva into the mouth to moisten food for swallowing. The tract continues down the throat to the esophagus, through the cardiac sphincter, and into the stomach. Acid and digestive enzymes are added to the food to produce chyme. The chyme passes through the pyloric sphincter to enter the small intestine. Digestive enzymes from the pancreas and bile from the liver are added to the chyme. The processes of digestion and absorption are completed in the small intestine. Wastes are carried through the ileocecal valve into the large intestine. The wastes are moved to the rectum, from where they can be expelled through the anus.

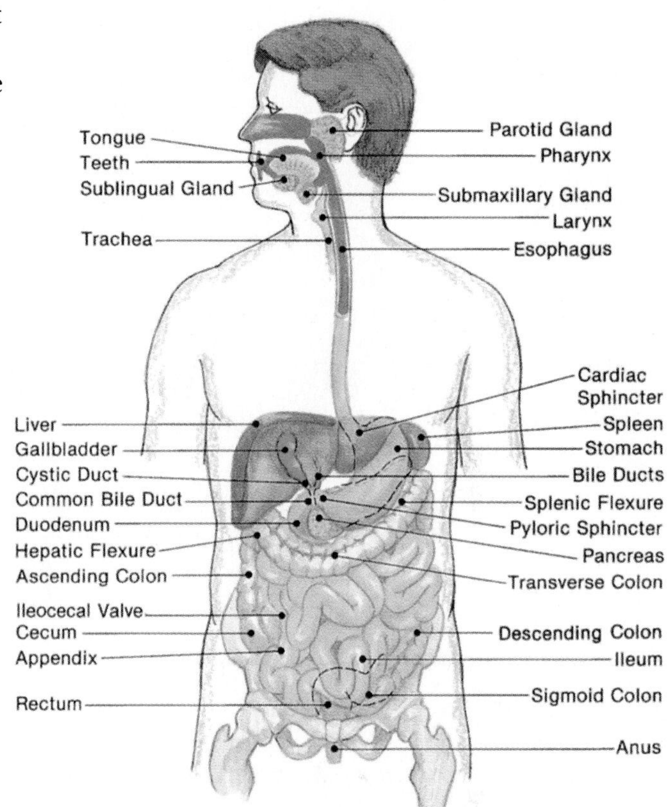

Organs of the Digestive System

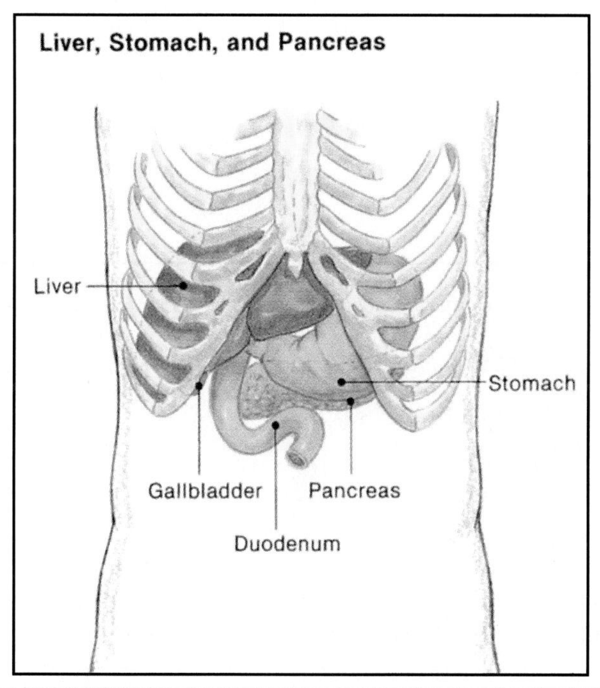

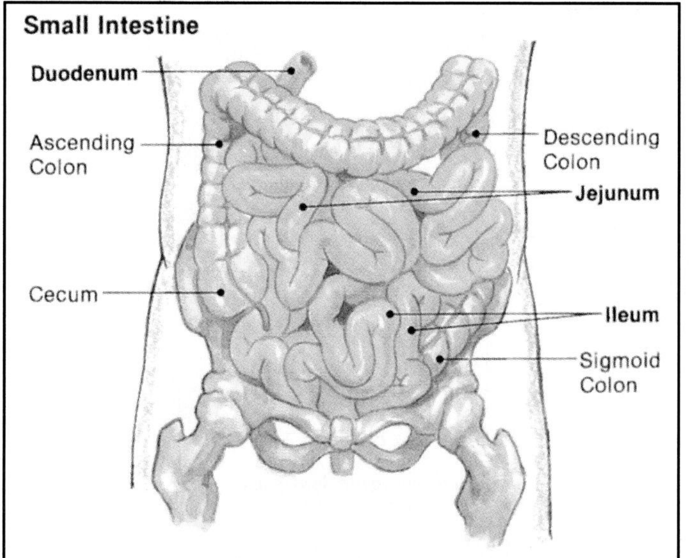

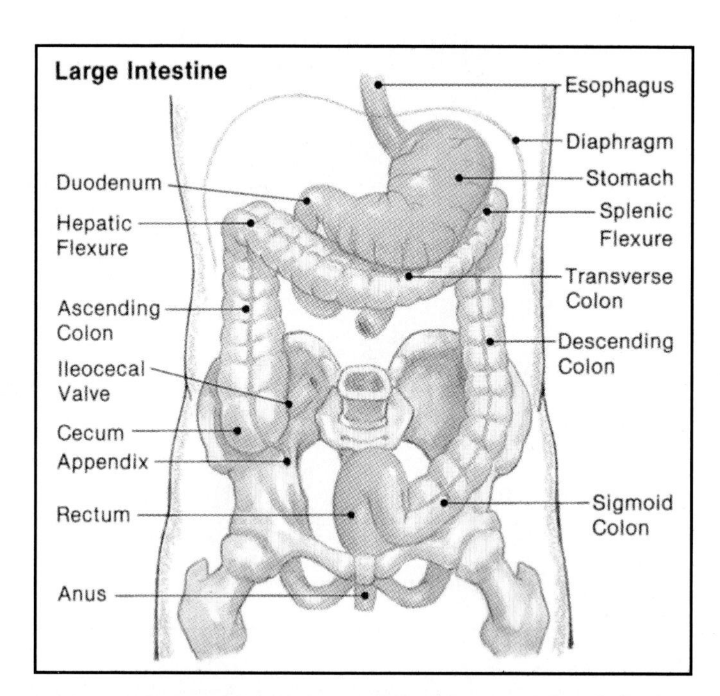

Urinary System

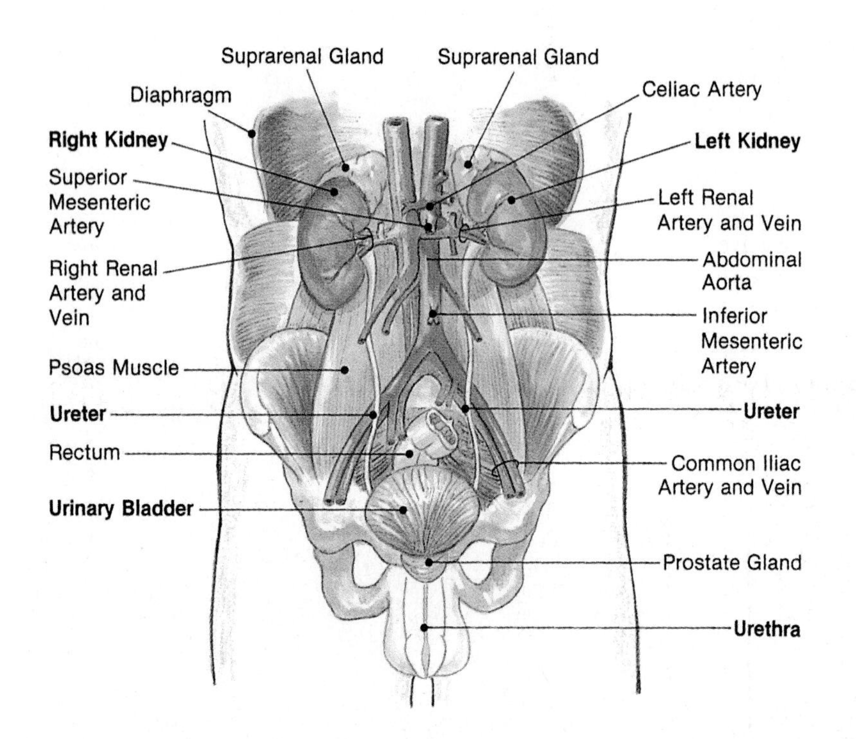

The urinary system is part of the body's excretory structures (urinary system, lungs, sweat glands, and intestine). The kidneys remove the wastes of chemical activities (metabolism) in the body. These wastes are removed from the blood to produce urine. At the same time, the kidneys remove certain excess compounds, regulate the blood pH (acid–base balance), and the concentration of sodium, potassium, chlorine, glucose, and other important chemicals.

The Nephron

Each kidney is made up of microscopic nephrons. Both wastes and needed chemicals are filtered from the blood. As these materials are passed through the nephron, the needed compounds (including water) are sent back into the blood. Wastes are collected as urine.

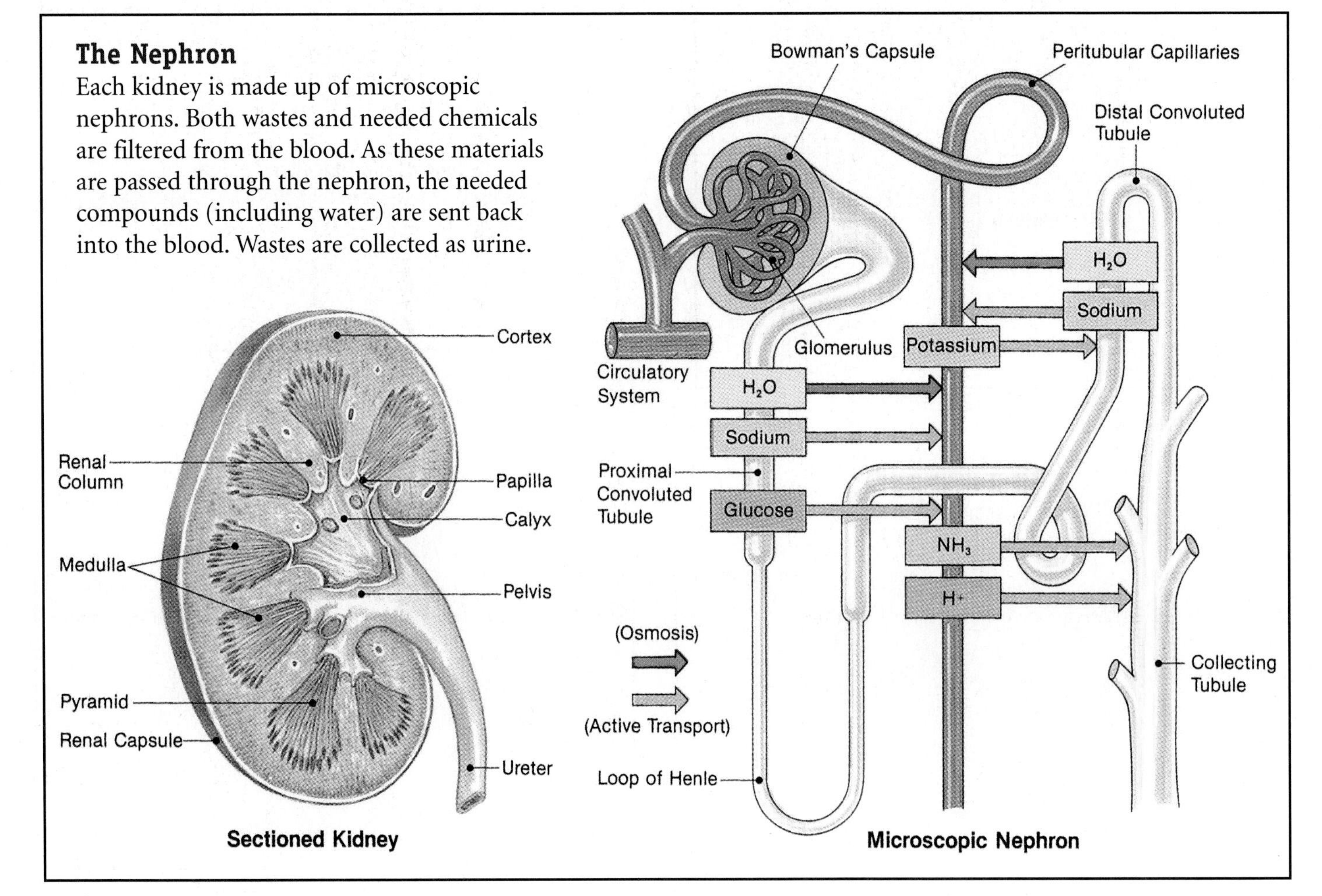

Reproductive System

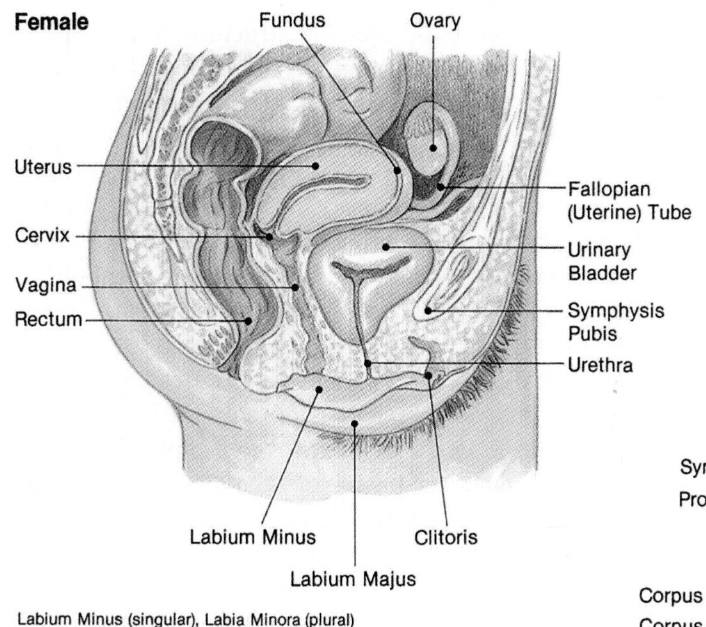

Labium Minus (singular), Labia Minora (plural)
Lablum Majus (singular), Labia Majora (plural)

The reproductive system consists of the organs, glands, and supportive structures that are involved with human sexuality and procreation. In the male, spermatozoa and the hormone testosterone are produced in the testes. The female produces ova (eggs) and the hormones estrogen and progesterone in her ovaries. The union of ovum and sperm produce a single cell called a zygote. Through growth, cell division, and cellular differentiation (the formulation of specialized cells) the new individual develops and matures.

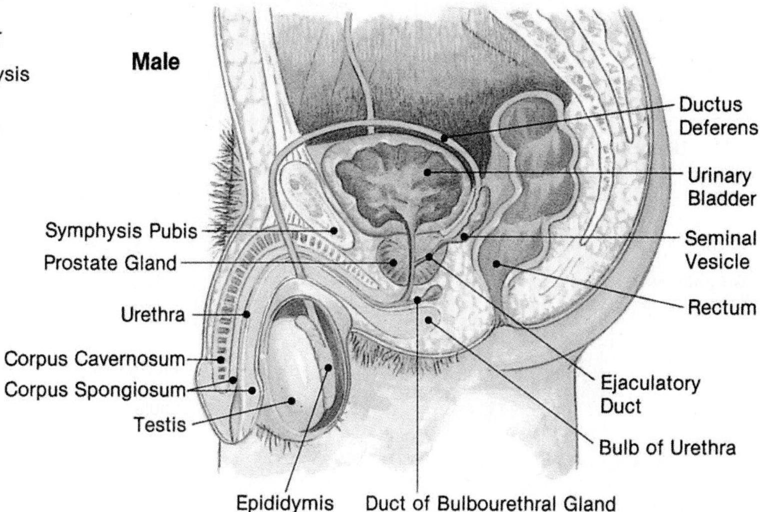

The Ovary

Suspensory Ligament of Ovary
End of Fallopian Tube
Released Ovum
Mature Follicle
Maturing Follicle
Primary Follicle (Ovum and Single Layer of Follicle Cells)
Ovum
Ovarian Ligament
Corpus Luteum (Produces Estrogen and Progesterone)
Egg Nest
Corpus Albicans

The developing ovum and its supportive cells are called a follicle. Each month, follicle-stimulating hormone (FSH) from the pituitary gland starts the growth of several follicles. Usually, only one will mature and release an ovum (ovulation). During its growth, the follicle produces estrogen. After ovulation, the remaining cells of the follicle form a specialized structure that produces both estrogen and progesterone.

The Breast

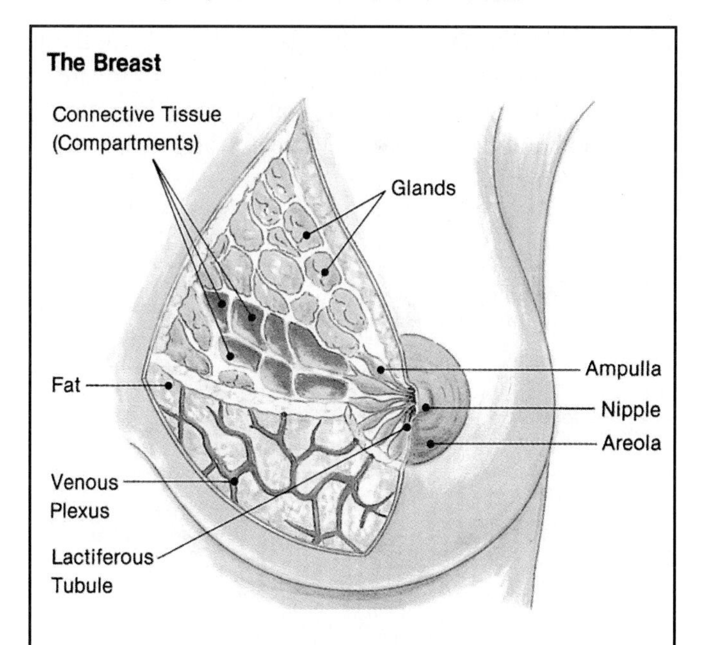

The breasts contain the mammary glands that produce milk (lactation). A mammary gland is a highly modified form of sweat gland. Estrogen stimulates the growth of the ducts, while progesterone stimulates the development of the secreting (milk-producing) cells. Lactic hormone from the pituitary stimulates milk production. Another pituitary hormone, oxytocin, stimulates the milk-producing cells to eject their milk into the ducts.

Integumentary System

Membranes

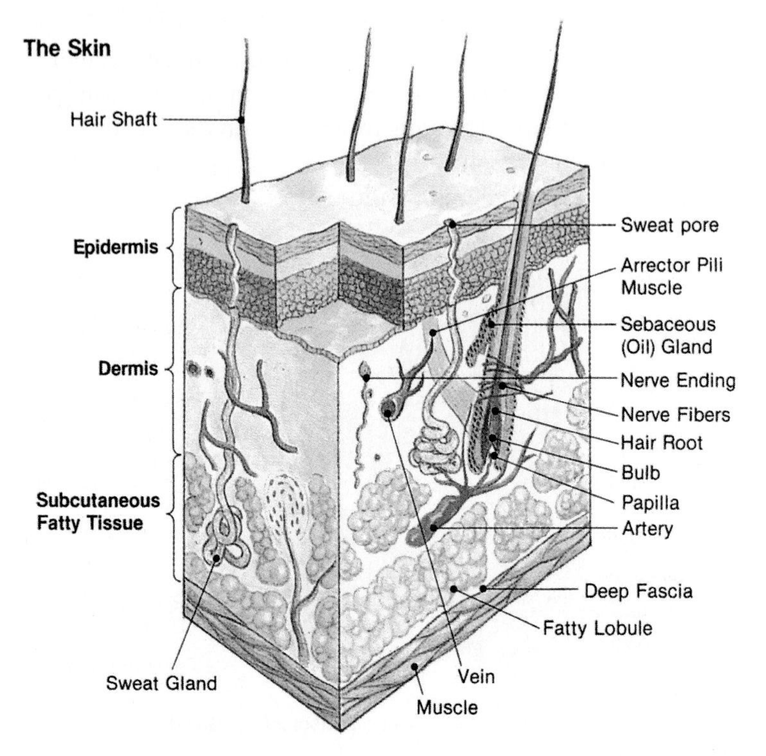

The skin is the largest organ of the body. In the adult the skin covers about 3000 square inches (1.75 square meters) and weighs about 6 pounds. It is involved with protection, insulation, thermal regulation, excretion, and the production of vitamin D.

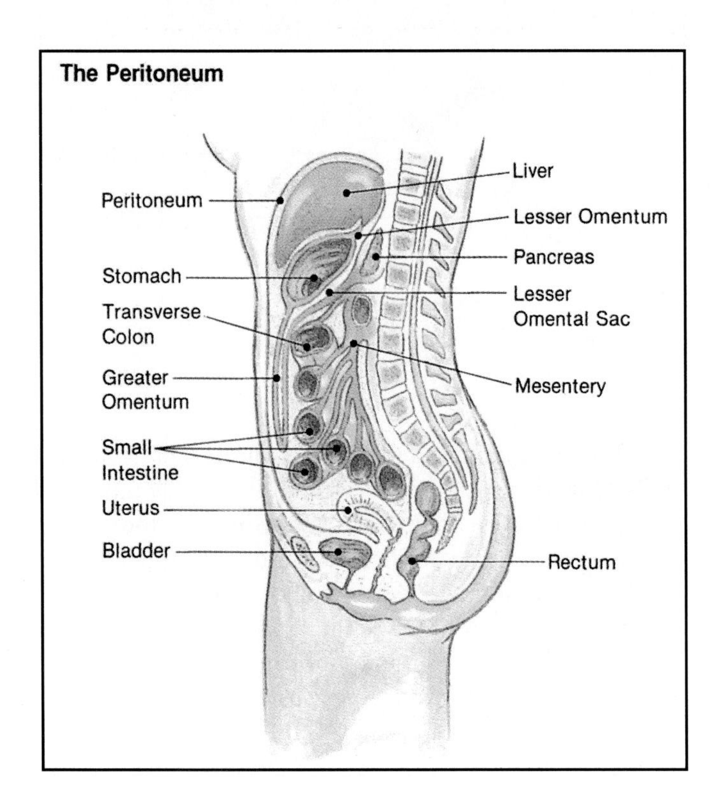

Membranes

Membranes cover or line body structures to provide protection from injury and infection. There are four major classes of membranes. Mucous membranes line those structures that open to the outside world (for example, the mouth, the airway, digestive tract, urinary tract, and vagina). Serous membranes line the closed body cavities and cover the outsides of organs. The cutaneous membrane is the skin. Synovial membranes line joints to reduce friction during movement.

A serous membrane that covers an organ is called a visceral layer. The term parietal layer is used for the part of the serous membrane that lines a cavity. The serous membrane in the thoracic cavity is called pleura (for example, the parietal pleura lines the chest cavity). In the abdominal cavity, it is called peritoneum (for example, the parietal peritoneum).

A double layer of peritoneum is called mesentery. The membrane that lines the sac surrounding the heart is pericardium.

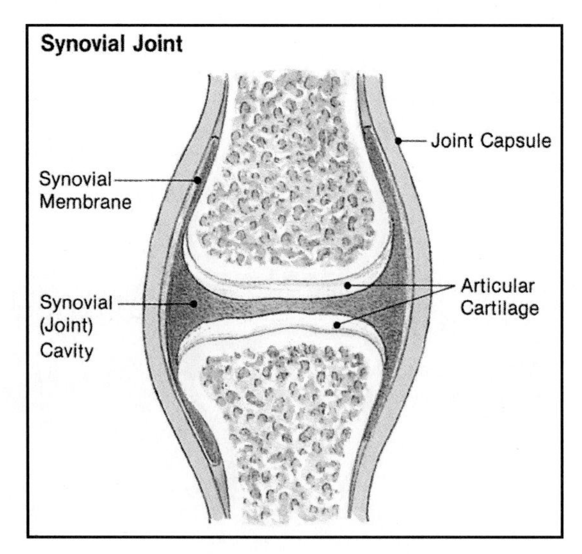

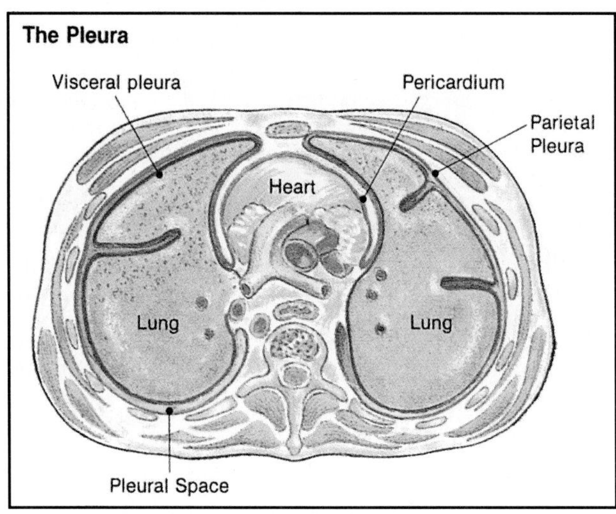

Senses

Eye and Ear

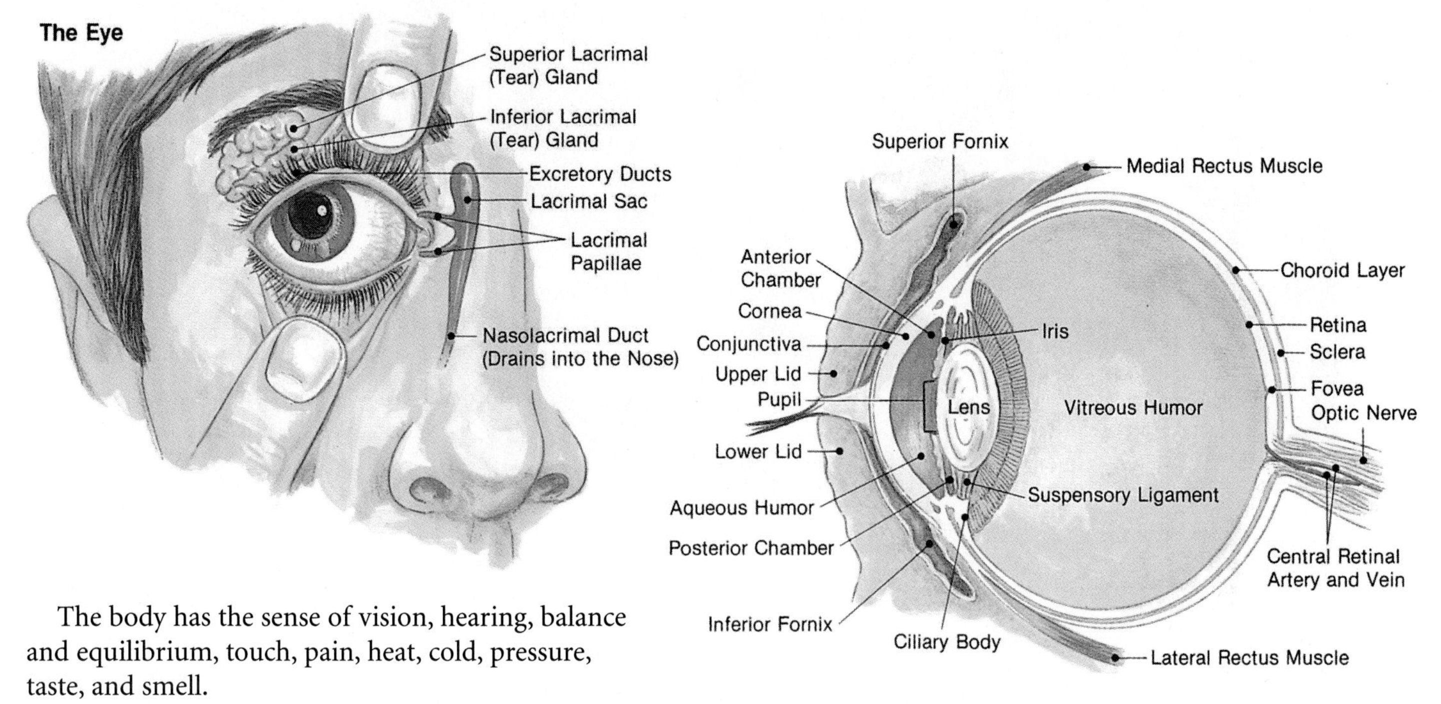

The body has the sense of vision, hearing, balance and equilibrium, touch, pain, heat, cold, pressure, taste, and smell.

The eye can receive and focus light and then convert this energy into nerve impulses to be sent to the brain. The nerve impulses originate from the retina. Visual receptors in the retina called rods can work in low intensity light. They have no color function. The visual receptors called cones operate in high intensity light and do receive colors.

The ear's functions include hearing, static equilibrium (balance while standing still), and dynamic equilibrium (balance when moving). The outer and middle ear are responsible for sound gathering and its transmission. The inner ear has the nerve endings for hearing and equilibrium.

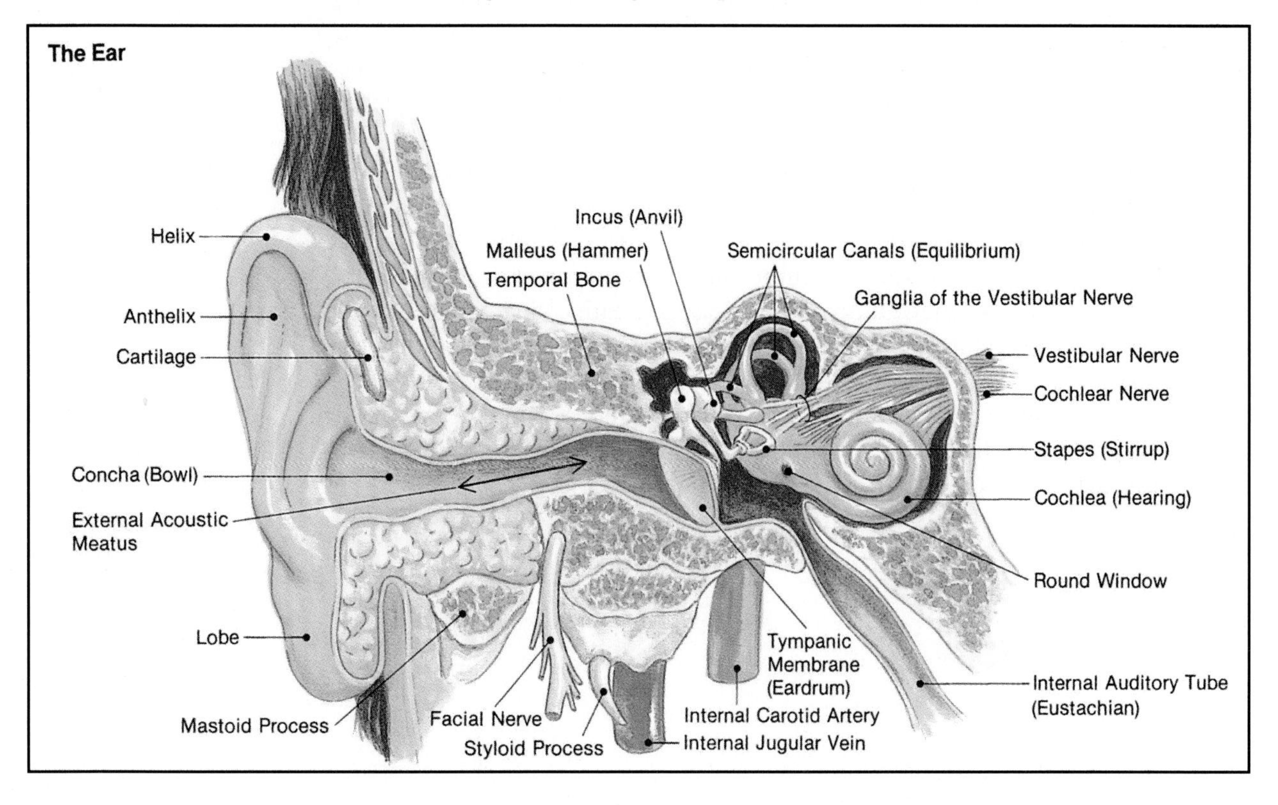

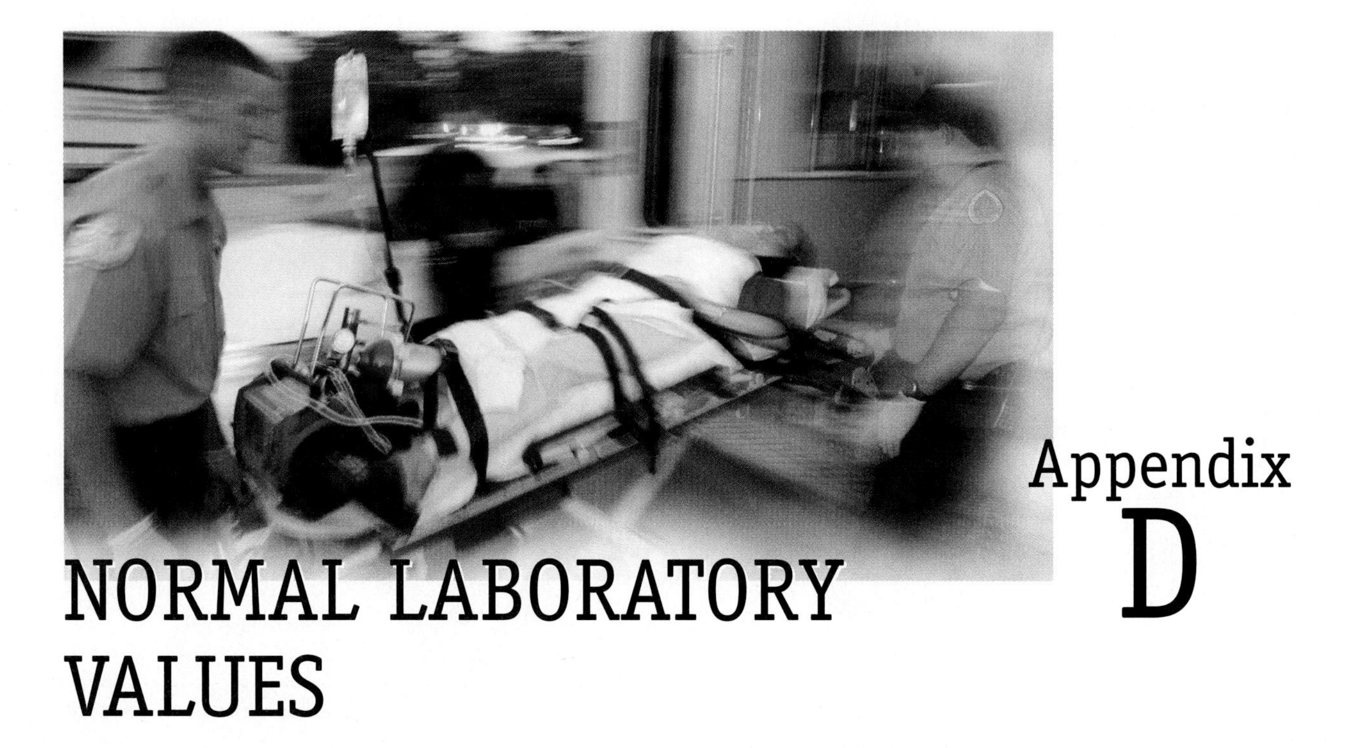

Appendix D

NORMAL LABORATORY VALUES

Normal lab values represent a range around the mean values in a healthy population. Each test is run independently of any other test, and it is unlikely that any individual will have totally normal results across a whole spectrum of lab tests. A number of factors, besides the presence or absence of disease, can contribute to an inodividual's test results, including sex, age, diet/malnutrition, drugs, time of day, measurement variations, and even the position the patient was in when the specimen was drawn.

Two key concepts in the use of lab test results to diagnose disease are sensitivity and specificity. *Sensitivity* refers to the proportion of patients with a given disease in whom the test is positive (called *percentage positive in disease*). *Specificity* refers to the proportion of patients who are free of the given disease in whom the test is negative (called *percentage negative in health*).

For any suspected disease, a variety of tests with useful sensitivity and/or specificity to that disease may be run. Conversely, a single test can be useful in discriminating more than one disease. For example, an increase in blood aspartate aminotransferase (AST/SGOT) is likely to be present with myocardial infarction, hepatic disease, pancreatitis, and seizures, among others. An increase in creatine kinase is likely to be present with myocardial infarction, meningitis, status epilepticus, and hyperthermia, among others.

Following are lists of normal values for lab tests commonly run. Keep in mind that the normal values listed by different hospitals and laboratories may vary slightly and that units will vary in some tests.

Blood Gases	
Partial pressure of carbon dioxide (PCO_2)	32–48 mmHg
Partial pressure of oxygen (PO_2)	83–108 mmHg
Bicarbonate (HCO_3)	22–28 mEq/l
pH	7.35–7.45

Blood/Plasma/Serum	
Chemistry	**Normal Values**
Alanine aminotransferase (ALT, SGPT)	0–35 U/l
Albumin	3.5–5.0 g/dl
Alkaline phosphatase	13–39 U/l
Aspartate aminotransferase (AST, SGOT)	0–35 U/l
Bilirubin, total **Direct bilirubin**	0.1–1.2 mg/dl 0.1–0.4 mg/dl
Blood urea nitrogen (BUN)	8–20 mg/dl
Calcium	8.5–10.5 mg/dl
Carbon dioxide	22–28 mEq/l
Chloride	98–107 mEq/l
Cholesterol, total **High density lipoprotein (HDL) cholesterol**	<200 mg/dl Male: 27–67 mg/dl Female: 34–88 mg/dl
Creatine	0.6–1.2 mg/dl
Creatine kinase (CK)	32–267 IU/l
Creatine kinase MB (CKMB)	<16 IU/l <4% total CK
Globulin	2.3–3.5 g/dl
Glucose	60–115 mg/dl
Iron binding capacity	250–460 μg/dl
Iron, total	50–175 μg/dl
Lactate dehydroginase (LDH)	88–230 U/l
Phosphorus	2.5–4.5 mg/dl
Potassium	3.5–5.0 mEq/l
Protein, total	6.0–8.4 g/dl
Sodium	135–145 mEq/l
Triglycerides	<165 mg/dl
Tropanin	0–1.5 ng/ml
Uric acid	Male: 2.4–7.4 mg/dl Female:1.4–5.8 mg/dl

Endocrine Tests	
Thyroids	**Normal Values**
Thyroid stimulating hormone (TSH)	0.5–5.0 μu/ml
Thyroxine-binding globulin capacity	15–25 μg T_4/dl
Total triodothyronine by radioimmunoassay (T_3)	75–195 ng/dl
Reverse diiodothyronine (rT_3)	13–53 ng/dl
Total thyroxine by radioimmunoassay (T_4)	4–12 μg/dl
T_3 resin uptake	25–35%
Free tyroxine index (FT_4I)	1–4

Hematology	
Coagulation Time	**Normal Values**
Prothrombin Time (PT)	11–15 sec or INR (international normalized ratio) 0.8–1.2
Partial thromboplastin time, activated (PTT)	25–35 sec
Hematological Results	**Normal Values**
White blood cell (WBC) count	3.4–10.0 thousand/μl
Red blood cell (RBC) count	4.2–5.6 million/μl
Hemoglobin, total (HGB)	Male: 13.6–17.5 g/dl Female: 12.0–15.5 g/dl
Hematocrit (HCT)	Male 39–49% Female 35–45%
Mean corpuscular volume (MCV)	80–100 fl
Mean corpuscular hemoglobin (MCH)	26–34 pg
Mean corpuscular hemoglobin concentration (MCHC)	31–36 g/dl
Platelets	150–450 thousand μl

Further Reading

For additional information about laboratory tests and normal values, you may consult the appropriate sections of the following, or newer editions as they become available:

1. BERKOW, R., A.J. FLETCHER, and M.H. BEERS, eds. *The Merck Manual.* 16th ed. Rahway, NJ: Merck Research Laboratories, 1992.
2. TIERNEY, L.M., JR., S.J. MCPHEE, and M.A. PAPADAKIS, eds. *Current Medical Diagnosis & Treatment.* 36th ed. Stamford, CT: Appleton & Lange, 1997.

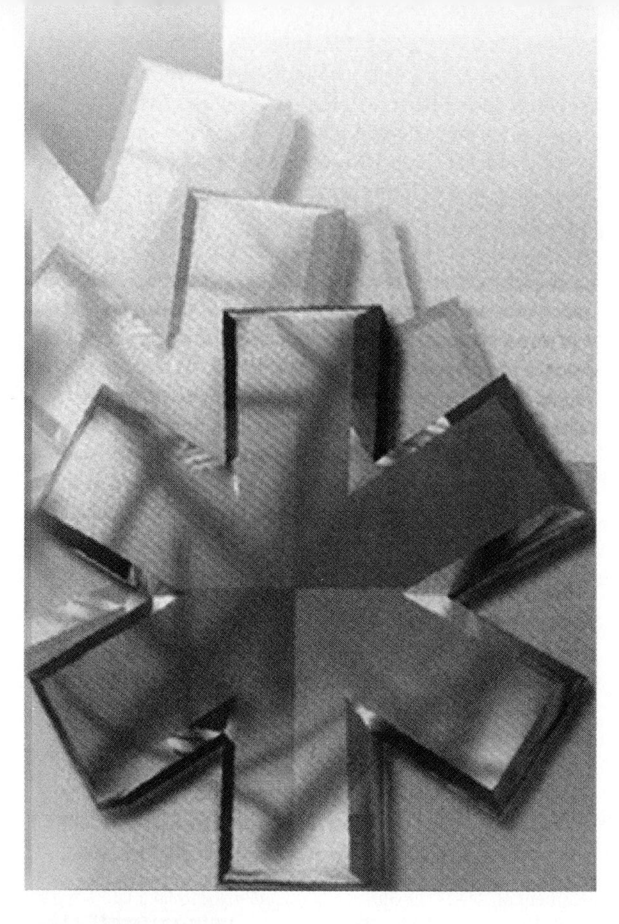

INDEX